Natural Immunomodulators: Promising Therapy for Disease Management

Edited By

Vandana S. Nikam

Department of Pharmacology, STES's Smt. Kashibai Navale College of Pharmacy, S. P. Pune University, Pune 411048, Maharashtra, India

Sujata P. Sawarkar

SVKM's Dr. Bhanuben Nanavati College of Pharmacy, V. M. Road, Mumbai University, Mumbai 400056, Maharashtra, India

Girish B. Mahajan

HiMedia Laboratories Pvt Ltd., Mumbai 400604, Maharashtra, India

&

Supriya G. Jagtap

Department of Pharmacognosy, STES's Smt. Kashibai Navale College of Pharmacy, S. P. Pune University, Pune 411048, Maharashtra, India

Natural Immunomodulators: Promising Therapy for Disease Management

Editors: Vandana S. Nikam, Sujata P. Sawarkar, Girish B. Mahajan & Supriya G. Jagtap

ISBN (Online): 978-981-5123-25-8

ISBN (Print): 978-981-5123-26-5

ISBN (Paperback): 978-981-5123-27-2

First published in 2023.

Bentham Science Publishers Pte. Ltd.
80 Robinson Road #02-00
Singapore 068898
Singapore
Email: subscriptions@benthamscience.net

BENTHAM SCIENCE

CONTENTS

PREFACE 1 i
PREFACE 2 ii

LIST OF CONTRIBUTORS iii

CHAPTER 1 INTRODUCTION: IMMUNE SYSTEM & MODULATION OF IMMUNE SYSTEM 1
Manali S. Dalvi, Sanjay D. Sawant and *Vandana S. Nikam*
INTRODUCTION 1
COMPONENTS OF THE IMMUNE SYSTEM 2
Bone Marrow 3
Thymus 4
Lymph Node 4
Spleen 5
IMMUNE SYSTEM IS COMPOSED OF TWO MAIN COMPONENTS, NAMELY 5
Innate Immunity 6
Anti-microbial Substance 6
Interferons 6
Iron Binding Proteins 7
Anti-Microbial Proteins (AMP) 7
Complement 8
Phagocytes 10
Natural Killer Cells 11
Mechanism of the Innate Response 12
Cell Involve in Innate Immunity 12
Granulocytes 13
Macrophages and Mast Cells 14
Dendritic Cells 14
Adaptive Immunity 15
Major Histocompatibility Complex Antigens 16
Clonal Selection 17
Cell-Mediated Response 18
Activation of T Cells 18
Humoral Response 20
Activation of B Cells 21
Immunological Memory 21
ALLERGY AND HYPERSENSITIVITY REACTION 21
Classification of Hypersensitivity Reactions 22
Type I Hypersensitivity Reaction Fig.(10) 23
Type II Hypersensitivity Reaction 24
Type III Hypersensitivity Reaction 26
Type IV Hypersensitivity Reaction 26
IMMUNOMODULATION 28
Microbiota and Prebiotic, Probiotics 29
Micronutrients 30
Natural Health Products 31
Vaccines 31
IMMUNOTHERAPY 32
CONCLUSION 33
CONSENT FOR PUBLICATION 34

CONFLICT OF INTEREST 34
ACKNOWLEDGEMENTS 34
REFERENCES 34

CHAPTER 2 DISEASES AND DISORDERS ASSOCIATED WITH IMMUNE SYSTEM 41
Pooja Shimpi, Smita Pillewan and *Vandana S. Nikam*
INTRODUCTION 41
CLASSIFICATION OF IMMUNE DISEASES AND DISORDERS 42
BROAD CLASSIFICATION OF IMMUNE DISEASES AND DISORDERS 42
Immunodeficiencies (IDs) 42
Classification of Immune Diseases and Disorders Based on Inborn Errors of Immunity 43
Phenocopies of Inborn Errors of Immunity 46
X-linked Agammaglobulinemia 46
Wiskott–Aldrich Syndrome (WAS) 46
Ataxia Telangiectasia (A-T) 47
DiGeorge Syndrome 47
Secondary Immunodeficiency Disorders 47
Allergic/ Hypersensitivity Reactions 48
Allergic Rhinitis 49
Atopic Eczema/ Atopic Dermatitis 49
Urticaria 51
Stevens-Johnson Syndrome 52
Autoimmune Disorders 53
CLASSIFICATION OF IMMUNE DISEASES BASED ON ORGAN SPECIFICITY 55
ORGAN-SPECIFIC (LOCALIZED) DISEASES FIG. (3) 56
Endocrinologic Diseases 56
Hashimoto's (autoimmune) thyroiditis 56
Neurological Disorders 57
Introduction 57
Alzheimer's Disease and Parkinson's Disease 58
Multiple Sclerosis 59
Auto-inflammatory Diseases/ Systemic Autoinflammatory Diseases (SAIDs) 60
Introduction 60
Classification Of Auto-Inflammatory Diseases 61
Monogenic Autoinflammatory Diseases 61
Polygenic Autoinflammatory Diseases 64
ROLE OF THE IMMUNE SYSTEM IN CANCER 65
IMMUNE CELLS AND CANCER PROGRESSION 65
CONCLUSION 68
CONSENT FOR PUBLICATION 68
CONFLICT OF INTEREST 69
ACKNOWLEDGEMENTS 69
REFERENCES 69

CHAPTER 3 NATURAL SOURCES OF IMMUNOMODULATORS 75
Vishal Bhange, Monika Kale, Ankita Dudhal, Nikhil Putta, Mukta Abhyankar, Supriya Jagtap and *Vandana S. Nikam*
INTRODUCTION 75
PLANTS AS SOURCE OF IMMUNOMODULATORS 77
Glycosides 77
Tannins 77
Coumarins 78

Anthocyanins 78
Saponins 78
Alkaloids 79
Volatile Oils and Terpenoids 79
MARINE-DERIVED IMMUNOMODULATORS 83
Immunomodulatory Compounds from Marine Origin 84
MICROBIOTA MODIFIERS 85
Prebiotics 85
Fructans (Fructo-oligosaccharide or FOS) 85
β-Glucan 86
Role of β-glucan Structure 86
Probiotic 86
Probiotic Augmentation Method in the Immune System 87
Mechanism of Action of Probiotics 87
VACCINES 90
Jennerian Vaccines 90
Live-attenuated Vaccines 91
Inactivated Vaccines 91
Toxoids 91
Subunit, Recombinant, Polysaccharide, and Conjugate Vaccines 92
Combination of Vaccine 92
Messenger RNA (mRNA) Vaccines 92
IMMUNOADJUVANTS 92
MICRONUTRIENTS 94
Vitamin A 94
Vitamin C 96
Vitamin D 97
Vitamin B 99
Vitamin E 99
TRACE ELEMENTS 100
Essential Elements 100
Zinc 100
Selenium 101
Copper 102
Omega-3 Fatty Acid 102
CONCLUDING REMARKS 103
CONSENT FOR PUBLICATION 103
CONFLICT OF INTEREST 103
ACKNOWLEDGEMENTS 103
REFERENCES 103

CHAPTER 4 STANDARDIZATION OF IMMUNOMODULATOR NATURAL DRUGS 108
Aishwarya R. Nale and *Supriya G. Jagtap*
INTRODUCTION 109
NEED FOR DRUGS FROM PLANT ORIGINS OVER SYNTHETIC DRUGS 110
STANDARDIZATION OF DRUGS FROM NATURAL ORIGINS 112
Need for Standardization: Producers' and Consumers' Outlook 113
Standardization of Natural Drugs Using Marker Compound Analysis 114
Processes and Procedures for Standardisation and Quality Control of Natural Drugs are Described 116
Authentication 117

Foreign Matter 117
Organic Evaluation 117
Microscopy 117
Volatile Matter 117
Ash Value 117
Extractive Values 118
Chromatographic Profile of Marker Compound 118
Pesticide Residues 118
Determination of Heavy Metals 119
Microbial Contamination 119
Radioactive Contamination 119
Current Natural Drug Standardization Regulations 119
IMMUNOMODULATING PLANT DRUGS 122
Importance of Natural Immunomodulators 122
Ayurveda Concept 122
PLANT TISSUE CULTURE 129
Advantages of Plant Tissue Culture for Standardization of Phytoconstituents 130
STANDARDIZATION OF NATURAL IMMUNOSTIMULANTS 130
A. Tinospora Crispa 130
Description 130
Collection and Extraction 130
Standardization 130
Immunomodulatory Assays 131
Results 132
Standardization 132
Immunomodulatory Assays 133
B. Mangifera Indica & Curcuma Domestica 133
Description 133
Collection and Extraction 133
Phytochemical Screening 133
Standardization 133
Immunomodulatory Assays 134
Results 135
Phytochemical Screening 135
Standardization 135
Immunomodulatory Assays 136
C. Stereospermum Suaveolens 136
Description 136
Collection and Extraction 136
Phytochemical Analysis 136
Standardization 136
Immunomodulatory Assays 137
Results 137
Phytochemical Analysis 137
Standardization 137
Immunomodulatory Assays 137
D. Barleria Prionitis 138
Description 138
Collection and Storage 138
Extraction 138
Phytochemical Screening 138

Standardization 138
Immunomodulatory Assays 139
Results 140
Phytochemical Screening 140
Standardization 140
Immunomodulatory Assays 140
STANDARDIZATION OF NATURAL IMMUNOSUPPRESSANTS 140
A. Phyllanthus Amarus 140
Description 140
Collection and Extraction 141
Standardization 141
Immunomodulatory Assays 142
Results 142
Standardization 142
Immunomodulatory Assays 143
B. Zingiber Zerumbet 144
Description 144
Collection and Extraction 144
Standardization 144
Reversed-phase HPLC 144
LC-MS/MS 146
Immunomodulatory Assays 146
Results 147
RP-HPLC 147
LC-MS/MS 147
Immunomodulatory Assays 148
C. Momordica Charantia 148
Description 148
Collection, Extraction and Standardization 149
Immunomodulatory Assays 149
Results 150
Standardization 150
Immunomodulatory Assays 150
D. Terminalia Chebula 150
Description 150
Collection, Extraction and Standardization 151
Immunosuppressive Effect as an Anti-arthritic Treatment 151
Results 152
Standardization 152
Immunosuppressive and Anti-arthritic Effects 152
STANDARDIZATION OF IMMUNOMODULATING TISSUE CULTURED PLANTS 152
Echinacea Angustifolia 152
Description 152
Cell Culture Formation & Extraction 153
Standardization 153
Immunomodulatory Assays 153
Helicteres Angustifolia 154
Description 154
Extraction of Callus Suspension Cultures 154
Standardization 154
FTIR Analysis 154

Phytochemical Screening ... 154
Quantitative Analysis ... 155
HPLC Analysis ... 155
Immunomodulatory Assays ... 156
RESULTS ... 156
Standardization ... 156
Ftir Analysis ... 156
Phytochemical Screening ... 156
Quantitative Analysis ... 157
HPLC Analysis ... 157
Immunomodulatory Assays ... 158
CONCLUDING REMARKS ... 158
CONSENT FOR PUBLICATION ... 159
CONFLICT OF INTEREST ... 159
ACKNOWLEDGEMENTS ... 159
REFERENCES ... 159

CHAPTER 5 IMMUNOMODULATORS: CHEMISTRY AND ANALYTICAL TECHNIQUES 165
Akalya Sendrayakannan and *Prashant S. Kharkar*
INTRODUCTION ... 165
IMMUNOMODULATORS ... 166
Immunomodulators from Natural Sources ... 168
PHYTOCHEMICALS AS IMMUNOMODULATORS ... 171
Emodin ... 171
Quercetin ... 172
Resveratrol ... 175
Genistein ... 177
SEARCH FOR NEWER, SAFER IMMUNOMODULATORS ... 178
ANALYTICAL TECHNIQUES FOR ISOLATION, PURIFICATION, QUANTIFICATION AND CHARACTERIZATION OF NATURAL IMMUNOMODULATORS ... 178
Chromatography ... 180
High-Performance Liquid Chromatography (HPLC) ... 180
High-Performance Thin Layer Chromatography (HPTLC) ... 180
Droplet Counter-Current Chromatography (DCCC) ... 180
High-Speed Counter-Current Chromatography (HSCCC) ... 181
High-Performance Capillary Electrophoresis (HPCE) ... 181
Spectroscopy ... 181
Ultraviolet/Visible (UV/Vis) Spectroscopy ... 182
Fourier-Transform Infra-Red (FT-IR) Spectroscopy ... 182
Mass Spectrometry (MS) ... 182
Nuclear Magnetic Resonance (NMR) Spectroscopy ... 182
BIOACTIVITY SCREENING METHODS FOR THE IMMUNOMODULATORS ... 182
CONCLUDING REMARKS ... 184
CONSENT FOR PUBLICATION ... 184
CONFLICT OF INTEREST ... 184
ACKNOWLEDGEMENTS ... 184
REFERENCES ... 184

CHAPTER 6 BIOASSAYS AND OTHER METHODS FOR IMMUNOMODULATORS IN PRECLINICAL AND CLINICAL SETTING ... 189
Priyanka P. Nigade, Pranjali S. Dhamane and *Vandana S. Nikam*
INTRODUCTION ... 189

ASSOCIATION OF INNATE IMMUNITY AND ADAPTIVE IMMUNITY AND THEIR MEASUREMENTS 190
Screening of Immunomodulators 192
Animal Models used for Immunomodulatory Studies 193
PRECLINICAL EVALUATION FOR IMMUNOMODULATORS 193
CELL CULTURE 193
IN VITRO METHODS FOR IMMUNOMODULATORS EVALUATION 193
Inhibition of Histamine Release from Mast Cells [20 - 22] 195
Mitogen-Induced Lymphocyte Proliferation /T Cell Proliferation Assay [17, 20, 23, 24] 196
Inhibition of T Cell Proliferation [20] 197
Phagocytosis Evaluation 197
Chemiluminescence in Macrophages [20] 197
Polymorphonuclear (PMN) Leucocyte's Function Test using Candida Albicans Spores [25, 26] 197
PFC (Plaque Forming Cell) Assay [27] 198
Inhibition of Dihydro-Orotate Dehydrogenase [20] 198
MTT Assay & Cyclic Voltammetry for Cell Viability and Proliferation 199
Cytokine ELISA and Biological Assay [31] 199
Nitrite Determination using Colorimetric Griess Reaction Assay [32] 200
Nitro-blue tetrazolium (NBT) Reduction Assay [33] 200
Myeloperoxidase Activity Assay [33] 200
A Flow Cytometry-Based Assay for Natural Killer Cell Activity Evaluation 201
IN VIVO METHODS FOR IMMUNOMODULATORS EVALUATION 201
Assessment of Cellular Immunity 202
Carbon-Clearance Test for Determination of Macrophage Phagocytic Index [35] 202
Neutrophil Adhesion Test [36] 203
Hypersensitivity Reaction [16] 203
Reversed Passive Arthus (RPA) Reaction [37] 204
Assessment of Humoral Immune Immunity [38] 204
Hemagglutination Antibody Titer Test 204
Mice Lethality Test 204
Determination of Immune Organ Index in Mice [35, 39] 205
Determination of Serum Hemolysin Level in Mice [35] 205
Systemic Anaphylaxis in Mice [40, 41] 205
Adjuvant Arthritis in Rats [42] 206
Collagen Type II Induced Arthritis in Rats [43] 207
Experimental Autoimmune Thyroiditis [44] 207
SPONTANEOUS AUTOIMMUNE DISEASE IN ANIMALS [20] 208
Anti-anaphylactic Activity (Schultz-Dale Reaction) [45] 208
Proteoglycan-Induced Progressive Polyarthritis in Mice [46] 209
Coxsackievirus B3-Induced Myocarditis [47] 209
Experimental Allergic Encephalomyelitis [20] 209
Prevention of Experimentally Induced Myasthenia Gravis in Rats [20] 209
Inhibition of Allogeneic Transplant Rejection [20] 210
Influence on SLE-like Disorder in MRL/lpr Mice [48, 49] 210
CONCLUSION 211
CONSENT FOR PUBLICATION 212
CONFLICT OF INTEREST 212
ACKNOWLEDGEMENTS 212
REFERENCES 212

CHAPTER 7 NATURAL IMMUNOMODULATORS IN CANCER THERAPY 216
Chaitrali Shevkar and *Abhijeet S. Kate*
INTRODUCTION 216
Curcumin 220
Resveratrol 221
Quercetin 222
Genistein 223
Betulinic Acid 224
Zerumbone 225
Berberine 226
Epigallocatechin Gallate 227
Miscellaneous 228
CONCLUDING REMARKS 231
CONSENT FOR PUBLICATION 231
CONFLICT OF INTEREST 231
ACKNOWLEDGEMENTS 232
REFERENCES 232

CHAPTER 8 NATURAL IMMUNOMODULATORS FOR INFECTIONS AND OTHER DISEASES 243
Aaliya Liyakath Ali, Namrata Nailwal, Sujata Sawarkar and *Gaurav Doshi*
INTRODUCTION 243
INFECTIOUS DISEASES 244
Curcumin 247
Antibacterial Activity 247
Antifungal Activity 247
Argyreia Speciosa 248
Antibacterial Activity 248
Antifungal Activity 248
Antiviral Activity 248
Antiparasitic Activity 249
Mangifera Indica 249
Antiviral Activity 249
Antiparasitic Activity 249
Antibacterial And Antifungal Activities 249
Tinospora Sinensis 250
Antimicrobial Activity 250
Antiviral Activity 250
Trigonella Foenum-gracium 250
Antifungal Activity 250
Antibacterial Activity 251
Antiparasitic Activity 251
Platycodon Grandiflorum 251
Antimicrobial Activity 251
Antiviral Activity 251
Resveratrol 252
Antibacterial Activity 252
Antifungal Activity 252
Antiparasitic Activity 252
Antiviral Activity 252
Epigallocatechin-3-Gallate 253

Antibacterial Activity ... 253
Antiviral Activity ... 253
Antifungal Activity ... 253
Antiparasitic Activity ... 253
Genistein ... 254
Antibacterial Activity ... 254
Antiviral Activity ... 254
Antiparasitic Activity ... 254
Quercetin ... 254
Antibacterial Activity ... 255
Antifungal Activity ... 255
Antiparasitic Activity ... 255
Antiviral Activity ... 255
Colchicine ... 255
Antibacterial Activity ... 256
Antiviral Activity ... 256
Capsaicin ... 256
Antibacterial Activity ... 256
Andrographolide ... 256
Antibacterial Activity ... 257
Antiviral Activity ... 257
Antiparasitic Activity ... 257
Tripterugium Wilfordii ... 257
Antibacterial Activity ... 257
Acorus Calamus ... 257
Antibacterial Activity ... 258
Antifungal Activity ... 258
Antiviral Activity ... 258
Antiparasitic Activity ... 258
Emblica Officinalis ... 259
Antibacterial Activity ... 259
Antifungal Activity ... 259
Antiviral Activity ... 260
Evolvulus Alsinoides ... 260
Antibacterial Activity ... 260
Antifungal Activity ... 260
CONCLUSION ... 260
CONSENT FOR PUBLICATION ... 261
CONFLICT OF INTEREST ... 261
ACKNOWLEDGEMENTS ... 261
REFERENCES ... 261

CHAPTER 9 DELIVERY OF IMMUNOMODULATORS: CHALLENGES AND NOVEL APPROACHES ... 275
Mansi Damani, Prabha Singh and *Sujata Sawarkar*
INTRODUCTION ... 275
NATURAL IMMUNOMODULATORS ... 277
CHALLENGES IN THE DELIVERY OF NATURAL IMMUNOMODULATORS ... 283
Standardization Challenges ... 283
Formulation Challenges ... 284
Administration Challenges ... 285

Regulatory Concerns ... 286
NOVEL APPROACHES FOR DELIVERY OF NATURAL IMMUNOMODULATORS ... 286
Nanoparticles ... 287
Polymeric Nanoparticless ... 287
Mesoporous Silica Nanoparticles ... 289
Lipid Nanoparticles ... 290
Metal Nanoparticles ... 293
Liposomes and Niosomes ... 294
Polymeric Micelles ... 296
Dendrimer ... 297
Nanoemulsion And Microemulsions ... 298
Transferosome ... 301
Ethosomes ... 302
CONCLUSION ... 307
CONSENT FOR PUBLICATION ... 307
CONFLICT OF INTEREST ... 307
ACKNOWLEDGEMENTS ... 308
REFERENCES ... 308

CHAPTER 10 MARKETING STRATEGY & REGULATORY PERSPECTIVE FOR NATURAL IMMUNOMODULATORS ... 323
Alveera Ansari, Namrata Nailwal, Sujata Sawarkar and *Gaurav Doshi*
INTRODUCTION ... 324
UNITED STATES OF AMERICA (USA) ... 328
Drugs & Biological Products ... 329
INDIA ... 330
AUSTRALIA ... 331
UNITED KINGDOM ... 331
CANADA ... 332
EUROPE ... 334
DENMARK ... 335
NEW ZEALAND ... 336
IRELAND ... 336
BRAZIL ... 337
THAILAND ... 339
SWEDEN ... 341
ITALY ... 343
GERMANY ... 344
CHINA ... 345
SOUTH KOREA ... 347
SWITZERLAND ... 349
HONGKONG ... 350
FRANCE ... 351
NIGERIA ... 351
UGANDA ... 354
MALAYSIA ... 354
NETHERLANDS ... 355
SINGAPORE ... 356
JAPAN ... 357
GULF COUNTRIES (SAUDI ARABIA, KUWAIT, THE UNITED ARAB EMIRATES, QATAR, BAHRAIN, OMAN) ... 358

Regulatory Agencies of the Gulf Cooperation Council 358
Procedure for Centralised Registration 358
Procedure for Registration that is not Centralised 359
SOUTH AFRICA 359
Application Number 359
Electronic Entries 359
Models of Reliance 360
GMP 360
Document SCoRE 360
ARMENIA, AZERBAIJAN, BELARUS, GEORGIA, KAZAKHSTAN, KYRGYZSTAN, TURKMENISTAN, MOLDOVA, RUSSIA, TAJIKISTAN, UKRAINE, UZBEKISTAN (THE COMMONWEALTH OF INDEPENDENT STATES) 360
VIETNAM, THAILAND, SINGAPORE, PHILIPPINES, BRUNEI, CAMBODIA, INDONESIA, LAOS, MALAYSIA, MYANMAR (ASSOCIATION OF SOUTH ASIAN NATIONS) 361
CONCLUSION 362
CONSENT FOR PUBLICATION 362
CONFLICT OF INTEREST 362
ACKNOWLEDGEMENTS 363
REFERENCES 363

CHAPTER 11 NATURAL *VS.* SYNTHETIC IMMUNOMODULATORS 368
Girish B Mahajan and *Lakshmi Balachandran*
INTRODUCTION 368
The Nature of the Immune Response 368
NATURAL IMMUNOMODULATORS (NI) 370
Rasayana [10] 370
CHEMICAL NATURE OF NATURAL IMMUNOMODULATORS 371
Propionibacterium Species as an Immunomodulator 372
Glucan 373
Curcumin [19] 373
Resveratrol 374
Glycosides [27] 375
Flavonoids [28] 375
Sapogenins 376
Alkaloids 376
Thiosulfinates 376
Volatile Oils and Terpenoids [32] 377
MECHANISM OF NATURAL IMMUNOMODULATORS 381
SYNTHETIC IMMUNOMODULATORS (SI) 383
Bacillus Calmette-Guerin (BCG) 383
Muramyl Dipeptide (MDP) 383
Lipopolysaccharide (LPS) [42] 383
Levamisole 384
Isoprenosine 384
Pyrimidine Derivatives [46] 384
Purine Derivatives [47] 384
Nitrogen Mustard Alkylating Agents [48] 385
Synthetic Corticosteroids [49] 385
Heterocyclic Structures 385
Aromatic Compounds 385

Simple Non-cyclic Chemicals 385
MECHANISM OF SYNTHETIC IMMUNOMODULATORS 385
MARKET ANALYSIS [54-56] 386
SIGNIFICANCE OF NATURAL IMMUNOMODULATORS AND SYNTHETIC IMMUNOMODULATORS 386
Role of Immunomodulators in Human Health and Animal Health 386
COMPARATIVE SIDE EFFECTS OF IMMUNOMODULATORS CONSIDERING THEIR NATURAL & SYNTHETIC ORIGIN [61] 387
INDUSTRIAL MANUFACTURERS [62, 63] 388
CONCLUSION 388
CONSENT FOR PUBLICATION 389
CONFLICT OF INTEREST 389
ACKNOWLEDGEMENTS 389
REFERENCES 389

CHAPTER 12 FUTURE PATH AND PERSPECTIVES OF IMMUNOMODULATORS 399
Megha Karne, Supriya G. Jagtap, Sujata Sawarkar and *Vandana S. Nikam*
INTRODUCTION 399
THE COMPLEXITY OF INNATE AND ADAPTIVE IMMUNITY 400
Approaches and Challenges in Standardization of Natural Immunomodulators 401
In-vitro, In-vivo Preclinical Models Development and Translating for Clinical Application 405
Novel Drug Delivery System of Natural Immunomodulators and Challenges, Future Outlook 406
Market and Regulatory Perspective of Natural Immunomodulators 408
CONCLUDING REMARKS 409
CONSENT FOR PUBLICATION 410
CONFLICT OF INTEREST 410
ACKNOWLEDGEMENTS 410
REFERENCES 410

SUBJECT INDEX 413

PREFACE 1

Immunomodulatory drugs, of both natural and synthetic origin, are increasingly being researched & developed for the treatment of human diseases, together with inflammatory disorders. In the post-SARS-CoV-2 pandemic of 2020, the research in immunomodulators has been found to be increased. The significance of such compounds, which focus on modulation of our immune status over remedial drugs, has been realized. Regardless of its extraordinary efficiency and specificity, the distortion of immune responses can be accountable for several disorders, such as autoimmune diseases, allergies, immunosuppression, and AIDS. Immunomodulators play a key role in diming such disorders too. In the past ten years (2011 to 2021), there have been several hundred reviews either on immunomodulators or combined with vaccines and adjuvants. However, a comprehensive book exclusively on all aspects of immunomodulators was needed for the clinicians, researchers, and Pharma & Biopharma professionals. Eminent and well-experienced professors, researchers, bioscience industry professionals, and technologists from India congregate to review this in the form of a comprehensive book. The book with the title "Natural Immunomodulators: promising therapy for disease management" encompasses all aspects such as ways of modulating immunity, diseases & disorders related to immunity, natural & synthetic immunomodulators, related analytical techniques, bioassays, and other methods for immunomodulators in the preclinical and clinical setting, delivery of immunomodulators: challenges and novel approaches, marketing strategy and regulatory perspectives, future path, and perspectives, *etc.* A glance through the twelve chapters reveals the vastness of the work on immunomodulators and their significance for mankind. The content of the book is like a crisp encyclopedia on the topic. The distinguished editorial team has refined the content to make it a ready one-stop reference for researchers, investors, bioscience & biotech professionals, vaccine developers, students, clinicians, *etc.* All the authors with decades of proficiency in the medical and clinical field put all their best effort to encompass the key literature in the past two decades along with representative historical aspects. I look upon this book as a high-impact reference.

Girish B. Mahajan
Senior Vice-President,
HiMedia Laboratories Pvt Ltd.,
Maharashtra, India

PREFACE 2

With the advancement and rapidly changing technology, information is accumulating in ever intimidating quantities with facts and figures that give logical reasoning, simple explanations about chaotic mechanisms, and the complexity of biology and life. Scientific knowledge is full of paradoxes, and with the addition of new information, it becomes easy and simple to unravel the unknown to known with rational justification.

Our book, entitled Natural Immunomodulators: promising therapy for disease management, is a small effort to gather recent updates in the field of immunology, pathology, and immunomodulatory therapies intended at harnessing the power of nature. Although the information is ever expanding in volume, we have taken intense efforts to conceptualize and summarize the information that emphasizes the significance of natural immunomodulators.

The immune system complexity is secondary to the nervous and endocrine systems. The immune system has a profound impact and involvement in emerging lifestyle-related chronic illnesses and infectious diseases. The outbreak of severe acute respiratory syndrome coronavirus 2 (SARS-CoV-2) in the year 2019 had underscored the significance of immunity. Moreover, the recent discovery of the brain lymphatic system in 2015 had stated the linkages of the immune system in neuropathology.

Our book provides a preview of the immune system and every aspect of natural immunomodulators, including their natural sources, standardization, novel drug delivery methods, marketing, regulatory requirements, challenges, and limitations to get them in mainstream in line with and parallel to modern medicines. The retrieved scientific information from literature is presented comprehensively without losing the essence of the research to readers, and the content is abstracted succinctly in simple, lucid language.

The successful completion of our book was possible due to the collective efforts and support from chapter authors, our research students, friends, and colleagues. We thank all of them for their sincere contributions in shaping this book. Finally, we are also grateful to the Bentham publishing team for their outstanding support and cooperation.

Vandana S. Nikam
Department of Pharmacology
STESs' Smt. Kashibai Navale College of Pharmacy
S. P. Pune University
Pune 411048 Maharashtra
India

List of Contributors

Ankita Dudhal	Department of Pharmacology, STES's Smt. Kashibai Navale College of Pharmacy, Kondhwa, S.P. Pune University, Pune 411048, Maharashtra, India
Aishwarya R. Nale	Department of Pharmacology, STES's Smt. Kashibai Navale College of Pharmacy, Kondhwa, S.P. Pune University, Pune, Maharashtra, India
Akalya Sendrayakannan	Department of Food Engineering and Technology, Department of Pharmaceutical Sciences and Technology, Institute of Chemical Technology (ICT), Nathalal Parekha Marg, Matunga, Mumbai 400 019, India
Abhijeet S. Kate	Department of Natural Products, National Institute of Pharmaceutical Education and Research, Ahmedabad, Gujarat, India
Aaliya Liyakath Ali	Department of Pharmacology, SVKM'S Dr. Bhanuben Nanavati College of Pharmacy, Mithibai Campus, Vile Parle (W), Mumbai-400056, India
Alveera Ansari	Department of Pharmacology, SVKM'S Dr.Bhanuben Nanavati College of Pharmacy, Mithibai Campus, Vile Parle (W), Mumbai-400056, India
Chaitrali Shevkar	Department of Natural Products, National Institute of Pharmaceutical Education and Research, Ahmedabad, Gujarat, India
Gaurav Doshi	Department of Pharmacology, SVKM'S Dr. Bhanuben Nanavati College of Pharmacy, Mithibai Campus, Vile Parle (W), Mumbai-400056, India
Girish B Mahajan	HiMedia Laboratories Pvt Ltd, Maharashtra, India
Lakshmi Balachandran	Freelance Medical Writer, Maharashtra, India
Manali S. Dalvi	Department of Pharmacology, STES's Smt. Kashibai Navale College of Pharmacy, Kondhwa, S.P. Pune University, Pune 411048, Maharashtra, India
Monika Kale	Department of Pharmacology, STES's Smt. Kashibai Navale College of Pharmacy, Kondhwa, S.P. Pune University, Pune 411048, Maharashtra, India
Mukta Abhyankar	Department of Pharmacognosy, STES's Smt. Kashibai Navale College of Pharmacy, Kondhwa, S.P. Pune University, Pune 411048, Maharashtra, India
Mansi Damani	Department of Pharmaceutics, SVKM's Dr. Bhanuben Nanavati College of Pharmacy, University of Mumbai, India
Megha Karne	Department of Pharmacology, STES's Smt. Kashibai Navale College of Pharmacy, Kondhwa, S.P. Pune University, Pune, Maharashtra, India
Nikhil Putta	Department of Pharmacognosy, STES's Smt. Kashibai Navale College of Pharmacy, Kondhwa, S.P. Pune University, Pune 411048, Maharashtra, India
Namrata Nailwal	Department of Pharmacology, SVKM'S Dr. Bhanuben Nanavati College of Pharmacy, Mithibai Campus, Vile Parle (W), Mumbai-400056, India
Pooja Shimpi	1Department of Pharmacology, STES's Smt. Kashibai Navale College of Pharmacy, Kondhwa, S.P. Pune University, Pune, Maharashtra, India
Prashant S. Kharkar	Department of Food Engineering and Technology, Department of Pharmaceutical Sciences and Technology, Institute of Chemical Technology (ICT), Nathalal Parekha Marg, Matunga, Mumbai 400 019, India
Priyanka P. Nigade	Department of Pharmacology, STES's Smt. Kashibai Navale college of Pharmacy, Kondhwa, S.P. Pune University, Pune, Maharashtra, India

Pranjali S. Dhamane	M. Pharm Pharmacology, STES's, Smt. Kashibai Navale College of Pharmacy, Kondhwa (Bk), Pune-411048, Maharashtra, India
Prabha Singh	Department of Pharmaceutics, SVKM's Dr. Bhanuben Nanavati College of Pharmacy, University of Mumbai, India
Sanjay D. Sawant	Department of Pharmaceutical Chemistry, STES's Smt. Kashibai Navale College of Pharmacy, Kondhwa, S.P. Pune University, Pune 411048, Maharashtra, India
Smita Pillewan	D.Y. Patil College of Pharmacy, Akurdi, S.P. Pune University, Pune, Maharashtra, India
Supriya Jagtap	Department of Pharmacognosy, STES's Smt. Kashibai Navale College of Pharmacy, Kondhwa, S.P. Pune University, Pune 411048, Maharashtra, India
Sujata Sawarkar	Department of Pharmaceutics, SVKM'S Dr. Bhanuben Nanavati College of Pharmacy, Mithibai Campus, Vile Parle (W), Mumbai-400056, India
Vandana S. Nikam	Department of Pharmacology, STES's Smt. Kashibai Navale College of Pharmacy, Kondhwa, S.P. Pune University, Pune 411048, Maharashtra, India
Vishal Bhange	Department of Pharmacology, STES's Smt. Kashibai Navale College of Pharmacy, Kondhwa, S.P. Pune University, Pune 411048, Maharashtra, India

CHAPTER 1

Introduction: Immune System & Modulation of Immune System

Manali S. Dalvi[1], **Sanjay D. Sawant**[2] and **Vandana S. Nikam**[1,*]

[1] *Department of Pharmacology, STES's Smt. Kashibai Navale College of Pharmacy, Kondhwa, S. P. Pune University, Pune 411048, Maharashtra, India*

[2] *Department of Pharmaceutical Chemistry, STES's Smt. Kashibai Navale College of Pharmacy, Kondhwa, S. P. Pune University, Pune 411048, Maharashtra, India*

Abstract: The immune system is a complex, intricate organ system with features like flexibility, recognition, discriminating potential between self from non-self, and memory to defeat notorious external and internal threats to human health functioning. Innate immunity is inborn, and acquired immunity develops through secondary education; they are interconnected, interdependent, and execute tasks with bi-directional communications. A deeper understanding of immune biology revealed a remarkable contribution of the immune system in several chronic illnesses, and has taken a central stage in pathophysiology. In essence, the weakened or overactivated immune system leads to these chronic illnesses. Modulation of the immune system is an efficient and valid approach to prevent the underlying pathophysiology of such diseases. A gamut of natural immunomodulators targeted at specific or non-specif immune cells has delineated their potential to achieve the equilibrated and balanced immune system. Preclinical and clinical studies demonstrated the implication of microbiota, nutrients, natural herbs, and micronutrients for immunostasis. The immune system's complexity, its close association with the endocrine and nervous system, target identification, and convenient, reliable tools to assess immune function and modulation are a few limitations that hampered the attainment of immunostasis. Despite these limitations, novel therapies targeted at immunomodulation in chronic diseases are promising and paving the future path to novel therapeutics.

Keywords: Adaptive Immunity, Immune System, Innate Immunity, Immunomodulation.

INTRODUCTION

The principal components of the immune system are innate and adaptive immunity. The immune system is an older system on the evolutionary scale, and among

* **Corresponding author Vandana S. Nikam:** Department of Pharmacology, STES's Smt. Kashibai Navale College of Pharmacy, Kondhwa, S. P. Pune University, Pune 411048, Maharashtra, India; Tel: +912026931322; E-mail: nikam_vandana@yahoo.com

Vandana S. Nikam, Sujata P. Sawarkar, Girish B. Mahajan and Supriya G. Jagtap (Eds.)

the two, the innate immune system is the ancestral one, present in both invertebrates and vertebrates [1]. The innate system is considered as the first line of defense for invading infection, growing neoplastic cells, or any other foreign matter in the body. The innate system lacks clonal expansion, memory, and antibodies and does not respond to changes in external stimuli. The innate system reacts and responds through its receptors to highly conserved microbial proteins like lipoteichoic acids and lipopolysaccharide of gram-negative and gram-positive bacteria, respectively [2, 3].

Immunity is the mechanism by which the body protects itself against diverse environmental agents, such as microorganisms or their product lines, food, chemical products, drugs, and pollen grains. The word 'Immunity' originated from the Latin word 'Immunis', which means 'exempt from public services' (from im-, in- not, un-, without+munus duty, task, service). The very first term was introduced in B.C. 430 during the plague of Athens. Thucydides noticed that people who had managed to recover from a prior bout of the disease were capable of treating the sick without becoming sick on the second contact [4]. Later Rhazes (880-932) termed the immunity as acquired immunity with an explanation of excess moisture being expelled from the blood and therefore preventing the subsequent occurrence of the disease. This theory explains the term acquired immunity as smallpox bout was effective in protecting its survivors from future infections and explains several terms about smallpox known during the 10th century. Louris Pasteur reconfirmed these observations in his germ theory of disease [5], which were later proven by Robert Koch in 1891 and awarded with Nobel prize. In the 19th century, Paul Ehrlich had a substantial contribution to immunology by proposing the side-chain theory, explaining the specificity of the antigen-antibody reaction.

The immune system can be defined as the bodily system that produces the immune response to protect the body from foreign materials, cells, and tissues. It is the body's defense mechanism to render foreign antigens and disease-causing bacteria from entering the body. It never attacks commensal flora that inhabits the gut, skin, and other tissues to the host's benefit and always differentiates between individual own cells and other harmful invading cells. All animals have nearly the same immune system, but it varies within individuals. It varies as a consequence of heritable and non-heritable influences [6].

COMPONENTS OF THE IMMUNE SYSTEM

Immune system differs from other systems in the body, as the cells involved in the system are highly motile. It specifically uses the blood vessels and lymphatic vessels to reach the infection site in order to move in and out of the lymphatic tissue.

Though the immune system is found all over the body, it still contains some specialized organs, which regulate the immune response and are capable of rapidly producing numerous cells that can stop spreading infection. Immune cells present in the reservoir can penetrate any cells in the body to combat the invasion. All the cells in the body originate from hematopoietic stem cells in the bone marrow as a precursor, but their site of origin and residence differ from each other [7]. The thymus and bone marrow are primary immune organs. Secondary immune organs include the lymph nodes, spleen, Peyer's patches, appendix, tonsil, adenoids and other mucosal-associated lymphoid tissue (MALT) [8] Fig.(**1**).

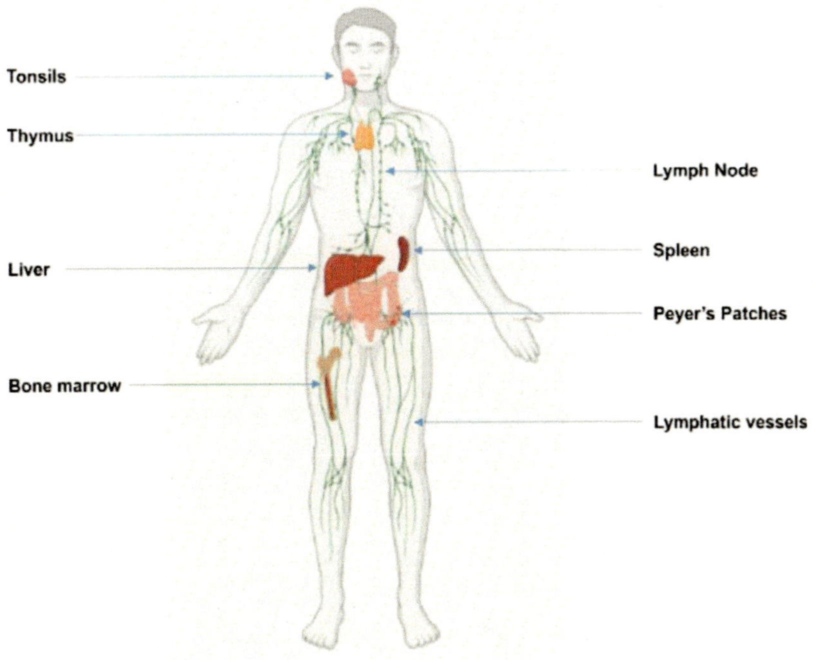

Fig. (1). Primary and secondary immune organs of human body.

Bone Marrow

It is the primary site for blood cell synthesis. It gives rise to all types of precursor blood cells. Red bone marrow is a connective tissue that is highly vascularized, having 0.05 to 0.1% pluripotent stem cells derived from mesenchyme. These cells proliferate; differentiate into lymphoid and myeloid stem cells, which give rise to lymphocytes and myeloid cells, respectively. These stem cells further differentiate and become committed progenitor cells, which give rise to specific blood cell types. Some progenitor cells are also referred to as colony-forming units (CFU) with abbreviations for a specific lineage. For instance, CFU-GM means progenitor cells committed to becoming neutrophils and monocytes cells [9].

Thymus

The thymus is bilobed, encapsulated and lymphocyte-rich organ located exactly above the sternum in the neck region. It plays a vital role in cell-mediated immunity, particularly in T cells, which are likely thymus-derived cells. Thymus activity is observed highly in early childhood and further decreases at puberty, although it never completely disappears. Cortical and medullary epithelial cells, stromal cells, interdigitating cells, and macrophages make up the thymus. Thymic epithelial cells produce thymosin and thymoproteins along with some cytokines like IL-7, which play an important role in the development and maturation of T cells [10]. The thymus is the site of T cells maturation, and they undergo a critical test. In the positive selection test, developing T cells are evaluated based on their ability to recognise major histocompatibility proteins (MHC, a set of proteins present on cells to distinguish self from foreign). The developing T cells, which fail to recognize self-cells, are eliminated for further development. In the next maturation stage, T cells are subjected to interactions with thymic dendritic cells. Those T cells that show high reactivity are omitted in order to avoid autoimmune reactions. This process is called the negative selection process. The highly selective maturation process in the thymus leads to the T helper and T killer cells development, which is critical for adaptive immune response.

Lymph Node

They are small, bean-shaped glands, strewn about the lymphatic vessels and they are also called lymph glands. They are of varying size and are most numerous in lymphatic organs. They are centered along the respiratory and gastrointestinal tracts, as well as in the mammary glands, axillae, and groyne. The lymph node's complex structure is divided into lobules, each of which contains an outer cortex, para cortex, and core medulla region. When challenged with an antigen, the outer cortex consists primarily of B cells arranged as follicles, which might also develop a germinal centre, and the deeper cortex primarily of T cells. Transient B and T lymphocytes, antigen processing and presenting cells, mimicking B and T lymphocytes (in response to an infection), persistent and transient final effector cells, and macrophages make up the normal or reactive lymph node. Each node's macrophages and reticular cells remove 99 percent of impurities as lymph moves from one node to the next. This is how virtually all impurities are normally removed [11].

Spleen

The spleen is the bean-shaped, encapsulated, large organ with an interior having a spongy interface, located on the opposite side of the abdomen, beneath the diaphragm. Spleen is enclosed in a fibro-elastic capsule that extends into the spleen, and they are called trabeculae. The cellular material between the trabeculae is called the splenic pulp, which is further subdivided into a white pulp and red pulp. The white pulp is the lymphatic tissue, which is lined with lymphocytes and macrophages along the splenic-central artery. The function of white pulp is to produce immune and blood cells. The red pulp has venous sinuses and splenic cords (Billroth's cord) and has plasma cells, granulocytes, and macrophages. The function of the red pulp is to filter antigens, micro - organisms, and damaged or worn-out red blood cells from the blood [12].

T cells defend the body against disease; the immune system should perform four tasks. The very first, the presence of the infection must be detected, which is called immunological recognition. This is done by the WBCs of innate immunity and lymphocytes of adaptive immunity. Second, the next task is to eliminate the infection completely and furthermore activate the immune effector functions, such as the complement system, lymphocyte-mediated antibodies productions, and destruction by lymphocytes. The most important task, however, is immune regulation, or the immune system's ability to self-regulate. The final task is to protect the body from recurring infection by building immunological memory [7].

IMMUNE SYSTEM IS COMPOSED OF TWO MAIN COMPONENTS, NAMELY

(a) Innate Immunity and

(b) Acquired Immunity

The innate and adaptive immune systems collaborate to keep the body protected from infection, cancerous cells, and any foreign bodies and work in coordination to protect and notify the body if injury occurs. The innate immune system is the inborn immune system that detects pathogenic organisms or injury and mounts an instantaneous, broad response. On the other hand, the adaptive immune system is an acquired and specific immunity. It creates a memory to enhance the body's response against future attacks. Both systems contain various cell-mediated and humoral components [13].

Innate Immunity

It is non-specific, naturally acquired defense mechanism of the body. It responds immediately to the exposure with the maximum response, either cell-mediated or humoral. It is considered the inborn defense mechanism, independent of previous exposure to the disease.

It includes two defense mechanisms. The skin and mucosa of the gastrointestinal, respiratory, and urogenital tracts provide a mechanical and physiological barrier, as well as continuously washing and cleansing the mucous surface and cilia, which aids in the removal of debris and foreign matter [14]. It is called physicochemical innate immunity. Pathogens and potential pollution are constantly present on our skin. Constant contact with exogenous stimuli and antigens more often results in the activation of resident immune cells [12, 13]. It is our intact skin, which prevents pathogens from entering the body. Its low pH and the presence of fatty acids make the environment non-conducive living for the pathogens, but the compromisation of skin continuity leads to secondary infection. Some barriers are found in the form of anti-microbial molecules, proteases, digestive enzymes, and lysozymes called innate humoral immunity. Lysozymes from the mucus secretion and tears contain hydrolytic enzymes and cause cleavage of peptidoglycan of the bacterial cell wall. Saliva contains hydrogen peroxide acting as an antibacterial. Also, the low pH environment of the stomach and vagina makes them inimical for bacteria to enter. Immunologically active factors of mucosal secretions in blood and in cerebrospinal fluid (the humors) also work as a humoral barrier.

Whenever the first-line defence fails to protect the body due to any acquired or congenital anomaly, the bacteria enter way deeper into the tissue causing activation of the second-line defence mechanism. The second line defense includes some anti-microbial proteins, phagocytes, NK cells, along with some inflammatory responses like fever and redness Fig. (**2**).

Anti-microbial Substance

Mainly four types of anti-microbial substances, which decrease microbial growth in the body, are discussed below.

Interferons

These are produced by various cells of the body as the inflammatory response produced by the virally infected macrophages, lymphocytes and fibroblast. After triggering, they produce some kind of molecular changes, which affect various cellular responses, including cell growth and in turn cause inflammation [15].

They can stop the replication of viral cells by producing antiviral protein in the neighboring uninfected cell. But, they cannot present the viral attachment to the host cell. There are particularly three types of interferons, Type 1 IFN-a, IFN-b, IFN-e, IFN-k, IFN-o, IFN-d, IFN-t, IFN-g, limitin, and type 2 IFN-g. Additional IFNs (IFN-like cytokines; IFN-λ subtype), interleukin-28A (IL-28A) and IL-28B, and IL-29 [16].

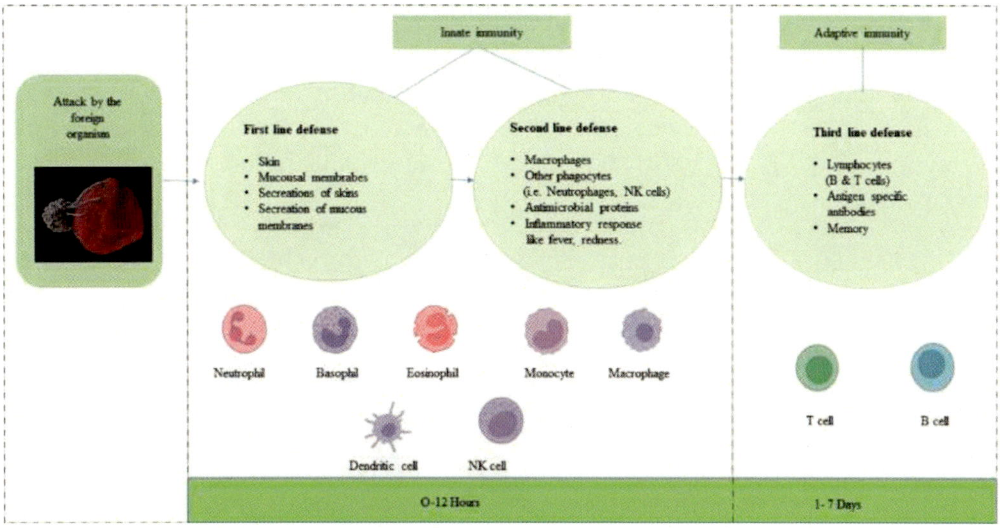

Fig. (2). Defense mechanisms of human body.

Iron Binding Proteins

They specifically inhibit bacterial growth by lowering the amount of iron available. Ferritin in the liver, spleen, and red bone is considered an intracellular iron storage protein. The ferritin inhibits the growth of hematopoietic progenitor cells and the proliferation of T lymphocytes, as observed in *in vitro* studies [17]. Lactoferrin, found in milk, saliva, and mucus; transferrin, found in blood and tissue fluid; and haemoglobin, found in RBCs, are all iron-binding proteins.

Anti-Microbial Proteins (AMP)

They are considered the main component of innate immunity and play an important role in the wedding of the pathogens forms the body. These are short peptides having potent anti-microbial properties. Some of the AMP are ubiquicidin, thrombocidin-1 (TC-1), hepcidin 25, RNase 7, RNase 5 (angiogenin), Substance P, Chemerin, Amylin, *etc* [18]. These small peptides not only kill the pathogens but also attract mast cells and dendrites cells, which take part in the further immune response.

Complement

Whenever the pathogens cross the barrier, the initial microbial defense gets into action along with the complement system. A complement is a group of heat-labile serum proteins, which complement antibodies in the destruction of organisms. Complement activation is a cascade (of the kinins and clotting cascades) composed of more than 30 proteins, including regulatory factors. Complement forms a protein cascade, with each activated component catalysing the activation of several molecules of the next, resulting in response amplification. Complement activation results in the production of pro-inflammatory mediators, cell lysis and the solubilization of antigen-antibody complexes. There are three pathways: classical and alternative pathways both activate the third common or membrane attack pathway [7].

The complement system serves several primary functions by:

(i) lysis of the bacterial cell (ii) production of peptide fragments, which participate in the inflammatory response; (iii) attracting the phagocytes; and (iv) opsonization and clearance of the infected cell from the site of the infection.

Classic Pathway

The classic pathway consists of various components numbered C1-C9, with the reaction sequence C1-C4-C2-C3-C5-C6-C7-C8-C9. Antigen-antibody complexes bind to C1q. C4 and C2 are cleared by the C1qr2s2 complex to form the classical pathway C3 convertase C4b2a. Following C3 cleavage, the CS convertase C4b2a3b is formed. Biologically active fragments C4a and C3a are generated. C3b has other actions and may also 'drive' forward activation of the alternative pathway Fig. (**3**) [19].

Alternative Pathway

Free C3b binds factor B, and the C3bB complex becomes the substrate of a circulating enzyme, factor D, which generates C3bBb by removing the fragment Ba from C3bB. The C3 convertase enzyme cleaves C3, detaching C3a from C3b, which can restart the activation process. The alternative pathway C3 convertase enzyme cleaves C3, detaching C3a from C3b, which can reinitiate the activation process. The complex C3bBb3b, analogous to C4b2b3,b is the alternative pathway C5 convertase, initiating the membrane attack pathway sequence (Fig. **4**).

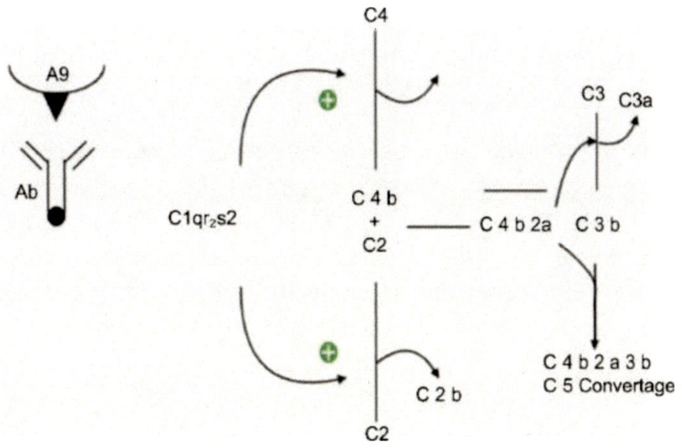

Fig.(3). Classic pathway of complement system.

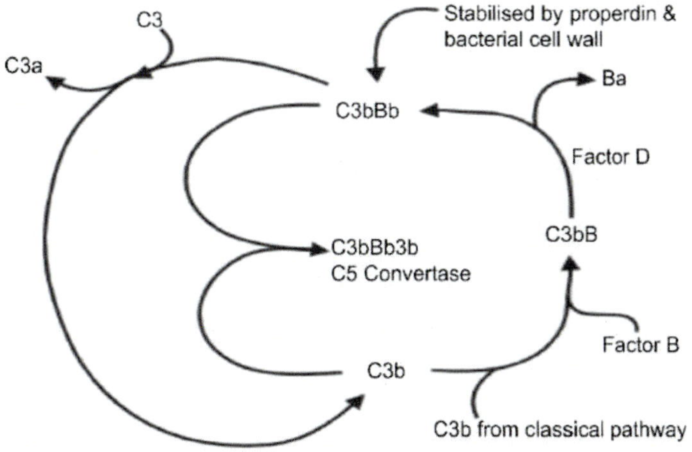

Fig.(4). Alternate pathway of complement system.

The Membrane Attack Pathway

The final common complement pathway produces another bioactive component C5a, but more interestingly, it results in the formation of the system's 'killer molecule.' As it causes membrane damage, this is known as the membrane attack complex (MAC) Fig. (**5**).

C5 convertase cleaves C5 into smaller fragments C5a and larger fragment C5b, which persists the reaction sequence by binding to C6 and provoking it to express an unstable, reactive site for C7. The C5b67 complex is lipophilic in nature and binds to the membrane surface, where it acts as a C8 receptor with high affinity. C8 has three chains that insert into the membrane, anchoring the C5b678 complex, which further binds and polymerizes C9, forming MAC, the system's final component. As many as 12-15 C9 molecules can congregate around a single

C5b678 complex inserting into and traversing the membrane. If a sufficient number of holes are made in the membrane, it results in cell death due to osmotic lysis.

Besides creating membrane lesions on target cells, complement components initiate phagocytosis and inflammatory reactions. C3b and C3bi are the reaction products of C3, which coat the surface of the microorganisms and thus, facilitate the adherence of these coated microbes to the surface of phagocytic cells. In delayed hypersensitivity reaction, antigen-antibody complexes fix complement. C3a fragment causes histamine release with increased vascular permeability and formation of oedema. C5a and C567 attract the neutrophils at the site, which in turn releases lysosomal enzymes, including collagenases leading to inflammation [20].

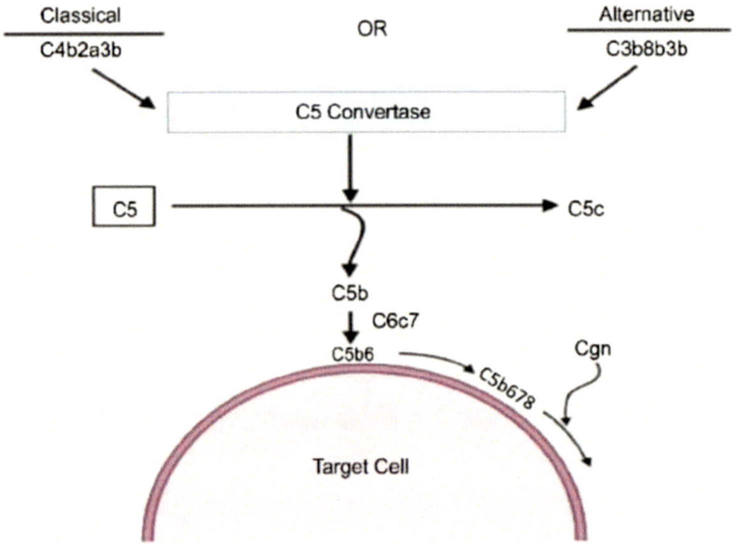

Fig. (5). The Membrane Attack Pathway.

Phagocytes

Phagocytes are a special type of leukocytes. These are the specialized group of cells, which work by finding and engulfing the virus, bacteria, or any other pathogens harmful to the body. The process of engulfing the bacteria is called phagocytosis, and the cells involved in this process are macrophages, neutrophils, and dendritic cells. Whenever foreign pathogens enter the body, the motile phagocytes search for and destroy them.

Phagocytosis is the multistep process by which the phagocytes remove the bacteria from the body. It involves different stages Fig. (**6**).

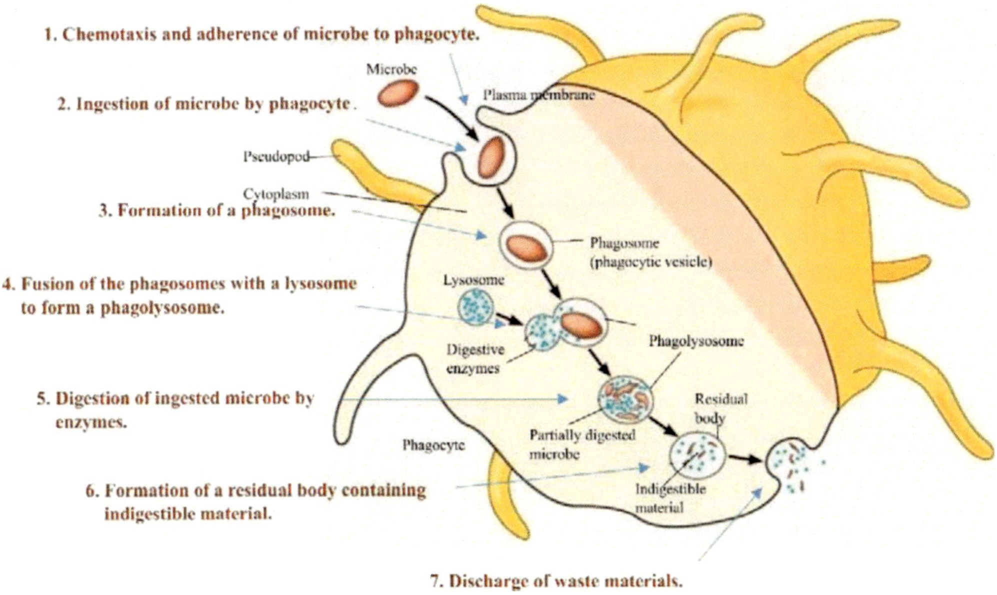

Fig.(6). Different stages of phagocytosis.

Phagocytes recognize the foreign microbes with the help of N- formylated peptides, which in turn activate different mediators of the inflammation and the complement system. The first step involves the margination, in which the leucocytes flow through the blood and get attached to the endothelial cell lining. The selectin and integrin are two sets of adherent molecules that carry out this process. Selectin initiates interaction, whereas integrin-mediated adhesive interaction causes the phagocytic movement in the direction of cell junction. Other chemoattractants are some microbial proteins like N-formyl methionine, which are present on their amino-terminal end. The process of attracting phagocytes to the site of infection is called chemotaxis. Additionally, phagocytic cells attach through the different receptors found on their surface, which help them to attach infectious agents (for example, Fc receptor, toll-like receptor). Moreover, the phagocytic cells can physically trap the microbes and start ingestion [20].

Natural Killer Cells

These are called NK cells, and NK cells are cytotoxic, and function by killing infected cells. Killer activation receptors (KARs) and killer inhibitory receptors (KIRs) are two types of receptors found on the surface of NK cells (KIRs). These are a small group of cells that look like lymphocytes but have a different lineage than T and B cells. Around 5- 10% of the blood lymphocytes are NK cells. Tumor cells and virally infected cells are also killed by NK cells with no need for prior sensitization. Cytokines (IFN-) secreted by NK cells promote a cellular immune response by activating phagocytic cells and recruiting T cells [21]. The toll-like receptor presented on NK cells activates cytokine production and, in turn, cytotoxicity.

Whenever there is a binding between the Nk cell and non-infected self-cell, Nk cells get the negative signal from the KIR. This happens due to the special recognition of MHC class 1 leader peptides presented on the MHC-like molecules by the KIR. The expression is reduced in the infected cells, which in turn decreases the loading of class 1 peptides in HLA-E (MHC class I antigen E). This further leads to activation through KARs and the killing of the infected cells by NK cells. It is an important mechanism by which Nk cells recognize infected and no infected cells [11]. The binding of the human infected cell with the Nk cell causes the release of a toxic substance containing granules, specifically the performin protein. The performin protein creates the channel on the surface of the cell membrane, increasing the extracellular flow. This process is known as cytolysis [13]. It also releases the digestive enzyme, Granzymes, which particularly induces apoptosis in infected cells. The killing of the cells causes the microbe to release from the cell environment, which is further killed by phagocytosis [10].

Mechanism of the Innate Response

Whenever any pathogens enter the body breaking physiological barriers, the innate immune system responds by migrating phagocytic innate cells to the lesion and releasing toxic mediators. On the innate immune cells' surface, highly specialized receptors called patterned recognition receptors (PRRs) interact with highly conserved molecules on microorganisms, which are referred to as "PAMPs" (pathogen-associated molecular patterns), particularly present on pathogens not in mammalian cells [22]. Activating innate defense mechanisms through these interactions results in phagocytosis and enzymatic degradation of the infectious organisms and eventually, inflammatory proteins secretion, secreting chemokines and cytokines, activating the complement system, and producing acute-phase proteins [23] (Fig. **7**).

Cell Involve in Innate Immunity

Innate Immunity produces the rapid response through granulocytes-neutrophils, basophils, eosinophils, macrophages, monocytes and mast cells, and dendritic cells.

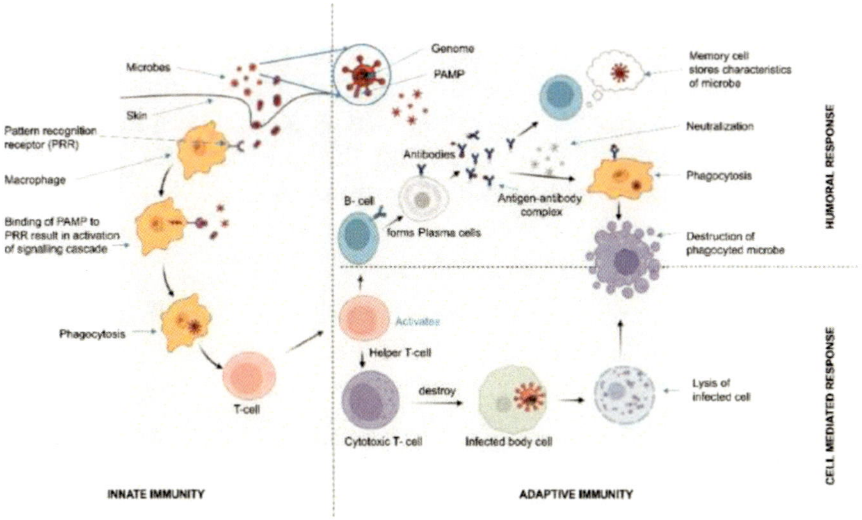

Fig. (7). Overview of Immune system.

Granulocytes

Granulocytes play a variety of roles in the immune response. These cells have a lifespan of more than 5 days, but they react quickly to parasites, extracellular bacteria, and tumours. The presence of these cells early in the healing process causes acute wound inflammation and dilation of surrounding blood vessels, which allows a rapid influx of inflammatory cells. Neutrophils along with their close relative cells, including basophils and eosinophils, are collectively called granulocytes. These are circulating cells, and do not reside in the tissue and wait for the signal so that it can permit into the peripheral tissue.

Neutrophils are short-lived polymorph nuclear granulocytic cells that play an important role in the cellular innate immune system by killing bacteria. They make up about 97% of the total population of granulocytes. Neutrophils reach very rapidly to the site of infections and activate numerous stimuli, and act rapidly through phagocytosis and killing target organisms [23]; some of the most described molecules involved in the signaling are cytokines, complement C5a, leukotriene (LTB4) interleukin - 8 (IL--S), N-formylated peptides. Each of these is likely to be released at the sites of infection and inflammation. Recently, it has been found that it undergoes suicidal extracellular traps composed of DNA and provides a physical barrier to trap the pathogens and spot spreading [24].

Basophils and eosinophils are rare in circulation and particularly bind to Ig E and produce defense against parasites. These are effective against parasites having tough outer shells like helminth worms. This contains specialized granules containing histamine, lipases, DNAases, peroxidase, proteases and the other major cytotoxic proteins. As the worms and parasites are multicellular organisms and cannot be phagocytosed by macrophages and neutrophils, the only way to destroy them is to bombard them with a large number of destructive proteins. In allergies and infestations, the number of eosinophils increases. The basophil and eosinophil are the important source of cytokines, and the cytokine, IL-4, is very much important in shaping the adaptive immune response [25].

Macrophages and Mast Cells

These are considered the tissue-resident cells and are the very first cells present in the body to detect pathogens. These cells play an essential role in sensing infection and amplifying immunological responses. In case of infection, they increase the production of cytokines, chemokines, and other soluble mediators, which facilitate the migration of other immune cells.

Macrophages are derived from the precursor of the monocyte, which at the time of the existing circulation resides on the cell surface and differentiates into the specialized tissue called macrophages. Both the Monocytes as well as free and fixed macrophages are involved in phagocytosis. Macrophages and neutrophils are together responsible for the destruction of pathogens [24]. Fig. **(3a)** Macrophages are more responsible for the initiation of an inflammatory response, destruction of the pathogen, and direct elimination of malignant cells and antigens by producing immune factors such as interleukin (IL)-1, tumour necrosis factor (TNF), and interferon (IFN)-, which can then activate and recruit additional immune cells. They also contribute to the activation of the adaptive immune response *via* antigen presentation [26]. There are different types of tissue macrophages present in the human body. For instance, Kuffer cells (liver), mesangial cells (kidney), microglial cells (brain), alveolar cells (lung), and osteoclast (bone). Mast cells promote vasodilation by the histamine release, which positively affects local vasculature [9]. These are similar in structure to the basophil and are bone marrow-derived cells specifically present on the skin and epithelial mucosa. These cells are not circulating in the blood but rather found on the tissue surface, adjacent to tiny blood vessels and nerves. They express the high-affinity plasma membrane receptor for IgE antibodies. When these antibodies get activated by binding to the antigens, it results in the induction of signaling event, releasing the cytoplasmic granules from the extracellular space. The granular content includes histamine. Mast cells also act as the sentinels in tissue where they produce cytokines in response to microbial products [27].

Dendritic Cells

Dendritic cells primarily function through phagocytosis and play an important role in cell activation for adaptive immunity. These are essential for both innate and adaptive immunity. They have extremely long membranous projections and can be found in lymphatic tissue, organ parenchyma, and mucosal epithelium. Dendritic cells are derived from a precursor that can differentiate into monocytes but not granulocytes because they belong to the myeloid lineage of hematopoietic cells. The maturation of these cells depends on the Cytokine, Flt3 ligand, which further binds to precursor cells through the Flt3 tyrosine kinase receptor. Because of their efficient ability to internalise pathogens and present pathogen peptides on their cell surface, both dendritic cells and macrophages are frequently referred to as antigen-presenting cells (APCs). These are characterized by highly characterized and elaborated dendrites through which they possess maximum contact with the surrounding.

There is two major part of dendritic cells, First-those cells particularly express a high level of MHC class 2 for antigen presentation to T cells; Second-those who do not express MHC class 2 but have a marker that can form interaction with B cells [12].

Dendritic cells usually migrate to lymph nodes of the lymphatic system. Dendritic cells recognise PAMPs and pack the antigenic peptide into the major histocompatibility complex (MHC) (human leukocyte antigens in humans), ensuring that virtually any non-self peptide is presented on T cells with optimal specificity and affinity for T cell receptors [28]. In doing so, stimulate the adaptive immune response.

Adaptive Immunity

Adaptive immunity is a specific type of acquired defense mechanism. The selection of the most appropriate receptor as a target for infecting pathogen is the first step, followed by the activation in response to pathogens or injury. Adaptive immunity maintains the pathogen-specific memory cells [8] and takes a few days or weeks for memory development.

The prime mediators of adaptive immunity are lymphocytes, which are of many types, but the main types include T-lymphocytes (T-cells) and B-lymphocytes (B-cells), and they are antigen-specific. They possess the immunological memory to respond to antigens on re-exposure very quickly. T-lymphocytes are of two types: helper T cells called regulatory cells, which mediate the innate response and produce efficient mediators. Secreted mediators help B lymphocytes and cytotoxic T cells in eliminating infected cells. B cells are predominantly involved in antibody generation in response to antigens.

Immunogenicity and reactivity are two properties of antigens. Immunogenicity refers to the ability to elicit an immune response by producing specific antibodies.

The term antigen comes from its function as an antibody-producing body. The ability to react specifically to antibodies or cells that it stimulates is referred to as reactivity. According to the immunologist, antigens are substances having reactivity. A substance having both reactivity and immunogenicity is considered a complete antigen. The small molecule, having reactivity but not immunogenicity, is called hapten. Haptens combined with small molecules stimulate the immune response [10].

Major Histocompatibility Complex Antigens

MHC antigens are the primary proteins involved in immune recognition and are found on the plasma membrane of somatic cells, where they are referred to as the self-antigen. These are human leukocyte antigens, which are transmembrane glycoproteins (HLA), and they were termed so because of their identification in Leukocytes. MHC is classified into three types: Class I, Class II, and Class III, with Class I and Class II playing critical roles in the adaptive immune system. Class I and class II MHC molecules are involved in the antigen-presenting process for T cell recognition.

MHC class I (MHC-I) - It is made up of two chains namely, alpha and beta chains, non-covalently bonded polypeptides. The immunogenic peptide complexes are likely to be present on the nucleated cells and recognized by the cytotoxic CD8+ T cell. CD8 antigens have a higher affinity toward alpha three molecules. Somatic cells plasma membranes, except red blood cells, have these molecules. MHC Class I Level 2 MHC - These are heterodimers and contain two chains of the non-covalently bonded polypeptide (alpha30kDa and beta26kDa). These (MHC-II) molecules are found on the surface of antigen-presenting cells (for example, macrophages, B cells, Dendrites cells, *etc.*). They activate CD4+T cells, resulting in effector cell coordination and regulation [8, 32]. Class 3 MHC molecules play no role in antigen presentation. Complement components C2, C4A, C4B, and factor B, among others, are involved in class 3MHC molecules. This category includes heat shock protein and tumour necrosis factor-alpha and beta.

The presence of the foreign antigen recognized by both T cells and B cells is required to be present to show an immune response. Antigens can be recognised and bound by B cells in blood plasma, lymph, and intestinal fluid. T cells, on the other hand, can recognise fragments of antigenic proteins that have been processed and presented in a specific manner. Antigen processing entails fragmenting the antigenic protein and then associating it with the MHC2 molecule. After that, the complex formation between the antigen and MHC 2 molecules is inserted into the plasma membrane of the cell body, which is known as antigen presentation. Peptide fragments from self-proteins are ignored by the T cells, and non-self-peptide fragments after recognition are taken for the immunogenic response.

Clonal Selection

Clonal selection theory explains why exactly lymphocytes can react to various types of antigenic responses Fig. (**8**). The immunologist Niels Jerne, in 1954, made a hypothesis that before the infection also, there were a large number of lymphocytes already present in the body. When the antigens enter the body, they specifically search for the lymphocytes specific for them and, in turn, produce antibodies to destroy antigens. A hypothesis states that lymphocytes, especially B cells, express the antigen-specific receptors even before the antibody encounter antigens and activate cells. It leads to the formation of the clone daughter cells. This hypothesis is commonly used to determine the immune system's response in immunogenic conditions, as well as the selection of T and B lymphocytes for the destruction of invading antigens [29].

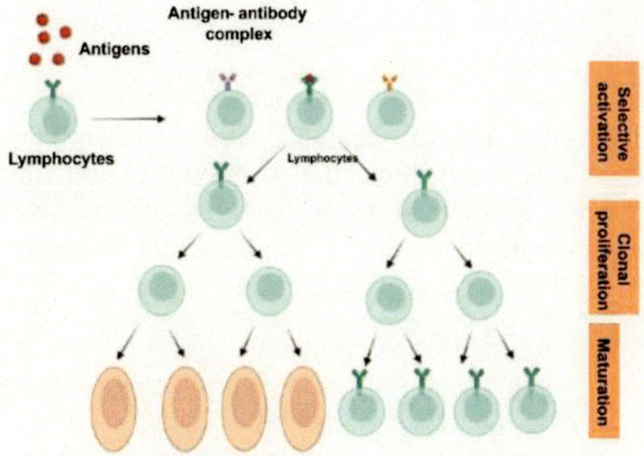

Fig. (8). Clonal selection.

In clonal selection, antigens are exposed to many circulation B cells and T cells *via* MHC. The secreted lymphocytes that match the antigens exactly are chosen to form memory and effector clones among themselves. This is referred to as clonal expansion. During this process, the cells divide to form daughter cells, which proliferate for several generations to form clones of the original cells. In the future attack of similar antigens, the preexisting lymphocytes which already bear the receptor for that antigens are merely selected because of their confirmed binding to the antigen.

Clonal selection is indeed useful even during the negative selection of T cell maturation, in which the infant lymphocyte is exposed to the body's epitopes rather than antigens. The lymphocytes which react to the body's antigen are called autoreactive and are destroyed before they form the cloned daughter cells and cause damage to the body. This happens due to random mutation, in which the lymphocytes attack to body's cells instead of non-self-antigens [30].

On the adaptive response of the immune system on the further antigen attacks, the memory cells respond more quickly as compared to the effector cells. It is because, during the clonal expansion and the clonal selection, a certain mutation in antigen-binding affinity in memory cells increases the binding affinity of the memory cells more than the effector cells in the first antigenic attack.

Adaptive immunity work in two ways.

Cell-Mediated Response

It is also called cell-mediated immunity. The cell-mediated immunity activates macrophage and NK cells to destroy intracellular pathogens and causes the release of various cytokines in response to an antigen [29]. It involves mostly immature T lymphocytes and related effector products, which bind antigens. It is also called cell-mediated immunity. The cell-mediated immunity activates macrophage and NK cells to destroy intracellular pathogens and causes the release of various cytokines in response to an antigen [31]. It primarily consists of immature T lymphocytes and related effector products that bind antigens.

T cells are classified into two types: helper T cells and cytotoxic T cells. Helper-T cells produce some chemicals, which aid B lymphocytes. They produce cytokines to activate phagocytes. These cells, which include a subset of helper T cells, express the protein from the CD (cluster of differentiation) family on their cell surface and are known as CD4+ cells (for example, Th-1, Th-2, and Th- 17). Cytotoxic T cells directly kill infected cells and, as CD8+ cells, express protein from the CD8 family on their cell surface. Other subsets of T-lymphocytes include T suppressors cells, called regulatory cells.

Activation of T Cells

T cells are produced in the thymus and are specifically programmed to eliminate foreign particles, antigens, which are commonly found in the inactivated form. T cell receptor refers to the antigen-binding receptor on the surface of T cells

(TCRs). This receptor binds *via* a specific receptor fragment present on the antigen MCH complex. T cells have the ability to produce $\sim 10^{13}$ different receptors [32]. Each different T cells have its specific and unique TCRs, but on 5the exposure of antigen, only a few receptors are able to recognize the antigen. This is when the action of surface protein takes place. The CD4 and CD8 proteins are considered as the co-receptor as these proteins interact with antigen MCH complex and help to maintain the coupling in between. These proteins are considered the first signal in the activation of T cells Fig. (**9**).

Additional secondary signals are too closely linked to activate both helper and cytotoxic T cells in response to antigens CD28 of Helper T cell and bind to the antigen-presenting complex *via* B7.1 (CD80) or B7.2 (CD86) and stimulate T cell proliferation. The resulting lymphocytes have the power to recognize the antigen, and the proliferative signal is controlled through CTA-4. Similarly, cytotoxic T cells require co-stimulatory molecules like CD70 and 4-1BB (CD137). Other molecules include LCOS, 4-1BB, and OX40, but these are not as predominant as CD28. TCR interaction with antigen MHC complex in the absence of the co-stimulatory molecule causes the T cells to switch off [31, 33].

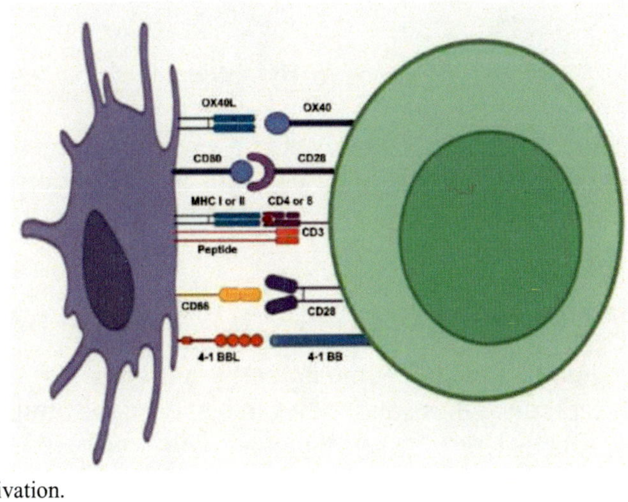

Fig. (9). T-cells activation.

Generally, after the invasion of antigen in the body, the T cells receive the response in the form of cytokines. Different cells presented at the site of inflammation, like mast cells, neutrophils, and epithelial cells, release cytokines and chemokines, which increases the activation as well as a proliferation of T cells [32, 34].

Helper T Cells

They are the key cell population in the adaptive immune system, activating B cells for antibody release, macrophages to destroy the pathogen, and stimulation of the cytotoxic T cells to completely kill the targeted cells. They have CD4 protein on their surface, useful for presenting APC MHC2 and activation. On activation, the Naïve T cells differentiate into Th1 and Th2 effector subsets, derived based on their cytokines secretion pattern and effector functions [42, 43]. After activation, these cells undergo clonal selection to generate helper and memory T cells [35].

Cytotoxic T Cells

The CD8 protein is found on the cell surface of cytotoxic T cells and are called T-killer cells or CD8+ cells. The cytotoxic T cells with MHC1 and TCR recognize antigens presented on the cell surface infected by tumor cells, microbes and tissue transplants. Moreover, helper T cells mediated costimulation by IL2 and cytokine is the critical step for cytotoxic T cells activation. The activation results in the clonal selection and further results in the formation of cytotoxic T cells and memory cytotoxic T cells.

Cytotoxic T cells destroy the pathogen by three main mechanisms. The first mechanism includes the secretion of Cytokines, initially TNF alpha and TNF gamma. The second mechanism involves the cytotoxic granules that contain perforin and Granzymes(serine proteases) and induce apoptosis. The third mechanism includes Fas/FasL interaction and stimulation of apoptosis cascade [36].

Humoral Response

It is also called humoral immunity, mediated by antibodies of different classes. The B lymphocytes produce these antibodies in response to stimulation by antigen in the presence of T cell-derived growth factors. During plasma cell formation, a clone of B lymphocytes does not undergo the formation of plasma cell but remains as a dormant B lymphocyte until activated by a new amount of the same antigens. Therefore, these lymphocytes are referred to as memory cells. As a result, subsequent exposure to the same antigen will result in a much stronger antibody response. The humoral immune system is made up of various components immunoglobulins from the acute phase (IgA, IgG, IgM, IgD, & IgE),(C-reactive proteins) + inflammatory mediators, Complement (C1-C9), factor B, factor D, properdin.

Activation of B Cells

B cells become activated by binding to B cell receptors (BCRs), and they can respond to both unprocessed and processed antigens, but the response to the processed antigen is always intense. Antigen processing occurs through the fragmentation of the antigen inside the B cell and combing them with MHC2 self-antigens. B cells-MHC2 complex moves toward the B cell plasma membrane and is essential for differentiation and B-cell proliferation.

B-cells undergo clonal selection, which results in the formation of plasma cells and memory B cells, and plasma cells aid the secretion of antibodies up to 4 - 5 days post-exposure. Interleukin 4 and interleukin 6 secreted from T cells help B cell proliferation, differentiation, and antibody secretion by plasma cells. When B cells are inactive, they express IgM/IgD, but when activated, they express IgA, IgE, IgG, or may remain in their IgM expression form. There are mainly two types of immune responses, T cells - independent immune response of B cells and T cells - dependent immune response of B cells.

Immunological Memory

The immune system remembers the previous antigen attack and produces long-lasting antibodies as well as the long-lived lymphocytes produced during clonal selection [37]. When an antigen enters the body, the immune system recognises it and prepares memory cells accordingly so that when the same antigen attacks again, the immune system is ready to fight. The immunogenic memory is quantified as antibody titer, the total amount of antibodies in the serum. After the initial attack, the antibody count decreases and thereafter, increases slowly, firstly IgM, then IgG. The primary response of the body is a gradual decrease in antibody titer. On the subsequent attack by the same antigen, the number of the antibodies increases resulting in a rapid increase in the memory cells. At some point, the antibody titer is observed to be greater than the primary response, specifically an increased amount of IgG antibodies, this is called the secondary response. Immunological memory provides the basis for immunization. There are various vaccines available for different diseases like polio.

ALLERGY AND HYPERSENSITIVITY REACTION

Allergic and hypersensitivity conditions (A/H) are multifaceted problems that can affect multiple organs and people of all ages, and they have a significant impact on the quality of life of patients and their families. “Hypersensitivity” is defined as “conditions clinically representing allergy that cause objectively repeatable symptoms or signs, introduced by exposure to a defined impulse at a dose tolerated by normal subjects,” while “allergy” is defined as “a hypersensitivity reaction initiated by proven immunologic mechanisms." [38]. "A/H are dangerous immune responses which cause tissue damage and can lead to serious diseases."

A/H accounts for even more than 17 million outpatient services in the United States alone each year [39]. The complexity and severity of all these conditions continue to rise, particularly among children and young people, who bear the brunt of the burden. Allergy symptoms are now the world's fourth most common chronic disease. According to the WHO, by 2050, one in every two people worldwide will suffer from allergies, with this Fig. expected to rise steadily, particularly in industrialised countries.

Clemens von Pirquet coined the term allergy in 1906, referring to an abnormal response by the adaptive immune system which may or may not involve allergen-specific Immunoglobulin (IgE). The substance which induces allergy is called an allergen which includes non-infectious components of certain infectious organisms. There are basically two types of allergens.

Fist type of allergens causes IgE production, in turn sensitizing the subject. This later causes an allergic reinduction reaction on re-exposure. Grass and tree pollens, animal dander (shedding from skin and fur), house dust mite faecal particles, certain foods (particularly peanuts, tree nuts, fish, shellfish, milk and eggs), latex, some medicines, and insect venoms are common allergen sources. Allergen-specific IgE targeting invading pathogens can actually recognise cross-reactive host antigens, but the clinical relevance of this is unclear. The second type of allergen is the non-infectious substance present in the environment that acts through local inflammation and induces adaptive immune response independently of IgE, like allergic contact dermatitis caused by exposure to nickel [40].

As the first exposure to the allergen causes a release of IgE antibodies which further attach to the mast cell, and on next exposure, with the help of a special mediator released by the mast cell, easily capture the allergen. These mediators, in turn, produce classic allergic symptoms such as swelling of body tissues, sneezing, wheezing, coughing, as well as other symptoms. Different types of allergy-related diseases include rhinitis, asthma conjunctivitis, contact dermatitis, atopic eczema, urticarial, anaphylaxis, food hypersensitivity, Hymenoptera, and other insect hypersensitivities [39].

Classification of Hypersensitivity Reactions

Hypersensitivity reactions are classified into four types depending upon the mechanism of the reaction.

1. Type I (immediate or immunoglobulin E [IgE] mediated)
2. Type II (cytotoxic or IgG/ IgM mediated)
3. Type III (immune complex-mediated)
4. Type IV (delayed-type or T-cell mediated)

Table 1. Types of hypersensitivity reactions and their characteristics.

Characteristics	Type I	Type II	Type III	Type IV
Common name	Immediate or immunoglobulin E [IgE] mediated	Cytotoxic or IgG/ IgM mediated	Immune complex mediated	Delayed type or T-cell mediated
Effector mechanism	Mast cell activation	Complement, ADCC, opsonization	Complement	Macrophage activation and cytotoxicity (perforin and granzyme)
Antibody	IgE	IgG, IgM	T cell mediated	None
Antigen	Exogeneous	Cell surface	Soluble	Tissue and Organ
Response time	15-30 min	Minute hour	3-8 hours	48-72 hour
Histology	Basophils and eosinophils	Antibody and complement	Complement and neutrophils	Monocytes and lymphocytes
Transfered with	Antibody	Antibody	Antibody	T- cells
Example	Anaphylaxis, urticarial, drug allergy, food allergy, dust allergy, asthma	Myasthenia gravis, haemolytic disease in new born, drug sensitivity	Arthus reaction, serum sickness reaction	Delayed hypersensitivity, allergic rhinitis, allergic rhinitis, acute generalized exanthematous pustulosis

Type I Hypersensitivity Reaction Fig.(10)

Type I hypersensitivities basically involve IgE antibodies that initiate a quick inflammatory response by sensitizing an individual to the different allergen upon subsequent exposure. It involves mast cells and basophils [41]. During the sensitization T helper (Th) cells along with their mediator, cause the isotopic switch to B cells while producing IgE antibodies. A portion of IgE remains bound on the surface of the high-affinity IgE receptor Fc RI found on mast cells and basophils, which releases mediator upon re-exposure. The release occurs in two phases; the early phase causes the release of histamine, lysosomal enzymes, and other mediators like protease. Furthermore, mast cells produce some lipid mediators that are released into the bloodstream in under 15 minutes of cross-reaction with IgE antibodies [42]. And this is the reason why it is called an immediate hypersensitivity reaction. Some examples are food allergies, anaphylaxis, drug allergies, and dust allergies. Whereas the late phase usually occurs after 4 to 8 hours of exposure due to *de novo* production of cytokines such as interleukin (IL)-1, IL-4, IL-5, IL-13, tumor necrosis factor (TNF) and granulocyte monocyte colony-stimulating factor (GM-CSF) by mast cells. The type I hypersensitivity reaction is a common anaphylaxis reaction [43]. Some of the hypersensitivity reactions are caused by IgE-independent non-specific activation of the mast cells and is called a subset of type I hypersensitivity reactions. Example Urticaria.

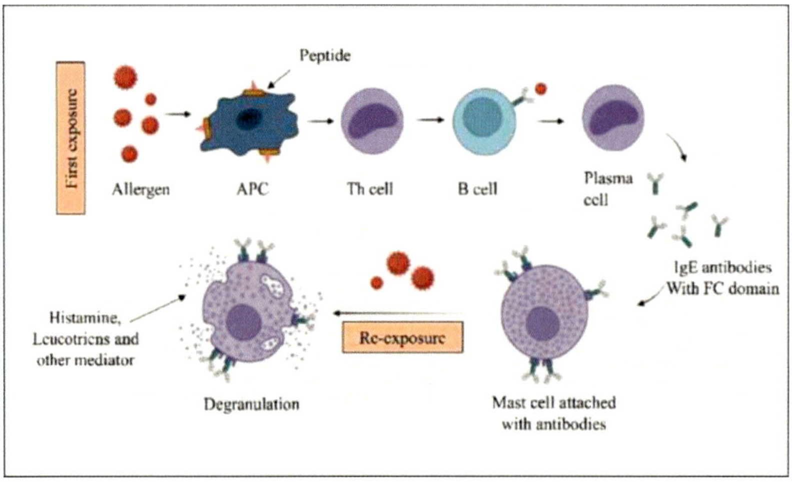

Fig. (10). Type I (immediate or immunoglobulin E [IgE] mediated).

Type II Hypersensitivity Reaction

Type II hypersensitivity refers to the overactivation of IgG and IgM antibody-mediated cytotoxic reactions against cell surface and extracellular matrix proteins Fig. (**11**). The immunoglobulins damage cells by complement system activation, interfering with normal cellular functions or phagocytosis [44, 45]. Immune thrombocytopenia, autoimmune hemolytic anaemia, and autoimmune neutropenia are all examples of type II hypersensitivity reactions. It normally involves exogenous chemicals like heptane.

Type II hypersensitivity reactions are of two types - type IIa and type IIb. They are distinguished by catalytic destruction of the targeted cells *via* IgG and IgM binding to the cell component, and three main mechanisms underline the hypersensitivity of this type [46].

1. Complement-mediated cell lysis: It is the system of lytic enzymes which only get activated by antigen-antibody complex by classic, alternate, and lectin pathways. The activation of the complement system on the cell's surface results in lysis.

2. Antibody-dependent cell-mediated cytotoxicity (ADCC): Once antibodies bind to its Fab portion, the Fc region has always had a binding site on cytotoxic cells, resulting in cross-linking between target and cytotoxic cells and, as a result, promoting killing. IgG on binding causes the release of perforin and granzyme directly killing cells and, along with IgM, initiates phagocytosis by binding the Fc receptor. In ADCC, the antibody does not kill or destroy cells directly, but rather mediates killing by presenting antigen to cytotoxic cells; the antibody's ability to bind antigen is dependent on its ability to bind antigen. As a result, the mechanism is referred to as antibody-dependent cell-mediated cytotoxicity.

3. Opsonisation: When the antigen-antibody complex forms, binding occurs *via* the Fab region, while the Fc regions of the antibody remain free, containing the FcR receptor to which neutrophils, macrophages, and monocytes can bind. The direct linkage of antigen with phagocytic cells results in the increased rate of phagocytosis, called opsonization.

Type IIb reactions directly stimulate the cells to create a pathogenic state, for example, Myasthenia gravis [42].

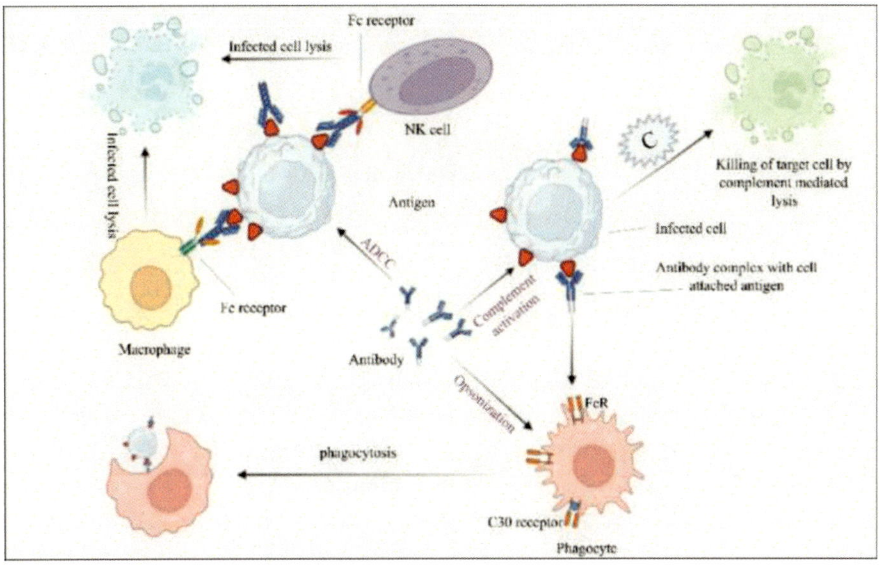

Fig. (11). Type II (cytotoxic or IgG/ IgM mediated).

Type III Hypersensitivity Reaction

Type III reactions are considered as immune-complex reactions containing IgG, IgM, and sometimes IgA antibodies Fig. (**12**). The antibodies form a complex with antigen and cause direct damage to the tissue by the complement system activation, leading to polymorph nuclear leukocytes (PMNs) chemotaxis [58]. Small arteries, renal glomeruli, and synovial capsules of joints are common sites of complex deposition, resulting in vasculitis, glomerulonephritis, and arthritis, respectively. Symptoms of this type of hypersensitivity reaction have been linked to the site of infection rather than the source of antigen. Example Serum sickness reaction [47].

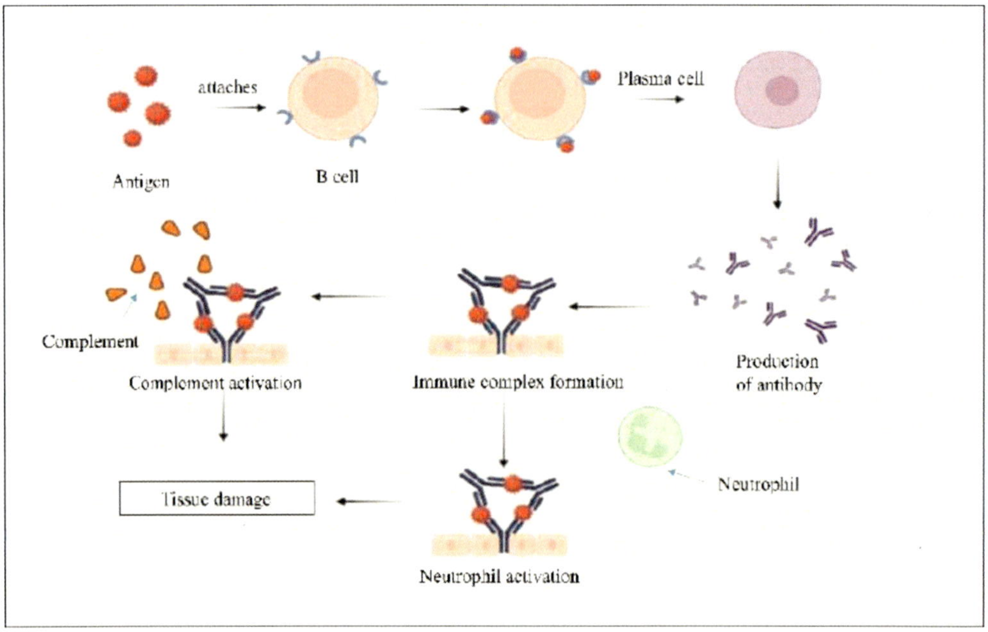

Fig. (12). Type III (immune complex-mediated).

Type IV Hypersensitivity Reaction

It is also known as cell-mediated delayed hypersensitivity, which usually takes about 12-24 hours to progress and remains for about 2 to 3 days. T lymphocytes induce a cell-mediated response, which is intermediated by effector T cells and macrophages [47]. In certain cases, monocytes, eosinophils, and neutrophils are also involved. It is divided into two phases: the sensitization phase, in which primary antigen exposure sensitises T memory cells (TH1 cells), and the effector phase includes activation of pro-inflammatory mediators on secondary exposure of pre-sensitized H1 cells with familiar antigens by stimulated T cells.

Then macrophages and monocytes engulf the antigens and become sensitized later, and cause tissue damage by cytokines and chemokines release, as depicted in Fig. (**13**). Based on the type of T cell (CD4 T-helper type 1 and type 2 cells) involved and the cytokines/chemokines produced, cell delayed hypersensitivity is classified as type IVa, IVb, IVc, and IVd [48]. Contact dermatitis, which can be caused by a variety of substances such as poison ivy and oak, is an example of this type. Type IVb reaction induces B cell production and eosinophilic inflammation by increasing the production of IL-4, IL-5, and IL-13 by Th2 cells. Example asthma or allergic rhinitis. Type IVc involves the direct killing of a targeted cell through CD8 T cells. Example, Stevens-Johnson syndrome and toxic epidermal necrolysis are conditions in which activated CD8 T cells cause keratinocyte apoptosis and/or necrosis. Type IVd responds by CXCL8 (IL-8) which recruits neutrophils at inflammatory tissue to create sterile neutrophilic inflammation. Example acute generalized exanthemata's pustulosis [42].

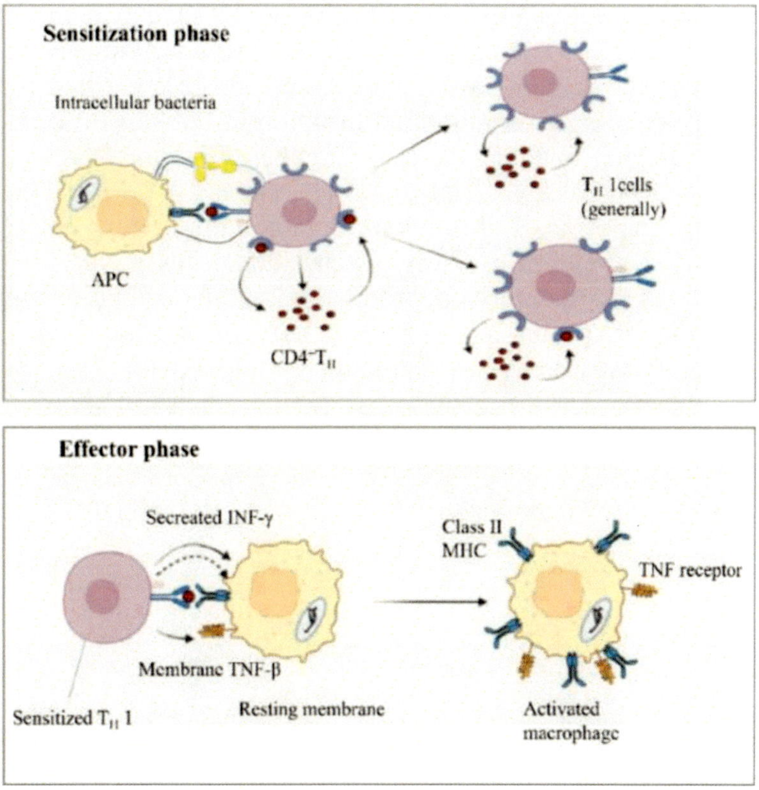

Fig. (13). Type IV (delayed type or T-cell mediated).

IMMUNOMODULATION

Immunity is an essential system of the human body, and the human body cannot escape from its surveillance. After birth, the immune system is naturally well-educated and trained to identify and eliminate external and internal threats to protect the human body. Immunity works in a coordinated manner for good health. We have learned that adaptive and innate immunity are interconnected and interdependent. Various mediators like cytokines, soluble anti-microbials, and other signaling molecules initiate, and modulate immune response with the help of immune cells. If the immune system is weakened or overactivated, it can lead to several diseases. In the last century, advancements in modern medicines have given therapies to curb infection, sanitation, and public health initiatives through discoveries of vaccines and drugs. However, the gamut of chronic illnesses remained untreated, and research in modern medicines to deal with these diseases is quite disappointing.

The research outcome throughout the last century provided evidence of weakened or imbalanced immune systems being one of the underlying causes for these chronic illnesses. The immune system is central to these chronic illnesses. The immune system requires the spatiotemporal interplay of several immune cells to suppress or stimulate, overactivated or weaken immunity, respectively and regulate immune homeostasis. The growing evidence of several modalities to restore immune homeostasis through immunomodulation is emerging and is currently receiving attention globally. These modalities include natural health products like herbs, marine-derived products, animal origin products, vaccines, antibodies, prebiotics, probiotics, and restoration of microbiota, micronutrients (vitamins, minerals, fatty acids), as enumerated in Fig. (**14**).

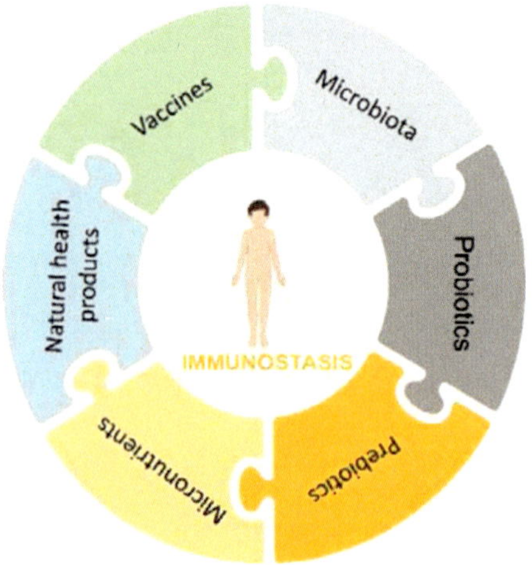

Fig. (14). Modalities of Immune System.

Microbiota and Prebiotic, Probiotics

The gastrointestinal tract (GIT) and skin are the physiological barriers that maintain systemic integrity and ward off external threats to the immune system. In particular, GIT is a complex, intricate immune organ having the highest number of lymph nodes. The GIT harbor a diverse spectrum of bacterial flora in infants right after birth and throughout their lifespan. There is a significant positive relationship between GIT mucosa microbiota and immunity. Prebiotics and probiotics directly or indirectly affect immune health, positively, and these positive effects ascribe to their immunomodulating capacity [49].

Prebiotics are non-digestible food ingredients that improve host health by stimulating one or more microbial flora in the GI tract. There are many types of prebiotics, and their definition and features were revised recently [61]. As per recent revision, prebiotics is classified based on several characteristics. Prebiotics are those substances that (i) are resistant to stomach acidic pH; (ii) are non-modifiable with digestive enzymes; (iii) are non-absorbable in GIT; (iv) undergo fermentation with microbial flora of the gut; (v) stimulate activity and/or growth of host-microbiota Prebiotics include fructans (fructo-oligosaccharide- FOS), galacto-oligosaccharides, starch and glucose-derived oligosaccharide (GOS), other oligosaccharides, and non-carbohydrate oligosaccharides. Prebiotics are naturally present in many food products like cereals, pulses, and fruits. Consuming prebiotics improves immunity in several ways and has been proven clinically. Prebiotics induce the expression of cytokines, and decrease the population of harmful pathogens in the GUT. FOr instance, mannose binds to salmonella and reduces their colonization in the GIT (Table **1**) [49, 50].

Probiotics are live bacteria, and they have manifold implications in boosting immunity. Probiotics principally exert their effect by replacing the pathogenic microbes with improving intestinal barrier function, restoring intestinal integrity in case of allergy or inflammation, lowering proinflammatory cytokines generation, and synthesizing vitamins, and folic acid [51]. The probiotic immunomodulatory and immunoregulatory capacity have provided clinical evidence in children and the elderly [51, 52]. The nutrigenomics study conducted in healthy human volunteers revealed bacteria-strain-specific responses when measuring the changes in the transcriptional profile of genes of duodenal mucosa following probiotic, Lactobacillus consumption [53]. The consistent responses of transcription profile were observed in all volunteers, and strain-specificity was also detected. Three strains of Lactobacilli were evaluated for immune responses, which showed a range of responses distinct to the respective strain. For instance, immune tolerance was observed with Lactobacillus Plantarum probiotic consumption; Lactobacillus acidophilus probiotic consumption showed stimulation of T-helper cells, whereas Lactobacillus casei probiotic induced Th1/Th2 balance immune response [50, 54]. On a similar note, several human studies delineated the immunomodulatory effect of probiotic consumption (Table **2**).

Table 2. Prebiotic and probiotic effects on the human immune system.

Prebiotic/Probiotic	Effect on Immune System	References
FOS (8 oz/day of an experimental formula containing FOS for 183 days)	Improvement in antibody responses toward viral vaccines Decrease in hospitalization due to influenza and side effects of influenza vaccines.	[55]
FOS (8 g/day Orafti® Synergy1 for 4 week)	Salivary IgA, immune cells in serum, activation, Proliferation of T and NK cell not changed.	[56]
GOS (5.5 g/day for 10 week)	Phagocytosis, NK cell activity, and IL-10 (an anti-inflammatory cytokine) level increased. Pro-inflammatory cytokines, such as IL-6, IL-1β, and tumor necrosis factor-α, levels decreased.	[57]
L. acidophilus and bifidobacteria in a fermented milk product	A significant elevations of total IgA, IgA specific for *Salmonella enterica* subsp. *enterica serovar Typhi*	[58]
Faecalibacterium prausnitzii and *L. paracasei*	Inhibit nuclear factor-κB (NF-κB) activation and ongoing inflammation in tissues from patients with inflammatory bowel disease (IBD)8	[59]
Bifidobacterium infantis 35624	An increase in the amount of IL-10 produced by peripheral blood mononuclear cells and the expression of the transcription factor forkhead box P3 (FOXP3) by TReg cells	[60]

Micronutrients

Several studies showed remarkable improvement in immune health with micronutrient intake and preventive, therapeutic benefits in chronic illness Table **3**. Micronutrients represented by different vitamins (Vitamin A, B, C, D, E) and trace elements (zinc, selenium, copper, magnesium) support the development of adaptive and innate immunity. Vitamin C has shown cognitive betterment in neurodegenerative disorders and effects linked with dysfunction in the immune component [61]. A meta-analysis of 9 clinical trials data revealed the shortened incidence of the common cold with the daily supplement of extra doses of vitamin C [51, 52]. Zinc deficiency adversely affects immune function. The Zinc deficiency in humans showed a decreased number of natural killer cells, T, B cells, and reduced cytokine production, leading to recurrent infectious diseases [62]. Vitamin A supports adaptive immunity, as evident from clinical trials in pediatric populations wherein an increase in the CD4 subpopulation of T cells was reported [63].

Table 3. Impact of micronutrients on immune health.

Micronutrients	Effect on the Immune System	References
Vitamin A	Treatment of respiratory syncytial virus infection with Vitamin A showed a shorter duration of hospitalization along with a more rapid resolution of tachypnea.	[64]
-	Vitamin A supplement along with retinol in pre-scool students, showed about 12% reduction in all-cause mortality.	[65]
Vitamin D	Risk of the acute lower respiratory infection is more in the children with lower vitamin D intake	[66]
-	Lower Vitamin D levels increase the possibility of having viral infections.	[67]
Zinc	Weekly zinc supplements to children with pneumonia and diarrhea reduce mortality	[68]
-	Zinc as adjuvant therapy in young children with severe pneumonia causes slightly faster recovery along with a lower risk of treatment failure.	[69]

Natural Health Products

Many herbal preparations or their phytoconstituents display an array of immunomodulatory effects on the immune system Table **4**. Immunomodulatory effects include cytokine secretion, class switching, immunoglobin production, increased lymphocytes and phagocytes count, and many more [53, 70]. The medicinal herbs constituents are a different class of compounds like flavonoids, terpenes, alkaloids, saponins, tannins, glucans, and polyphenols and have been reported their activity in many preclinical and clinical studies. The food, spices, and herbs showed promising results against various cancers [71]. The consumption of green tea and Brassica vegetables (broccoli, cabbage) depicted a lower risk of cancers observed in epidemiological studies). A random screening method and ethnopharmacology approach are two major bioprospecting of natural product strategies. The random screening method is a classic method and depends on the random screening of phytochemical factors and herbs. The ethnopharmacology approach is time-consuming and lengthy with traditional knowledge and practices as a drug discovery search engine [61, 72].

Vaccines

Vaccination works by triggering host immunity with the safe version of infectious agents without causing severe illness to the host. Several vaccines are prepared with an attenuated strain of pathogens or heat-killed preparation, whereas recombinant vaccines are designed in several ways. Some vaccines are produced in cell culture, challenging the cells with the epitope of the pathogen (*e.g.* hepatitis and human papillomavirus vaccines). The vaccine with immunomodulators is a promising modality to boost immune response. Vaccine adjuvants are a key component in the vaccine design for sharpening or enhancing the antigen-specific-immune response. The immunomodulators are considered an effective adjuvant for vaccine efficacy Table **5.**

Table 4. Immunoactive leads from natural origin.

Phytoconstituents	Effect on Immune System	References
Artemisinin (*Artemisia annua*)	Shows synergistic immune suppressive effect on inflammation and autoimmune disease	[73]
Shatavarin (*Asparagus racemosus*)	Shows immunostimulatory activity	[74]
Sinomenine (*Sinomenium acutum*)	Improves immunosuppression	[75]
Apocynin (*Picrorhiza kurroa*)	Stimulates humoral as well as a cell-mediated component of the immune system	[76]
Ginsan (*Panax ginseng*)	Enhance resistance and maintain the homeostasis of the Immune system	[65]
Piperine (*Piper longum*)	Shows immunomodulatory response by inhibition of MHC-II	[77]

Table 5. Vaccine adjuvants from natural origin.

Adjuvants	Immune Response	References
Saponins (for example, QS21)	Ab, TH1,TH2, CD8+ T cells	[78]
C-type lectin ligands (for example, TDB)	Ab, TH1, TH17	[79]
Polysaccharide adjuvant inulin, derived from the roots of the Asteraceae	Humoral and cellular immune response	[80]
Tomatine is a glycoalkaloid derived from *Lycopersicon pimpinellifolium*	Significantly upregulated interferon (IFN)-γ	[81]

IMMUNOTHERAPY

Immunotherapy is the therapeutic approach targeting multiple factors of the immune system. The vaccine is the first effective immunotherapy discussed in the above section. But then, immunotherapy extends beyond vaccine technology and includes the use of antibodies, recombinant proteins, *ex-vivo* edited autologous cells, and many more. The first example of the clinical application of immunotherapy was the diphtheria vaccine. Behring and his group immunized guinea pigs with attenuated diphtheria toxin, and serum isolated from immunized animals was used for the virulent strain of diphtheria. Such anti-toxin benefited children with diphtheria disease worldwide.

An exaggerated immune response against the self is characteristic of autoimmune disorders. The goal of immunotherapy is to switch off an exaggerated immune response. However, targeting autoantigen without damaging other self-cells is a challenging task. In the absence of effective auto-antigen-specific immunotherapy, different strategies are explored. One example is a neutralizing mediator, cytokine TNF, in rheumatoid arthritis patients (infliximab (IFX), etanercept (ETN), adalimumab (ADA), golimumab (GOLI) and certolizumab pegol (CZP)) [82]. Other cytokine antibodies like anti-IL1, IL 10 and anti-IL-6 are employed for autoinflammatory diseases.

Immunity has become instrumental in several chronic illnesses, like cancer, neurodegenerative diseases, and metabolic disorders, apart from infectious diseases, owing to advancements in technology and a deeper understanding of the diseases.

Many-fold interactions exist between immune cells and cancer cells, and these interactions were well-defined in 1909 by Paul Ehrlich in his immunization experiments with tumor cells. Innovative strategies are being investigated and implemented for cancer immunotherapy that encompasses passive and active immunotherapy. Passive immunotherapy elicits anti-tumor response with monoclonal antibodies, small molecule inhibitors, and Chimeric Antigen Receptor (CAR) T cell therapy, while active immunotherapy evokes anti-tumor response through vaccine, immunomodulation, or targeting antigen receptor of tumor cells [62, 83 - 87]. Immunotherapy for neurodegenerative diseases emerged as a new facet in modern therapeutics with the discovery of the brain lymphatic system and cross-talk between CNS biology and the immune system. Though the proposed approach of immunotherapy for neurodegenerative diseases remains in its initial stage, the rejuvenating immune system with immunotherapy in combination with other treatment modalities would be a promising potential strategy to prevent and cure neurodegenerative diseases [88].

CONCLUSION

The immune system comprises innate and acquired immunity, innate being the oldest one on an evolutionary scale. The immune system includes white blood cells, lymphocytes, and various soluble mediators and provides defense against invading infection or any cells that become a threat to the host, as in the case of cancer or autoimmune disorders. As the immune system works in close association with the nervous system and endocrine system, its complexity and depth make it difficult to reach the girth of the system and identify the precise target for modulation. The progress in research over the last century and advancement in genomics and proteomics have shown the significant contribution and involvement of the immune system in several chronic illnesses.

Immunomodulation is a strategic approach to correct dysfunction of the immune system. It can be achieved through natural immunomodulators. The maintaining microbiota of host with prebiotics, probiotics, and natural health products usage have proven their benefits in preclinical and clinical studies. The deficiency of micronutrients leads to impaired immunity. Immunotherapy in cancer and autoimmune disorders has depicted encouraging results in the clinical setting. Taken together, the precise maneuvering of the immune system with tools of advanced science and technology revives the hope of scientists to unravel the potential of natural immunomodulators in the service of human health.

CONSENT FOR PUBLICATION

Not applicable.

CONFLICT OF INTEREST

The authors declare no conflict of interest, financial or otherwise.

ACKNOWLEDGEMENTS

Declared none.

REFERENCES

[1] Cooper EL. Commentary on *CAM and NK Cells* by Kazuyoshi Takeda and Ko Okumura. Evid Based Complement Alternat Med 2004; 1(1): 29-34. [http://dx.doi.org/10.1093/ecam/neh011] [PMID: 15257323]

[2] Kiessling R, Klein E, Wigzell H. "Natural" killer cells in the mouse. I. Cytotoxic cells with specificity for mouse Moloney leukemia cells. Specificity and distribution according to genotype. Eur J Immunol 1975; 5(2): 112-7. [http://dx.doi.org/10.1002/eji.1830050208] [PMID: 1234049]

[3] Herberman RB, Nunn ME, Lavrin DH. Natural cytotoxic reactivity of mouse lymphoid cells against syngeneic and allogeneic tumors. I. Distribution of reactivity and specificity. Int J Cancer 1975; 16(2): 216-29. [http://dx.doi.org/10.1002/ijc.2910160204] [PMID: 50294]

[4] Retief FP, Cilliers L. The epidemic of Athens, 430-426 BC. S Afr Med J 1998; 88(1): 50-3. [PMID: 9539938]

[5] Plotkin SA. Vaccines: past, present and future. Nat Med 2005; 11(S4) (Suppl.): S5-S11. [http://dx.doi.org/10.1038/nm1209] [PMID: 15812490]

[6] Brodin P, Davis MM. Human immune system variation. Nat Rev Immunol 2017; 17(1): 21-9. [http://dx.doi.org/10.1038/nri.2016.125] [PMID: 27916977]

[7] Gulati P. Janeway's Immunobiology, 7th Edition by Kenneth Murphy, Paul Travers, and Mark Walport. Biochemistry and Molecular Biology Education 2009; 37(2): 134-4. https://onlinelibrary.wiley.com/doi/abs/10.1002/bmb.20272

[8] McComb S, Thiriot A, Akache B, Krishnan L, Stark F. Introduction to the Immune System. In: Fulton KM, Twine SM, editors. Immunoproteomics [Internet]. New York, NY: Springer New York; 2019 [cited 2021 Nov 17]. p. 1–24. (Methods in Molecular Biology; vol. 2024). Available from: http://link.springer.com/10.1007/978-1-4939-9597-4_1

[9] Delves PJ, Martin SJ, Burton DR, Roitt IM. Roitt's Essential Immunology. NY: Wiley-Blackwell 2017.

[10] Derrickson BH, Tortora GJ. Tortora's Principles of anatomy & physiology. Wiley 2017.

[11] Hall J. Guyton and Hall Textbook of Medical Physiology. Elsevier 2015.

[12] Lydyard P, Whelan A, Fanger M. Understanding the Purpose of Lymph Nodes in the Body [Internet]. Verywell Health. [cited 2021 Nov 29]. Available from: https://www.verywellhealth.com/understanding-the-purpose-of-lymph-nodes-2249122

[13] Totsch SK, Sorge RE. Immune system involvement in specific pain conditions. Mol Pain 2017; 13. [http://dx.doi.org/10.1177/1744806917724559] [PMID: 28741433]

[14] Doran KS, Banerjee A, Disson O, Lecuit M. Concepts and mechanisms: crossing host barriers. Cold Spring Harb Perspect Med 2013; 3(7): a010090-0. [http://dx.doi.org/10.1101/cshperspect.a010090] [PMID: 23818514]

[15] Graber JJ, Dhib-Jalbut S. Interferons.Encyclopedia of the Neurological Sciences. 2nd ed. Oxford: Academic Press 2014; pp. 718-23. [Internet] [http://dx.doi.org/10.1016/B978-0-12-385157-4.00182-2]

[16] Pestka S, Krause CD, Walter MR. Interferons, interferon-like cytokines, and their receptors. Immunol Rev 2004; 202(1): 8-32. [http://dx.doi.org/10.1111/j.0105-2896.2004.00204.x] [PMID: 15546383]

[17] Morikawa K, Oseko F, Morikawa S. A role for ferritin in hematopoiesis and the immune system. Leuk Lymphoma 1995; 18(5-6): 429-33. [http://dx.doi.org/10.3109/10428199509059641] [PMID: 8528049]

[18] Wang G. Human antimicrobial peptides and proteins. Pharmaceuticals (Basel) 2014; 7(5): 545-94. [http://dx.doi.org/10.3390/ph7050545] [PMID: 24828484]

[19] Role of the Complement System in Immunity," Medicine LibreTexts, Jul. 22, 2018. https://med.libretexts.org/Bookshelves/Anatomy_and_Physiology/Book%3A_Anatomy_and_Physiology_(Boundless)/20%3A_Immune_System/20.6%3A_Humoral_Immune_Response/20.6C%3A_Role_of_the_Complement_System_in_Immunity

[20] Phagocytes Process in Immune System. https://www.ukessays.com/essays/biology/essay- on-phagocytes-and-infection-biology-essay.php2021.

[21] Diefenbach A. Natural Killer Cells.Antibody Fc. Boston: Academic Press 2014; pp. 75-93. [Internet] [http://dx.doi.org/10.1016/B978-0-12-394802-1.00004-2]

[22] Medzhitov R, Janeway C Jr. Innate Immunity. N Engl J Med 2000; 343(5): 338-44. [http://dx.doi.org/10.1056/NEJM200008033430506] [PMID: 10922424]

[23] Müller L, Di Benedetto S, Pawelec G. The Immune System and Its Dysregulation with Aging. Subcell Biochem 2019; 91: 21-43. http://link.springer.com/10.1007/978-981-13-3681-2_210.1007/978-98--13-3681-2_2

[24] Medina E. Neutrophil extracellular traps: a strategic tactic to defeat pathogens with potential consequences for the host. J Innate Immun 2009; 1(3): 176-80. [http://dx.doi.org/10.1159/000203699] [PMID: 20375575]

[25] Nicholson LB. The immune system. Essays Biochem 2016; 60(3): 275-301. [http://dx.doi.org/10.1042/EBC20160017] [PMID: 27784777]

[26] Oishi Y, Manabe I. Macrophages in age-related chronic inflammatory diseases. NPJ Aging Mech Dis

2016; 2(1): 16018.
[http://dx.doi.org/10.1038/npjamd.2016.18] [PMID: 28721272]

[27] Abbas AK, Lichtman AH, Pillai S. Cellular and molecular immunology. 8th ed., Philadelphia, PA: Elsevier Saunders 2015.

[28] Yatim KM, Lakkis FG. A Brief Journey through the Immune System. Clin J Am Soc Nephrol 2015; 10(7): 1274-81. https://cjasn.asnjournals.org/lookup/doi/10.2215/CJN.10031014
[http://dx.doi.org/10.2215/CJN.10031014]

[29] "11.7C: Clonal Selection of Antibody-Producing Cells," Biology LibreTexts, Jun. 23, 2018. https://bio.libretexts.org/Bookshelves/Microbiology/Book%3A_Microbiology_(Boundless)/11%3A_Immunology/11.07%3A_Antibodies/11.7C%3A_Clonal_Selection_of_Antibody-Producing_Cells (accessed Dec. 02, 2021).

[30] "Clonal Selection - Immune System - MCAT Content," Jack Westin, Mar. 19, 2020. https://jackwestin.com/resources/mcat-content/immune-system/clonal-selection (accessed Dec. 02, 2021).

[31] "14.1: Cell-Mediated Immunity - An Overview," Biology LibreTexts, Mar. 18, 2016. https://bio.libretexts.org/Bookshelves/Microbiology/Book%3A_Microbiology_(Kaiser)/Unit_6%3A_Adaptive_Immunity/14%3A_Cell-Mediated_Immunity/14.1%3A_Cell-Mediated_Immunit-_-_An_Overview (accessed Nov. 20, 2021).

[32] Smith-Garvin JE, Koretzky GA, Jordan MS. T cell activation. Annu Rev Immunol 2009; 27(1): 591-619.
[http://dx.doi.org/10.1146/annurev.immunol.021908.132706] [PMID: 19132916]

[33] Chaplin DD. Overview of the immune response. J Allergy Clin Immunol 2010; 125(2) (Suppl. 2): S3-S23.
[http://dx.doi.org/10.1016/j.jaci.2009.12.980] [PMID: 20176265]

[34] Mohanty SK, Sai Leela K. Textbook of immunology. 2nd ed., New Delhi, Philadelphia: Jaypee Brothers Medical Pub 2014.
[http://dx.doi.org/10.5005/jp/books/11991]

[35] Turk JL. Almroth Wright--phagocytosis and opsonization. J R Soc Med 1994; 87(10): 576-7.
[http://dx.doi.org/10.1177/014107689408701002] [PMID: 7966100]

[36] https://www.immunology.org/public-information/bitesized-immunology/cells/cd8-t-cells

[37] Charles A, Janeway J, Travers P, Walport M, Shlomchik MJ. "The components of the immune system," Immunobiology: The Immune System in Health and Disease. 5th edition, 2001, Accessed: Nov. 18, 2021. [Online]. Available: https://www.ncbi.nlm.nih.gov/books/NBK27092/

[38] Tanno LK, Calderon MA, Smith HE, Sanchez-Borges M, Sheikh A, Demoly P. Dissemination of definitions and concepts of allergic and hypersensitivity conditions. World Allergy Organ J 2016; 9: 24.
[http://dx.doi.org/10.1186/s40413-016-0115-2] [PMID: 27551327]

[39] Krishna MT, Mahesh PA, Vedanthan PK, Mehta V, Moitra S, Christopher DJ. The burden of allergic diseases in the Indian subcontinent: barriers and challenges. Lancet Glob Health 2020; 8(4): e478-9.
[http://dx.doi.org/10.1016/S2214-109X(20)30061-9] [PMID: 32199115]

[40] Galli SJ, Tsai M, Piliponsky AM. The development of allergic inflammation. Nature 2008; 454(7203): 445-54.
[http://dx.doi.org/10.1038/nature07204] [PMID: 18650915]

[41] https://www.thoughtco.com/types-of-hypersensitivity-reactions-4172957

[42] Dispenza MC. Classification of hypersensitivity reactions. Allergy Asthma Proc 2019; 40(6): 470-3.
[http://dx.doi.org/10.2500/aap.2019.40.4274] [PMID: 31690397]

[43] G. Thapa, "Hypersensitivity and its Types – The Science Notes." https://www.thesciencenotes.

com/hypersensitivity-introduction-and-classification-types-of- hypersensitivity/ (accessed Nov. 24, 2021).

[44] A. A. Justiz Vaillant, R. Vashisht, and P. M. Zito, "Immediate Hypersensitivity Reactions," in StatPearls, Treasure Island (FL): StatPearls Publishing, 2021. Accessed: Nov. 24, 2021. [Online]. Available: http://www.ncbi.nlm.nih.gov/books/NBK513315/

[45] Aryal S. "Hypersensitivity- Introduction, Causes, Mechanism and Types," Microbe Notes, Mar. 12, 2021. https://microbenotes.com/hypersensitivity-introduction-causes-mechanism-and-types/ (accessed Nov. 24, 2021).

[46] Adkinson NF, Bochner BS, Burks AW, Busse WW, Holgate ST, Lemanske RF, *et al.* Middleton's Allergy: Principles and Practice. 8th ed. Elsevier Inc 2013; Vol. 1–2. [Internet]

[47] Basu S, Banik BK. Hypersensitivity: An Overview. Immunol Curr Res 2018; 2:1.

[48] Marwa K, Kondamudi NP. Type IV Hypersensitivity Reaction.StatPearls. Treasure Island, FL: StatPearls Publishing 2021.http://www.ncbi.nlm.nih.gov/books/NBK562228/ Internet

[49] Zoetendal EG, Raes J, van den Bogert B, *et al.* The human small intestinal microbiota is driven by rapid uptake and conversion of simple carbohydrates. ISME J 2012; 6(7): 1415-26. [http://dx.doi.org/10.1038/ismej.2011.212] [PMID: 22258098]

[50] Gibson GR, Scott KP, Rastall RA, *et al.* Dietary prebiotics: current status and new definition. Food Sci Technol Bull 2010; 7(1): 1-19. [http://dx.doi.org/10.1616/1476-2137.15880]

[51] Resta-Lenert S, Barrett KE. Live probiotics protect intestinal epithelial cells from the effects of infection with enteroinvasive Escherichia coli (EIEC). Gut 2003; 52(7): 988-97. [http://dx.doi.org/10.1136/gut.52.7.988] [PMID: 12801956]

[52] Oyofo BA, DeLOACH JR, Corrier DE, Norman JO, Ziprin RL, Mollenhauer HH. Prevention of Salmonella typhimurium colonization of broilers with D-mannose. Poult Sci 1989; 68(10): 1357-60. [http://dx.doi.org/10.3382/ps.0681357] [PMID: 2685797]

[53] van Baarlen P, Troost F, van der Meer C, *et al.* Human mucosal *in vivo* transcriptome responses to three lactobacilli indicate how probiotics may modulate human cellular pathways. Proc Natl Acad Sci USA 2011; 108(Suppl 1) (Suppl. 1): 4562-9. [http://dx.doi.org/10.1073/pnas.1000079107] [PMID: 20823239]

[54] Amani Denj K, Razeghi Ma M, Akrami R. Ghobadi Sh, Jafarpour SA, Mirbeygi SK. Effect of [Dietary Prebiotic Mannan Oligosaccharide (MOS) on Growth Performance, Intestinal Microflora, Body Composition, Haematological and Blood Serum Biochemical Parameters of Rainbow Trout (Oncorhynchus mykiss) Juveniles. Su Ürün Derg 2015; 10(4): 255-65. [Internet].

[55] Langkamp-henken B, Bender BS, Gardner EM, *et al.* Nutritional formula enhanced immune function and reduced days of symptoms of upper respiratory tract infection in seniors. J Am Geriatr Soc 2004; 52(1): 3-12. [http://dx.doi.org/10.1111/j.1532-5415.2004.52003.x] [PMID: 14687308]

[56] Lomax AR, Cheung LVY, Tuohy KM, Noakes PS, Miles EA, Calder PC. β2-1 Fructans have a bifidogenic effect in healthy middle-aged human subjects but do not alter immune responses examined in the absence of an *in vivo* immune challenge: results from a randomised controlled trial. Br J Nutr 2012; 108(10): 1818-28. [http://dx.doi.org/10.1017/S0007114511007276] [PMID: 22244014]

[57] https://academic.oup.com/ajcn/article/88/5/1438/4648926

[58] Link-Amster H, Rochat F, Saudan KY, Mignot O, Aeschlimann JM. Modulation of a specific humoral immune response and changes in intestinal flora mediated through fermented milk intake. FEMS Immunol Med Microbiol 1994; 10(1): 55-63. [http://dx.doi.org/10.1111/j.1574-695X.1994.tb00011.x] [PMID: 7874079]

[59] Sokol H, Pigneur B, Watterlot L, *et al.* *Faecalibacterium prausnitzii* is an anti-inflammatory commensal bacterium identified by gut microbiota analysis of Crohn disease patients. Proc Natl Acad Sci USA 2008; 105(43): 16731-6.
[http://dx.doi.org/10.1073/pnas.0804812105] [PMID: 18936492]

[60] Konieczna P, Groeger D, Ziegler M, *et al.* *Bifidobacterium infantis* 35624 administration induces Foxp3 T regulatory cells in human peripheral blood: potential role for myeloid and plasmacytoid dendritic cells. Gut 2012; 61(3): 354-66.
[http://dx.doi.org/10.1136/gutjnl-2011-300936] [PMID: 22052061]

[61] Martin A. Antioxidant vitamins E and C and risk of Alzheimer's disease. Nutr Rev 2003; 61(2): 69-73.
[http://dx.doi.org/10.1301/nr.2003.febr.69-73] [PMID: 12674439]

[62] Sazawal S, Black RE, Jalla S, Mazumdar S, Sinha A, Bhan MK. Zinc supplementation reduces the incidence of acute lower respiratory infections in infants and preschool children: a double-blind, controlled trial. Pediatrics 1998; 102(1): 1-5.
[http://dx.doi.org/10.1542/peds.102.1.1] [PMID: 9651405]

[63] Villamor E, Fawzi WW. Effects of vitamin a supplementation on immune responses and correlation with clinical outcomes. Clin Microbiol Rev 2005; 18(3): 446-64.
[http://dx.doi.org/10.1128/CMR.18.3.446-464.2005] [PMID: 16020684]

[64] Dowell SF, Papic Z, Bresee JS, *et al.* Treatment of respiratory syncytial virus infection with vitamin A: a randomized, placebo-controlled trial in Santiago, Chile. Pediatr Infect Dis J 1996; 15(9): 782-6.
[http://dx.doi.org/10.1097/00006454-199609000-00009] [PMID: 8878221]

[65] Awasthi S, Peto R, Read S, Clark S, Pande V, Bundy D. Vitamin A supplementation every 6 months with retinol in 1 million pre-school children in north India: DEVTA, a cluster-randomised trial. Lancet 2013; 381(9876): 1469-77.
[http://dx.doi.org/10.1016/S0140-6736(12)62125-4] [PMID: 23498849]

[66] Larkin A, Lassetter J. Vitamin D deficiency and acute lower respiratory infections in children younger than 5 years: identification and treatment. J Pediatr Health Care 2014; 28(6): 572-82.
[http://dx.doi.org/10.1016/j.pedhc.2014.08.013] [PMID: 25441970]

[67] Jartti T, Ruuskanen O, Mansbach JM, Vuorinen T, Camargo CA Jr. Low serum 25-hydroxyvitamin D levels are associated with increased risk of viral coinfections in wheezing children. J Allergy Clin Immunol 2010; 126(5): 1074-1076.e4, 1076.e1-1076.e4.
[http://dx.doi.org/10.1016/j.jaci.2010.09.004] [PMID: 21050947]

[68] Brooks WA, Terebuh P, Bridges C, *et al.* Influenza A and B infection in children in urban slum, Bangladesh. Emerg Infect Dis 2007; 13(10): 1507-8.
[http://dx.doi.org/10.3201/eid1310.070368] [PMID: 18257997]

[69] Srinivasan MG, Ndeezi G, Mboijana CK, *et al.* Zinc adjunct therapy reduces case fatality in severe childhood pneumonia: a randomized double blind placebo-controlled trial. BMC Med 2012; 10(1): 14.
[http://dx.doi.org/10.1186/1741-7015-10-14] [PMID: 22316073]

[70] Plaeger SF. Clinical Immunology and Traditional Herbal Medicines. Clin Diagn Lab Immunol 2003; 10(3): 337-8.
[http://dx.doi.org/10.1128/CDLI.10.3.337-338.2003]

[71] Béliveau R, Gingras D. Green tea: prevention and treatment of cancer by nutraceuticals. Lancet 2004; 364(9439): 1021-2.
[http://dx.doi.org/10.1016/S0140-6736(04)17076-1] [PMID: 15380952]

[72] Ran L, Zhao W, Wang J, *et al.* Extra Dose of Vitamin C Based on a Daily Supplementation Shortens the Common Cold: A Meta-Analysis of 9 Randomized Controlled Trials. BioMed Res Int 2018; 2018: 1-12.
[http://dx.doi.org/10.1155/2018/1837634] [PMID: 30069463]

[73] Hou L, Huang H. Immune suppressive properties of artemisinin family drugs. Pharmacol Ther 2016;

166: 123-7.
[http://dx.doi.org/10.1016/j.pharmthera.2016.07.002] [PMID: 27411673]

[74] Gautam M, Saha S, Bani S, *et al.* Immunomodulatory activity of Asparagus racemosus on systemic Th1/Th2 immunity: Implications for immunoadjuvant potential. J Ethnopharmacol 2009; 121(2): 241-7.
[http://dx.doi.org/10.1016/j.jep.2008.10.028] [PMID: 19038322]

[75] Yan LC, Bi EG, Lou YT, *et al.* Novel sinomenine derivative 1032 improves immune suppression in experimental autoimmune encephalomyelitis. Biochem Biophys Res Commun 2010; 391(1): 1093-8.
[http://dx.doi.org/10.1016/j.bbrc.2009.12.028] [PMID: 20004644]

[76] Sharma ML, Rao CS, Duda PL. Immunostimulatory activity of Picrorhiza kurroa leaf extract. J Ethnopharmacol 1994; 41(3): 185-92.
[http://dx.doi.org/10.1016/0378-8741(94)90031-0] [PMID: 8176958]

[77] Bae G-S, Jong-Jin K, Park K-S, et al., Piperine inhibits lipopolysaccharide-induced maturation of bone-marrow-derived dendritic cells through inhibition of ERK and JNK activation. Phytother Res. 2012; 26(12): 1893-7.
[http://dx.doi.org/10.1002/ptr.4649]

[78] Agnandji ST, Lell B, Soulanoudjingar SS, *et al.* First results of phase 3 trial of RTS,S/AS01 malaria vaccine in African children. N Engl J Med 2011; 365(20): 1863-75.
[http://dx.doi.org/10.1056/NEJMoa1102287] [PMID: 22007715]

[79] Henriksen-Lacey M, Devitt A, Perrie Y. The vesicle size of DDA:TDB liposomal adjuvants plays a role in the cell-mediated immune response but has no significant effect on antibody production. J Control Release 2011; 154(2): 131-7.
[http://dx.doi.org/10.1016/j.jconrel.2011.05.019] [PMID: 21640145]

[80] Aguilar JC, Rodríguez EG. Vaccine adjuvants revisited. Vaccine 2007; 25(19): 3752-62.
[http://dx.doi.org/10.1016/j.vaccine.2007.01.111] [PMID: 17336431]

[81] Morrow WJW, Yang YW, Sheikh NA. Immunobiology of the Tomatine adjuvant. Vaccine 2004; 22(19): 2380-4.
[http://dx.doi.org/10.1016/j.vaccine.2004.03.022] [PMID: 15193398]

[82] Ma X, Xu S. TNF inhibitor therapy for rheumatoid arthritis. Biomed Rep 2013; 1(2): 177-84.
[http://dx.doi.org/10.3892/br.2012.42] [PMID: 24648915]

[83] Zhao YD, Chu L, Lin K, Granton E, Yin L, Peng J, et al. A Biochemical Approach to Understand the Pathogenesis of Advanced Pulmonary Arterial Hypertension: Metabolomic Profiles of Arginine, Sphingosine-1-Phosphate, and Heme of Human Lung. Plos One 2015; 10(8). https://dx.plos.org/10.1371/journal.pone.0134958

[84] Sathyanarayanan V, Neelapu SS. Cancer immunotherapy: Strategies for personalization and combinatorial approaches. Mol Oncol 2015; 9(10): 2043-53.
[http://dx.doi.org/10.1016/j.molonc.2015.10.009] [PMID: 26548534]

[85] Feltkamp MCW, Smits HL, Vierboom MPM, *et al.* Vaccination with cytotoxic T lymphocyte epitope-containing peptide protects against a tumor induced by human papillomavirus type 16-transformed cells. Eur J Immunol 1993; 23(9): 2242-9.
[http://dx.doi.org/10.1002/eji.1830230929] [PMID: 7690326]

[86] Bagarazzi ML, Yan J, Morrow MP, *et al.* Immunotherapy against HPV16/18 generates potent T_H1 and cytotoxic cellular immune responses. Sci Transl Med 2012; 4(155) 155ra138.
[http://dx.doi.org/10.1126/scitranslmed.3004414] [PMID: 23052295]

[87] Trepiakas R, Pedersen AE, Met Ö, Svane IM. Addition of interferon-alpha to a standard maturation cocktail induces CD38 up-regulation and increases dendritic cell function. Vaccine 2009; 27(16): 2213-9.
[http://dx.doi.org/10.1016/j.vaccine.2009.02.015] [PMID: 19428835]

[88] Zella M, Metzdorf J, Ostendorf F, *et al.* Novel Immunotherapeutic Approaches to Target Alpha-Synuclein and Related Neuroinflammation in Parkinson's Disease. Cells 2019; 8(2): 105. [http://dx.doi.org/10.3390/cells8020105] [PMID: 30708997]

CHAPTER 2

Diseases and Disorders Associated with Immune System

Pooja Shimpi[1], **Smita Pillewan**[2] and **Vandana S. Nikam**[1,*]

[1] *Department of Pharmacology, STES's Smt. Kashibai Navale College of Pharmacy, Kondhwa, S. P. Pune University, Pune, Maharashtra, India*

[2] *D.Y. Patil College of Pharmacy, Akurdi, S. P. Pune University, Pune, Maharashtra, India*

Abstract: The human immune system is one of the complex systems of the body, which works against both external and internal invasion. It has two parts: the innate and the acquired immune systems. We have been born with the innate system which gives a quick response for the invading pathogen non-specifically. To deal with the typical environmental antigens, immune system adapts to changes. The acquired (or adaptive) component develops over time and produces antibodies that "remember" invaders to fight them if they return. Failure of it could be due to genetic defect (weak natural immunity), inability to adapt to the change, hyper-responsiveness, or inability to distinguish self from foreign, leading to various diseases and disorders. Various genetic defects of the immune system are at the core of Primary Immune disorders (PIDs), while overactivity is responsible for allergic diseases. Autoimmune diseases are mostly due to malfunction of the adaptive immune system, while in Systemic Auto-inflammatory Disorders (SAIDs), the innate immune system is affected. Advancements in technology and genetics have improved our understanding of the pathogenesis, diagnosis, and management of these diseases.

Keywords: Autoimmunity, Allergic Diseases, Auto-inflammation, Cancer Immunotherapy, Immunological Disorders, Immunodeficiency, Neuro-immune System.

INTRODUCTION

The immune system is an efficient complex network of cellular elements, molecules, and pathways that is evolved to protect the host or multicellular organisms against external offends or invaders, and its balance functioning is essential to avoid the development of various disorders. In a normal infectious state, the infectious agent activates the innate immune response, which causes symptoms followed by an adaptive immune response that leads to clear infections

* **Corresponding author Vandana S. Nikam:** Department of Pharmacology, STES's Smt. Kashibai Navale College of Pharmacy, Kondhwa, S. P. Pune University, Pune, Maharashtra, India; E-mail: nikam_vandana@yahoo.com

Vandana S. Nikam, Sujata P. Sawarkar, Girish B. Mahajan and Supriya G. Jagtap (Eds.)

and develops a protective immunity state. But in several circumstances, this will not happen, and there can be a failure of the host Immune response against the invasive agents. The failure of the host immune system can be due to avoidance of a normal immune response by pathogens; genetic defects give rise to failures of defence mechanisms, immunodeficiency syndromes, autoimmunity, allergic responses, *etc.* The prevalence of Immune disorders is on the rise, as many new rare disorders have been identified in the last few decades. Autoimmune Diseases (ADs) account for about 3–5% of the world population, whereas a 30 to 40% rise in allergic disorders is seen. Major advancements in technology and genetics have improved our understanding of the pathogenesis, diagnosis, and management of these diseases [1 - 3].

CLASSIFICATION OF IMMUNE DISEASES AND DISORDERS

When we talk about immunological diseases and immunological disorders, we can sketch a marked line between these two terms. The term immunological disease is ascribed to the situation in which the part, organ, or organ systems of the body get affected by various internal or external factors, whereas immunological disorders are characterized by irregularity or failure of organ function or organ system. The immunological disorders can be physical, structural, genetic, and behavioural. The immune diseases and disorders can be classified based on Organ-specific and organ-non-specific, or we can classify them as Phenotypic diseases or disorders according to the Inborn Errors of Immunity Committee (IEIC). The immune system works for the protection of the body.

BROAD CLASSIFICATION OF IMMUNE DISEASES AND DISORDERS

I. Immunodeficiency disorders
II. Allergic/ Hypersensitivity reactions
III. Autoimmune disorders
IV. Auto-inflammatory disorders

Immunodeficiencies (IDs)

A person with immune deficiency syndromes has lost the ability of one or more components of the immune system to respond protectively to a pathogen. Immunodeficiencies (IDs) are a group of diseases with alterations in either inborn or adaptive immune responses. They are classified as primary when of genetic origin, more recently called inborn errors of immunity (IEI), and secondary when they are acquired [4]. Primary immunodeficiencies (PIDs) include approximately 420 monogenic diseases that are more susceptible to infections and non-infectious complications, including allergies, malignancies and autoimmune diseases (ADs), which also include developmental disorders, autism, intellectual disability, epilepsy, gastroenteropathies, pneumopathies, dermatoses, skeletal and renal abnormalities [5]. There are two types of PIDS. Monogenic immunodeficiencies occur because of mutations in genes responsible for immunological tolerance, thus triggering autoimmunity, including poly-autoimmunity and polygenic immunodeficiencies with a complex pathophysiology and having a multifactorial etiology.

Classification of Immune Diseases and Disorders Based on Inborn Errors of Immunity

Inborn errors of immunity are also known as primary Immunodeficiencies. All types of inborn errors of immunity are compiled by the International Union of Immunological Societies Expert Committee. The important manifestations of primary immunodeficiency are the increased sensitivity to auto-inflammatory diseases, autoimmunity, and allergic diseases. According to the ISEC committee, primary Immunodeficiencies can be classified into 10 classes Table **1.**

Table 1. Classification of immunodeficiency disorders.

Immunodeficiency Disorders		
Class	**Subclass**	**Disease/Disorder**
Immunodeficiencies Affecting Cellular and Humoral Immunity	T-B+ severe combined immune deficiency (SCID)	i. CD45 deficiency ii. L7Rα deficiency iii. AK3 deficiency iv. Coronin-1A deficiency
	T-B- SCID	i. RAG deficiency ii. AK2 defect iii. DCLRE1C (Artemis) deficiency iv. DNA ligase IV deficiency v. Adenosine deaminase (ADA) deficiency
	Combined immunodeficiency (CID), generally less profound than SCID	i. CD40 ligand (CD154) deficiency ii. CD40 deficiency iii. D3γ deficiency iv. ICOS deficiency

(Table 1) cont.....

Immunodeficiency Disorders		
Class	**Subclass**	**Disease/Disorder**
Combined Immunodeficiencies with Associated or Syndromic Features	Immunodeficiency with congenital thrombocytopenia	i. Wiskott-Aldrich syndrome (WAS LOF) ii. WIP deficiency iii. Arp2/3-mediated filament branching defect
	DNA repair defect	i. Ataxia-telangiectasia ii. Ligase I deficiency iii. Nijmegen breakage syndrome iv. PMS2 deficiency
	Thymic defects with additional congenital anomalies	i. Winged helix nude FOXN1 deficiency ii. Chromosome 10p13-p14 deletion syndrome (10p13-p14DS) iii. FOXN1 haploinsufficiency
	Immuno-osseous dysplasias	i. Cartilage hair hypoplasia ii. Schimke immuno-osseous dysplasia iii. MOPD1 deficiency (Roifman syndrome)
Predominantly Antibody Deficiencies	Severe reduction in all serum immunoglobulin isotypes with profoundly decreased or absent B cells, agammaglobulinemia	i. μ heavy chain deficiency ii. Ig-α deficiency iii. Igβ deficiency iv. Hoffman syndrome/TOP2B deficiency v. p85 deficiency
	Severe reduction in at least 2 serum immunoglobulin isotypes with a normal or low number of B cells, CVID phenotype	i. CD19 deficiency ii. Activated p110δ syndrome iii. Mannosyl-oligosaccharide glucosidase deficiency
	Severe reduction in serum IgG and IgA with normal/elevated IgM and normal numbers of B cells, hyper IgM	i. AID deficiency

(Table 1) cont.....

Immunodeficiency Disorders		
Class	**Subclass**	**Disease/Disorder**
Diseases of Immune Dysregulation	Familial hemophagocytic lymph histiocytosis (FHL syndromes)	i. Perforin deficiency
	FHL syndromes with hypopigmentation	i. Griscelli syndrome, type 2 ii. Chediak-Higashi syndrome
	Regulatory T cell defect	i. CD25 deficiency ii. IPEX, immune dysregulation, polyendocrinopathy, enteropathy X-linked
	Autoimmunity with or without lymphoproliferation	i. Tripeptidyl-peptidase II deficiency ii. Prolidase deficiency iii. APECED (APS-1), autoimmune polyendocrinopathy with candidiasis and ectodermal dystrophy
Congenital Defects of Phagocyte Number or Function	Congenital neutropenias	i. Elastase deficiency (Severe congenital neutropenia [SCN] 1) ii. Glycogen storage disease type 1b iii. X-linked neutropenia/myelodysplasia
Defects in intrinsic and Innate Immunity	Mendelian susceptibility to mycobacterial disease (MSMD)	i. IL-12 and IL-23 receptor β1 chain deficiency ii. IFN-γ receptor 1 deficiency iii. Macrophage gp91 pho x deficiency iv. JAK1 deficiency
	Herpes simplex encephalitis (HSE)	i. TLR3 deficiency ii. TRAF3 deficiency
	Predisposition to invasive fungal diseases	i. CARD9 deficiency
	TLR signaling pathway deficiency with bacterial susceptibility	i. IRAK4 deficiency ii. TIRAP deficiency
Autoinflammatory Disorders	Type 1 interferonopathies	i. STING-associated vasculopathy, infantile-onset (SAVI) ii. ADA2 deficiency iii. TREX1 deficiency, Aicardi-Goutieres syndrome 1 (AGS1)
	Defects affecting the Inflammasome	i. Familial Mediterranean fever ii. Mevalonate kinase deficiency (Hyper IgD syndrome
	Non-inflammasome-related conditions	i. Pyogenic sterile arthritis, pyoderma gangrenosum, acne (PAPA) syndrome

(Table 1) cont.....

Immunodeficiency Disorders		
Class	**Subclass**	**Disease/Disorder**
Complement Deficiencies	-	i. C1q deficiency due to defects ii. Thrombomodulin deficiency iii. Membrane Cofactor Protein (CD46) deficiency
Bone Marrow Failure	-	i. Fanconi anemia ii. Coats plus syndrome
Phenocopies of Inborn Errors of Immunity	Associated with somatic mutations	i. Autoimmune lymphoproliferative syndrome (ALPS–SFAS) ii. RAS-associated autoimmune leukoproliferative disease (RALD
	Associated with autoantibodies	i. Chronic mucocutaneous candidiasis ii. Acquired angioedema iii. Adult-onset immunodeficiency with susceptibility to mycobacteria

Phenocopies of Inborn Errors of Immunity

X-linked Agammaglobulinemia

Bruton's or X-linked agammaglobulinemia is a primary immunodeficiency disorder characterized by repetitive infections in early childhood of affected males. Low immunoglobulin levels make them susceptible to infections. Before diagnosis, recurrent otitis media is the most common infection. Also conjunctivitis, sinus infections, diarrhoea, and skin infections are frequently observed. Gamma globulin substitution therapy remains mainline of treatment. Antibiotics can be added to prevent secondary complications.

Wiskott–Aldrich Syndrome (WAS)

WAS is a rare X-linked primary immunodeficiency disorder affecting males. Characteristic features include eczema, thrombocytopenia, and severe infections. Immunodeficiency, autoimmunity and malignancy are associated with the disorder. Mutations in the WAS gene, which is located on the short arm of X chromosome Xp11.22–p11.23 is responsible for the disorder. X-linked thrombocytopenia (XLT) and X-linked neutropenia are the phenotypic variations of WAS. It is inherited in an X-linked manner. Intravenous Ig (IVIG) is the mainline treatment for WAS, along with its symptomatic treatment that need to be given like prophylactics of antibiotics. Autologous gene-modified HSCT (hematopoietic stem cell transplantation) is emerging as a new therapy option [6].

Ataxia Telangiectasia (A-T)

Also known as Louis-Bar syndrome is a rare genetic form of early-onset autosomal recessive cerebral ataxia. Mutation of the ataxia-telangiectasia mutated (ATM) gene is responsible for the neurological and systemic symptoms. Ataxia is poor coordination, and telangiectasia refers to small dilated blood vessels, which are the hallmarks of the disease. Also, progressive cerebellar degeneration, immunodeficiency, pulmonary infections, radiation sensitivity, and risk of cancer development, mostly for the lymphatic system, are other features. Treatment of A-T is symptomatic and supportive due to the variety of manifestations. For neurologic defects, along with physical or occupational therapy, antiparkinsonian drugs or anti-epileptic drugs can be given for symptomatic relief. Antibiotics and modified cancer treatment as per symptoms are suggested. New therapies like antioxidants, antisense morpholino oligonucleotides (AMO) and aminoglycoside antibiotics affecting ATM protein are under investigation [7].

DiGeorge Syndrome

DiGeorge syndrome (DGS) is a type of 22q11 deletion syndrome. It is a congenital disorder with characteristic features like hypoplastic thymus or aplasia, cardiac anomalies, and hypocalcaemia appearing in early childhood. Also, recurrent infections, craniofacial deficits, cleft palate, and developmental delay are observed. T-box transcription factor 1 (TBX1) gene is found to be associated with DGS. Signs and symptoms presented by DGS range from mild to life-threatening, and the therapy line is decided accordingly. For Immunodeficiency, intravenous IgG, antibiotic prophylaxis, and either thymic or hematopoietic cell transplant (HSCT) can be given. Cardiothoracic surgery, calcium and vitamin D supplementation, speech therapy, and psychiatric care may be required according to the severity of the disease [8].

Secondary Immunodeficiency Disorders

Secondary Immunodeficiency Disorders are quite common as compared with PID's. External factors adversely affect the immune system to develop secondary immunodeficiency disorders and consequent increased risk of infections. These immunodeficiencies can arise from a few conditions, such as treatment with immunosuppressive drugs, surgery and trauma, prolonged illness, extreme environmental conditions, and systemic infections, such as those caused by HIV. Immunodeficiency can also result from loss of serum proteins (particularly IgG and albumin) through the kidneys in nephrotic syndrome; the skin in severe burns or dermatitis, and the gastrointestinal (GI) tract in enteropathy [9].

The list of Secondary Immunodeficiency Disorders based on causes is summarised in Table **2**.

Table 2. Secondary Immunodeficiency Disorders.

Category	Examples
Endocrine	Diabetes mellitus
Gastrointestinal	Hepatic Insufficiency, Hepatitis, protein-losing enteropathy
Hematologic	Aplastic anemia, cancers (*e.g.*, chronic lymphocytic leukaemia, multiple myeloma, Hodgkin lymphoma), sickle cell anaemia, splenectomy
Iatrogenic	Drugs, like chemotherapeutic drugs, immunosuppressants, corticosteroids; radiation therapy; splenectomy
Infectious	Viral infections (*e.g.*, cytomegalovirus, HIV, Measles virus, Varicella-zoster virus), bacterial infections, rare bacterial infections (mostly *Staphylococcus aureus*), mycobacterial infections
Nutritional	Alcohol abuse, Malnutrition
Physiologic	Physiologic immunodeficiency in infants due to immaturity of the immune system, pregnancy
Renal	Nephrotic syndrome, uremia
Rheumatologic	Systemic Lupus Erythematosus (SLE)
Other	Burns, chromosomal abnormalities (*e.g.*, Down syndrome), congenital asplenia, critical and chronic illness like histiocytosis, sarcoidosis

Allergic/ Hypersensitivity Reactions

Allergic diseases and disorders are always a socioeconomic burden with increasing widespread presence. Regardless of considerable efforts to identify safe and efficacious treatment, the lack of validated biomarkers remains the main challenge to advance the preciseness of treatments [10]. Allergic diseases, including Allergic rhinitis, Atopic dermatitis, Urticaria, Steven Johnson's syndrome, and many others, are chronic immunological diseases that affect children and adults. The environmental and developmental factors play an important role in the pathogenesis of these diseases. Genetic or phenotypic mechanisms are the arbitrator of some effects evoked by the environment for allergic diseases. Epigenetic modifications, including DNA methylation, non-coding RNAs, and histone modifications, disclose new insights into the mechanisms involved and have the potential to be used as novel biomarkers for the treatment of heterogeneous allergic diseases [11].

Allergic Rhinitis

Allergic rhinitis(AR), also called "hay fever," is an atopic disease characterized by rhinorrhea, itching, sneezing fits, nasal congestion and nasal pruritis and is caused by immunoglobulin E (IgE) mediated reactions to inhaled allergens [12]. Allergic rhinitis is the most common type of chronic rhinitis, affecting 20 to 30% of adults and 40% of children [13]. Allergic rhinitis can be classified as seasonal (intermittent) and perennial (chronic), with approximately 20% of cases being seasonal, 40% perennial, and 40% with features of both. AR can also be classified based on etiology as IgE-mediated (allergic), autonomic, infectious, and idiopathic (unknown) [14].

Pathophysiology of allergic rhinitis includes the various inflammatory cells, including mast cells, macrophages, CD4-positive T cells, B cells, and eosinophils. The process is initiated by exposure to the allergens like pollen, mites, animal dander and faecal particles that are identified by antigen-specific immunoglobulin E (IgE) receptors located on mast cells and basophils in hosts. The early phase is associated with mast cell degranulation followed by histamine release from mast cells in nasal mucosa leading to acute nasal symptoms and ocular symptoms. In this phase, other potent pro-inflammatory cytokines, such as interleukin [IL]-3, IL-4, IL-5, and IL-13 and eicosanoids like prostaglandins, and kinins, increase vascular permeability. Cytokines release is also initiated by T cells, predominantly T helper (Th2), which infiltrates nasal mucosa in an early phase of AR. Late-phase reaction progression is recognized by cellular recruitment of basophils, neutrophils, T-lymphocytes, eosinophils, and monocytes by the release of mediators such as cytokines, prostaglandins, leukotrienes showing inflammatory response which contribute to bronchial hyper-responsiveness. Allergic rhinitis management includes avoidance of exposure to triggers and allergens, which require significant lifestyle changes that may not be acceptable to patients. The pharmacological therapies, such as intranasal corticosteroids (beclomethasone, ciclesonide, budesonide), antihistamines (Bilastine, cetirizine, desloratadine), immunotherapy (Allergen-specific therapy), leukotrienes receptor antagonists (montelukast, zafirlukast, pranulukast), *etc.* [12, 15, 16] are available.

Atopic Eczema/ Atopic Dermatitis

Atopic eczema is the most common chronic inflammatory disease characterized by dry skin, highly pruritic skin, and eczematous lesions. Atopy can be defined as an inherited propensity to produce immunoglobulin E (IgE) antibodies in response to minute amounts of common environmental proteins, such as pollen, house dust, mites, and food allergens. Dermatitis derives from the Greek "derma", which means skin, and "itis" which means inflammation. Dermatitis and eczema are often used synonymously, even though the term eczema is sometimes reticent for the acute phenomenon of the disease (from Greek, eczema, to boil over); here, no variance is made [17]. Atopic dermatitis affects approximately 10% to 30% of children and 2% to 10% of adults in developed countries. This widespread presence has increased two to three-fold in recent decades. Atopic dermatitis has a higher occurrence at higher latitudes, which may be due to decreased sun exposure and lower humidity levels [18]. The pathophysiology of atopic dermatitis is not fully understood, but the hypothesis has been proposed as a complex interaction between defects in skin barrier function, immune dysregulation, and infectious agents. Mutations or impaired expression of the filaggrin gene, which encodes a structural protein required for skin barrier formation, lead to skin barrier abnormalities [19].

Several theories of immunological imbalance proposed that atopic dermatitis originates from dysregulation of T helper cells 1,2,17 and 22 as well as regulatory T cells. The abnormal skin barrier may allow allergens and irritants to penetrate the skin, which activates the Th2 response in acute lesions and Th1 response in chronic lesions, which results in the production of chemokines and proinflammatory cytokines (*e.g.*, interleukin [IL]- 4, IL-5, and tumor necrosis factor) and further enhances IgE production *via* signal transducer and activator of transcription (STAT) pathway to cause inflammatory responses and pruritis [20].

The currently available therapy for atopic eczema includes two primary objectives, prevention, and actual treatment. Prevention aims to reduce the dryness of skin, avoid hot baths, and keep the epidermis moist. The pharmacological treatment aims to maintain an intact skin barrier. Various pharmacological agents include emollients, topical corticosteroids, calcineurin inhibitors, and systemic immunosuppressants. Emollients can form an occlusive layer on top of the epidermis, resulting in increased skin hydration *via* reducing evaporation. Topical corticosteroids of 4 classes are used such as type I (Hydrocortisone), type II (hydrocortisone-17-butyrate), type III (betamethasone, fluocinonide), and type IV (Clobetasol propionate) which shows vasoconstrictive effects. Furthermore, calcineurin inhibitors like pimecrolimus and tacrolimus are also used to treat atopic eczema [17]. Novel therapies such as monoclonal antibodies targeting IL-5, IL-13, IL-17, IL-22, IL-23, IL-31, and TSLP are currently under investigation in patients having moderate to Severe Atopic Dermatitis. Also, small molecules like anti-PDE4 and JAK inhibitors may represent other potential treatments [21].

Urticaria

Urticaria is a common dermatological condition characterized by pruritic and raised wheals, erythematous, oedematous, itchy, and ephemeral or temporary urticarial plaques which lasts for a couple of hours not exceeding 48 hrs. Approximately 12–22% of the general population can suffer at least one sub-type of urticaria during life. In the adult population, there is a female predominance (about 60%), while this gender difference is less significant in children. In 40-50% of patients, urticaria and angioedema are seen in combination. The Urticaria can be classified as Acute Spontaneous urticaria (lasts less than 6 weeks), Chronic spontaneous urticaria (lasts for more than 6 weeks), and Episodic chronic urticaria (lasts more than 6 weeks but recurs twice a week) [22, 23]. The common causes of urticaria include allergens, food pseudo-allergens, infectious agents such as viruses, bacteria, parasites and several medications like opiates, NSAID, *etc.* [24].

Pathogenesis of urticaria involves infiltrating cells' immunophenotypes and related cytokines, adhesion molecules, and chemokine receptors. Several hypotheses of the pathogenesis of urticaria include mast cell degranulation, infiltration, up-regulation of various adhesion molecules and cells, and autoimmunity. One of the key features of urticaria, wheal, results from perivascular infiltration of mononuclear cells preponderantly CD4+ lymphocytes, monocytes, eosinophils, and neutrophils, among which neutrophils are more significant. Mast cells get degranulated and activate unsuitably, releasing several cellular contents such as cytokines, chemokine, and adhesion molecules. This cellular content regulates vasoactivity and cellular infiltration. Regulatory T-cells (T(REG)), particularly the naturally occurring CD4(+) CD25(+) subset of T (REG), provide a substantial component of autoimmune balance. An increase in T cells can be an evident mechanism of autoimmunity [25]. As a result, histamines, protease, prostaglandins D2, LT4 and interleukin 4 (IL-4), IL - 8, and tumor necrosis factor (TNF - a) are released, which further leads to activation of substance P and expression of adhesion molecules like P selectin and E selectin amplifying wheeling reaction. Furthermore, IL-8 causes the accumulation of neutrophils, and IL-4 activates T-lymphocytes differentiation and Immunoglobulin production [26].

Current approaches to therapy of urticaria aim, symptomatic pharmacotherapy, and patient education to avoid known triggers. The stepwise therapeutic approach is developed by American practice parameters, which include step-1 as monotherapy with second-generation H1 antihistamines (loratadine, bilastine, fexofenadine), step-2 consists of either 4 times increasing dose of H1 anti-histamines or adding H2 anti-histamines (ranitidine, famotidine). Also adding Leukotriene receptor antagonists (Monelukast, zafirlukast). Step-3 includes adding potent H1 anti-histamines (doxepin, hydroxyzine), and further, those patients having inadequate controlled symptoms recommend step-4 to follow consisting of Omalizumab, cyclosporin, and corticosteroids. Novel therapeutics aim to target IL-1β-ligand/IL-1 receptors, development of molecules inhibiting the expression of an apoptosis-related speck-like protein containing a caspase recruitment domain (ASC), the expression of NLRP3, and/or the formation of the NLRP3 inflammasome complex by using diacerein or its analogues [27].

Stevens-Johnson Syndrome

Stevens-Johnson syndrome (SJS) is a rare, emergency and immune-mediated disease characterized by a prodromal illness followed by severe mucocutaneous symptoms comprising toxic epidermal necrolysis (TEN), inflammatory vesiculobullous reactions. The commencing presentation of SJS/TEN may include non-specific symptoms such as fever, discomfort with swallowing, and stinging eyes. Generally, the cutaneous manifestations of SJS/TEN are usually preceded by these non-specific symptoms. The mortality rate of Stevens-Johnson syndrome is estimated as 1-10%. SJS was classically related to a medication-induced hypersensitivity reaction. Nevertheless, infectious aetiologies are increasingly recognized as arousing agents. The most common pathogens causing SJS are Mycoplasma pneumoniae, Enterovirus, hepatitis B virus, Yersinia enterocolitica, Epstein–Barr virus, group A streptococcus, and Mycobacterium tuberculosis [28]. As mentioned earlier, SJS can be induced by medications, including antibiotics (amoxicillin/clavulanate, cephalosporin), and anticonvulsants (carbamazepine, lamotrigine, and levetiracetam), NSAIDs (acetaminophen), Carbonic anhydrase inhibitors (acetazolamide, methazolamide, and dorzolamide) [29]. Among the antibiotics, the most incriminated high-risk reason for SJS/TEN is the sulphonamides, especially Trimethoprim-Sulfamethoxazole, which accounts for about 69% of cases. Genetic factors comprising human leukocyte antigen (HLA) allotypes may lead to a bigger risk of Stevens-Johnson syndrome/toxic epidermal necrolysis when expose to aromatic anticonvulsants and xanthine oxidase inhibitor (allopurinol). Furthermore, Tyrosine kinase inhibitors (Vandetanib, Imatinib, Sunitinib), Immunosuppressants/ immunomodulators (Thalidomide, Lenalidomide, Mizoribine) are also one of the key molecules leading the development of SJS [30].

As far as the Pathophysiology is concerned, the initial step may be the binding of drug-associated antigen or metabolite to the major histocompatibility complex (MCH) type 1 to form an immunogenic compound. The Stevens-Johnson syndrome/toxic epidermal necrolysis is a rare and uncertain reaction to medication that includes drug-specific CD8+ cytotoxic lymphocytes, the Fas-Fas ligand (FasL) pathway of apoptosis, and granule-mediated exocytosis and tumor necrosis factor-alfa (TNF–alpha)/death receptor pathway. The key compound of cytotoxic granules, granulysin, is a major cause of keratinocyte apoptosis. Cytotoxic T cells may exocytose perforin and granzyme B, creating channels in target cell membranes and activating caspases. CD40 ligand cells are also present and may initiate the release of TNF–alpha, nitrous oxide, interleukin 8 (IL8), and cell adhesion antibodies. TNF–alpha also initiates apoptosis. Other cells involve in the pathogenesis of SJS are macrophages, neutrophils, and natural killer cells [31]. Systematic approaches to treat SJS include supportive care and medications such as cyclosporine, plasmapheresis, IV immune globulin, and TNF-γinhibitors. (Infliximab and etanercept). Prophylactic systemic antibiotics are contentious and frequently avoided [32]. Rapid withdrawal of the convict drugs and intensive supportive care is the keystone for the treatment of SJS/TEN. The use of systemic corticosteroids and IVIG is still controversial. Nevertheless, recently, there has been an increasing number of studies suggesting the efficacy of cyclosporine or TNF-α inhibitors [33].

Autoimmune Disorders

Autoimmune diseases (AI) are characterized by dysfunction of the immune system tolerance against self-tissues, due to the presence of autoreactive T and B cells, thus failing to distinguish self from non-self. Until now, 100 autoimmune disorders are known to us Fig. (**1**) [34]. In healthy individuals, by the mechanism of immunological tolerance; autoantibodies and autoreactive T cells are regulated. Regulatory mechanisms include clonal deletion, clonal energy (clonal paralysis), clonal ignorance, and T cells with regulatory functions (Tregs). An autoimmune response is only initiated when such regulated immune responses are pathologically activated by a certain trigger of genetic predisposition and environmental factors [35].

Genetically, human leucocyte antigens (HLAs) and non-HLA loci (*e.g.* the protein tyrosine phosphatase non-receptor type 22 (PTPN22) gene, expressed by hematopoietic cells) are found to be associated with autoimmune disorders. HLAs are the gene products of the major histocompatibility complex (MHC) residing on the short arm of chromosome 6 and are responsible for antigen presentation critical for differentiating self from non-self.

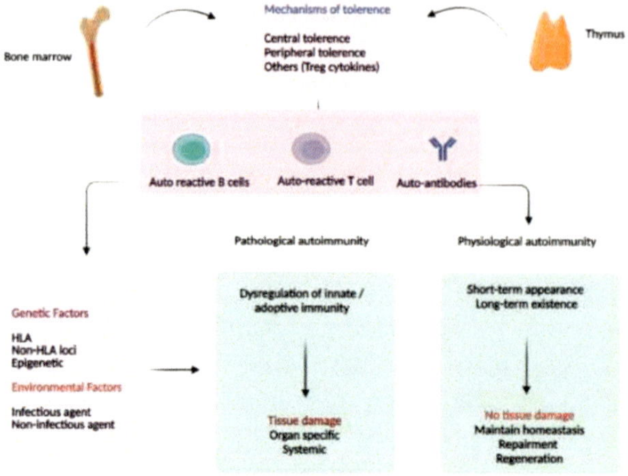

Fig. (1). Summary for development of autoimmune disease. Few autoreactive T and B cells 'leak out' into the periphery in normal individuals, despite strict central and peripheral checks. Only when genetic predisposition rules out tolerance and an environmental trigger or triggers stimulate; the autoimmune reaction begins.

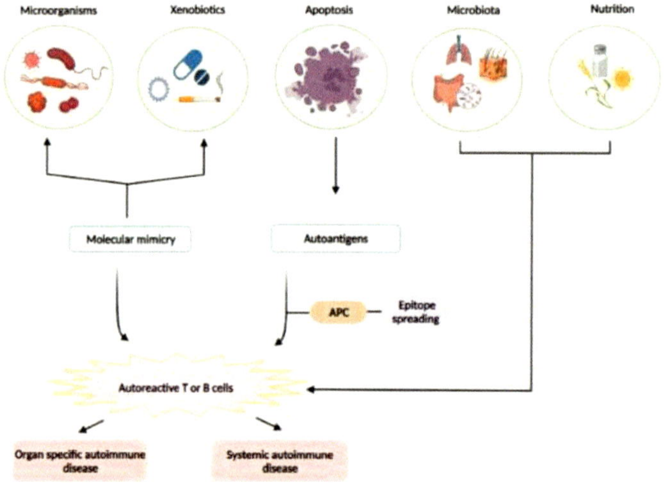

Fig. (2). Environmental factors in autoimmunity. Various environmental factors act as triggers for autoimmunity by activating autoreactive T and B cells, thus losing tolerance.

Environmental factors, which could be infectious (microbiota) or non-infectious (nutrition, xenobiotics like tobacco smoke, pharmaceutical agents, *etc.*) nature act as triggers for autoimmune reactions, leading to loss of tolerance Fig. (**2**).

Following are the mechanisms involved with infection-related autoimmunity.

i. Molecular mimicry: Sequence of pathogen-derived peptides and self-peptides are similar.
ii. Epitope spreading: Primary epitope changes to other epitopes.
iii. Bystander activation: Pre-existing autoreactive immune cells get activated.

Viral persistence and polyclonal activation: Constant presence of viral antigen driving the immune response or epitope spreading [36]. Autoimmune conditions may be systemic (targeting multiple organs and tissues), as is the case of lupus, or tissue-specific, as is the case of multiple sclerosis (against myelin) or type 1 diabetes (against pancreatic beta cells) [37]. Majorly immunotherapeutic strategies are used to treat autoimmune diseases, which include conventional immunosuppressive drugs like corticosteroids, azathioprine (AZA) and methotrexate (MTX) and targeted biologic agents for B cells, T cells, TNFα, IL-6, *etc.* Also, novel therapies have been introduced, like costimulatory molecule blockade and cytokine-directed therapies. Non-pharmacological options of Surgery (thymectomy, splenectomy), Plasma Exchange and Intravenous Immunoglobulin, Gene therapy, Autologous Haematopoietic Stem Cell Transplantation (AHSCT), and Antigen-specific immunotherapy are the new strategies adopted to combat autoimmune disorders.

CLASSIFICATION OF IMMUNE DISEASES BASED ON ORGAN SPECIFICITY

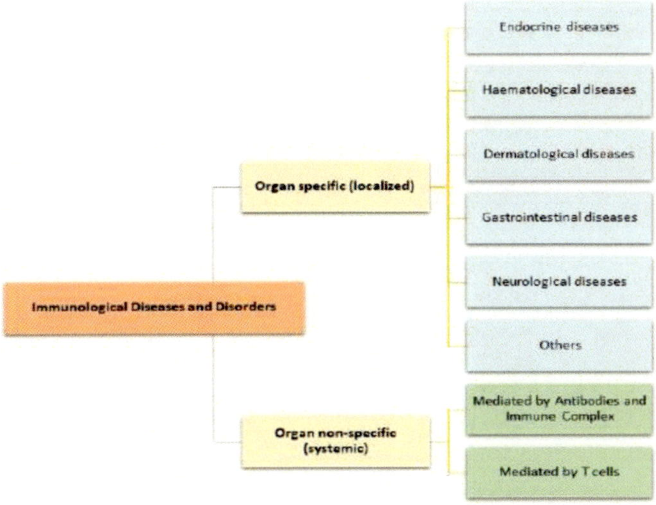

Fig. (3). Classification of Immune diseases based on organ specificity.

ORGAN-SPECIFIC (LOCALIZED) DISEASES FIG. (3)

Endocrinologic Diseases

Hashimoto's (autoimmune) thyroiditis

Fig. (**4**) is a thyroid-affecting disorder, especially in genetically susceptible women with hypothyroidism without goiter. Genetic, immune, and environmental factors are supposed to contribute together to the pathogenesis of HT. Environmental factors like improved hygiene, raised dietary iodine consumption, modified treatment, chemical agents, stress, climate, age, and gender shows linkage in HT [38]. Cellular and humoral immunity both play a significant role in HT pathogenesis. The altered function of T regulatory cells and hyperactive follicular helper T cells stimulates the immune system causing infiltration of lymphocytes which produces a cytotoxic effect on thyroid follicular cells (TFC), modulating their metabolic and immune function. Thyroid peroxidase and thyroglobulin antibodies are majorly seen in HT patients, and sometimes sodium iodide symporter and pendrin are present too. In recent studies, it is found that the DNA fragments generated due to cell death and micro RNA also contribute to the HT pathogenesis. [39, 40]. Compromised function to T regulatory (Treg) cells, increased activity of follicular helper T cells (Tfh), DNA fragments (frag) released following cell death, and altered microRNA (miRNA) profile triggers the autoimmune process. T and B cells infiltration results in cell cytotoxicity, apoptosis, and antibody production. Cytokines produced *via* infiltration further enhance the inflammatory process and gland destruction.

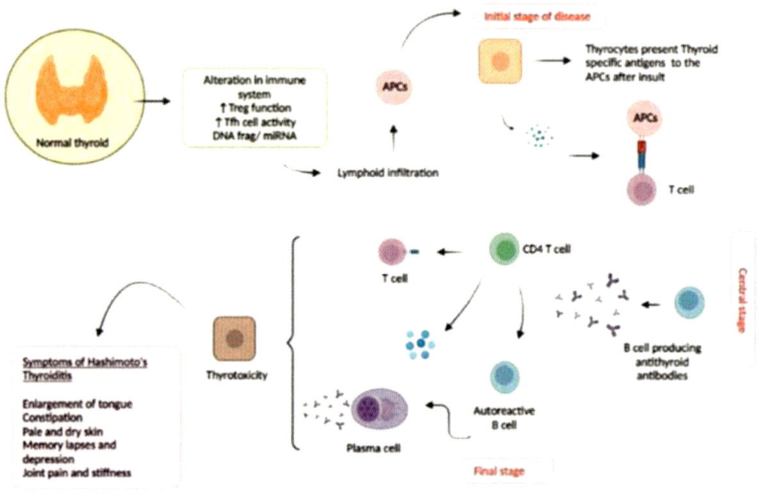

Fig. (4). Summary of the pathogenic mechanisms in Hashimoto's thyroiditis.

In a nutshell, lymphocytic infiltration and autoantibodies production against TSHR, thyroglobulin, thyroid peroxidase, and sodium symporter are characteristic of the disorder [39]. Signs and symptoms include fatigue, increased sensitivity to cold, constipation, pale and dry skin, a puffy face, brittle nails, hair loss (alopecia), enlargement of the tongue, unexplained weight gain, muscle aches (myalgia), joint pain (arthralgia), muscle weakness, heavy menstrual bleeding (menorrhagia), irregular menstruation (oligomenorrhea), depression, lapses in memory ("brain fog"), low sex drive, growth delay in children. Also, miscarriage is seen as an altered menstrual cycle and ovulation. Goiter appears to compensate for thyroxine deficiency. Hyperproliferation of the glandular cells may lead to the tumor of the thyroid, in later stages. HT Therapy aims to control hypothyroidism with drugs and supplementary measures. Oral administration of a synthetic hormone, the Levo-Thyroxine 4 (L-T4), at a dosage of 1.6–1.8 micrograms per kilo needs to be prolonged for a lifetime to maintain normal circulating thyrotropin (TSH) levels. Glucocorticoids like prednisolone can be given for a limited duration. HT Patients with selenium deficiency would be benefited from oral administration of selenium in the form of seleno-methionine. Diet can be modified to support treatment with the addition of vitamin D and calcium supplements and the limitation of iodine content. Thyroidectomy is preferred for HT patients with cancer. Thyroid gland transplantation still needs validation [41].

Neurological Disorders

Introduction

Neurological disorders such as Parkinson's disease, Alzheimer's disease, Multiple sclerosis, Amyotrophic lateral sclerosis is affecting a million peoples worldwide, leading to a major socioeconomic burden [42]. The central nervous system is privileged with the immune system, and immune cells are increasingly known to involve in both the health and disease state of the CNS [43]. The innate immune system, as well as the adaptive immune system, contribute to the development of neurodegenerative diseases. Clinical observation and biomedical research have revealed that inflammatory cytokines, chemokines, and other arbitrators are upregulated in neuroinflammation in various neurodegenerative diseases. Neuroinflammation is a term used to express the situation when injury, infection, or disease stimulate the resident immune cells to produce the inflammatory responses and production of the cytokines and chemokines at the injured site. The neuroinflammation also contributes to the proliferation and activation of glial cells, astrocytes, and microglia and additional immune responses [44]. The immune cells such as microglia, B cells, T cells, astrocytes, and the inflammatory mediators such as classical cytokines, and chemokines are major players in the pathogenesis of neurodegenerative diseases.

Alzheimer's Disease and Parkinson's Disease

Alzheimer's Disease

Aging may lead to various changes in the central nervous system as well as the other physiological systems such as the immune system resulting in more susceptibility to infectious diseases and contributing to cardiovascular, metabolic, autoimmune, and neurodegenerative diseases of aging. The detrimental alterations in the immune system that occurs with human aging are known as immunosenescence which is a multistage process consisting of various interrelated changes that lead to unidirectional damage to the immune system. [45]. Immune system dysregulation can be a cause of Alzheimer's disease pathogenesis and progression. In CNS, the deposition of an amyloid peptide can activate the immune cascades in microglia and astroglia, and this activation primarily initiates the phagocytic clearance response. The activation of microglial response may lead to inflammation which can be chronic, harmful, and contribute to a succession of diseases. Chronic inflammatory initiation of microglia results in pyroptosis, which further results in the release of apoptosis-associated speck-like protein containing CARD (ASC) complexes, also called ASC specks. And in the peripheral system, the production of ASC may cause the rapid responses of the innate immune system [46].

Parkinson's Disease

Parkinson's disease is described by James Parkinson's in his "Essay on the shaking palsy", and is characterized by motor and non-motor symptoms such as bradykinesia, rigidity, tremors, *etc.* Pathological hallmarks of Parkinson's disease may include Lewy bodies (intracytoplasmic inclusions) and deficiency of dopamine due to degeneration of dopaminergic neurons in substantia nigra. α-synuclein is a major component of Lewy bodies, and various studies show that the pathology of it is involved in the peripheral, olfactory bulb and then propagates from the caudal brainstem [47].

Aging is the most common factor in the development of Parkinson's disease. The aging process has a normal part, the decreasing function of the immune system. Henceforth due to a weakened immune system elderly population loses the strength to maintain the critical balance leading to increased susceptibility to various diseases. The patients with Parkinson's disease have demonstrated an increase in heterogeneity of immune function resulting in an imbalance of autoimmune reactions towards endocrine insulin and astrocytic S100B [48].

Parkinson's disease also has one marker, the inflammation in the brain and periphery, which is caused due to the autoreactive T cells, autoantigens, and activation of microglia and lymphocytes. A recent study has demonstrated the α-synuclein specific T cells specified with the α- synuclein misprocessing which can be a possible hypothesis saying that PD is an autoimmune disorder. Increased levels of proinflammatory cytokines such as IL-2,6,8, Monocyte chemoattractant proteins, and normal T-cells were seen in the patients with PD. The increased T cell populations lead to the activation of the circulatory cytokines and chemokines such as TH17+, CD4+, IFN -γ, TNF α, and IL-17 [49].

The local immune cells microglia get activated in the brain to protect the CNS by clearing the debris and are responsible for maintaining homeostasis in the CNS. Healthy microglia have a phagocytic activity to clear the α- synuclein *via* antibody mediation. Several toxic forms of α- synuclein activates microglia, and activated microglia shows deleterious effects on dopaminergic neurons *via* various pathways, including direct phagocytic activity on dopaminergic neurons, activating the direct antigen-presenting cells, which further activates T cells, activating the cytokines and complement cascades such as astrocytes and spreading of toxic forms of the α- synucleins to healthy neurons [50].

Multiple Sclerosis

Multiple Sclerosis (MS) is a chronic, progressive immune-mediated disease of the central nervous system (CNS) characterized by damage to normal-appearing white matter (NAWM), multifocal demyelination, axon degeneration, and brain atrophy Fig. (**5**). The location of sclerotic plaques and neurodegeneration within the CNS results in variable clinical manifestations of MS, which may include sensory and motor deficits, visual disturbances, autonomic dysfunction, cognitive impairment, and pain. It predominantly affects young adults and women are three times more at risk to develop MS than men [51, 52]. There are four clinical forms of MS: relapsing-remitting MS (RRMS), secondary progressive MS (SPMS), primary progressive MS (PPMS), and progressive relapsing MS (PRMS); of which relapsing-remitting type is the most common [53]. Lesions of the CNS white matter, with loss of myelin, neuronal axons, and myelin-producing oligodendrocytes, are the pathophysiologic characteristic of MS. The relapses are said to start when peripherally activated leukocytes enter the CNS through blood-brain barrier gaps, as shown in Fig. (**5**) [54].

MS therapy aims to prevent relapse and progressive disability. From the early 1990s, immunomodulator classes of drugs were preventing the relapses of MS. Recently, "disease-modifying therapies" (DMTs) with 10 approved drugs are used for the MS treatment: four forms of interferon (IFN) beta, glatiramer acetate, natalizumab, fingolimod, alemtuzumab, teriflunomide, and dimethyl fumarate (BG-12), along with new therapies on its way [51].

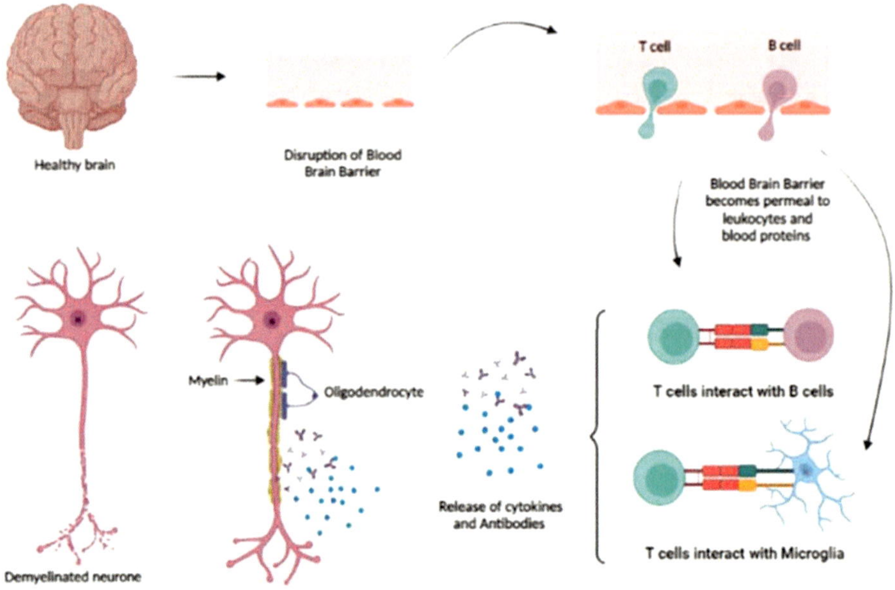

Fig. (5). Pathogenesis of Multiple sclerosis.

Auto-inflammatory Diseases/ Systemic Autoinflammatory Diseases (SAIDs)

Introduction

Autoinflammatory diseases or SAIDs, earlier called periodic fever syndromes, are a group of heterogeneous, rare, hereditary, recurrent type of clinical disorders which arise from the innate immune system and are distinguished by the periodic episodes of localized or systemic inflammation at disease-prone sites, with no autoreactive T cells and high autoantibody titers. Rashes, fever, arthritis, serositis, lymphadenopathy, central nervous system, and other organ involvement can be the manifestations of auto-inflammatory diseases.

The causative factors for these diseases can be single-gene mutations or multifactorial polygenic origin, with environmental influence modulating the phenotype. Inflammasome proteins have majorly been encoded by AIDs genes. HIDS/MKD is the only exception, as it occurs due to a mutation in the mevalonate kinase gene. All genes associated with AIDs have common structural patterns and functions which are involved with cytokine signaling pathways. Monogenic forms are quite frequent as compared to polygenic disorders [55, 56].

Classification Of Auto-Inflammatory Diseases

Auto-inflammatory diseases can be classified on the basis of gene mutations as monogenic auto-inflammatory diseases and polygenic auto-inflammatory diseases, as depicted in Fig. (**6**) [57].

Monogenic Autoinflammatory Diseases

Mevalonate Kinase Deficiency or Hyper-Immunoglobulin D Syndrome (MKD/HIDS)

Mevalonate kinase deficiency is a hereditary autosomal recessive transmission disease characterized by the elevation of serum immunoglobulin D, which is the distinct biochemical marker of MKD and reduced activity of the mevalonate kinase enzyme. This disease was first described in 1984 and is known as hyper IgD syndrome. Symptoms may include fever (can exceed 39^0 C), inflammatory attacks that last for 7 days which relapse every 4-8 weeks, abdominal pain, diarrhea, and arthralgia. Mucocutaneous symptoms may include urticarial lesions, erythematous macules, and oral ulcers [58].

Mutations in the MVK gene are the hallmark of the MKD. These mutations are mostly single-nucleotide polymorphisms that result in missense mutations and impairment of Mevalonate kinase stability. Afterward,>120 sequential mutations or variations of the MVK gene are reported which are associated with the MKD. Mevalonate kinase deficiency Syndrome has two phenotypic forms, namely mevalonic aciduria (MA), which is the most severe end of the syndrome, and HIDS, characterized by the self-limited bouts of multi-system inflammation.

The MA phenotypic MVK variations clump together in the core of proteins leading to very low enzyme activity. Loss of this mevalonate kinase enzyme activity results in cellular isoprenoid deficiency leading to initiation of the RhoA activity and increase in IL-Iβ gene expression along with Rac I. Rac I is responsible for activation of the procaspase-I. Simultaneously, monocytes and macrophages are activated by toll-like receptors ligands followed by proinflammatory gene expression and inflammasome priming. Inflammasomes activate caspase-I, which leads to the processing of pyroptosis and the release of inflammatory cytokines, including IL-I. Isoprenoid deficiency also leads to the impairment of mitochondrial function and stability and clearance of the damaged mitochondria through an autophagic process which further results in hypersecretion of IL-Iβ [59]. Gene therapies, inhibition of pyrin inflammasomes, altering isoprenoid biochemistry, enzyme replacement, replacement of affected cells, blocking of IL-Iβand other cytokines can be targets for the treatment of MKD [60].

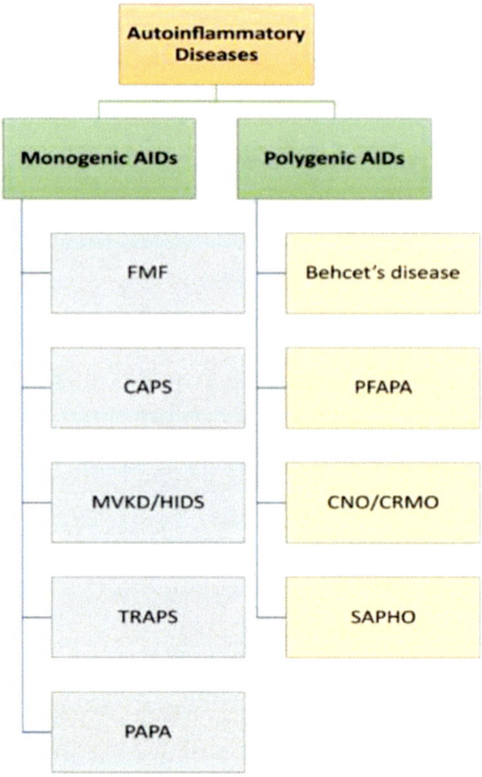

Fig. (6). Classification of Autoinflammatory diseases.

Pyogenic Arthritis, Pyoderma Gangrenosum, and Acne (PAPA)

Pyogenic arthritis, pyoderma gangrenosum, and acne (PAPA) syndrome is an autosomal dominant auto-inflammatory disorder. This disorder is distinguished by the trinity of Pyogenic sterile arthritis, Pyoderma gangrenosum, and Acne. The mutation of the Proline-Serine-Threonine Phosphatase-Interacting Protein 1 (PSTPIP1) gene, which is also known as the CDBP1 gene, is a hallmark of this disorder. Particularly A230T, E250K and E250Q mutation at the PSTPIP1 is responsible for the symptoms of PAPA syndrome [61]. Chromosome 15q encodes the proline-serine-threonine phosphatase interacting protein-1 and contains extended Fes-CIP4 homology domain, also known as F-BAR at N-terminal, SH3 domain at the C-terminal end. The F-BAR binds to the PTP-PEST and CD2, where the mutations for PAPA syndrome take place. Termination of the interaction of the PSTPIP1 and PTP-PEST results in hyperphosphorylation of the PSTPIP1, which further leads to initiation of inflammasome assembly followed by IL-aB release.

Caspase 1 mediated and NALP3 inflammasome-driven proinflammatory signaling pathways cleave pro- IL-1-β into active IL-1-β, but the loss of activity of pyrin leads to the failure of an inhibitory effect of pyrin on this pathway followed by an overproduction of IL-1-β which further accelerate neutrophil-mediated inflammation. The other role of PSTPIP1 is participation in Wiskott-Aldrich Syndrome Protein (WASP) biogenesis which regulates the podosome formation and cell migration. The mutation of PSTPIP1 at R450 may lead to a drastic increase in the macrophage levels and increased matrix degradation [62].

Familial Mediterranean Fever (FMF)

FMF is the most common monogenic AID, mainly affecting populations of Mediterranean origin living in Arabic or Turkish coasts, South Europe, and North Africa [63]. Its prevalence is high among Sephardic Jews (100-400 every 100000 inhabitants) and quite low among west Europeans (2.5 per 100000). The characteristic features include recurrent episodes of short-lasting fever (12–72 h), serositis (peritonitis, synovitis, or pleuritis)), non-erosive acute arthritis of large joints, erysipelas-like lower extremity erythematous rash which can lead to potentially fatal amyloidosis. The most significant complication of FMF is Amyloidosis causing the deposition of serum amyloid A protein (SAA) mostly in the kidney, which leads to renal disease. Triggers may include stress, menstrual cycle, even drugs (metaraminol, cisplatin), exercise, and subclinical infections [64].

The disease is caused by mutations in the MEFV gene, which is located on the short arm of chromosome 16 (16p13.3) and consists of 10 exons encoding a protein of 781 amino acids, called pyrin (also named marenostrin or TRIM20). Wild-type pyrin has an anti-inflammatory effect through suppression of inflammasome-mediated IL-1b production and an antiapoptotic role through inhibition of NF-kB nuclear transcription factor [64]. The Pyrin inflammasome is regulated by RhoA-dependent phosphorylation. Ras homolog gene family member A (RhoA) GTPase activates two serines. Threonine kinases called protein kinase N (PKN1 and PKN2) bind and phosphorylate pyrin: phosphorylated pyrin interacts with the regulatory protein 14-3-3 to block pyrin inflammasome activity. Mutations that primarily occur in the B30.2 domain result in dysregulated interaction between PKN1, PKN2, and 14-3-3, causing activation of pyrin inflammasome.

The most commonly reported mutations of the MEFV gene are M694V, M680I, and V726A. M694V mutation has been associated with more severe disease courses and specifically with the development of amyloidosis. More than 300 different mutations of the *MEFV* gene have been identified, of which only four have clear pathogenicity [65]. The diagnosis of FMF is based on either Tel Hashomer or Yalcinkaya-Ozen clinical criteria and can be supported by genetic analysis [56].

Colchicine has been the drug of choice since 1970 for FMF. Patients who are resistant to colchicine or other disease treatments can be given drugs as per requirement. Intravenous methylprednisolone for acute phase, alpha interferon, IL-1 cytokine antagonist, IL1 alpha and IL-1 beta-blocker, anti-TNF, and dapsone can be effective measures [66].

Polygenic Autoinflammatory Diseases

Bechet's Disease (BD)

Behcet's disease (BD) is a rare, severely debilitating, systemic inflammatory vasculitis characterized by a range of clinical manifestations, including oral aphthae, genital ulcers, skin lesions, ocular, vascular, articular, gastrointestinal, urogenital, pulmonary, and neurologic involvement [67]. Oral and genital ulcers are the hallmarks of the disease, seen in up to 97% and 60–90% of patients, respectively [68]. BD is associated along the old silk route among Japan to Turkish population than Caucasians. BD mostly starts at the ages of 20–40 and is equally distributed between men and women [67].

The triad of genetics, environment, and immunity is interwoven in the pathogenesis of BD. External environmental factors trigger the innate immune inflammatory response which is further maintained by the adaptive immune system. HLA-B51 is the most important gene with a key role in BD. Also, interleukin (IL)-10, IL23R/IL12RB2, STAT4, and endoplasmic reticulum aminopeptidase1 (ERAP1) genes are reported to be associated with BD (S. Demir 2018). Altered T cell balance with Th1/Th17 activation and Tregs suppression is significantly contributing to the pathogenesis of BD. Inflammatory mediators invade through Th1 and Th-17 pathways while Tregs (responsible to control autoimmunity) and IL-10 (an anti-inflammatory cytokine) are suppressed [67].

Multisystem involvement develops complexity in BD; hence type and severity of clinical manifestations decide the treatment line. Colchicine is widely used in the treatment of BD. Corticosteroids alone or in combination with immunosuppressant drugs or Disease-modifying drugs like Azathioprine, Methotrexate, Sulfasalazine, Prednisolone, Cyclophosphamide along with Tumor necrosis factor (TNF)-blocking agents such as Infliximab (an anti-TNFα chimeric monoclonal antibody), Etanercept, Adalimumab, *etc.* are the mainline drugs for BD. Novel targeted biotherapies such as Apremilast – phosphodiesterase-4 inhibitor, Anakinra – interleukin (IL)-1 receptor antagonist, Canakinumab –

human monoclonal immunoglobulin G1 inhibitor of IL-1β, Tocilizumab – IL-6 inhibitor, Ustekinumab – IL-12/23 inhibitor is under consideration [68].

ROLE OF THE IMMUNE SYSTEM IN CANCER

Cancer is a global health problem responsible for one in six deaths worldwide. In 2020, cancer cases reached up to 19.3 million, and 10 million death were reported globally. Cancer is a complicated succession of disease conditions that gradually progresses to a generalized loss of growth control [69]. The development of cancer processes *via* eight steps, namely sustained proliferation, evasion of growth suppressors, cell death resistance, replicative immortality, angiogenesis, metastasis, reprogrammed metabolism, and evasion of the immune system. Several studies were conducted to establish a link between cancer and the immune system, and the term immunoediting was described to all phases of cancer and immune system interactions or interlinks [70].

IMMUNE CELLS AND CANCER PROGRESSION

The number of mechanisms controls cellular growth and death. Failure in this mechanism caused due to DNA mutations is the main reason behind the development of the cellular aberrant, which accumulates and further forms tumors. Cancer is diverse masses of various types of cells, including immune cells, fibroblasts, tumor cells, and pericytes. This niche consists of cells, and by-products of this cell comprise the Tumor microenvironment (TME) [71].

Innate and adaptive immunity plays an important role in the progression of cancer *via* selecting the aggressive clones comprising the immunosuppression and stimulating the cancer cell proliferation along with metastasis. During the elimination phase, the natural killer cells and CD4+ cells detect the more immunogenic cells, and this phase selects the proliferation of the less immunogenic cells henceforth, the system cannot detect the cancerous cells [72].

As discussed earlier, immune cells, including macrophages, natural killer cells, neutrophils, T cells, and B cells, play an important role in cancer development and progression. Macrophages play a crucial role in tissue homeostasis, cancer development, and tumor promotion in established cancer. Tumor-associated macrophages are important factors in the tumor micro-environment. Macrophages can promote tumor-associated inflammation by secreting the pro-inflammatory cytokines, such as IL-6, IL-1β, and TNF –α, which leads to activation of the Nuclear factor- κ B (NF- κ B) pathway by THF-α and activation of JAK/STAT 3 pathway by pro-inflammatory cytokines followed by initiation of cell proliferation, differentiation, and apoptosis [73].

Neutrophils are the foremost white blood cells in the circulatory system, which play a major role in cancers, most linked to inflammation and active participation in metastasis. Granulocyte colony-stimulating factor (G-CSF) is a cytokine secreted by various cells, such as macrophages, endothelial cells, and cancer cells responsible for the recruitment of neutrophils in tumor micro-environment. Another important factor leading the neutrophil recruitment is IL- 17. Neutrophils have two polarization states, N1 and N2, where N1 is anti-tumor activity, and N2 is pro-tumor neutrophil. N1, after exposure to the regulatory factors like G-CSF and TNF-β, gets transformed into the N2 phenotype, which constitutes a higher number of pro-tumor factors which initiate the immunosuppression in the tumor micro-environment. In this tumor micro-environment, neutrophils induce the reactive oxygen species, and some enzymes, such as matrix metalloprotease 9 (MMM-9), CG, and NE (serine proteases), also secret the chemokines and cytokines [74].

Furthermore, the B cells also play a key role in the tumor progression *via* several mechanisms, including the modulation of the immune response towards cancer, production of the autoantibodies, indirectly and directly suppressing the Th1 and CD4+ cytolytic T cell responses. It has been studied that the production of IL-21 by Tregs may also result in making B cells more "regulatory" in nature, as IL-21 enhances the upregulation of IL-10, IDO, and granzyme B in B cells [75].

So, overall, the immune system greatly impacts cancer development and progression.

Chemotherapy is said to be the most widely used and effective therapy for cancer, along with Radiotherapy. The novel drug development for cancer treatment depends on the various pathways and characteristics of the various tumors. One can divide the cancer treatment ways into Conventional and Modern / Novel categories. Conventional cancer treatment involves the surgical resection of tumors followed by chemotherapy and radiotherapy and modern or novel cancer treatment. The novel drug development for cancer treatment depends on the various pathways and characteristics of the various tumors. In the current scenario, various therapies are emerging to treat the different types of cancer, and Immunotherapy is one of the attractive therapies for cancer [69].

Cancer Immunotherapy utilizes the components of the immune system of the host and modifies it to treat cancer. Immunotherapy has fewer side effects and is target-specific compared to conventional cancer treatment. As shown in Fig. (**7**). it can be classified as active (stimulates the immune system) and passive Immunotherapy (which does not stimulate the immune system but increases the anti-Tumor activity), both of which are further subdivided as specific and non-specific Immunotherapy [76].

One of the Active Immunotherapeutic agents, Monoclonal antibodies, targets specific Signal transduction pathways, which are dysregulated in cancer. Naked, Conjugated and Bispecific are types of monoclonal antibodies used to treat various cancer types. Naked mAbs get attached to antigens on Tumor cells and block them. (Alemtuzumab binds to the CD52 antigen on lymphocytes and is hence used to treat chronic lymphocytic leukemia). Conjugated antibodies get attached to chemotherapeutic agents and directly get them to cancerous cells. (Brentuximab vedotin, an antibody that targets CD30 antigen om lymphocytes and is hence used to treat Hodgkin lymphoma and anaplastic large cell lymphoma).

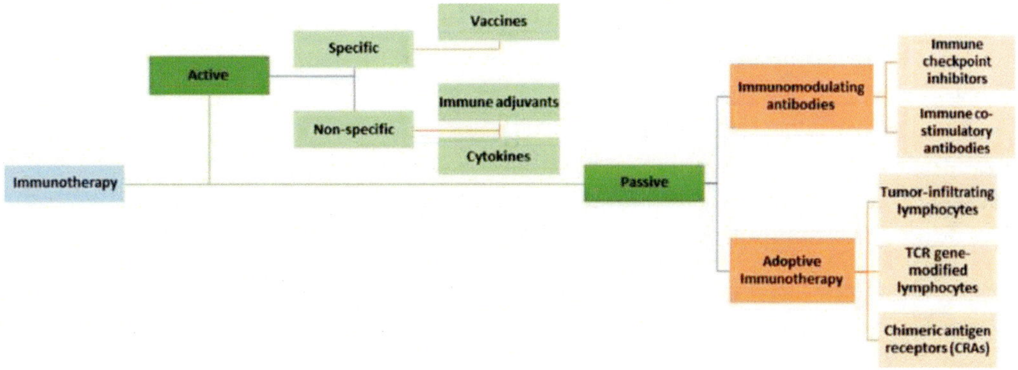

Fig. (7). Classification of Immunotherapy.

Bispecific Antibodies have 2 parts of 2 different antibodies (Blinatumomab binding to both CD3 and CD19 used to treat acute lymphocytic leukemia (ALL)). Several other antibodies have already been tested and accepted by FDA for immunotherapy, such as rituximab, ibritumomab, tiuxetan, trastuzumab, emtansine, nivolumab, and pembrolizumab [77, 78].

Another fascinating key approach to treat cancer is cancer vaccines which stimulate the active immune response toward the tumor. Adenoviral, dendritic cell, tumor cell, adoptive T-cell transfer, and peptide are types of cancer vaccines under development. In a Phase III trial for Sipileucel-T (Provenge®, Dendreon Corporation), which is the first autologous vaccine consisting of activated dendritic cells consisting of granulocyte-macrophage colony-stimulating factor (GM-CSF) and prostatic acid phosphatase (PAP) approved by the FDA for treatment of advanced prostate cancer. This vaccine comprises a large proportion of antigen-presenting cells, which were infused back into the patient to stimulate antitumor T-cell responses [79]. Another example is Mucin 1 (MUC1), which is highly shown in adenocarcinomas. A lot of vaccines for MUC1 have been developed and tested in preclinical and clinical studies. In the past 2 decades, vaccines for cancer have shown potential in pre-clinical and human clinical trials [80]. Administration of antitumor immune cells using adoptive cell therapy (ACT) is another effective cancer treatment. The ACT treatment aims to initiate the immune-mediated antitumor responses *via* infusion of ex *et al* manipulated T cells [81].

Immuno-checkpoint inhibitors are also one of the developing and promising therapy to treat different types of cancers. Cancer immuno-editing is the process by which numerous immune system components protect the host against primary tumor development by forming tumor immunogenicity or diminishing anti-tumor immune responses. This process is strictly regulated by the immune checkpoints and immune surface receptors. Immune checkpoint inhibitors such as CTLA-4 inhibitors (Ipilimumab), PD-1 inhibitors (Pembrolizumab), PD-L1 inhibitors (Atezolizumab Avelumab, Durvalumab) are approved for advanced-stage cancers by Health Canada. Numerous agonistic and antagonistic immune checkpoint inhibitors are currently under investigation, such as Utomilumab, ARGX-110 (cusatuzumab), Mogamulizumab, Lirilumab, Ciforadenant, Indoximod, Epacadostat, Rintatolimod, AM0010 (pegilodecakin), *etc.* [82].

CONCLUSION

The immune system is the body's defense mechanism to protect from all types of infections. The innate immune system is the first-line defense mechanism that responds immediately against foreign bodies, injuries, and pathogens. To combat specific antigens or changed body cells, the adaptive immune system is expressed. Both innate and acquired immune system works together against invaders. The defense mechanism of the body collapse due to defects and/or imbalance of the immune system and thus leads to various disorders and diseases of the immune system. Understanding the genetics and molecular level pathogenesis has paved the way for the accurate diagnosis and new immuno-modulating therapies for immune system-related disorders. Immuno-modulating therapy is not only restricted to immune system-related disorders but becoming a major focus of the mainline therapeutic intervention for all major diseases.

CONSENT FOR PUBLICATION

Not applicable.

CONFLICT OF INTEREST

The authors declare no conflict of interest, financial or otherwise.

ACKNOWLEDGEMENTS

Declared none.

REFERENCES

[1] Janewayr C. Immunobiology: the immune system in health and disease. animated CD-ROM inside. 5 Ed.. New York, NY: Garland Publ. 2001; 732.

[2] Tolentino Júnior DS, de Oliveira CM, de Assis EM. Population-based Study of 24 Autoimmune Diseases Carried Out in a Brazilian Microregion. J Epidemiol Glob Health 2019; 9(4): 243-51. [http://dx.doi.org/10.2991/jegh.k.190920.001] [PMID: 31854165]

[3] Catanzaro M, Corsini E, Rosini M, Racchi M, Lanni C. Immunomodulators Inspired by Nature: A Review on Curcumin and Echinacea. MDPI molecules 2018; (23): 1-17.

[4] Amaya-Uribe L, Rojas M, Azizi G, Anaya JM, Gershwin ME. Primary immunodeficiency and autoimmunity: A comprehensive review. J Autoimmun 2019; 99: 52-72. [http://dx.doi.org/10.1016/j.jaut.2019.01.011] [PMID: 30795880]

[5] Barreto ICDP, Barreto BAP, Cavalcante EGN, Condino Neto A. Immunological deficiencies: more frequent than they seem to be. J Pediatr (Rio J) 2021; 97 (Suppl. 1): S49-58. [http://dx.doi.org/10.1016/j.jped.2020.10.009] [PMID: 33238140]

[6] Buchbinder D, Nugent D, Fillipovich A. Wiskott–Aldrich syndrome: diagnosis, current management, and emerging treatments. Appl Clin Genet 2014; 7: 55-66. [http://dx.doi.org/10.2147/TACG.S58444] [PMID: 24817816]

[7] Riboldi GM, Samanta D, Frucht S. Ataxia Telangiectasia, in StatPearls, Treasure Island (FL): StatPearls Publishing, 2021. http://www.ncbi.nlm.nih.gov/books/NBK519542/

[8] Lackey AE, Muzio MR. DiGeorge Syndrome, in StatPearls, Treasure Island (FL): StatPearls Publishing 2021. http://www.ncbi.nlm.nih.gov/books/NBK549798/

[9] Chinen J, Shearer WT. Secondary immunodeficiencies, including HIV infection. J Allergy Clin Immunol 2010; 125(2) (Suppl. 2): S195-203. [http://dx.doi.org/10.1016/j.jaci.2009.08.040] [PMID: 20042227]

[10] Layhadi JA, Palmer E, Sharif H, Shamji MH. Current Drug Treatments for Allergy. In: Janes SM, Ed. Encyclopedia of Respiratory Medicine. 2nd ed. Oxford: Academic Press 2022; pp. 477-90. https://www.sciencedirect.com/science/article/pii/B9780081027233002365 [http://dx.doi.org/10.1016/B978-0-08-102723-3.00236-5]

[11] Akhtari M, Mahmoudi M. Chapter 6 - Epigenetic biomarkers of asthma and allergic disorders," in Prognostic Epigenetics, vol. 15, S. Sharma, Ed 2019.https://www.sciencedirect.com/science / article/ pii/ B9780128142592 000078

[12] Bousquet J, Anto JM, Bachert C, *et al.* Allergic rhinitis. Nat Rev Dis Primers 2020; 6(1): 95. [http://dx.doi.org/10.1038/s41572-020-00227-0] [PMID: 33273461]

[13] Hoyte FCL, Nelson HS. Recent advances in allergic rhinitis. F1000 Res 2018; 7(1333): 1-10. [PMID: 30210782]

[14] Akhouri S, House SA, Doerr C. Allergic Rhinitis (Nursing). StatPearls. Treasure Island, FL: StatPearls Publishing 2021.http://www.ncbi.nlm.nih.gov/books/NBK568690/ Internet

[15] Small P, Keith PK, Kim H. Small P, Keith PK, Kim H. Allergic rhinitis Allergy Asthma Clin

Immunol. 2018; 51: pp. (2)31-41.

[16] Bjermer L, Westman M, Holmström M, Wickman MC. The complex pathophysiology of allergic rhinitis: scientific rationale for the development of an alternative treatment option. Allergy Asthma Clin Immunol 2019; 15(1): 24. [http://dx.doi.org/10.1186/s13223-018-0314-1] [PMID: 31015846]

[17] Thomsen SF. Atopic dermatitis: natural history, diagnosis, and treatment. ISRN Allergy 2014; 2014: 1-7. [http://dx.doi.org/10.1155/2014/354250] [PMID: 25006501]

[18] Kolb L, Ferrer-Bruker SJ. Atopic Dermatitis. StatPearls. Treasure Island, FL: StatPearls Publishing 2021.http://www.ncbi.nlm.nih.gov/books/NBK448071/ Internet

[19] Kapur S, Watson W, Carr S. Atopic dermatitis. Allergy Asthma Clin Immunol 2018; 14(S2) (Suppl. 2): 52. [http://dx.doi.org/10.1186/s13223-018-0281-6] [PMID: 30275844]

[20] Langan SM, Irvine AD, Weidinger S. Atopic dermatitis. Lancet 2020; 396(10247): 345-60. [http://dx.doi.org/10.1016/S0140-6736(20)31286-1] [PMID: 32738956]

[21] Pescitelli L, Rosi E, Ricceri F, Pimpinelli N, Prignano F. Novel Therapeutic Approaches and Targets for the Treatment of Atopic Dermatitis. Curr Pharm Biotechnol 2020; 22(1): 73-84. [http://dx.doi.org/10.2174/1389201021666200611112755] [PMID: 32525769]

[22] Aslan Kayıran M. Diagnosis and Treatment of Urticaria in Primary Care. North Clin Istanb. 2018; v.6(1). [http://dx.doi.org/10.14744/nci.2018.75010]

[23] Nettis E, Foti C, Ambrifi M, *et al.* Urticaria: recommendations from the Italian Society of Allergology, Asthma and Clinical Immunology and the Italian Society of Allergological, Occupational and Environmental Dermatology. Clin Mol Allergy 2020; 18(1): 8. [http://dx.doi.org/10.1186/s12948-020-00123-8] [PMID: 32390768]

[24] Schaefer P. Acute and Chronic Urticaria: Evaluation and Treatment. Am Fam Physician 2017; 95(11): 717-724, 717-724. [PMID: 28671445]

[25] Jain S. Pathogenesis of chronic urticaria: an overview. Dermatol Res Pract 2014; 2014: 1-10. [http://dx.doi.org/10.1155/2014/674709] [PMID: 25120565]

[26] Prasad PS. Urticaria. Indian J Dermatol Venereol Leprol 2001; 67(1): 11-20. https://ijdvl.com/urticaria/ [Internet]. [PMID: 17664692]

[27] Hon KL, Leung AKC, Ng WGG, Loo SK. Chronic urticaria: an overview of treatment and recent patents. Recent Pat Inflamm Allergy Drug Discov 2019; 13(1): 27-37. [http://dx.doi.org/10.2174/1872213X13666190328164931] [PMID: 30924425]

[28] Sah R, Neupane S, Khadka S, *et al.* A case study of stevens–johnson syndrome-toxic epidermal necrolysis (SJS-TEN) overlap in *mycoplasma pneumoniae* -associated tracheobronchitis. Case Rep Infect Dis 2019; 2019: 1-5. [http://dx.doi.org/10.1155/2019/5471765] [PMID: 31275674]

[29] Kim MK, Yoon KC, Yoon SH, Seo KY. Clinical aspects of stevens-johnson syndrome and toxic epidermal necrolysis with severe ocular complications in south korea. Front Med (Lausanne) 2021; 8: 640360. [http://dx.doi.org/10.3389/fmed.2021.640360] [PMID: 33693020]

[30] Fakoya AOJ, Omenyi P, Anthony P, *et al.* Stevens - johnson syndrome and toxic epidermal necrolysis; extensive review of reports of drug-induced etiologies, and possible therapeutic modalities. Open Access Maced J Med Sci 2018; 6(4): 730-8. [http://dx.doi.org/10.3889/oamjms.2018.148] [PMID: 29731949]

[31] Oakley AM, Krishnamurthy K. Stevens Johnson Syndrome. StatPearls. Treasure Island, FL: StatPearls Publishing 2021.http://www.ncbi.nlm.nih.gov/books/NBK459323/ Internet

[32] Kirchhof MG, Miliszewski MA, Sikora S, Papp A, Dutz JP. Retrospective review of Stevens-Johnson syndrome/toxic epidermal necrolysis treatment comparing intravenous immunoglobulin with cyclosporine. J Am Acad Dermatol 2014; 71(5): 941-7. [http://dx.doi.org/10.1016/j.jaad.2014.07.016] [PMID: 25087214]

[33] Hasegawa A, Abe R. Recent advances in managing and understanding Stevens-Johnson syndrome and toxic epidermal necrolysis. F1000 Res 2020; 9: 612. [http://dx.doi.org/10.12688/f1000research.24748.1] [PMID: 32595945]

[34] Bigley T M, Cooper M A. ScienceDirect Monogenic autoimmunity and infectious diseases: the double-edged sword of immune dysregulation. Current Opinion in Immunology 2021; 72: 230-8.

[35] K Yamamoto. Mechanisms of Autoimmunity Recent concepts. Japan Medical Association; 2004; 403-6. Internet https://www.med.or.jp/english/pdf/2004_09/403_406.pdf

[36] Wang L, Wang FS, Gershwin ME. Human autoimmune diseases: a comprehensive update. J Intern Med 2015; 278(4): 369-95. [http://dx.doi.org/10.1111/joim.12395] [PMID: 26212387]

[37] Arakelyan A, Nersisyan L, Poghosyan D, *et al.* Autoimmunity and autoinflammation: A systems view on signaling pathway dysregulation profiles. PLoS One 2017; 12(11): e0187572. [http://dx.doi.org/10.1371/journal.pone.0187572] [PMID: 29099860]

[38] Mak TW, Saunders ME. The immune response: basic and clinical principles. Amsterdam, Boston: Elsevier/Academic 2006. http://www.dawsonera.com/abstract/9780080534480 Internet

[39] Ajjan RA, Weetman AP. The pathogenesis of hashimoto's thyroiditis: further developments in our understanding. Horm Metab Res 2015; 47(10): 702-10. [http://dx.doi.org/10.1055/s-0035-1548832] [PMID: 26361257]

[40] Ramos-Leví AM, Marazuela M. Pathogenesis of thyroid autoimmune disease: the role of cellular mechanisms. Endocrinol Nutr 2016; 63(8): 421-9. [http://dx.doi.org/10.1016/j.endonu.2016.04.003] [PMID: 27234136]

[41] Ralli M, Angeletti D, Fiore M, *et al.* Hashimoto's thyroiditis: An update on pathogenic mechanisms, diagnostic protocols, therapeutic strategies, and potential malignant transformation. Autoimmun Rev 2020; 19(10): 102649. [http://dx.doi.org/10.1016/j.autrev.2020.102649] [PMID: 32805423]

[42] Lindestam Arlehamn CS, Garretti F, Sulzer D, Sette A. Roles for the adaptive immune system in Parkinson's and Alzheimer's diseases. Curr Opin Immunol 2019; 59: 115-20. [http://dx.doi.org/10.1016/j.coi.2019.07.004] [PMID: 31430650]

[43] Sabatino JJ Jr, Pröbstel AK, Zamvil SS. B cells in autoimmune and neurodegenerative central nervous system diseases. Nat Rev Neurosci 2019; 20(12): 728-45. [http://dx.doi.org/10.1038/s41583-019-0233-2] [PMID: 31712781]

[44] Frost GR, Jonas LA, Li YM. Friend, Foe or Both? Immune Activity in Alzheimer's Disease. Front Aging Neurosci 2019; 11: 337. [http://dx.doi.org/10.3389/fnagi.2019.00337] [PMID: 31920620]

[45] Müller L, Di Benedetto S, Pawelec G. The Immune System and Its Dysregulation with Aging. Biochemistry and Cell Biology of Ageing: Part II Clinical Science 2019; vol. 91: 21-43.http://link.springer.com/10.1007/978-981-13-3681-2_2 [http://dx.doi.org/10.1007/978-981-13-3681-2_2]

[46] Bettcher BM, Tansey MG, Dorothée G, Heneka MT. Peripheral and central immune system crosstalk in Alzheimer disease — a research prospectus. Nat Rev Neurol 2021; 17(11): 689-701. [http://dx.doi.org/10.1038/s41582-021-00549-x] [PMID: 34522039]

[47] Jankovic J, Tan EK. Parkinson's disease: etiopathogenesis and treatment. J Neurol Neurosurg Psychiatry 2020; 91(8): 795-808.
[http://dx.doi.org/10.1136/jnnp-2019-322338] [PMID: 32576618]

[48] Immune System and Parkinson's Disease. Arch Med (Oviedo) 2016; 8(2): 6.

[49] Garretti F, Agalliu D, Lindestam Arlehamn CS, Sette A, Sulzer D. Autoimmunity in Parkinson's Disease: The Role of α-Synuclein-Specific T Cells. Front Immunol 2019; 10(303): 303.
[http://dx.doi.org/10.3389/fimmu.2019.00303] [PMID: 30858851]

[50] Tan EK, Chao YX, West A, Chan LL, Poewe W, Jankovic J. Parkinson disease and the immune system — associations, mechanisms and therapeutics. Nat Rev Neurol 2020; 16(6): 303-18.
[http://dx.doi.org/10.1038/s41582-020-0344-4] [PMID: 32332985]

[51] Finkelsztejn A. Multiple sclerosis: overview of disease-modifying agents. Perspect Medicin Chem 2014; 6: PMC.S13213.
[http://dx.doi.org/10.4137/PMC.S13213] [PMID: 25336899]

[52] Thomas RH, Wakefield RA. Oral disease-modifying therapies for relapsing-remitting multiple sclerosis. Am J Health Syst Pharm 2015; 72(1): 25-38.
[http://dx.doi.org/10.2146/ajhp140023] [PMID: 25511835]

[53] Ghasemi N, Razavi S, Nikzad E. Multiple Sclerosis: Pathogenesis, Symptoms, Diagnoses and Cell-Based Therapy. Cell J 2017; 19(1): 1-10.
[PMID: 28367411]

[54] Lassmann H, Brück W, Lucchinetti CF. The immunopathology of multiple sclerosis: an overview. Brain Pathol 2007; 17(2): 210-8.
[http://dx.doi.org/10.1111/j.1750-3639.2007.00064.x] [PMID: 17388952]

[55] Doria A, Zen M, Bettio S, *et al.* Autoinflammation and autoimmunity: Bridging the divide. Autoimmun Rev 2012; 12(1): 22-30.
[http://dx.doi.org/10.1016/j.autrev.2012.07.018] [PMID: 22878274]

[56] Krainer J, Siebenhandl S, Weinhäusel A. Systemic autoinflammatory diseases. J Autoimmun 2020; 109: 102421.
[http://dx.doi.org/10.1016/j.jaut.2020.102421] [PMID: 32019685]

[57] Demir S, Sag E, Dedeoglu F, Ozen S. Vasculitis in Systemic Autoinflammatory Diseases. Front Pediatr 2018; 6: 377.
[http://dx.doi.org/10.3389/fped.2018.00377] [PMID: 30560109]

[58] Georgin-Lavia S, Ducharme-Benard S, Sarrabay G, Savey L, Grateau G, Hentgen V. Systemic autoinflammatory diseases: Clinical state of the art. Best Pract Res Clin Rheumatol 2020; 34(4): 101529.
[http://dx.doi.org/10.1016/j.berh.2020.101529] [PMID: 32546426]

[59] Schulert G, Favier L. Mevalonate kinase deficiency: current perspectives. Appl Clin Genet 2016; 9: 101-10.
[http://dx.doi.org/10.2147/TACG.S93933] [PMID: 27499643]

[60] Jeyaratnam J, Frenkel J. Management of Mevalonate Kinase Deficiency: A Pediatric Perspective. Front Immunol 2020; 11: 1150.
[http://dx.doi.org/10.3389/fimmu.2020.01150] [PMID: 32582214]

[61] Punaro MG, Wise CA. Pyogenic Arthritis Pyoderma Gangrenosum and Acne (PAPA) Syndrome. In: Hashkes PJ, Laxer RM, Simon A, Eds. Textbook of Autoinflammation. Eds. Cham:: Springer International Publishing 2019; pp. 405-15.

[62] Cugno M, Borghi A, Marzano AV. PAPA, PASH and PAPASH Syndromes: Pathophysiology, Presentation and Treatment. Am J Clin Dermatol 2017; 18(4): 555-62.
[http://dx.doi.org/10.1007/s40257-017-0265-1] [PMID: 28236224]

[63] Lucherini OM, Rigante D, Sota J, *et al.* Updated overview of molecular pathways involved in the most common monogenic autoinflammatory diseases. Clin Exp Rheumatol 2018; 36(1) (Suppl. 110): 3-9. [PMID: 29742053]

[64] De Sanctis S, Nozzi M, Del Torto M, *et al.* Autoinflammatory syndromes: diagnosis and management. Ital J Pediatr 2010; 36(1): 57. [http://dx.doi.org/10.1186/1824-7288-36-57] [PMID: 20813071]

[65] El-Shanti H. Familial Mediterranean Fever. NORD Guide to Rare Disorders. Philadelphia, PA: Lippincott Williams & Wilkins 2003; p. 19.

[66] Bashardoust B. Familial Mediterranean fever; diagnosis, treatment, and complications. J Nephropharmacol 2015; 4(1): 5-8. [PMID: 28197466]

[67] Leccese P, Alpsoy E. Behçet's Disease: An Overview of Etiopathogenesis. Front Immunol. 2019; (1067): 1-8.https://www.frontiersin.org/articles/10.3389/fimmu.2019.01067/full [http://dx.doi.org/10.3389/fimmu.2019.01067]

[68] Nair JR, Moots RJ. Behcet's disease. Clin Med (Lond) 2017; 17(1): 71-7. [http://dx.doi.org/10.7861/clinmedicine.17-1-71] [PMID: 28148585]

[69] Debela DT, Muzazu SG, Heraro KD, Ndalama MT, Mesele BW, Haile DC, *et al.* New approaches and procedures for cancer treatment: Current perspectives. SAGE Open Med (10): 1-10. [http://dx.doi.org/10.1177/20503121211034366] [PMID: 34408877]

[70] Abbott M, Ustoyev Y. Cancer and the Immune System: The History and Background of Immunotherapy. Semin Oncol Nurs 2019; 35(5): 150923. [http://dx.doi.org/10.1016/j.soncn.2019.08.002] [PMID: 31526550]

[71] Barbosa AM, Gomes-Gonçalves A, Castro AG, Torrado E. Immune system efficiency in cancer and the microbiota influence. Pathobiology 2021; 88(2): 170-86. [http://dx.doi.org/10.1159/000512326] [PMID: 33588418]

[72] Gonzalez H, Hagerling C, Werb Z. Roles of the immune system in cancer: from tumor initiation to metastatic progression. Genes Dev 2018; 32(19-20): 1267-84. [http://dx.doi.org/10.1101/gad.314617.118] [PMID: 30275043]

[73] Cendrowicz E, Sas Z, Bremer E, Rygiel TP. The role of macrophages in cancer development and therapy. Cancers (Basel) 2021; 13(8): 1946. [http://dx.doi.org/10.3390/cancers13081946] [PMID: 33919517]

[74] Wu L, Saxena S, Singh RK. Neutrophils in the Tumor Microenvironment. Adv Exp Med Biol 2020; 1224: 1-20. [http://dx.doi.org/10.1007/978-3-030-35723-8_1] [PMID: 32036601]

[75] Yuen GJ, Demissie E, Pillai S. B lymphocytes and cancer: a love-hate relationship. Trends Cancer 2016; 2(12): 747-57. [http://dx.doi.org/10.1016/j.trecan.2016.10.010] [PMID: 28626801]

[76] Trends in nonparenteral delivery of biologics, vaccines and cancer therapies. Novel Approaches and Strategies for Biologics, Vaccines and Cancer Therapies 2015. 89-122. Available from https://linkinghub.elsevier.com/retrieve/pii/B9780124166035000055 [http://dx.doi.org/10.1016/B978-0-12-416603-5.00005-5]

[77] Zhang H, Chen J. Current status and future directions of cancer immunotherapy. J Cancer 2018; 9(10): 1773-81. [http://dx.doi.org/10.7150/jca.24577] [PMID: 29805703]

[78] Innovative approaches for cancer treatment: current perspectives and new challenges. Ecancer medical science. 2019 13: 961. Available from https://ecancer.org/journal/13/full/961-innovative-approach-s-for-cancer-treatment-current-perspectives-and-new-challenges.php

[http://dx.doi.org/10.3332/ecancer.2019.961]

[79] Anassi E, Ndefo UA. Sipuleucel-T (provenge) injection: the first immunotherapy agent (vaccine) for hormone-refractory prostate cancer. P T Peer-Rev J Formul Manag 2011; 36(4): 197-202. [http://dx.doi.org/21572775]

[80] Apostolopoulos V. Cancer Vaccines: Research and Applications. Cancers (Basel) 2019; 11(8): 1041. [http://dx.doi.org/10.3390/cancers11081041] [PMID: 31344788]

[81] Met Ö, Jensen KM, Chamberlain CA, Donia M, Svane IM. Principles of adoptive T cell therapy in cancer. Semin Immunopathol 2019; 41(1): 49-58. [http://dx.doi.org/10.1007/s00281-018-0703-z] [PMID: 30187086]

[82] Esfahani K, Roudaia L, Buhlaiga N, Del Rincon SV, Papneja N, Miller WH Jr. A review of cancer immunotherapy: from the past, to the present, to the future. Curr Oncol 2020; 27(12) (Suppl. 2): 87-97. [http://dx.doi.org/10.3747/co.27.5223] [PMID: 32368178]

CHAPTER 3

Natural Sources of Immunomodulators

Vishal Bhange[1], Monika Kale[1], Ankita Dudhal[1], Nikhil Putta[2], Mukta Abhyankar[2], Supriya Jagtap[2] and **Vandana S. Nikam[1,*]**

[1] *Department of Pharmacology, STES's Smt. Kashibai Navale College of Pharmacy, Kondhwa, S. P. Pune University, Pune 411048, Maharashtra, India*

[2] *Department of Pharmacognosy, STES's Smt. Kashibai Navale College of Pharmacy, Kondhwa, S. P. Pune University, Pune 411048, Maharashtra, India*

Abstract: Nature is replete with an arsenal of compounds that can be investigated for their therapeutic potential. The immune system involvement in severe chronic illnesses or emerging infectious diseases has provided clinical evidence. The prevention and treatment of these diseases targeted at the immune system with natural immunomodulators are gaining momentum, owing to their diverse array of activities. Treating acute illnesses with modern medicines has been successful; however, treating chronic illness treatment remains elusive and disappointing. Notably, this chapter reviews the natural resources of immunomodulators. Natural immunomodulators from plants, marine, and animals are of prime importance, and they possess many pharmacological activities. Similarly, microbiota modifiers - prebiotics, probiotics, and micronutrients- are imperative in restoring immune homeostasis. This chapter summarizes these natural immunomodulators and their power to boost immunity and human well-being.

Keywords: Alkaloids, Glycosides, Micronutrients, Microbiota, Natural Immunomodulators, Prebiotics, Probiotics.

INTRODUCTION

Immunopharmacology, the most upcoming and rapidly developing branch of pharmacology, deals with pharmacology, immunology and pathology. It holds considerable potential for the prophylaxis and treatment of various spectrum of immune system illnesses and disorders. The etiology and pathophysiology of many diseases are known to be influenced by the host's immune system's specific and non-specific defences. Almost every culture has a history of herbalism, depending on the natural flora and vegetation and evidence of harnessing the power of natural remedies to heal human diseases and disorders. Ayurveda (Ayu:

* **Corresponding author Vandana S. Nikam:** Department of Pharmacology, STES's Smt. Kashibai Navale College of Pharmacy, Kondhwa, S. P. Pune University, Pune 411048, Maharashtra, India; Tel: +9130806361; E-mail: vandananikam@sinhgad.edu

Vandana S. Nikam, Sujata P. Sawarkar, Girish B. Mahajan and Supriya G. Jagtap (Eds.)

(Ayu: Life Veda: Knowledge), 'the science of life, is the world's oldest system of medicine and has enlisted various indigenous herbal and herbo-mineral formulations (for example, Shilajit) for human well-being.

Regulation of immune response to alleviate illnesses has piqued interest for many years, and the Ayurvedic notion of Rasayana is built on similar concepts. Many factors, such as medications and stress hormones, can affect the immune system's function and efficiency, resulting in either immunostimulation or immunosuppression. The healthy state is thought to be the result of a complex fine-tuning of immunoregulatory mechanisms. Immunomodulators are agents that maintain the homeostasis of the host immune system either by immunostimulation or by immunosuppression.

In light of the current context where the emergence of viral diseases like AIDS, hepatitis, and Severe Acute Respiratory Syndrome CoronaVirus (SARS-CoV) are viewed, and host defenses are compromised, the concept of Rasayana in Ayurveda as we understand, it seems to be imperative as it elevates the host defenses. Immunomodulatory medications may be used in clinical settings to restore immunological insufficiency, as in AIDS and other viral diseases, or to reduce normal or excessive immune efficiency, as in transplant rejection and autoimmune disorders.

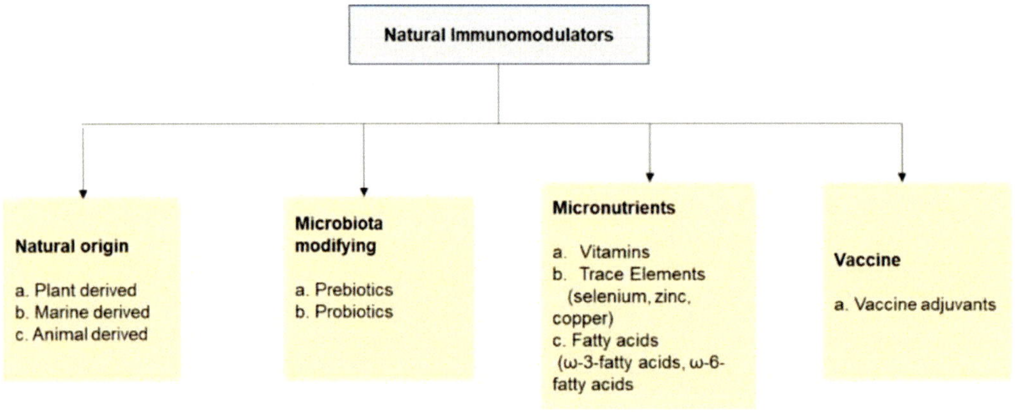

Fig. (1). Classification of natural immunomodulators.

The literature is replete with a plethora of natural immunomodulators derived from several sources like plants, animals and marines. The cross-talk between immune cells and natural microbial flora also has a significant role in immunity, and disturbed immune function can be corrected with the use of microbiota-modifying reagents like prebiotics and probiotics. Based on their sources and role, natural immunomodulators are broadly classified into many groups, as depicted in Fig. (**1**) [1 - 4].

PLANTS AS SOURCE OF IMMUNOMODULATORS

Herbal medicine is one of the most ancient forms of remedial treatment evolving with humanity. A retrospection of the healing power of plants and a return to natural remedies is an absolute need of our times. Herbal medicine is based upon the principles that plants contain. As research on herbals continues, an increasing number of plants is becoming recognized as immunomodulators. Table **1** and Fig. (**2**).

Glycosides

These organic compounds from plant sources are degraded by enzymes, yielding one or even more glucose molecules. They are acetals, or sugar elixirs, which are formed when the hydroxy groups of glucose and non-sugar molecules come in contact with the loss of a hydroxyl group. A number of glycosides have been shown to have immunomodulatory properties. *Picrorhiza scrophulariiflora* iridoid glycosides [1] and *Andrographis paniculata* anthraquinone glycosides [2] are two examples of them. Dendroside A and dendronobilosides A and B, three novel sesquiterpene glycosides, have been identified in the stem of *Dendrobium nobile*, a plant used in traditional Chinese medicine. Dendroside A and dendronobilosides A were known to increase the proliferation of murine T and B lymphocytes *in vitro*, although dendronobiloside B inhibited it [5].

These are some of the widely spread organic compounds in plants, present as free-state glycosides. They are mostly made up of water-soluble chemicals. The carbon skeleton of their molecular structure is C6-C3-C6. Flavonoids are powerful water-soluble strong antioxidants as well as free radical scavengers that protect cells from oxidative damage. They also have great anti-cancer properties, which protect against all phases of carcinogens. Flavonoids in the blood have been related to a decreased risk of heart disease [5]. They impede the initiation, propagation, and advancement of malignancies in terms of anti-cancer action. Plant flavonoids, with chemoprotective agents, have recently garnered the attention of many researchers as a highly essential dietary supplement for people with cancer [6, 7].

Tannins

Tannins are amorphous, seldom crystalline compounds that are astringent and bitter in taste. They are soluble in water and alcohol. They are phenolic compounds, classified chemically based on the hydrolysis product.

They are common in vascular plants but only found in woody tissues in angiosperms. Hydrolysable tannins are made up of several esters of gallic acid with D-glucose, whereas condensed tannins (typically proanthocyanides) are made up of flavonoid monomers. Tannins have been associated with phagocytic cell stimulation, host-mediated tumour activity, and anti-infective action, among other physiological functions [8].

Coumarins

Furanocoumarins are made by joining a furan ring to a coumarin at the 6 and 7 position, or the 7 and 8 position, respectively. These glycosides are benzo--pyrone derivatives. These glycosides have immunomodulatory properties as well.

For example, Auraptene from *Citrus natsudaidai*, *Achillea millefolium*, *Heracleum persicum, Artemisia capillaries*, *Citrus limonia*, and *Euphorbia lathyris,* all contain escultin (6,7-dihydroxycoumarin), a coumarin derivative.

It exhibits pleiotropic biological activities, including lipoxygenase inhibition, free radical scavenging activity, suppressive effect on oxidative DNA damage, tyrosinase inhibition, cancer chemopreventive activity, and anticancer activity. The root of *Angelica dahurica* contains cytotoxic coumarins [9, 10].

Anthocyanins

The bioflavonoid phytochemicals anthocyanins are the most well-known and conspicuous of bioflavonoid phytochemicals. Anthocyanin may protect against DNA cleavage, estrogenic activity (altering the advancement of hormone-dependent disease symptoms), enzyme inhibition, cytokine production (thereby trying to regulate immune function), anti-inflammatory activity, lipid peroxidation, capillary permeability and fragility, and membrane strengthening [11, 12].

Saponins

Saponins are found in the roots, tubers, leaves, flowers, and seeds of plants. Based on their carbon skeletons, saponins were divided into triterpenes and steroids. Their glycone components were largely oligosaccharides, which were organized as linear or branched structures and linked to hydroxyl groups by acetal linkage.

Saponins have an anticancer effect on a variety of cancer cells researched by modern researchers. With IC50 values as low as 0.2 mM, some saponins suppress tumor cell proliferation by cell cycle arrest, including death. Saponins can improve the therapeutic success rate when used in conjunction with traditional tumour therapy procedures [13, 14].

Alkaloids

Alkaloids are among the most potent and significant medicinal chemicals found in plants, with over 5,500 alkaloids that are well-known in medicines for their pharmacological activities. Nitrogen atoms are frequently utilised in conjunction as a component of a cyclic structure. Nicotine, cocaine, morphine and codeine, quinine, and reserpine are just a few examples. Alkaloids have anti-tumor (vinblastine and vincristine), antibacterial (cepharanthine), analgesic (morphine) and immunostimulatory effects, and a wide range of alkaloids are being studied for their immunostimulatory qualities [15, 16].

Volatile Oils and Terpenoids

Isoprenoids are natural materials with a structure that may be separated into isoprene units, such as volatile oils and terpenoids. Triterpenoids have a carbon skeleton made up of six isoprene units, a cyclic C30 hydrocarbon. They are colourless, crystalline, and optically active compounds with high melting points.

Saponins, steroids, and cardiac glycosides, which are mostly glycosides, are essential triterpenoids. Triterpenes are found in the waxy coverings of leaflets and on fruit, such as apples and pears, and they may act as a repellent against insects or microbial attacks. Several terpenoids have antiarthritic or antiphlogistic properties, and their biological actions appear to be mediated *via* immunological mechanisms.Various terpene-containing plant components include eugenol from *Ocimum sanctum*, diterpenes from *Andrographis paniculata*, *Achillea millefolium*, *Alternanthera tenella*, triterpenes from *Ganoderma lucidum*, lupeol, and amyrine from *Bauhinia variegate*, show immunomodulatory activity [17].

Table 1. Different classes of phytoconstituents in medicinal plants.

Class	Plants	Mechanism of Action
Glycosides Isorhamnetin-3- O-glucoside Mangiferin	*Salicornia herbacea* Leaves of mango	Immuno-modulatory potential [18]. Enhances the production of immunoglobulins IgG1 and IgG2 [19]
Flavonoids Centaurein Orientin	*Bidenspilosa* *Vitex grandifolia*	Increasing activity of Interferon [21]. The immune system's humoral and cell-mediated responses are triggered.
Tannins Chebulagic acid Coraline	*Terminalia chebula*	Reduction in level of TNF-α, IL-6 [20]. Neuroprotection.
Anthocyanins Cyanidin-3-glycoside Peonidin	Blackberry Roses	Antioxidant and anti-inflammatory mechanism [21, 22].

(Table 1) cont.....

Class	Plants	Mechanism of Action
Saponins Asiaticoside Glycyrrhizin	*Centellaasiatica* Roots of *Glycyrrhiza glabra* L.	Enhances phagocytic index and total WBC count [23]. Inhibits classical complement pathway [24].
Alkaloids Piperine Berberine	Roots of *Piper nigrum* L. European barberry	Total WBC count, bone marrow cellularity, and total antibody production are all enhanced [25]. Plasma TNF, IFN, and NO levels were significantly reduced [26].
Volatile oils and terpenoids Andrographolide Eugenol	*A. paniculata* Nees Clove buds, cinnamon bark	Increases IL-2 expression and inhibits NO production in endotoxin-stimulated macrophages [7, 27]. LPS activity is inhibited, which has an effect. Eugenol's regulation of the nuclear factor-B pathway was most likely one of the mechanisms of action [28].

Mangiferin Isorhamnetin-3-O-glucoside.

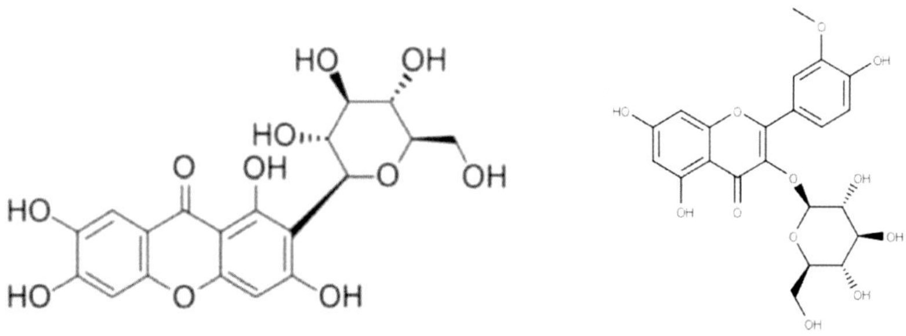

Fig. (2a). Glycosides derived from plants (Mangiferin and Isorhamnetin-3-O-glucoside).

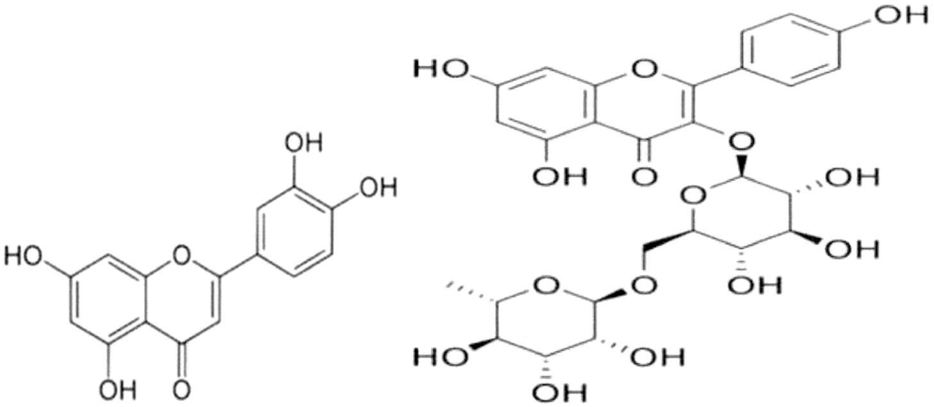

Fig. (2b). Flavonoids derived from plants (Luteolin and Kaempherol-3-O-rutinoside).

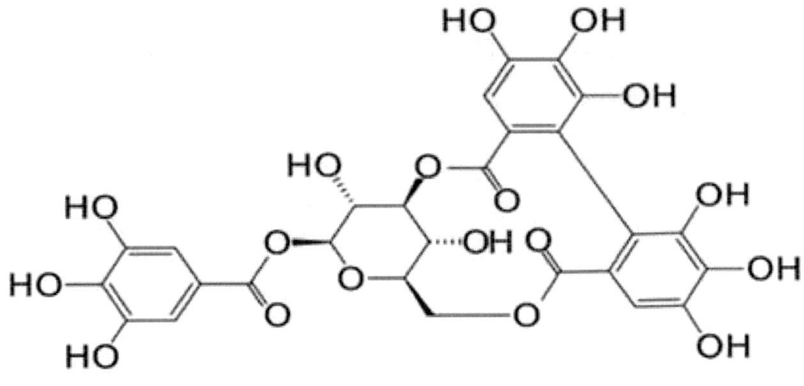

Fig. (2c). Tannins derived from plants (Corilagin).

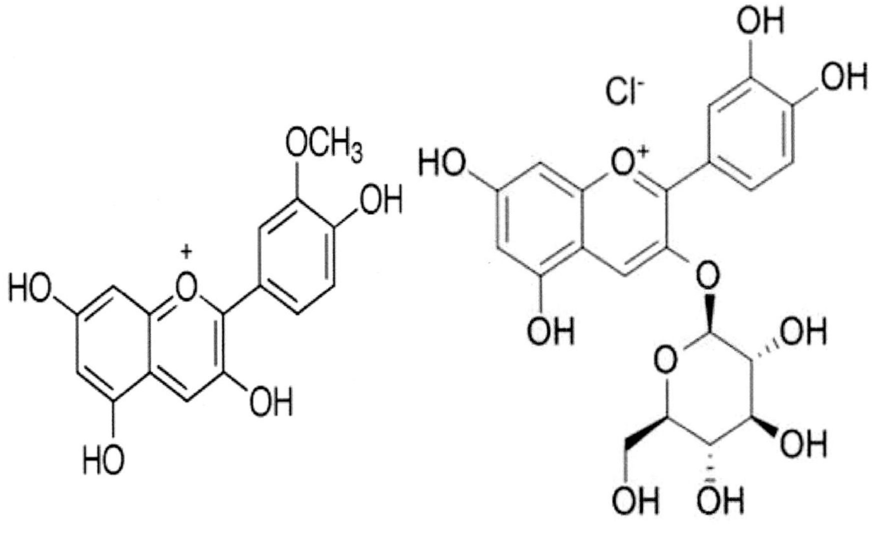

Fig. (2d). Anthocyanins derived from plants (Peonidin and Cyanidin-3-glycoside).

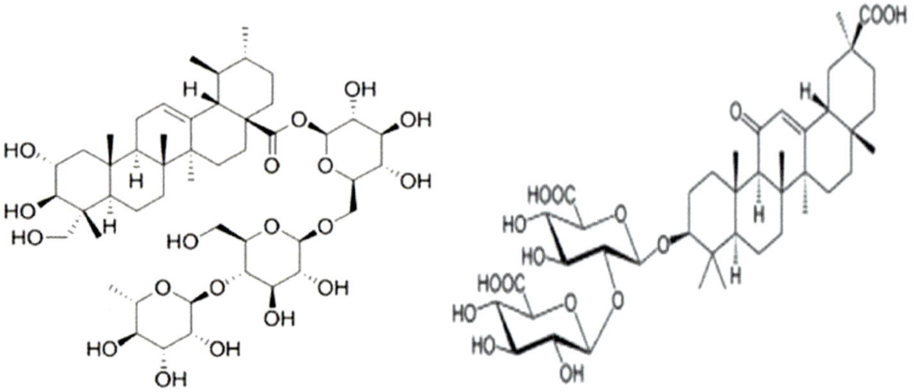

Fig. (2e). Saponins derived from plants (Asiaticoside and Glycyrrhizin).

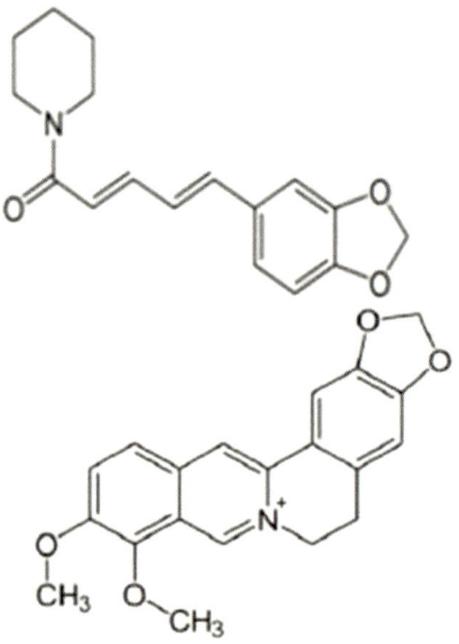

PiperineBerberine

Fig. (2f). Alkloids derived from plants (Piperine and Berberine).

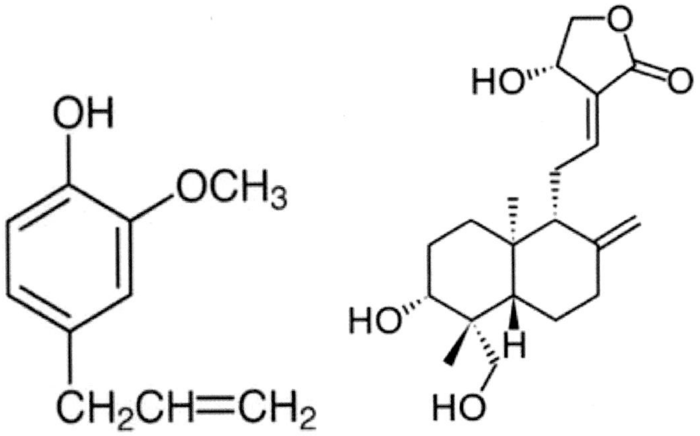

Fig. (2g). Volatile oils and terpenoids (Eugenol and Andrographolide).

MARINE-DERIVED IMMUNOMODULATORS

Marine immunomodulators are produced mostly from bacteria, cyanobacteria, sponges, algae, fungi, and marine creatures found in the ocean. The oceans offer a great source of structurally and chemically new bioactive chemicals with unique biological capabilities Table **2**.

Natural products play an important role in medicine, and in particular marine metabolites have a role in recent drug discovery. It totally depends on the structurally unique molecules produced by marine organisms, which contain a significant number of stereogenic centres and halogen atoms, the latter introduced by metabolic processes of the inorganic species present in seawaters.

New trends in drug development from natural sources involve research into the marine ecosystem to uncover chemical entities that can be used to treat a variety of ailments, including cancer, AIDS, and inflammatory conditions. A wide range of viral, bacterial, and fungal illnesses are also present. Marine compounds have new structures with strong biological and pharmacological activity Fig. **(3).**

Natural items from the sea have a lot of potentials. The first marine-derived medications were produced in the 1950s, and two of them are still being used today. About 15,000 natural goods have been described, with sponges accounting for around 30% of all these natural items. Ara-C is an anticancer medicine that is used to treat non-lymphoma Hodgkin's and acute myelocytic leukaemia, while Ara-A is an antiviral drug that is used to treat herpes [29].

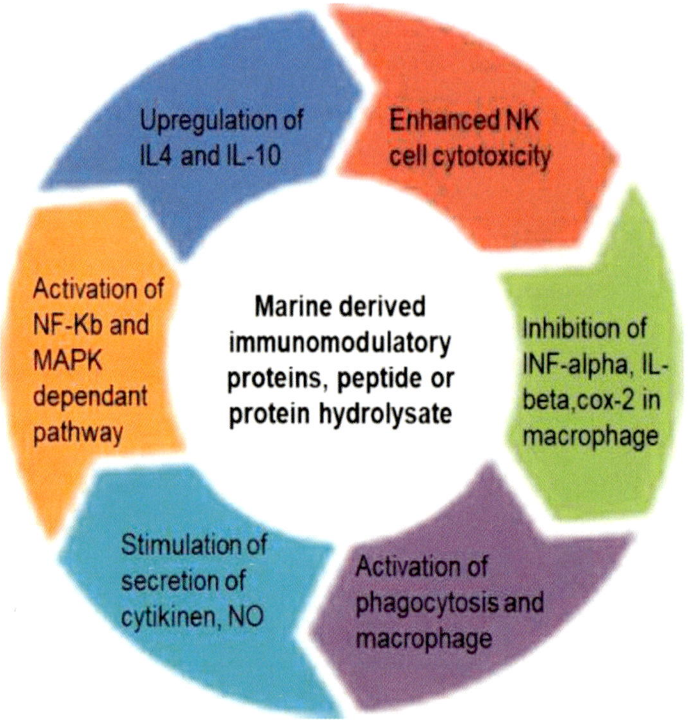

Fig. (3). Mechanism of action of marine derived immunomodulators.

Immunomodulatory Compounds from Marine Origin

There are three main types of immunomodulatory compounds which are derived from marine, namely (i) Proteins and amino acids, (ii) Antimicrobials and immunomodulatory peptides, (iii) Immunomodulatory protein hydrolysates Table **2**.

Table 2. Bioactive compounds derived from Marine Sources.

Name of Compound	Source	Mechanism of Action	Reference
Immunomodulatory Proteins and Amino Acid Hemocyanin	*Concholepas concholepas*, *Megathura crenulata*, and *Fissurellalati marginata* are mollusks.	Immunostimulatory chara cteristics without side effects against various cancers; interact with T cells, monocytes, macro phages, and polymorphonuclear lymphocytes to increase the immunological response of the host	[30 - 33]

(Table 2) cont.....

Name of Compound	Source	Mechanism of Action	Reference
Antimicrobial and Immunomodulatory Peptides Callinectin	Blue crab: *Callinectes sapidus*, Mediterranean mussel: *Mytilus galloprovincialis*	Antibacterial activity against gram-negative bacteria and antibodies binding to anti-callinectin-like peptides antibodies in blue crab hemocytes	[34, 35]
Immunomodulatory Protein Hydrolysates *Paphiaundulata* meat protein hydrolysate	Paphiaundulata PHTC, VGYT, EF, LF, and EGAL, WI, or WL mollusc.	*Ex vivo* increased the ability of mice spleen lymphocytes to proliferate	[36]

MICROBIOTA MODIFIERS

Microbiota is an important factor for nutrition, immunity, and its effects on the brain and behaviour. Modulation of the gut microbiota is a unique method for preventing and treating colorectal cancer (CRC). Microbiota modifiers include probiotics, prebiotics, postbiotics, and antibiotics, among other things.

There is a significant positive relationship between GIT mucosa microbiota and immunity. Prebiotics and probiotics directly or indirectly affect immune health. Elements that are normally present in food give the health-beneficial features of functional foods. Ingredients are categorized into three parts: Probiotics (microorganisms), prebiotics (compounds such as fiber), and antioxidants have become more popular in food markets, due to their immunomodulating properties.

Prebiotics

Prebiotics are fermenting nutrients that allow for differences in the composition and activities of the gastrointestinal microflora, resulting in health advantages for the host. Among the prebiotics, fructans are the best ones, which are fructose-derived oligo-polysaccharides of 15% flowering plants. They are water-soluble.

Fructans (Fructo-oligosaccharide or FOS)

Wheat, rye, oat, barley, leek, Belgian endives, lettuce, and salsify, all contain fructans. Regular consumption of fructans (such as inulin) promotes overall health and well-being by (i) improving blood parameters, (ii) increasing resistance to intestinal and extraintestinal infections, (iii) modifying immunological responses, and (iv) reducing allergies.

The colonic environment is altered by the fermentation of fructans (such as inulin and FOS). Lower pH and FOS result in the proliferation of beneficial bacteria like *bifidobacteria* and *lactobacilli*. Moreover, inulin and FOS consumption boost mineral absorption in the gut.

Our human digestive system is unable to hydrolyze the β-linkages of FOS. The hydrolytic enzymes of colon microflora catalyze the reaction; thus, microflora-assisted FOS metabolism helps to build the immune health of the colon.

Inulin-type fructans with a lower degree of polymerization enhanced the ratio of interleukin 10 to interleukin 12 (IL-10/IL-12) in HPBM cells and also induced a more anti-inflammatory balance. TLR2, and to a lesser extent TLR4, 5, 7, and 8, regulate the activities of human peripheral blood mononuclear (HPBM) cells through different DP classes of inulin-type fructans.

In monocyte, it shows proinflammatory cytokine production; in eukaryotic, it maintains homeostasis.Fructans also have antiviral activity. Fructans stimulate IL-1β, IL-6, IL-10, IFN-γ and TNF-α factors [37].

β-Glucan

Beta-glucan is normally obtained from several plants and foods. The main sources are oats, mushrooms, yeast, algae, and barley.They show GI and metabolic effects and alter the lipid and glucose metabolism, regulating the diet. They also have immune-modulating properties, which have led to research into using them as adjuvants for cancer, and immune-mediated illnesses to improve wound healing [40]. The action of β-glucan can be separated into two categories: a. metabolic/GI effects, and b. immune-modulatory effects. Functional impacts will be determined by molecular and structural properties. β-glucans operate in a variety of ways and have a well-defined structure-activity link.

Role of β-glucan Structure

For biological activity, 1,3 backbone of beta-glucan is necessary. The degree of biological activity depends on its structure. The frequency and length of side chains are essential, with a larger extent of branching linked to greater biological activity. Most biologically active beta-glucans have branching frequencies between 0.20 and 0.33. The length and frequency of side-chains are important factors in immunomodulatory action. The total size of the beta-glucans molecule also impacts the activity, with greater molecular weight fractions having a significant effect.

Probiotic

In 1974, Parker coined the term probiotics to describe organisms and substances that aid in the balance of intestinal microbes. They affect the host animal by improving the microbial balance in the intestine. Probiotics are live cultures of bacteria and fungi that benefit health when introduced through the feed. Probiotics are 'live microorganisms that, when administered in adequate amounts, impart a health benefit' as per the current FAO/WHO definition. A few currently reside in individuals' digestive tracts, while others come from some external origin. They are also known as direct-fed microbial (DFM).

Probiotics can also be used to promote growth as well as for therapeutic purposes. In the digestive tract, a diverse population of microorganisms exists, which is influenced by many factors such as diet,age, stress, environment, and medication. *Lactobacilli*, *streptococci*, and *bifidobacteria* are the most widely used organisms in probiotic preparations. Probiotics include *Bacillus spp*., *Saccharomyces spp*., yeasts, and filamentous fungi (*Aspergillus oryzae*). Tablets, capsules, pastes, powders, or sprays are the different preparations available for probiotics.

Probiotic Augmentation Method in the Immune System

Probiotic micro-organisms in the gastrointestinal tract induce host immune responses in two different ways. They can translocate as viable cells through the intestinal walls, expanding to a small extent, or antigens produced by the dead organisms are absorbed and directly stimulate the immune response. Probiotics are commonly used in aquafeed because they improve growth rate, feed consumption, and resistance to disease. Probiotics boost the host immune response besides increasing macrophage action, as evidenced by increased phagocytosis of organisms or carbon particles, elevation in production of systemic antibodies including IgM and interferon, and improved effects of local antibodies on mucosal membranes like the intestinal walls. Probiotics have immune-boosting properties.

The digestive system is one of the most microbiologically efficient ecosystems, so it is important to function as a mucosal immune system (MIS). In this ecosystem, the ingested probiotics trigger an immune response as well as elicit connectivity of transmitters facilitated by the whole bacteria as well as their cell wall structure. The immune mechanisms of probiotics and also their advantageous effects on the host are mentioned.

Mechanism of Action of Probiotics

Probiotic bacteria found inside the intestinal mucosa have immunomodulatory effects Fig. (**4**). Particular receptors on probiotic bacteria enable them to connect to and stimulate IECs. IECs release cytokines and chemokines, creating a micro-environment in the gut basal lamina, tracheae, and mammary glands, allowing B cells to clonally broaden and produce IgA.

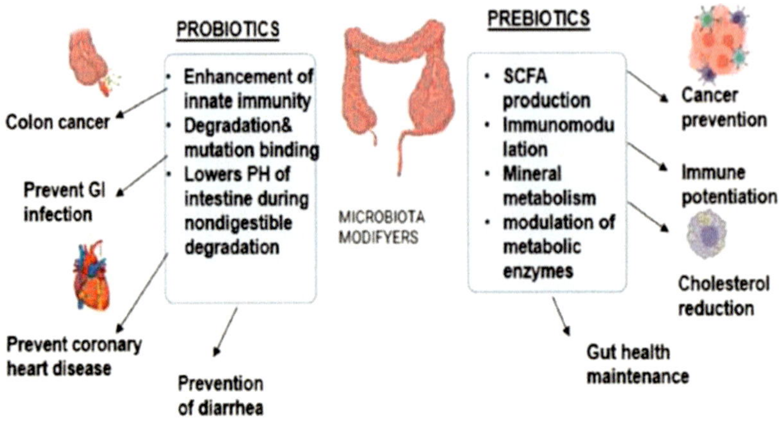

Fig. (4). Mechanism of action and applications of pre and probiotics.

Concurrently, probiotic bacteria-stimulated cytokines induce the production of Treg cells (Foxp3+), which also maintain immune homeostasis inside the gut mucosa. After being stimulated by probiotic bacteria, PPs macrophages discharge cytokines. They do, though, exhibit a characteristic hyporesponsive to commensal microbes. Furthermore, as a result of probiotic stimulation, macrophages in places other than the GT, such as the peritoneum and spleen, increase their features (cytokines production, microbic activity, and phagocytic), bolstering the innate immune response. Probiotic bacteria administration induces a Th1 response with elevated amounts of IL-10 and IFN, both of which are important in immunomodulation. PP (Peyer patch), and Treg (T regulator).

IECs are affected by probiotics. Because of one's prominent position inside the GT, such cells act as active sensors, establishing a dialogue between the host and the environment. Internalization of probiotic bacterial fragments in to the IECs stimulates immune cells associated with the gut.This finding leads to the conclusion that the immune system, *via* TLRs, activates the cell wall of probiotic bacteria.

Paneth cells are other vital cells that have greater importance in the epithelial barrier. Probiotic bacteria significantly impact such cells, raising their amount in the intestinal crypts and thus strengthening the epithelial barrier. The existence of probiotic bacteria in the intestinal lumen (72 hours) is sufficient to produce changes in gut immune cells, raising the number of macrophages and DCs inside the lamina propria and improving their functionality, as demonstrated by cytokine production.

Interestingly, stimulation of immune cells has no effect on intestinal homeostasis, which is likely due to the activation of regulatory cells, which maintain an innate and adaptive immunity environment. These facts highlight the importance of ensuring that probiotics can be ingested for long periods without harming people. The cytokine micro-environment formed by immune cells to respond to probiotics encourages the growth of IgA+ cells inside the intestines. Moreover, cytokines affect the activity of immune cells that are not located inside the intestines, including such macrophages from the spleen and peritoneum, and other mucosa sites including such lung tissue and mammary glands.

Probiotic administration in malnutrition processes helps in restoring thymus histopathology and stimulates the adaptative immune response [38].

The administration of probiotics orally stimulates immune mechanisms that regulate allergic response at the pulmonary level. Oral ingestion of probiotics stimulates DCs (dendritic cells) in the intestines, leading to the release of IL-12, which also helps balance the bronchial adaptative response to the Th1 profile. Increased CD4 and IFN expression on Th1 cells result in an increase in IgG production instead of IgE production. Treg cells did not go up, suggesting that the probiotic's regulation impact has been mediated by IL-10, which Th1 and Th2 cells start producing. Mast cells are also stimulated in order to facilitate tissue regeneration. Concurrently, the Th2 response was significantly reduced, as was the manufacturing of IL-4, IL-13, and IgE. DC (dendritic cell) and Treg (T regulatory cell) Fig. **(5).**

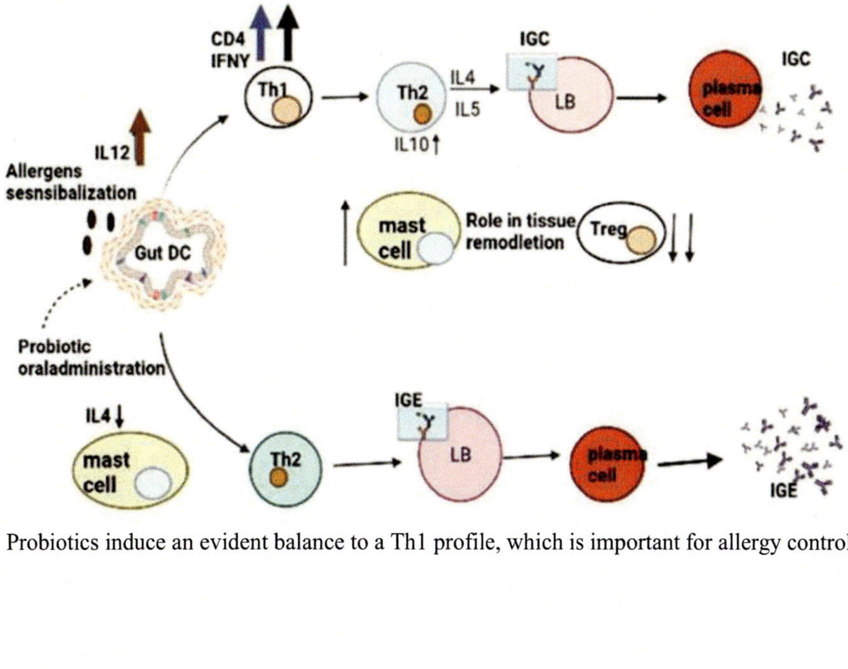

Fig. (5). Probiotics induce an evident balance to a Th1 profile, which is important for allergy control.

Probiotic bacteria and their cellular membranes enhance transmissions in the intestinal wall, which improves the system's immune actions and host wellness. Probiotics mainly target IECs, which would, in combination with innate immune cells connected to the intestinal wall, reduce oral mucosa and systemic immunity. Probiotic bacteria have proven to be an efficient method of preserving intestinal homeostasis and encouraging the mucosal immune system in both the gut and elsewhere. Probiotic bacteria are gaining popularity as a natural, risk-free allergy prevention and treatment strategy [39].

VACCINES

Nowadays, vaccination is the most important medical treatment for the prevention of infectious diseases. Microorganism elimination in the community is a challenging goal to achieve, but effective protection against serious disease is generally possible. Age, immunological status, dietary health, genetic polymorphisms, and environmental exposures are all factors that affect vaccine responses. The various types of vaccines are used for boosting the immune response towards infectious diseases Fig. **(6).**

Passive immunisation is the process of giving antibodies to inexperienced receivers in order to impart temporary humoral immunity. Active immunisation is the process of directly vaccinating people to develop adaptive immune responses defined by memory. The main approach for the development of an effective vaccine is to understand the etiology or pathogenesis of the disease and then correlate the disease [40].

Jennerian Vaccines

Jenner developed the method, which involves infecting humans with an animal microbe to trigger cross-protective immunological responses. The smallpox vaccine was similarly multiply passaged and developed using this approach [40, 41]. By using a modified Jennerian approach, combining genes (from animal and human viruses), a chimeric virus is created that contains human antigens and animal genes that affect the viral replication, resulting in attenuation. Because these organisms frequently multiply to some degree in their hosts, they can often elicit both T- and B-cell responses, making them highly immunogenic.

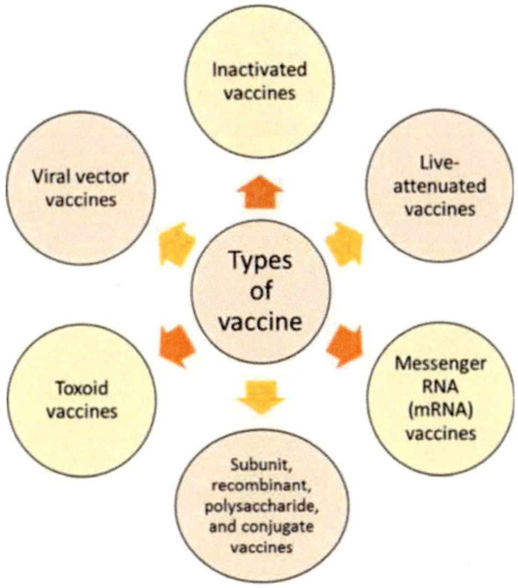

Fig. (6). Vaccine strategies.

Live-attenuated Vaccines

In the vaccine, the live or attenuated form of the organism is used that causes a disease. It produces a strong immune response for a long duration of time. Example, smallpox, and yellow fever.

Inactivated Vaccines

Inactivated vaccinations use a dead form of the disease-causing organism. They are inactivated by using beta propiolactone, formalin, UV irradiation, and other techniques, *e.g.* Salk polio vaccine.

If a virulent strain is utilised to make the virus stock, insufficient inactivation can result in iatrogenic illness, as happened in the so-called Cutter case. A handful of infants suffered paralytic poliomyelitis after being inoculated with just an inactivated poliovirus vaccine that contained insufficiently inactivated Mahoney poliovirus [40].

Toxoids

Bacterial toxins, mainly endotoxins, produce disease, and it is addressed by the formation of toxoids. The toxin's pathogenicity is decreased or eliminated in some way, yet the immunogenicity of the resultant protein is preserved. Examples of this method are tetanus toxoid and diphtheria toxoid.

Subunit, Recombinant, Polysaccharide, and Conjugate Vaccines

In these vaccines, a specific portion of an organism, such as protein, sugar, or capsid, is used. Antibodies to type-specific capsular polysaccharide antibodies provide immunity to most of these species. As a result, immunisation with pure polysaccharides from the organism is immunogenic and safe in older people. *H.influenza* type B (Hib), a previously major cause of sepsis and meningitis in children, was the target of the first conjugate vaccines. In young children, the polysaccharide Hib vaccine was ineffective, but the conjugate vaccination has effectively eliminated the disease in the United States.

Combination of Vaccine

In recent years, vaccines have been combined to minimize injections, visits, and administration expenses. Diphtheria and pertussis toxoids are commonly given in combination with pertussis antigens, but Hib conjugate vaccination and trivalent inactivated poliovirus can also be given.

Messenger RNA (mRNA) Vaccines

For decades, scientists have been researching and conducting experiments with mRNA vaccines, and many of the COVID-19 vaccines have been established using this new technology. The messenger RNA vaccines generate proteins that stimulate an immune response. The advantages of these vaccines are that they require a short time for development, and no risk of sickness in the individual getting vaccinated because they do not contain a live virus.

IMMUNOADJUVANTS

Adjuvants are substances used to boost antibody formation or to control the adaptive response Table **3.** Immunoadjuvants improve vaccine performance, allowing for a lower antigen dose to be necessary. Adjuvants can improve vaccine action, and adjuvant research is currently receiving a lot of attention as a way to significantly improve the performance of vaccines energy against a variety of diseases.

The type of adjuvant used will be determined by the characteristics of the required CD4+T cell response. Organic adjuvants, such as those based on proteins, polysaccharides, and lipopeptides, peptides, lipids enable more tailored immune responses and are an important topic in the development of novel vaccines [41].

The immunologic substance combines with a specific vaccine antigen, increasing the magnitude, induction, or durability of antigen-specific immune responses. In the absence of vaccine antigen, the adjuvants are not antigenic. In the past, only aluminium salt or alum are used as an adjuvant by a human. Vaccine adjuvants with antigens boost the immune response.

Table 3. Classification of adjuvants based on their effector mechanisms.

Types of Adjuvants	Examples	Mechanism of Action
Type A	CpG ODN, Monophosphoryl lipid A	Agonists of the Pattern Recognition Receptor (PRR).
Type B	Toxin-derived adjuvants, nanoparticles Alum hydroxide, MF59, Freund's adjuvant.	The depot effect occurs when APCs and antigens interact in an unspecific manner.
Type C	CD28 superagonist antibody TGN1412	Interact with APC co-stimulatory molecules.

The various plants and proteins are used for the formation of an adjuvant, such as saponins, heat shock proteins, polysaccharides and lectins *etc.* Table **4.**

Table 4. Adjuvants derived from plant sources and proteins.

Class and Plant Name	Adjuvant	Immune Response	Mechanism of Action
Saponins and Saponin-Derived Compounds *Quillaja saponaria* *Quillaja brasiliensis* *Panax ginseng*	Quil A, QS-21 QB-90 Rg1 and Rb1	Humoral and cellular responses to co-administered antigens, with Th1 and cytotoxic T lymphocytes (CTLs) responses.	Binds to and activates particular Receptors on APCs.
Polysaccharides	Soy-lecithin adjuvant, Providean-AVECR, AdvaxTM	Proliferation of T cells (CD8+ and CD4+) Cytokine response Th1/Th2 cytokine response	Binding of specific carbohydrate receptors present on Antigen-presenting cells (APCs)
Lectins *e.g.*(*Canavalia ensiformis*) jack bean (*Artocarpus integrifolia*) Jackfruit *Viscum album* *Lycopersicum esculentum* *Ulex europaeus*	Canavalin A (ConA) ArtinM and Jacalin Mistletoe lectin 1; ML-1 Tomato lectin; LEA UEA-1	Induce Th1 immunity IFN- γ production stimulates Th2 immunity Th1, IL-12 Anti-bystander effect (serum IgG and IgA)	Glycosylated TLR receptors on macrophages and DCs interactions
Heat Shock Proteins	Hsp110, Hsp90, Hsp70, Hsp60, Hsp40, and small Hsps	CD8+ T cells, Th1 response	It binds to antigenic peptides and presents them to APC

Lipopeptides are lipidated peptides formed by combining peptides with lipids. Peptides and lipopeptides are useful in developing the vaccine as antigens and as adjuvants. Antigenic protein sequences can be utilised to create peptide and lipopeptide antigens, which can be employed to excite surface receptors in a very particular fashion [40 - 42].

MICRONUTRIENTS

It is well known that the immune system depends on the host's nutritional status. Some vitamins (like Retinol, Pyridoxine, Folate, Cobalamine, Ascorbic acid, Calcitriol and Tocopherol), trace minerals (such as zinc, iron, selenium, copper), and omega-3 long-chain polyunsaturated fatty acids (such as N3 PUFA) have been shown to help the immune systems (innate as well as adaptive).

Micronutrient deficit or inadequate circumstances might harm immune function and infection resistance Fig. **(7).** Certain trace elements and metals are essential cofactors for critical enzymes and antioxidant compounds, and they play a role in humoral and cell-mediated immune responses [43]. It is well known that good nutrition supports immune function and reduces the severity of illness. Some vitamins and trace elements play essential roles in maintaining immune system cells, increasing disease resistance. Other nutrients support optimal immune system performance, like omega-3 fatty acids. Micronutrients such as vitamins A, B, C, D, and E and trace minerals (zinc, selenium, copper, magnesium) boost the immune system. Therefore, deficiency can increase the host's sensitivity to infectious diseases.

Vitamin A

Retinol (Vitamin A1) is a fat-soluble vitamin found primarily in guts, milk, cheese, green vegetables, and yellow fruits. All trans-retinoic acids regulate the expression of multiple genes by binding to specific nuclear transcription factors and help support the integrity of the gastrointestinal epithelium [3].

Vitamin A affects inflammation and congenital reactions in our body. It regulates the number and function of natural killer cells, macrophages, and neutrophils. It plays an essential role in promoting Foxp3 + Treg production, phagocytic and oxidative burst activity, antibody production, and early differentiation of natural killer cells. Vitamin A deficiency adversely affects the secretion of inflammatory cytokines such as IL-12 and IL-23 and the function of B cells [44, 45].

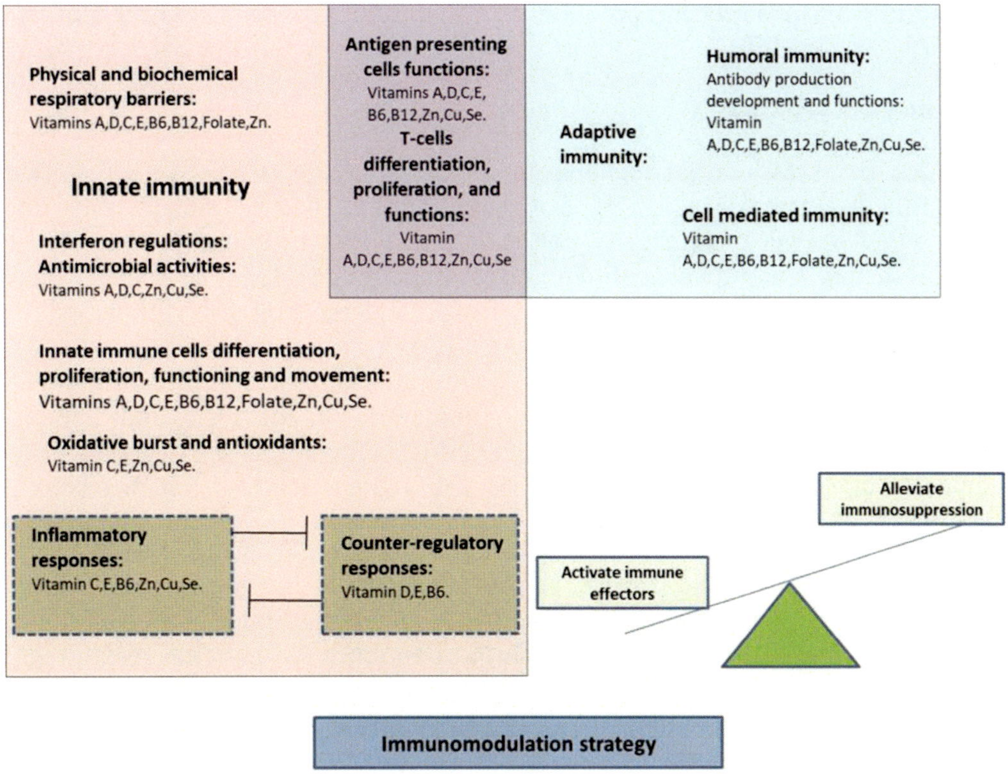

Fig. (7). Role of micronutrients in immune modulation.

Adequate levels of folic acid and vitamin A are required to produce the optimal antibody response to the antigen. For example, B cells are stimulated by retinoic acid (a vitamin A metabolite) produced by gut-associated lymphoid tissue. Dendritic cells (DC) have high intestinal homing receptors. It is a substance that could help with gut immunity and tolerance. IgA antibody responses to bacterial antigens are mediated by B cells, and the process requires vitamin A.Vitamin A is required for Th1 and Th2 cell growth and differentiation because it promotes the anti-inflammatory response of Th2 by reducing the synthesis of IL-12, TNF, and IFN by Th1 lymphocytes [45].

Vitamin A also supports adaptive and cell-mediated immunity and is an essential cofactor for T cell activation. Pediatric studies with vitamin A have shown potential effects on the growth of the CD4 subpopulation of T cells [44].Vitamin A supplements (50,000-200,000 IU per 4-6 months) have been shown to decrease the incidence of measles and diarrhea. However, other studies in children found no evidence that vitamin A minimised the risk of lower respiratory tract infections or pneumonia. Vitamin A supplements should be taken within the suggested safety limits, especially in potentially vulnerable groups like pregnant and childbirth women [45].

Vitamin C

Tomatoes, potatoes, citrus fruits and green leafy vegetables are all good sources of vitamin C (ascorbic acid). It is a water-soluble vitamin and an important nutrient that affects the integrity of the immune system barrier and leukocyte function. Vitamin C impacts cellular and immune processes in the hematopoietic system because it increases non-heme iron, converts iron from transferrin to ferritin, and synthesizes tetrahydrofolic acid [44]. In response to chemotherapy drugs, vitamin C helps phagocytic cells (neutrophils and macrophages) migrate to sites of infection. When neutrophils commence phagocytosis and generate reactive oxygen species (ROS) to remove antigens during the early stages of the immune response, vitamin C shields them from oxidative stress, which acts as an antioxidant [46].

Vitamin C treatment has been shown to reduce the production of the proinflammatory cytokines TNF, IL-6, and IL-1. According to *in vitro* studies, ascorbic acid is a potent immuno-stimulator of antibody formation (IgM and IgG) in humans, and intracellular levels of ascorbic acid are an essential parameter in determining the immune response of peripheral blood cells. Vitamin C has been shown to promote T-cell maturation in other *in vitro* experiments. New research suggests that ascorbic acid may play a role in regulating T-cell development through epigenetic mechanisms such as ten-eleven translocation (TET) and histone demethylation [44]. Vitamin C has been shown to support Treg cell function by allowing constant Foxp3 expression. Vitamin C supplementation may play some role in other recently revealed neutrophil functions, such as developing the neutrophil extracellular trap (NET), which forms when the harmful intracellular compounds are released after neutrophil necrosis. Ascorbic acid may decrease NET production by minimizing tissue damage. Vitamin C also plays a role in IFN-γ production, apoptosis, and removal of macrophage-depleted neutrophils from sites of infection and regeneration of antioxidants such as vitamin E and glutathione about their operating status. Vitamin C supplementation has been shown to reduce the incidence of pneumonia in children and adults, especially when food intake is low (poor to intermediate quality studies). Finally, there is some evidence that taking 100 mg of vitamin C per day during pregnancy may decrease the prevalence of urinary tract infections.

In adults and children with colds, ascorbic acid supplementation (0.2 g/day or therapeutic dose 4-8 g/day) can considerably lessen the length and intensity of the illness and reduce cold symptoms such as chest pain, fever, and chills, based on most of the high-quality evidence. Although there are no therapeutic trials of vitamin C in treating the common cold in children, there have been no consistent advantages in treatment-specific studies in adults. Vitamin C can significantly reduce disease severity and mortality risk in older adults with pneumonia, particularly if low baseline plasma concentrations (poor-to-intermediate quality evidences). Vitamin C supplements can also shorten the duration of pneumonia [45]. Vitamin C may help prevent and treat severe viral respiratory illness caused by SARSCoV2 during the COVID-19 outbreak.

Vitamin D

Nutritional sources, ultraviolet B (UVB)-dependent endogenous synthesis, and supplementation are all possible sources of vitamin D. Vitamin D is primarily generated in human skin after UVB exposure, with only a tiny amount acquired from food sources. Few natural, non-fortified foods, such as fatty fish (sardines, salmon, mackerel, cod liver oil) and some types of mushrooms (Shiitake), especially if sundried, contain significant levels of one of the two principle forms of vitamin D, cholecalciferol (vitamin D3) or ergocalciferol (vitamin D2) [47].

Calcitriol (vitamin D's active form) increases the production of antimicrobial peptides in epithelial cells, such as those lining the respiratory system, which protects them from infection. Vitamin D reduces T helper and cytotoxic T cell effector functions, but stimulates the formation of Tregs, which reduce immune-mediated inflammation [45].

The vitamin D receptors (VDRs) are found on the surface of most immune cells, such as monocytes, macrophages, DCs, T- and B-lymphocytes, and these cells also express the enzyme 25-(OH)-D-1-hydroxylase (CYP27B1), which allows 25-(OH)-vitamin D (25-(OH)-D) to be converted to its active form. 1,25-dihydrox--vitamin D (1,25-(OH)2-D) is a type of vitamin D. Vitamin D deficiency has been linked to various inflammatory and autoimmune disorders, including diabetes mellitus type 1, inflammatory bowel disease, Hashimoto thyroiditis, and multiple sclerosis, among others [47]. By upregulating MAPK phosphatase-1 and suppressing p38 activation, vitamin D lowers the production of proinflammatory cytokines and promotes the production of anti-inflammatory cytokines by macrophages [45].

Vitamin D inhibits cell proliferation, induces cell differentiation and death, and reduces proinflammatory cytokine production in typical human cell types (average human bronchial epithelial cells, monocyte-derived macrophages), according to *in vitro* research. Vitamin D also boosts the production of antiviral proteins [48].Vitamin D has also been shown to suppress T cell cytokines such as IL-2 and IL-17, as well as monocyte toll-like receptors [49].

Vitamin D increases monocyte-to-macrophage differentiation and enhances phagocytosis, superoxide generation and bacterial killing. Vitamin D also can influence adaptive immunity by inhibiting T helper type 1 (Th1) cell function and lowering the expression of proinflammatory cytokines such as IL-2 and interferon-gamma (INF- γ) [50, 51]. Calcitriol has been shown to directly affect B cell homeostasis, including suppression of memory and plasma cell formation and stimulation of immunoglobulin-producing B cell death [49].

Vitamin D supplements have been shown to reduce the occurrence and severity of viral illness, and there is an inverse connection between blood 25-hydroxyvitamin D levels and upper respiratory tract infection. COVID-19 patients have been observed to have decreased vitamin D levels, with mean plasma concentrations half that of controls, albeit the research group was unclearly selected, and the results were uncorrected for significant confounders, making their conclusions imprecise. As a result, vitamin D administration may be beneficial in boosting COVID-19 immunity and lowering human mortality [50]. Vitamin D insufficiency is a persistent factor in several illnesses, including influenza, respiratory syncytial virus (RSV), and TB [52].

In vitro studies have revealed that vitamin D boosts airway epithelial cells' antiviral and anti-inflammatory responses during respiratory viral infections. Strong evidence links vitamin D deficiency to an increased risk of pulmonary exacerbations in chronic airway illnesses like asthma. Clinical studies of vitamin D supplementation in preventing or treating RTIs, on the other hand, have had mixed outcomes [48]. Vitamin D (300–3653 IU per day) in children and adults can lower the incidence of RTI, according to 5 meta-analyses of generally high-quality research.

So there are reports showing inconsistency in the outcome of vitamin D supplementation advantages in children and adults with TB, upper RTI or influenza. Supplementing children with vitamin D as an adjuvant to antibiotics had ambiguous results; there was a significant decrease in the length of hospitalization, but only minor improvements in the resolution of acute infection and death rate, and no favorable effects on fever [45].

Several research looked at the relationship between maternal vitamin D status during pregnancy and/or cord blood vitamin D levels and baby respiratory illness. Vitamin D levels were consistently linked to a lower incidence of lower respiratory tract infection (LRTI) in newborns worldwide. Vitamin D is particularly well known for its ability to suppress the "cytokine storm" that plays a role in the development of viral illness, including COVID-19 [44].

Vitamin B

Folate (Vitamin B9) is important for nucleic acid and protein synthesis since it provides one-carbon units in conjunction with vitamins B6 and B12, resulting in a shortfall. Folate deficiency can impair the immune system by preventing CD8+ T-lymphocyte cells from proliferating in response to mitogen stimulation [53]. A vitamin B1 (thiamin) shortage in the diet might impact host immunological responses by regulating immune cell development and proliferation, affecting the gut microbiota.

When a short-term dietary vitamin B2 (riboflavin) deficit was produced in mice, the gut microbiota could supply compensatory riboflavin. Vitamin B3 (Niacin) is a potent anti-inflammatory agent and antioxidant that regulates intestinal barrier function and bacterial endotoxin generation. These findings imply that niacin may have a beneficial influence on human gut microbial composition [54]. The findings suggest that vitamin B12 may serve as a cellular immunity modulator, particularly with respect to CD8+ and NK cells [53].

Vitamin B12 boosts the number of cytotoxic T cells, whereas vitamin B6 keeps NK cells active. Vitamin B6, B12, and Folate are all involved in gut immune regulation, supporting the gut barrier (for example, vitamin B6 mediates lymphocyte migration into the intestine, while vitamin B9 is required for the survival of regulatory T cells in the small intestine, and human gut microbes use cobalamine as a cofactor for metabolic pathways). Vitamin B6 is involved in lymphocyte differentiation, proliferation, maturation, and activity; it maintains the Th1 immune response while inhibiting the function of Th2 cytokine receptors [45].

Vitamin E

Vitamin E is made up of eight different compounds (tocopherols and tocotrienols), with α-tocopherol having the highest bioavailability and being the most well-studied [55]. Vitamin E is a lipid-soluble antioxidant that protects cell membranes from oxidative damage and keeps respiratory epithelial barriers intact.

Supplementing with vitamin E enhances general immune function, decreases the severity of respiratory tract infections, lowers viral load in lung tissues, and raises antibody titers, especially in the elderly [56]. Vitamin E has shown impacts on various immune system branches, from phagocytosis to T cell proliferation and differentiation and antibody production. Vitamin E blocks the effects of PGE2 by lowering its activity but not its transcription.

Vitamin E supplementation increased lymphocyte proliferation in response to mitogens, IL-2 production, NK cell cytotoxic activity, and phagocytic activity by alveolar macrophages, as well as increased resistance to infectious agents, indicating that higher vitamin E intake promotes a Th1 cytokine-mediated response while suppressing a Th2 response. In addition to its role as a protective antioxidant, vitamin E is associated indirectly by decreasing the expression of the T-cell-suppressive factors such as PGE 2 by macrophages [53].

Vitamin E also counters the release of proinflammatory cytokines, including IL-1, IL-6, TNF, and the chemokine IL-8, by monocytes and macrophages. It is also involved in the production of IFN-γ and interleukin-2. Vitamin E has protective effects on animal models of atherosclerosis and ischemia-reperfusion injury (IRI) [55, 56].

TRACE ELEMENTS

Trace elements are found in trace concentrations in the human body, usually less than 0.01 percent. They are crucial for healthy growth, development, maintenance, and recovery. Some metals are poisonous in even minute amounts, whereas others are required for cell activity. Based on their potential nutritional significance, the World Health Organization (WHO) divided trace elements into 3 groups:

1. Lead (Pb), cadmium (Cd), fluorine (F), mercury (Hg), arsenic (As), aluminium (Al), barium (Ba), lithium (Li), and tin(Sn) are examples of potentially poisonous elements.

2. Manganese (Mn), silicon (Si), nickel (Ni), boron (B), and vanadium (V) are examples of possible physiologically essential elements.

3. Copper (Cu), zinc (Zn), selenium (Se), molybdenum (Mb), cobalt (Co), Chromium (Cr), and iodine (I) are all crucial elements [43].

Essential Elements

Zinc

Meat, milk, beans, eggs, fish, and grains are all excellent sources of Zinc in the diet [43]. Zinc is necessary for more than 300 enzymes' catalytic activation and is engaged in a variety of critical catalytic, structural, and regulatory physiological activities [43, 57].

It is a cofactor of multiple transcription factors [47], that modulates zinc-sensitive genes' expression and is involved in DNA, RNA, and protein synthesis, activating

T cells and controlling the generation of Th1 cytokines [53], B lymphocytes and antibodies mediate innate immunity and modulate acquired immunity. Macrophages need it for phagocytosis and cytokine generation as well. Low zinc levels exacerbate immune abnormalities linked to starvation. A systemic zinc shortage, in particular, is linked to inflammation, which impacts the immune system.

Zn lowers the expression of reactive oxygen species (ROS) involved in the activation of NF-kB, an immune response modulator whose malfunction can lead to autoimmune disorders and malignancies. Inhibition of NF-kB causes a decrease in the production of inflammatory cytokines and adhesion molecules [43].

Zn demonstrated antiviral efficacy against hepatitis C and rhinovirus by inhibiting RNA-dependent RNA polymerase (RdRp) and other cellular cofactors. In SARS-CoV, zinc reduces the elongation phase of RNA synthesis, which might be owing to its influence on template binding. In a case report, Sattar *et al.* indicated that combining zinc with azithromycin and chloroquine improves the recovery rate in COVID-19 patients [58].

The Zn ionophore pyrrolidine dithiocarbamate suppresses SARS-CoV-2 multiplication by inhibiting the RNA-dependent RNA polymerase enzyme [56]. It can also interfere directly with viral multiplication and protein synthesis, providing antiviral and therapeutic advantages. Studies have demonstrated zinc supplementation to reduce COVID-19-related symptoms such as lower respiratory tract infection.These side effects might be linked to COVID-19 and are produced by viral uncoating, binding, and replication being suppressed [50]. Copper/zinc superoxide dismutase (Cu/ZnSOD) and manganese superoxide dismutase (MnSOD) are necessary antioxidant enzymes that protect cells from oxidative stress-induced damage [59].

Selenium

Selenium (Se) is required for reductive-oxidative equilibrium, protein folding, calciumflux, immune cell activation, proliferation, and differentiation [58]. Selenium is a cellular antioxidant that helps the body's immunological response and is best recognized as a cofactor in glutathione peroxidase and selenoprotein.This antioxidative function makes selenium a vital component of the immune system because it protects immune cells such as phagocytes from oxidative stress, such as that caused by a respiratory burst, while also allowing for the physiological roles of ROS as signal transducers and microbicidal agents [47].

Selenium deficiency reduced IgM and IgG immunoglobulin titers, hindered neutrophil chemotaxis and lymphocyte antibody production, increased Coxsackie virus virulence, and increased CD4+ T cells while decreasing CD8+ and CD4–/ CD8– thymocytes. As a result, a sufficient selenium level may be required to combat some viral infections [53].

There is a correlation between regional selenium levels and COVID-19 cure rates in different Chinese areas, according to studies. Both vitamin E and selenium function through antioxidant pathways to increase T cell numbers, enhance mitogenic lymphocyte responses, increase IL-2 cytokine production, increase NK cell activity, and reduce infection risk. Supplementing with selenium and vitamin E has also been proven to increase resistance to respiratory illness [46].

Copper

The primary sources of copper sulphate exposure for the population are food, beverages, and water. Meat, liver, and kidneys, as well as cereals, mollusks, and some fruits, contain higher levels of copper (avocado, walnuts, hazelnuts, and dried grapes).

After iron and zinc, copper (Cu) is the third most prevalent necessary trace metal in the human body, accounting for 75–100 mg of the total amount. Copper is required in the diet in amounts of 1.6 mg per day for men, 1.3 mg per day for women, and 1 mg per day for children. Copper has antibacterial, antifungal, antiviral, and anti-inflammatory properties, which can help the host's immune system fight against germs.

Copper is required to form the myelin sheath; hence a deficit can result in myelopathy [43]. Reduced antibody-forming cell response and increased susceptibility to a range of viral infections are caused by copper deficiency [58].

Omega-3 Fatty Acid

Eicosapentaenoic and docosahexaenoic fatty acids, which make up omega-3 fatty acids, are polyunsaturated fatty acids that have been demonstrated to benefit immunity and inflammationby reducing influenza virus replication.Omega-3 fatty acids have antiviral properties [50].

The presence of a double bond at the omega-3 carbon atom distinguishes omega-3 fatty acids from other polyunsaturated fatty acids (PUFAs). An essential omega-3 fatty acid is α-linolenic acid, which is produced through desaturation, catalyzed by delta-15 desaturase, from the omega-6 fatty acid linoleic acid.

Immune-regulatory actions are critical for both omega-3 and omega-6-derived metabolites. PUFAs serve as substrates for the enzymatic creation of molecules known as specific pro-resolving mediators, which play a vital role in the resolution of inflammation (SPMs). These molecules differ from immunosuppressive medicines in that they not only aid in the explanation of inflammatory responses but also have antibacterial properties that aid in host defense. Resolvins, which are metabolites of omega-3 fatty acids, are efficient at inhibiting neutrophil migration and decreasing the future neutrophil entrance into the inflammatory region [44].

CONCLUDING REMARKS

The immune imbalance in various emerging infectious diseases or severe chronic illnesses gained the attention of natural immunomodulators, and modulation of immune response with natural immunomodulators had been of great interest to alleviate these diseases. The vaccine gives protection against infection and that immunoadjuvant plays a critical role in boosting antigen-specific immune response. Microbiota-immune cell linkages reflect immune health, and the dysfunction of microbial flora adversely affects it. The microbiota modifiers to restore immunity had provided ample evidence in clinical outcomes. Prebiotics and probiotics are commonly used as immune modifiers. Additionally, micronutrients and trace elements play a crucial role in enhancing immunity.

CONSENT FOR PUBLICATION

Not applicable.

CONFLICT OF INTEREST

The authors declare no conflict of interest, financial or otherwise.

ACKNOWLEDGEMENTS

Declared none.

REFERENCES

[1] Singh N, Tailang M, Mehta SC. A review on herbal plants as immunomodulators. Int J Pharm Sci Res 2016; 7(9): 3602.

[2] Kumar D, Arya V, Kaur R, Bhat ZA, Gupta VK, Kumar V. A review of immunomodulators in the Indian traditional health care system. J Microbiol Immunol Infect 2012; 45(3): 165-84. [http://dx.doi.org/10.1016/j.jmii.2011.09.030] [PMID: 22154993]

[3] Hofmeyr SA. An Interpretative Introduction to the Immune. Design principles for the immune system and other distributed autonomous systems 2001; 3.

[4] Nagoba B, Davane M. Natural Immunomodulators. J Immunol Microbiol 2018; 2(1): 2.

[5] Hertog MGL, Hollman PCH, van de Putte B. Content of potentially anticarcinogenic flavonoids of tea infusions, wines, and fruit juices. J Agric Food Chem 1993; 41(8): 1242-6. [http://dx.doi.org/10.1021/jf00032a015]

[6] Elangovan V, Sekar N, Govindasamy S. Chemopreventive potential of dietary bioflavonoids against 20-methylcholanthrene-induced tumorigenesis. Cancer Lett 1994; 87(1): 107-13. [http://dx.doi.org/10.1016/0304-3835(94)90416-2] [PMID: 7954363]

[7] Kandaswami C, Perkins E, Soloniuk DS, Drzewiecki G, Middleton E Jr. Antitproliferative effects of citrus flavonoids on a human squamous cell carcinoma *in vitro*. Cancer Lett 1991; 56(2): 147-52. [http://dx.doi.org/10.1016/0304-3835(91)90089-Z] [PMID: 1998943]

[8] Halder S, Bharal N, Mediratta PK, Kaur I, Sharma KK. Anti-inflammatory, immunomodulatory and antinociceptive activity of Terminalia arjuna Roxb bark powder in mice and rats. Indian J Exp Biol 2009; 47(7): 577-83. [PMID: 19761042]

[9] Leung KN, Leung PY, Kong LP, Leung PK. Immunomodulatory effects of esculetin (6,7-dihydroxycoumarin) on murine lymphocytes and peritoneal macrophages. Cell Mol Immunol 2005; 2(3): 181-8. [PMID: 16212885]

[10] Thanh PN, Jin W, Song G, Bae K, Kang SS. Cytotoxic coumarins from the root of Angelica dahurica. Arch Pharm Res 2004; 27(12): 1211-5. [http://dx.doi.org/10.1007/BF02975883] [PMID: 15646793]

[11] Lazzé M, Pizzala R, Savio M, Stivala LA, Prosperi E, Bianchi L. Anthocyanins protect against DNA damage induced by tert-butyl-hydroperoxide in rat smooth muscle and hepatoma cells. Mutat Res Genet Toxicol Environ Mutagen 2003; 535(1): 103-15. [http://dx.doi.org/10.1016/S1383-5718(02)00285-1] [PMID: 12547288]

[12] Rossi A, Serraino I, Dugo P, *et al.* Protective effects of anthocyanins from blackberry in a rat model of acute lung inflammation. Free Radic Res 2003; 37(8): 891-900. [http://dx.doi.org/10.1080/1071576031000112690] [PMID: 14567449]

[13] Sparg SG, Light ME, van Staden J. Biological activities and distribution of plant saponins. J Ethnopharmacol 2004; 94(2-3): 219-43. [http://dx.doi.org/10.1016/j.jep.2004.05.016] [PMID: 15325725]

[14] Sulaiman SM, Rajashekha G, Prakash PJ, Singh DS, Saleem C. Immunoprophylactic activity of immunol, a polyherbal formulation against dexamethasone induced immunosuppression in rats. J Pharmacol Toxicol 2010; 5(6): 275-87. [http://dx.doi.org/10.3923/jpt.2010.275.287]

[15] Herborne JB. Phytochemical methods A guide to modern techniques of plantanalysis 1973; 2: 5-11.

[16] Okwu DE. Phytochemicals, vitamins and mineral contents of two Nigerian medicinal plants. Int J Mol Med Adv Sci 2005; 1(4): 375-81.

[17] Khare CP. Centella asiatica (Linn.) Urban Indian Medicinal Plants: An Illustrated Dictionary. Verlag Berlin/Heidelberg: Springer 2007.

[18] Akbay P, Basaran AA, Undeger U, Basaran N. *in vitro* immunomodulatory activity of flavonoid glycosides from Urtica dioica L. Phytother Res 2003; 17(1): 34-7. [http://dx.doi.org/10.1002/ptr.1068] [PMID: 12557244]

[19] García D, Leiro J, Delgado R, Sanmartín ML, Ubeira FM. *mangifera indica* L. extract (Vimang) and mangiferin modulate mouse humoral immune responses: modulation of antibody responses by vimang and mangiferin. phytother res 2003; 17(10): 1182-7. [http://dx.doi.org/10.1002/ptr.1338] [PMID: 14669253]

[20] Reddy DB, Reddanna P. Chebulagic acid (CA) attenuates LPS-induced inflammation by suppressing NF-κB and MAPK activation in RAW 264.7 macrophages. Biochem Biophys Res Commun 2009; 381(1): 112-7. [http://dx.doi.org/10.1016/j.bbrc.2009.02.022] [PMID: 19351605]

[21] Rechner AR, Kroner C. Anthocyanins and colonic metabolites of dietary polyphenols inhibit platelet function. Thromb Res 2005; 116(4): 327-34. [http://dx.doi.org/10.1016/j.thromres.2005.01.002] [PMID: 16038718]

[22] Wang LS, Stoner GD. Anthocyanins and their role in cancer prevention. Cancer Lett 2008; 269(2): 281-90. [http://dx.doi.org/10.1016/j.canlet.2008.05.020] [PMID: 18571839]

[23] Punturee K, Wild CP, Kasinrerk W, Vinitketkumnuen U. Immunomodulatory activities of Centella asiatica and Rhinacanthus nasutus extracts. Asian Pac J Cancer Prev 2005; 6(3): 396-400. [PMID: 16236006]

[24] Chang Y, Chen C, Kuo CL, Chen B, You J. Glycyrrhetinic acid inhibits ICAM-1 expression *via* blocking JNK and NF-κB pathways in TNF-α-activated endothelial cells. Acta Pharmacol Sin 2010; 31(5): 546-53. [http://dx.doi.org/10.1038/aps.2010.34] [PMID: 20418897]

[25] Sunila ES, Kuttan G. Immunomodulatory and antitumor activity of Piper longum Linn. and piperine. J Ethnopharmacol 2004; 90(2-3): 339-46. [http://dx.doi.org/10.1016/j.jep.2003.10.016] [PMID: 15013199]

[26] Li F, Wang H, Lu D, *et al.* Neutral sulfate berberine modulates cytokine secretion and increases survival in endotoxemic mice. Acta Pharmacol Sin 2006; 27(9): 1199-205. [http://dx.doi.org/10.1111/j.1745-7254.2006.00368.x] [PMID: 16923341]

[27] Varma A, Padh H, Shrivastava N. Andrographolide: a new plant-derived antineoplastic entity on horizon. Evid Based Complement Alternat Med 2011; 2011: 1-9. [http://dx.doi.org/10.1093/ecam/nep135] [PMID: 19752167]

[28] Singh S, Taneja M, Majumdar DK. Biological activities of Ocimum sanctum L. fixed oil—An overview. Indian J Exp Biol 2007; 10. [PMID: 17569280]

[29] Arya V, Gupta VK. A review on marine immunomodulators. Life Sci 2011; 2(5): 8.

[30] Dolashka-Angelova P, Stefanova T, Livaniou E, *et al.* Immunological potential of Helix vulgaris and Rapana venosa hemocyanins. Immunol Invest 2008; 37(8): 822-40. [http://dx.doi.org/10.1080/08820130802403366] [PMID: 18991098]

[31] Zhong TY, Arancibia S, Born R, *et al.* Hemocyanins Stimulate Innate Immunity by Inducing Different Temporal Patterns of Proinflammatory Cytokine Expression in Macrophages. J Immunol 2016; 196(11): 4650-62. [http://dx.doi.org/10.4049/jimmunol.1501156] [PMID: 27183578]

[32] Lammers RJM, Witjes WPJ, Janzing-Pastors MHD, Caris CTM, Witjes JA. Intracutaneous and intravesical immunotherapy with keyhole limpet hemocyanin compared with intravesical mitomycin in patients with non-muscle-invasive bladder cancer: results from a prospective randomized phase III trial. J Clin Oncol 2012; 30(18): 2273-9. [http://dx.doi.org/10.1200/JCO.2011.39.2936] [PMID: 22585689]

[33] McFadden DW, Riggs DR, Jackson BJ, Vona-Davis L. Keyhole limpet hemocyanin, a novel immune stimulant with promising anticancer activity in Barrett's esophageal adenocarcinoma. Am J Surg 2003; 186(5): 552-5. [http://dx.doi.org/10.1016/j.amjsurg.2003.08.002] [PMID: 14599624]

[34] Noga EJ, Stone KL, Wood A, Gordon WL, Robinette D. Primary structure and cellular localization of callinectin, an antimicrobial peptide from the blue crab. Dev Comp Immunol 2011; 35(4): 409-15. [http://dx.doi.org/10.1016/j.dci.2010.11.015] [PMID: 21115038]

[35] Li C, Haug T, Moe MK, Styrvold OB, Stensvåg K. Centrocins: Isolation and characterization of novel dimeric antimicrobial peptides from the green sea urchin, Strongylocentrotus droebachiensis. Dev Comp Immunol 2010; 34(9): 959-68.

[http://dx.doi.org/10.1016/j.dci.2010.04.004] [PMID: 20438753]

[36] He XQ, Cao WH, Pan GK, Yang L, Zhang CH. Enzymatic hydrolysis optimization of *Paphia undulata* and lymphocyte proliferation activity of the isolated peptide fractions. J Sci Food Agric 2015; 95(7): 1544-53.
[http://dx.doi.org/10.1002/jsfa.6859] [PMID: 25087732]

[37] Dobrange E, Peshev D, Loedolff B, Van den Ende W. Fructans as Immunomodulatory and Antiviral Agents: The Case of *Echinacea.* Biomolecules 2019; 9(10): 615.
[http://dx.doi.org/10.3390/biom9100615] [PMID: 31623122]

[38] Ganguly S, Paul I, Mukhopadhayay SK. Immunostimulant, probiotic and prebiotic–their applications and effectiveness in aquaculture: A Review. Isr J Aquacult Bamidgeh 2010; 62(3): 130-8.

[39] Maldonado Galdeano C, Cazorla SI, Lemme Dumit JM, Vélez E, Perdigón G. Beneficial effects of probiotic consumption on the immune system. Ann Nutr Metab 2019; 74(2): 115-24.
[http://dx.doi.org/10.1159/000496426] [PMID: 30673668]

[40] Crowe JE Jr. Prevention of Fetal and Early Life Infections Through Maternal–Neonatal Immunization. In Infectious Diseases of the Fetus and Newborn WB Saunders 2011; 1212-30.
[http://dx.doi.org/10.1016/B978-1-4160-6400-8.00038-9]

[41] Hamley IW. Lipopeptides for Vaccine Development. Bioconjug Chem 2021; 32(8): 1472-90.
[http://dx.doi.org/10.1021/acs.bioconjchem.1c00258] [PMID: 34228433]

[42] Sander VA, Corigliano MG, Clemente M. Promising Plant-Derived Adjuvants in the Development of Coccidial Vaccines. Front Vet Sci 2019; 6: 20.
[http://dx.doi.org/10.3389/fvets.2019.00020] [PMID: 30809529]

[43] Cannas D, Loi E, Serra M, Firinu D, Valera P, Zavattari P. Relevance of essential trace elements in nutrition and drinking water for human health and autoimmune disease risk. Nutrients 2020; 12(7): 2074.
[http://dx.doi.org/10.3390/nu12072074] [PMID: 32668647]

[44] Pecora F, Persico F, Argentiero A, Neglia C, Esposito S. The role of micronutrients in support of the immune response against viral infections. Nutrients 2020; 12(10): 3198.
[http://dx.doi.org/10.3390/nu12103198] [PMID: 33092041]

[45] Gombart AF, Pierre A, Maggini S. a review of micronutrients and the immune system–working in harmony to reduce the risk of infection. Nutrients 2020; 12(1): 236.
[http://dx.doi.org/10.3390/nu12010236] [PMID: 31963293]

[46] Cerullo G, Negro M, Parimbelli M, *et al.* The long history of vitamin C: from prevention of the common cold to potential aid in the treatment of COVID-19. Front Immunol 2020; 11: 574029.
[http://dx.doi.org/10.3389/fimmu.2020.574029] [PMID: 33193359]

[47] Elmadfa I, Meyer AL. The role of the status of selected micronutrients in shaping the immune function. Endocr Metab Immune Disord Drug Targets 2019; 19(8): 1100-15.
[http://dx.doi.org/10.2174/1871530319666190529101816] [PMID: 31142256]

[48] Zdrenghea MT, Makrinioti H, Bagacean C, Bush A, Johnston SL, Stanciu LA. Vitamin D modulation of innate immune responses to respiratory viral infections. Rev Med Virol 2017; 27(1): e1909.
[http://dx.doi.org/10.1002/rmv.1909] [PMID: 27714929]

[49] Prietl B, Treiber G, Pieber T, Amrein K. Vitamin D and immune function. Nutrients 2013; 5(7): 2502-21.
[http://dx.doi.org/10.3390/nu5072502] [PMID: 23857223]

[50] Shakoor H, Feehan J, Al Dhaheri AS, *et al.* Immune-boosting role of vitamins D, C, E, zinc, selenium and omega-3 fatty acids: Could they help against COVID-19? Maturitas 2021; 143: 1-9.
[http://dx.doi.org/10.1016/j.maturitas.2020.08.003] [PMID: 33308613]

[51] Sassi F, Tamone C, D'Amelio P. Nutrient, Hormone, and Immunomodulator. Nutrients 2018; 10(11):

1656.
[http://dx.doi.org/10.3390/nu10111656] [PMID: 30400332]

[52] Kumar R, Rathi H, Haq A, Wimalawansa SJ, Sharma A. Putative roles of vitamin D in modulating immune response and immunopathology associated with COVID-19. Virus Res 2021; 292: 198235.
[http://dx.doi.org/10.1016/j.virusres.2020.198235] [PMID: 33232783]

[53] Wintergerst ES, Maggini S, Hornig DH. Contribution of selected vitamins and trace elements to immune function. Ann Nutr Metab 2007; 51(4): 301-23.
[http://dx.doi.org/10.1159/000107673] [PMID: 17726308]

[54] Uebanso T, Shimohata T, Mawatari K, Takahashi A. Functional roles of B-Vitamins in the gut and gut microbiome. Mol Nutr Food Res 2020; 64(18): 2000426.
[http://dx.doi.org/10.1002/mnfr.202000426] [PMID: 32761878]

[55] Mora JR, Iwata M, von Andrian UH. Vitamin effects on the immune system: vitamins A and D take centre stage. Nat Rev Immunol 2008; 8(9): 685-98.
[http://dx.doi.org/10.1038/nri2378] [PMID: 19172691]

[56] Gasmi A, Tippairote T, Mujawdiya PK, *et al.* Micronutrients as immunomodulatory tools for COVID-19 management. Clin Immunol 2020; 220: 108545.
[http://dx.doi.org/10.1016/j.clim.2020.108545] [PMID: 32710937]

[57] Goswami TK, Bhar R, Jadhav SE, Joardar SN, Ram GC. Role of dietary zinc as a nutritional immunomodulator. Asian-Australas J Anim Sci 2005; 18(3): 439-52.
[http://dx.doi.org/10.5713/ajas.2005.439]

[58] Dharmalingam K, Birdi A, Tomo S, *et al.* Trace elements as immunoregulators in SARS-CoV-2 and other viral infections. Indian J Clin Biochem 2021; 36(4): 416-26.
[http://dx.doi.org/10.1007/s12291-021-00961-6] [PMID: 33613002]

[59] Andreou A, Trantza S, Filippou D, Sipsas N, Tsiodras S. COVID-19: the potential role of copper and N-acetylcysteine (NAC) in a combination of candidate antiviral treatments against SARS-CoV-2. *In Vivo.* 2020; 34(3 suppl) (Suppl.): 1567-88.
[http://dx.doi.org/10.21873/invivo.11946] [PMID: 32503814]

CHAPTER 4

Standardization of Immunomodulator Natural Drugs

Aishwarya R. Nale[1] and **Supriya G. Jagtap**[2,*]

[1] *Department of Pharmacology, STES's Smt. Kashibai Navale College of Pharmacy, Kondhwa, S.P. Pune University, Pune, Maharashtra, India*

[2] *Department of Pharmacognosy, STES's Smt. Kashibai Navale College of Pharmacy, Kondhwa, S. P. Pune University, Pune, Maharashtra, India*

Abstract: Natural medications are gaining popularity as people become more aware of their benefits and accept their use in modern medicine. Natural drugs have demonstrated extensive suitability as curative agents for various disorders due to their fewer side effects and toxicity. Scientists face a tremendous problem in developing accurate analytical techniques that can efficiently profile the contents of phytochemicals. This is in addition to quantitative studies of marker or bioactive chemicals and some other important ingredients. Natural medicines, on the other hand, lack standardized parameters. Standardization is a vital step towards the formation of a constant chemical profile, consistent biological activity, or just a quality assurance programme for the production and manufacturing of natural products. As a requirement for global harmonization, the WHO criteria for assessing the safety, efficacy, and quality of natural drugs are extremely important. Scientific research of some of the natural origin plants regarded in Ayurvedic Rasayana for their beneficial potential has generated good results. The number of plants with a potential immunomodulatory activity that has been cultivated using conventional or cell culture methods is standardized. This can help to portray and validate their usage in folk medicine in the early days, as well as give an establishment for future investigation. The goal of this chapter is to showcase the findings of research evidence on standardized natural plant-origin immunomodulators. The chapter also goes through biological screening strategies for diverse plant medications with the goal of revealing the immunomodulation mechanism. Researchers will hopefully be encouraged to pursue more research on medicinal plants with immunomodulatory potential as a result of this study.

Keywords: Immmunomodulators, Immunostimulants, Immunosuppressants, Natural Drugs, Plant Tissue Culture, Standardization.

* **Corresponding author Supriya G. Jagtap:** Department of Pharmacognosy, STES's Smt. Kashibai Navale College of Pharmacy, Kondhwa, S. P. Pune University, Pune, Maharashtra, India; Tel:+918888837747; E-mail: supriyashinde2003@gmail.com

Vandana S. Nikam, Sujata P. Sawarkar, Girish B. Mahajan and Supriya G. Jagtap (Eds.)

INTRODUCTION

Natural drugs are the use of plants and plant remedies in the prevention and control of diseases. Plants have been utilized medicinally by societies all over the globe for more than thousands of years and contains a primary resource of drugs throughout human history. The fact that they are still extensively used nowadays is not a relic of the Dark Ages, but rather a sign that natural-origins plants are becoming an element of current high-tech medicine. Natural drugs act as an imperative role in the scientific structures of a few countries, like Ayurvedic medicine in India and Traditional Chinese Medicine (TCM), which, along with various complementary therapies, are seeing renewed interest. Natural drugs are recognized by the WHO as an essential component of primary health care and are 3 to 4 times more widely used than traditional medicine worldwide. According to the WHO, traditional medicine is used by 65–80% of the worldwide population as a primary resource of healthcare, and 40% of the worldwide population relies directly on traditional medicine for healthcare (WHO, 2003). It has also been discovered that nearly 15,000 plant species out of 45,000 are used for their precise medicinal value, demonstrating the significant diversity of plant species [1, 2].

According to the report, more than 130 compounds derived from approximately 100 plant species can be considered important drugs, with 77 percent presently utilized in one or more countries. Phytomedicines are flooding the markets of developed countries, and consumers all over the world have demonstrated a desire for natural drugs and their formulations. The emphasis is on 'natural is better' [3].

Today, Ayurveda has evolved into a scientific system of holistic healing that is now recognised all over the world [4].

Ayurveda is the Sanskrit word for "life science". It is not merely a system of medicine, however, but a general philosophical technique for maintaining good health, living a long life, and treating diseases. It provides a sole blend of science and philosophy that balances the physical, emotional, mental, and spiritual components required for lasting health. This healing system believes in treating the entire person, not just the part affected by the disease. Furthermore, the emphasis is on prevention rather than cure [5].

Ayurveda evolved in tandem with religion and mythology. It can be thought of as a stream of knowledge that has been passed down from time immemorial and has been reinterpreted and brought along with it. Ayurveda is possibly the only organized science that directs ecological development, medicinal plant cultivation, and the use of specific plant parts [6].

More than 2000 drugs are listed in the "Charaka" and "Sushruta" samhitas, with 70% of them being herbal. The importance of this science will continue to grow due to its biomedical implications and place in cultural beliefs. Despite its ability to treat a wide range of diseases, medicinal plant therapy was developed in preindustrial times [6].

Besides Ayurveda, a variety of healthcare systems have been practised around the world, including Siddha, Unani, and Homeopathy, the majority of which are based primarily on herbs and diet. Globally, the early twentieth century saw a decline in the popularity of natural drugs of plant origin due to the evolution of the pharmaceutical industry (synthetic medicines), as well as a lack of interest in medicinal plant research [5].

However, the pendulum has recently dangled back, and there is a reappearance of awareness in the study and application of plant-based drugs. Natural drugs are in high demand, particularly those scientifically validated, such as Garlic, Echinacea, Ginseng *etc.* 'Herbalism' refers to the more recent perception of using herbs or plants in a more scientific way [7, 8]. Since the origin of civilization, plants and plant compounds have been utilized as natural drugs. They are used to care for a wide range of acute and chronic illnesses, from the common cold to complex human problems, and they're regarded as the cornerstone of indigenous drugs [9]. As per WHO opinion, approximately 80% of the worldwide population anticipates using natural products for health care owing to their fewer side effects and the high price of modern medicine [10].

As the environment becomes more polluted, life becomes more stressful, and food becomes contaminated by chemicals, there is a greater need to reconnect with nature. Although allopathy and modern medicine are unquestionably effective and necessary in certain situations, there are some pitfalls where an alternative system of medicine offers some advantages.

NEED FOR DRUGS FROM PLANT ORIGINS OVER SYNTHETIC DRUGS

Allopathic treatment entails the administration of drugs that introduce toxins into the body. The body may be unable to eliminate or cope with them, resulting in adverse effects. Herbal medicines, which are based on a traditional system of natural cure, cleanse the body, increasing its ability to heal itself and defend against invaders while causing virtually no side effects.

Allopathic treatments are incapable of providing long-term solutions. Its most prevalent strategy is to suppress both physical and mental signs and symptoms. Natural drugs treat the symptoms as an indication or evidence of a deeper instability within the human being, attempting to restore physical and mental balance in order to lessen the symptoms. As a result, herbal drugs weed out disease at its source and provide a long-term cure rather than a quick fix.

Furthermore, despite great strides in technology and advances in medical science, some diseases still do not yield to treatment under the allopathic system, despite the fact that treatment for the same is claimed to be available in indigenous medicine. In addition, there have already been notable successes with botanical medicines. A few notable examples are quinghaosu, artemisinin from TCM, Rauwolfia, Neem, and Turmeric from Ayurvedic [11].

Today, demand for plant-based medicines is rising in both developing and developed nations as a result of increasing gratitude that natural drugs are non-toxic, have fewer side effects and are more easily obtainable at low prices than synthetic drugs [12].

There is a resurgence of interest in natural medicine these days, owing to a growing awareness of the well-being risks linked with the random use of modern medicine, and natural drug manufacturing is currently a very speedy rising sector in the worldwide market. Medicines of natural origin are in huge urging for both developed and developing nations, including India, due to their wide range of biological activities, higher safety margins than allopathic drugs, and lower cost [13].

Ayurveda suffered a setback as a result of a lack of communication and proper documentation. Much knowledge appears to have been lost as a result of the secrecy observed by Ayurvedic practitioners. Even what has been published is not readily available at the moment. Documentation of all medicinal plant information, including research work, is critical for future progress [14].

The modern system of medicine's reluctance to accept herbal remedies is primarily due to a lack of scientifically focused research and documentation regarding the so-called "scientific validity and quality."

It is therefore critical to incorporate the use of herbal remedies into an existing framework of rational scientific approach, which includes one of the basic quality control (standardization) criteria for both raw materials and finished products [15]. It is possible to save time and money on drug development by combining ethnobotany, medicine, and plant natural product chemistry. More people accept quantum acceptance as quality improves through the use of standardized natural products. Natural medicine is increasingly recognised for its ability to complement and coexist with modern science.

A number of pharmacopoeias, like the British Herbal Pharmacopoeia, the German E Commission, the British Herbal Compendium, the United States Pharmacopoeia, the Japanese pharmacopoeia, and others, establish monographs to ensure quality in their respective countries. The Indian government has also published an Ayurvedic Pharmacopoeia of India, which suggests essential quality parameters for 80 common Ayurvedic natural drugs [16].

Most natural drugs are generally thought to be safe to consume. However, some herb's bioactive constituents may be harmful and cause objectionable adverse effects. Because of hereditary, cultural, and ecological factors, the unpredictability of constituents in plants and their preparations has made the utilization of natural drugs more difficult than it would have been otherwise.

Raw material accessibility and quality, for example, are frequently issues; active principles in plants are varied and might be unfamiliar, and the quality of diverse sets of preparations may be complicated to control and determine. In most parts of the world, natural products typically enter the marketplace devoid of any restrictions such as safety and toxicological studies. There is currently no efficient device for regulating manufacturing preparations and quality standards. These products are available for purchase by consumers without a prescription and may be unaware of the risks associated with a subpar product. One of the vital requirements for the manufacturing of a luxurious-quality drug is, therefore, a definite and consistent drug composition. Natural drugs that are given by nature are not always consistent and are affected by a variety of issues. Ensuring consistent product quality is critical for the industry's continued existence and achievement.

STANDARDIZATION OF DRUGS FROM NATURAL ORIGINS

In general, whether synthetic or natural, all medicines must be both safe and efficacious. (EMEA, 2005; WHO, 2002c, 1998c, 1996, 1991a, b, 1990, 1988). Natural substances are plants or parts of plants that have been converted into phytopharmaceuticals through harvesting, drying, and storage methods (EMEA, 1998). As a result, they are versatile. Diversities in growth, geographical location, and harvesting time all contribute to unpredictability. Standardization of natural drugs refers to the procedure of recommending a set of standards or intrinsic characteristics, constant factors, and best qualitative and quantitative significance that carry an assurance of quality, efficiency, safety, and reproducibility. It is the method used to develop and approve the scientific specifications [17].

The standardization of natural drugs is intended to provide an opportunity to use herbs in a more rational manner for scientifically predetermined therapeutic goals. This includes the assurance of a consistently strong product as well as the guarantee of delivering an efficacious product on a consistent basis. Standardization is a very important aspect of herbal drug manufacturing and supply [18].

Some crises are not appropriate for synthetic drugs since they frequently impact the quality of natural drugs.

For example,

1. Natural drugs are basically blends of many constituents.
2. In most cases, the bioactive constituent (s) is (are) unknown.
3. Specific analytical methods or reference compounds may not be commercially obtainable.
4. Plant resources are chemically and naturally variable.
5. Chemo-varieties and chemo cultivars exist.
6. The source and quality of the raw material are uneven.

The impact on the quality of natural drugs is mainly due to factors like cultivation, collection, harvesting, drying, storage, transportation, and processing methods such as methods of extraction, selection of polarity extracting solvent, constituent instability, and many more. There are currently no official standards for natural drug preparations. At present, the industrialists involved in manufacturing are testing the preparations by their own parameters, many of which are very introductory. At the moment, determining the presence of all the compositions ascertained in preparation is extremely difficult. As a result, the first vital mission is to develop a parameter that can determine the presence of the whole component. Different chromatography and spectrophotometry methods, and the evaluation of Physico-chemical properties can be tried to develop a prototype to determine the presence of different components. Such methods can be used to quantify a bioactive set of compounds such as glycosides, alkaloids, polyphenolic components, flavonoids, or a specific compound [19].

Need for Standardization: Producers' and Consumers' Outlook

Today's worldwide outlook is a shift towards the use of medicine of natural origin, as the risks and deficiencies of allopathy medicine are becoming more obvious. It is the basic accountability of the regulatory bodies to make sure that end users get the medication with complete assurance of purity, safety, potency, and efficacy. The regulatory bodies strictly follow the different standards of quality mentioned for raw materials and finished products in pharmacopoeias, formularies, and manufacturing processes through statutory inflicts on good manufacturing practices (GMP). These methods would be relevant to all categories of medicine, whether they are integrated into the medicine of the modern era or the ancient era. Although natural products have become more widely accepted around the world, one of the barriers to their acceptance is a lack of standard quality assurance profiles.

The quality of natural medicine, *i.e.*, the composition of the final product, has consequences for efficacy and safety. Because of the complex nature and inherent unpredictability of plant-based drug constituents, it is difficult to establish quality control parameters, despite the fact that modern analytical techniques are expected to aid in avoiding this problem. Besides this, the constituents responsible for the asserted therapeutic effects are frequently unknown or simply partially explained. This is complicated further by the use of a combination of natural ingredients, as is common in conventional practice. A single product is likely to contain at least five phytoconstituents. In the absence of a standard reference for identification, batch-to-batch variation begins with the raw material collection. These variations become more pronounced during storage and subsequent analysis. standardisation for natural drugs and their products should include a comprehensive study of the field, from plant-based drug cultivation to its clinical trials [15].

Plant resources and natural therapies obtained from them account for a sizable part of the global marketplace, necessitating the use of worldwide identified guidelines for quality assurance and control.

There are several limitations that cause serious problems when attempting to build quality into a herbal product. For example, while each herb can contain a large number of compounds, overall pharmacological effects are caused by several compounds working together to cause synergistic effects rather than single compounds. All of these compounds cannot be analysed qualitatively or quantitatively for their presence or absence.

So, the logical approach is to use modern analytical techniques such as GC, HPLC, or HPTLC to analyze for the presence or absence of one or more active principles. This method is known as "marker compound testing," and it can only help in monitoring the presence or absence of a group of compounds from herbs. The lack of a validated marker compound that can be used as a reference substance, as well as the lack of standardization methods for detecting or quantifying the marker, add to the problems, which can be overcome by using techniques such as fingerprinting [20, 21].

Standardization of Natural Drugs Using Marker Compound Analysis

Chromatography is the most excellent method of standardizing plant origin drugs and their formulation, which is based on modern scientific tools. This method aids in establishing the correct botanical identity and also in regulating the chemical purity of the natural drugs. The technique recommended is marker compound testing and fingerprint analysis [22].

Chemical profiling (finger printing) is a versatile technique that can be useful in standardization. Fingerprinting refers to the process of establishing a distinctive chemical outline for a plant material, its fraction, or extract, which consists of well-known categories of chemical components such as primary metabolites (carbohydrates, lipids, proteins), secondary metabolites (alkaloids, coumarins, flavonoids, terpenoids, and so on), and inorganic salts and metals [21].

With the help of modern, sophisticated tools, various chromatographic techniques are used to analyze the marker compounds in plants, as mentioned in Table **1**. The most commonly used technique, High Performance Thin Layer Chromatography (HPTLC), is employed for fingerprinting the natural drug without quantifying the compounds, although the same can also be quantified using a densitometer. High-Pressure Liquid Chromatography (HPLC) is generally preferred for quantitative work. However, standardization is a time-consuming exercise in this technique due to the scarcity of literature for individual compound analysis.

Gas chromatography is primarily used to analyse volatile materials like aroma oils and perfumes. In terms of phytochemical studies, medicinal plants in India have been extensively studied, and at least the major components have been identified. As a result, based on the methods of isolation of these compounds, there is an opportunity to select compounds that can be used for standardization purposes. The current state of marker testing in various herbs, as well as the plants in which these tests can be performed to assure the quality and purity of the natural drugs, is described [23].

Table 1. Marker work achieved and required in medicinal plants [23].

Sr. No.	Name of the Herb	Marker Compounds
1.	*Acacia arabica*	Arabic acid
2.	*Acacia catechu*	Catechin
3.	*Aconitum heterophyllum*	Aconitin
4.	*Aegle marmelos*	Aegelin
5.	*Andrographis paniculata*	Andrographolides
6.	*Asparagus racemosus*	Shatawarine
7.	*Boerhaavia diffusa*	Punarnavine
8.	*Boswellia serrate*	Boswellic Acids
9.	*Cassia angustifolia*	Sennosides

(Table 1) cont.....

Sr. No.	Name of the Herb	Marker Compounds
10.	*Cassia fistula*	Fistuline
11.	*Centella asiatica*	Asiaticoside
12.	*Cinnamomum tamala*	Eugenol
13.	*Commiphora mukul*	Guggulusterones
14.	*Crocus sativus*	Crocetin
15.	*Curculigo orchioides*	Lycorine
16.	*Curcuma longa*	Curcuminoides
17.	*Cyperus rotundus*	Cypeerotundone
18.	*Embeliaribes*	Embelin
19.	*Eugenia caryophylata*	Eugenol
20.	*Evolvulus alsinoides*	Evolvine
21.	*Ferula asafoetida*	Ferulic acid
22.	*Glycyrrhiza glabra*	Glycyrrhizin
23.	*Holarrhena antidysenterica*	Kurchine/Kurchicine
24.	*Hyoscyamus niger*	Hyoscyamine
25.	*Melia azadirachta*	Nimbidine
26.	*Mentha arvensis*	Menthol
27.	*Ocimum basilicum*	Eugenol
28.	*Phyllanthus emblica*	Phylembelin
29.	*Phyllanthus niruri*	Phyllanthin
30.	*Picrorrhiza kurrroa*	Kutkin
31.	*Piper longum*	Piperine

Processes and Procedures for Standardisation and Quality Control of Natural Drugs are Described

In light of the widespread use of herbal drugs, WHO has highlighted the importance of ensuring quality control of plant-based drugs through the use of modern techniques and the application of appropriate standards. As a result, this association has issued guidelines to ensure the dependability and reproducibility of plant-based formulations.

The following are some of the major parameters recommended by WHO for ensuring the quality of herbal drugs, as depicted in Fig. (**1**) [20, 21]:

Authentication

Plant materials collected from a suitable area of the country at the appropriate stage of growth are thoroughly authenticated by taxonomical study, and the correct botanical characteristics is recognised.For example, a number of Phyllanthus species like *P. simplex, P. maderaspatensis, P. amarus, P. fraternus,* and *P. urinaria* grows in almost identical agro-climatic conditions in India, and only *P. amarus* with its distinct taxonomic characteristics, has been selected for clinical trials.

Foreign Matter

Plant drugs that are not drug constituents are classified as foreign matter. Soil, dust, stones, insects, and other animal contamination, such as animal excreta, should be completely removed from medicinal plant material.

Organic Evaluation

Organoleptic assessment refers to sensory evaluation and includes the macroscopy characteristics, color, odor, taste, fracture, and feel of the drug. *P. amarus* leaves are extremely bitter, *P. maderaspatensis* leaves are mildly bitter, and *P. fraternus* leaves are not bitter.

Microscopy

The examination of plant drugs under a microscope is not required for the study of adulterants, but it is required for accurate identification. *P. amarus* and *P. fraternus* have epidermal parenchyma with wavy walls, whereas *P. maderaspatensis* has straight-walled epidermal parenchyma. Furthermore, only anisocytic stomata were observed in *P. fraternus* and *P. maderaspatensis*, while both paracytic and anisocytic stomata were observed in *P. amarus*. Such diagnostic microscopic features are extremely functional in the standardization of plant drugs. Quantitative microscopy, such as stomatal number, stomatal index, and palisade ratio, can aid in distinguishing between intimately related species.

Volatile Matter

Steam distillation of the plant drug determines the volatile matter, if present.

Ash Value

The existence of ash in plant materials is quantified as total ash, acid insoluble ash, and sulphated ash. When plant drugs are incinerated, they produce an inorganic ash that varies within fairly broad limits in the case of many drugs, and these values are important for the purpose of plant evaluation.

Extractive Values

The amount of constituents extracted with solvents from a known quantity of plant-based material is referred to as "extractable matter." These extractive values indicate the proportion of polar, medium polar, and non-polar components in the plant-based material.

Chromatographic Profile of Marker Compound

Thin layer chromatography (TLC) has turned out to be widely accepted among the many chromatographic methods. This is currently available for the rapid and positive analysis of plant drugs because the time required for TLC to show most of the characteristic constituents is very short and provides qualitative results. TLC also provides semiquantitative data on the major constituents of the plant drug, allowing for drug quality evaluation. TLC focuses on providing a drug fingerprint. As a result, it is appropriate to examine the identity and purity of drugs, and also for the detection of adulteration and substitution. A TLC profile of *Phyllanthus* and *Curcuma* extracts has been demonstrated.

In clinical trials, TLC-densitometer scanners were used to obtain fingerprint profiles of extracts of many drugs, and representative fingerprint profiles of *P. amarus, P. maderaspatensis*, Ksharsootra, Shereesh, Varun, and others were developed. The quantification of plant drugs such as *Andrographis paniculata*, which contains the hepatoprotective bioactive compound andrographolide, has been carried out by High-Performance Liquid Chromatography (HPLC). Similarly, two lignans, phyllanthin and hypophyllanthin, have been quantified in *P. amarus* in various parts of the plant. A reverse phase HPLC method for analysing vasicine, the main active alkaloidal component of *Adhatoda vasica*, was used to standardize two polyherbal formulations used in the Ayurvedic medicine system for the treatment of bronchial asthma.

Pesticide Residues

Pesticides, which are biocidal agricultural chemicals, have significantly minimized the existence of insects, fungi, and molds in food. Plants-based medicines are thus vulnerable to pesticide residues accumulated from agricultural practices like spraying, soil treatment during cultivation, and fumigant use during storage. Because many plant-based medicine preparations are engaged for extended periods of time, pesticide residue limits should be recognized in accordance with the Food and Agriculture Organization's (FAO) and World

Health Organization's (WHO) recommendations. These recommended guidelines include pesticide residue analytical methodology. Pesticides containing Hg, DDT, HCH (BHC), dieldrin, aldrin, melipax, and toxaphene are not permitted for plant-based medicines.

Determination of Heavy Metals

Contamination of plant-based materials with arsenic and heavy metals like cadmium and lead can be associated with a variety of factors, like environmental pollution and pesticide residues.Heavy metal limits (ppm, parts per million) in plant-based medicines should be kept within specifications.

Microbial Contamination

Plant-based materials usually contain an immense number of bacteria and molds, frequently of soil origin. Whereas the naturally existing microflora of plants contains a diverse range of bacteria and fungi, aerobic spore-forming bacteria often prevail. Current harvesting, handling, and production lines frequently lead to additional contamination and microbial growth. The presence of *E. coli* and mould may indicate high-quality production and harvesting practices. Furthermore, the presence of aflatoxins in plant material can pose health risks if even trace amounts are absorbed. As a result, they must be determined after an appropriate clean-up procedure.

Radioactive Contamination

Irradiation could have been used to sterilize plant-based materials after harvesting, packaging materials, intermediate products, bulk materials, and finished products, as well as to decontaminate microorganisms. For this aspect, W.H.O. guidelines may be followed.

Current Natural Drug Standardization Regulations

The United States Herbal Pharmacopoeia Committee, the Chinese Herbal Pharmacopoeia, the British Herbal Compendium, the British Herbal Pharmacopoeia, the Ayurvedic Pharmacopoeia of India, and the Japanese Standards for Herbal Medicine are among the pharmacopeias to protect the quality of natural drugs and their products in their respective countries and establish a monograph. The Ayurvedic Pharmacopoeia of India, published by the Indian government, sets fundamental quality requirements for eighty major Ayurvedic herbal medications. The Ayurvedic Pharmacopoeia of India, published by the Indian government, sets fundamental quality requirements for eighty major Ayurvedic herbal medications. Traditional and herbal remedies are encouraged, recommended, and promoted by the World Health Organization (WHO) in national healthcare programmes because they are inexpensive, safe, and people trust them. In a number of decisions, the WHO has underlined the significance of adopting modern techniques and implementing appropriate standards to assure quality control of natural products [24, 25].

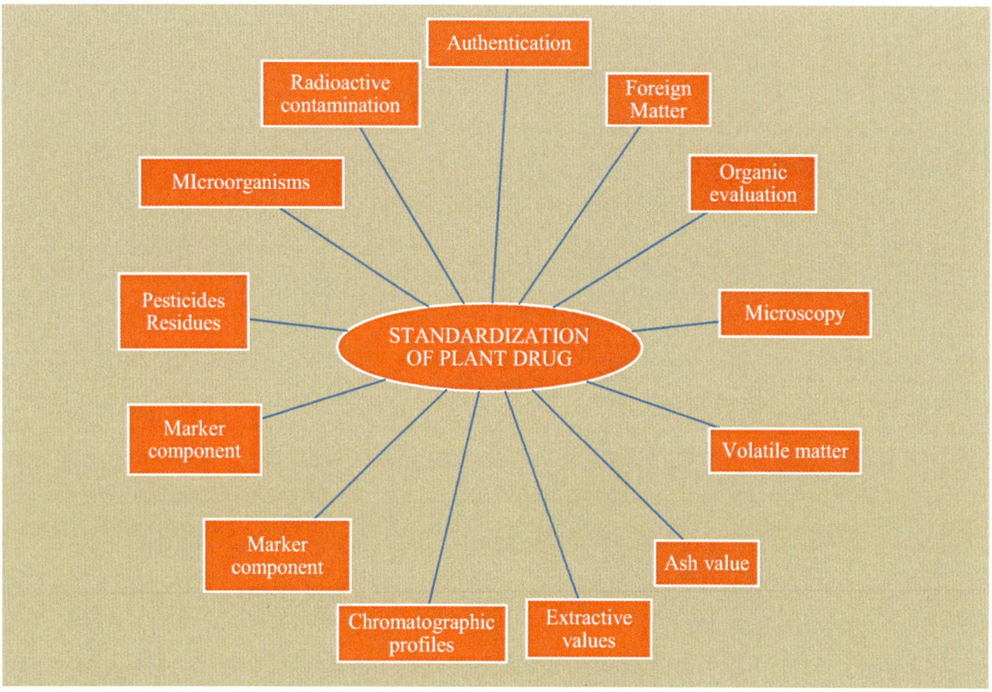

Fig. (1). Natural crude drug authentication and standardization [20, 21].

WHO Guidelines for QualityStandardized Plant-based Drug Formulations [24]:

1. Raw drug materials, plant preparations, and finished goods quality control.
2. Evaluation of stability and shelf life.
3. Safety evaluation; safety information based on experience or toxicological studies.
4. Ethnomedical data and biological activity are used to determine efficacy.

Apart from the WHO guidelines, it has made tremendous efforts to promote herbal drugs. Thus, WHO endorsement has encouraged a reexamination of traditional medicine in most developing countries, resulting in a new cultural awareness of, and pride in, traditional values. WHO collaborating centres have continued to support national research development efforts [26].

Natural medicines have always been regarded as a useful, safe, and effective mode of treatment in India. In terms of medicinal plants, India also has a rich heritage of its own. India has approximately 45,000 plant species, and because of its diverse soil and climatic conditions, as well as its rich flora and fauna, India has the capability to become a worldwide supplier of natural products that meet worldwide standards. Natural drug export potential has been estimated to be Rs 2840 million per year for India and Rs 16,000 million per year for China.

The consumption of natural drugs is in full stream, and the marketplace is rising day by day. The yearly income of India from plant-based manufacturing was estimated at around the US $300 million in plant-based medicines. The export of plant-based medicines and plants from India is around US $80 million [27].

Exploring conventional natural medicines in the context of modern sciences requires the need for optimum and proper use of conventional drugs. Ayurveda appears to offer remedies for the prevention and cure of ailments or when there is a need for new drugs, as the modern system has either no or only insufficient drugs. One of the most important areas is the use of health-promoting drugs. Ayurvedic drugs that "promote vigour in the healthy" are distinguished from curative drugs and are referred to as "Rasayana," which presumably aid in the development of non-specific body resistance to infection.

Rasayana therapy, according to Sushruta, stops ageing (Vaya-sthapan), increases lifespan (Ayushxarm), intelligence (Medha), strength (Bala), and allows one to prevent disease (Rogapharanasamarthan). This concept has received special attention in Ayurveda, and a variety of products that are widely used as Rasayanas are available.

A number of plants are highly valued for their ability to alleviate stress, age, memory, and learning. Withania, Galo, Tulsi, Brahmi (both varieties), Shankhpushpi, and Jatamansi are some of the important Rasayana drugs that have provided preliminary evidence validating Ayurvedic claims [23, 28].

In Ayurveda, a particular problem associated with natural drugs is the actual material used. In some cases, controversial identities crop up related to taxonomical descriptions and also due to their origin in different geographical regions. Through the commercialization of these natural medicines, it has turned out to be increasingly important to conduct comprehensive studies to assess their quality in order to ensure their safety and effectiveness levels.

IMMUNOMODULATING PLANT DRUGS

Plants and natural products have been used for fitness and life preservation for a long time. The most authentic, ancient Indian scripture, Vedic literature, provides references to many floras for various diseases and their prevention.

A natural immunomodulator is a substance that either stimulates or suppresses immune system factors, such as intrinsic and adaptive immune responses.

It can either stimulate effector cells or increase the production of their metabolic inducers to cause immunostimulation, or it can inhibit the immunity limiting factor.

Importance of Natural Immunomodulators

1. Natural immunomodulators are useful in the treatment of immune deficiencies, inflammations, infections, and cancer.

2. They have been shown to affect cytokines, interleukins, lymphocytes, *etc.*

3. They may indeed act as immunoadjuvants, immunosuppressive agents, or immunostimulants.

4. They enhance vaccine efficacy by continuing to act on cell-mediated immunity and increase muscle rigidity, in both, by responding with both arms of immune system function.

Ayurveda Concept

The Indian traditional medical system (Ayurveda) explains several modalities concerned with the prevention and treatment of diseases, with a focus on diet, lifestyle, and medications as pillars of therapy. The following Ayurvedic 'Sutra' highlights the concept that vitalization therapy is beneficial. “Vitalizers provide long life, greater memory and intelligence, disease-free youth, excellence of lustre, skin, voice, and body and mind strength,” the verse states. These “Rasayana” components could be inducers of enzymes, hormones, and other substances that the body needs for adaptability and survival in health, stress, and disease [29].

Rasayana is a Sanskrit word that applies to the flow of Rasa, or nutrition. Rasayana works to improve the nutrient flow to all parts of the body's functioning, even if they are systems, tissues, or even a unicellular organism.

Rasayana is a group of thirty-four plants in the Ayurvedic medical system. These plants also have immunostimulant, antibacterial, antiviral, anti-inflammatory, anti-cancer, anti-rheumatic, and other pharmacological characteristics. In addition to these, several other Ayurvedic therapeutic herbs that are not in the class of Rasayana have been found to have immunomodulation properties [29]. A list of them is contained in Table **2**.

Table **2a** and **2b**. Medicinal Plants from India (Rasayana and Non-Rasayana).

Table 2a. Rasayana Drugs [29].

Sr. No.	Botanical Name	Ayurvedic Name
1.	*Acorus calamus*	Vacha
2.	*Abutilon indicum*	Atibala
3.	*Aloe vera*	Ghrit-Kumari
4.	*Argyreia speciosa*	Vriddhadara
5.	*Asparagus racemosus*	Satavari
6.	*Azadirachta indica*	Nimba
7.	*Bacopa monnieri*	Nir-Brahmi
8.	*Boerhaavia diffusa*	Sothaghni
9.	*Cissampelos pareira*	Paatha
10.	*Commiphora mukul*	Guggulu
11.	*Convolvulus pluricauhs*	Shankhpushpi
12.	*Curcuhgoorchioides*	Krishna Musalee
13.	*Curcuma longa*	Haridra
14.	*Desmodium gangeticum*	Shalapami
15.	*Dioscorea bulbifera*	Raktalukum
16.	*Embhca officinalis*	Aamalaki
17.	*Embeliaribes*	Vidanga
18.	*Glycerrhiza glabra*	Yashtimadhu
19.	*Gmelina arborea*	Kasmari
20.	*Hemidesmus indices*	Anantamula
21.	*Ipomoea digitata*	Vidaree
22.	*Leptadenia reticulata*	Jeevantee
23.	*Piper longum*	Pippali
24.	*Psoralea coryhfolia*	Vakuchibheda
25.	*Pterocarpus marsupium*	Bijasar

(Table 2a) cont.....

Sr. No.	Botanical Name	Ayurvedic Name
26.	*Semecarpus anacardium*	Bhallatak
27.	*Sida spinosa*	Nagbala
28.	*Sida cordifolia*	Bala
29.	*Solanum nigrum*	Kakamachi
30.	*Sphaeranthus indie us*	Mundi
31.	*Terminalia bellirica*	Bibhitaka
32.	*Terminalia chebula*	Haritaki
33.	*Tinospora cordifolia*	Guduchi
34.	*Withania somnifera*	Ashwagandha

Apart from Rasayana, there is also one more principle in Ayurveda that may demonstrate the natural plants' immunostimulant potential. "Ama" is an immunologically active compound produced in the intestine as a result of improper food digestion, which is the reason for pathogenesis for a number of disorders, such as rheumatoid arthritis, liver disease, and ulcerative colitis, which all have an immune basis.

Table 2b. Non-Rasayana Drugs [29].

Sr. No.	Botanical Name	Ayurvedic Name
1.	*Abrus precatorius*	Gunja
2.	*Aconitum heterophyllum*	Ativisha
3.	*Albizzia lebbeck*	Shirisha
4.	*Amoorarohituka*	Rohitaka
5.	*Andrographis paniciaata*	Bhuinimba
6.	*Aristolochia indica*	Isharmula
7.	*Artocarpus lakoocka*	Lakucha
8.	*Astragalus multiceps*	Sarmul
9.	*Bauhania variegata*	Kachanara
10.	*Berberis aristata*	Daaruharidra
11.	*Blechnum onentah*	Rajhans
12.	*Bombax malabaricnm*	Raktashalmali
13.	*Bupleurum falcatum*	Sipil
14.	*Butea monosperma*	Palasha
15.	*Butea superba*	Latapalasha

(Table 2b) cont.....

Sr. No.	Botanical Name	Ayurvedic Name
16.	*Calotropis procera*	Alarka
17.	*Canssacarandus*	Karamarda
18.	*Calharanthus roseus*	Sadapushpa
19.	*Celastrus paniculatus*	Malkangni
20.	*Centella asiatica*	Mandukparni
21.	*Cicer arietinum*	Chanaka
22.	*Citrullus colocyntfus*	Indravaruni
23.	*Clerodendrum infortunatum*	Bhandira
24.	Chtoriaternatea	Aparajita
25.	*Costusspeciosus*	Kemuka
26.	*Cucumis sativus*	Aindri
27.	*Cumimum cyminum*	Jirak
28.	*Cymbopogon maritinu*	Dhymakah
29.	*Dryopteris cochlea'a*	Jatashankar
30.	*Elephantopus scaber*	Gojihwaa
31.	*Elytraria acaulis*	Sahustramuli
32.	*Eupatorium cannabinum*	Tongollati
33.	*Flacourtia indica*	Svadukantaka
34.	*Gymnema sylvestre*	Gurmar
35.	*Hibiscus esculentus*	Dindish
36.	*Holarrhena antidysenterica*	Kutaja
37.	*Hyoscyamus niger*	Parasikaya
38.	*Jasminum sambac*	Vrittamallika
39.	*Lawsonia inermis*	Madayanita, Mehendi
40.	*Luffa acutangula*	Krtavedhkna
41.	*Hoppea dichotoma*	Kuki
42.	*Luffa cylindrical*	Mahajalini
43.	*Mallotus philippensis*	Kampillaka
44.	*Magnifera indica*	Amra
45.	*Manilkara kauki*	Khireeni
46.	*Melia azadirachtc*	Mahanimba
47.	*Mentha spicata*	Pootihaa
48.	*Mucuna pruriem*	Kapikacchu
49.	*Nardostachys jatamansi*	Jatamansi

(Table 2b) cont.....

Sr. No.	Botanical Name	Ayurvedic Name
50.	*Nelsomacampestrs*	Pattakamraj
51.	*Ocimum canum*	Ajaka
52.	*Ocimum sanctum*	Tulsi, Bhutaghni
53.	*Ougeinia oojeinense*	Tinisha
54.	*Picrorrhiza kurroa*	Katurohim
55.	*Piper aurantiacum*	Shambhatuka
56.	*Piper betel*	Tambuli
57.	*Pluchea lanceolata*	Rasana
58.	*Prosopis spicigera*	Shami
59.	*Randia dumetorum*	Madanah
60.	*Saraca indica*	Ashoka
61.	*Selaginella bryoptens*	Amarbooti
62.	*Solanum trilobatum*	Alarka
63.	*Syzygium cumini*	Jambu
64.	*Valeriana wallichii*	Tagar
65.	*Viscum album*	Banda
66.	*Vitex negundo*	Sinduvara
67.	*Woodfordia fruticosa*	Dhataki
68.	*Zingiber officinalis*	Ardraka

Drugs like *Ferula narthex, Garcima pedunculata, Piper longum, Piper retro fractum, Plumbago zeylanica, Semicarpus anacardium, Trachys permum ammi* and *Zingiber officinalis* increases digestive capacity and prevent formation of 'Ama' (Deepak) while another group of drugs which digest 'Ama' (Pachak) are *Aconitum heterophyllum, Berberis aristata, Cissampelos pareira, Curcuma longa, Cyperus rotundus, Elettaria cardamomum, Emblica officinalis, Picrorr hizakurroa, Plumbago zeylanica, Saus surealappa, Semicarpus anacardium, Terminalia bellerica* and *Terminalia chebula*. Several other plants have anti-allergic properties and can be classified as 'immunomodulators', such drugs stimulate the formation of T- suppressor cells, *e.g., Picrorrhiza kurroa, Piper longum.*

In ancient Ayurvedic texts, "MedhyaRasayana" is described as counteracting the symptoms of psychological strain by tranquillizing consumers and enhancing their memory span and intelligence. *Centella asiatica, Bacopa monmera, Convolvulus pluricauhs, Nardostachys jatamansi, Acorus calamus,* and *Withania sommfera.*

Tinospora cordifolia improves phagocytic activity without affecting humoral or cell-mediated immunity [28].

Rasayana and non-rasayana plants contain immunomodulatory substances of a varying chemical structures and molecular sizes.

Some of the immunomodulator drugs have provided preliminary leads validating the claims made in Ayurveda and are enlisted in Table **3**.

Table 3. Immunomodulatory Effects of Some of the Indigenous Plants [29].

Sr. No.	Plants	Immunomodulatory Effects
1.	*Acorus calamus* (Bach)	Inhibits carageenin-induced inflammation in the rat paw Inhibits human carcinoma cell
2.	*Albizia labbek* (Shirisha)	Immunomodulatory activity Anticancer activity
3.	*Allium sativum* (Lahsuna)	Enhances fibrinolytic activity Antiinflammatory activity Antiarthritic activity Modulates the activity of chemical carcinogens
4.	*Aloe vera* (Ghrit-Kumari)	Inhibits inflammation Improves wound healing Proliferation-promoting activity on human and hamster cells
5.	*Andrographis paniculata* (Kalmegh)	Stimulates macrophage migration and *E. coli* phagocytosis, as well as antibody and DTH response to SRBC in mice. Spleen lymphocyte proliferation Effect on cell-mediated phagocytosis and cell-mediated immune response
6.	*Argyreia speciosa* (Samandar Ka Pat)	Inhibits growth of tumour Antifilarial activity
7.	*Asparagus racemosus* (Satavar)	Inhibits ochratoxin A induced suppression of IL-1, TNF-2 and macrophage chemotaxis Improves the humoral and cell-mediated immunity Induces lag in tumour development
8.	*Azadirachta indica* (Neem)	Attenuates stress and xenobiotic-induced suppression of humoral and cell-mediated immunity Improves anti-ovalbumin antibody, DTH response, macrophage migration inhibition Stimulates IL-1 IFN-a, TNF-y production, Improves proliferative response of spleen cells to con A and tetanus toxoid
9.	*Boerhaavia diffusa* (Punamava)	Augments antibody production and has restorative activity Antifibrinolytic activity Increases immunoglobulins and lowers immune-complex in nephrotic syndrome

(Table 3) cont.....

Sr. No.	Plants	Immunomodulatory Effects
10.	*Boswellia serrata* (Salai-Gum)	Effect on cell-mediated and humoral components of the immune response. Enhances phagocytic function, increases leucocyte count and humoral antibody litres Inhibits lipooxygenase production in stimulated PMN58 Inhibits human leukaemia HL-60 cells *in-vivo*
11.	*Celastrus paniculatus* (Malkangni)	Anti-inflammatory activity
12.	*Centella asiatica* (Brahmi)	Increases leucocytic and PMN counts Enhances circulating antibody against SRBC61 Immimostimulant property Antifilarial activity
13.	*Convolvulus pluricaulis* (Shankhpusphi)	Antiinflammatory activity
14.	*Commiphora mukul* (Guggul)	Inhibits carageenin-induced rat paw edema
15.	*Curcuma longa* (Haidar)	Increases phagocytic capacity by Anti-inflammatory activity
16.	*Emblica officinalis* (Amla)	Improves NK cells and antibody-dependent cellular cytotoxicity against Dalton's lymphoma ascites tumour Inhibitory effect on HIV reverse transcriptase Inhibits methyl eholanthrene-induced sarcoma Antitumour activity
17.	*Glycyrrhiza glabra* (Yashtimadhu)	Antiinflammatory and Antiallergic activity Antiinflammatory and Antiphlogistic activity
18.	*Nyctanthes arbor-tristis* (Har-singhar)	Protects mice against *Candida albicans* as a result of improved humoral, DTH and macrophage activity
19.	*Ocimum sanctum* (Tulsi)	Induces lag in tumour development in mice Prevents milk-induced leucocytosis in mice Adaptogenic (anti-stress) activity of dried powder on rat and mice
20.	*Picrorrhiza kurroa* (Kutaki)	Inhibits ochratoxin A-induced suppression of IL-1, TNF-a and macrophage chemotaxis. Protects animals against Leishmania and Filarial infection
21.	*Piper longum* (Long pepper)	Anti inflammatory activity 'Immimostimulant activity Antiallergic activity
22.	*Plucea lanceolata* (Surahi)	Antiinflammatory activity Anticandidal activity
23.	*Plumbago zeylamca* (Chita)	Anticandidal activity Antitumour activity
24.	*Pterocarpus marsupnum* (Bijasar)	Antitumour activity
25.	*Semecarpus anacardium* (Bhilawa)	Antitumour activity Antiinflammatory activity Antiarthritic activity

(Table 3) cont.....

Sr. No.	Plants	Immunomodulatory Effects
26.	*Terminalia chebula* (Haritaki)	Inhibition of chemiluminescence of human leucocytes induced by TPA / Prevention of DNA breaks of human leucocytes induced by TPA
27.	*Tinospora cordifolia* (Guduchi)	Increases proliferation in bone marrow Modulation of alveolar macrophage function Increase In the number and function of neutrophils, monocytes and macrophages Induces leucopoenia and myelosuppression Stimulatory action on granulocyte-macrophage Improves MHC Class II expression and antigen-presenting ability of macrophage; Improves antigen-specific antibody, Inhibits ochratoxin A-induced suppression of IL-1, TNF-a and macrophage chemotaxis, Improves IgG antibody and macrophage activation. Anticomplementary, immunomodulatory activities and inhibition of immune-haemolysis of antibody-coated sheep erythrocytes by guinea pig serum Antitumour activity against Dll and Ehrlich ascites carcinoma cells
28.	*Viscum album* (Banda)	Immunomodulatory activity
29.	*Vitex negundo* (Nirgundi)	Anti-tumour activity against Ehrlich ascites carcinoma cells Anti-inflammatory activity Anti-arthritic activity
30.	*Withania sommfera* (Ashwagandha)	Exhibits immunomodulatory activity by preventing myelosuppression induced by cyclophosphamide, azathioprine or prednisolone. Inhibits ochratoxin A-induced suppression of IL-1, TNF-a and macrophage chemotaxis. Suppress ovalbumin-specific IgE antibody production in mice by passive cutaneous anaphylaxis 1,1 Enhances radiosensitization for V97 Chinese hamster cell Inhibits inflammation m carrageenan-induced paw oedema in the rat. Induces a lag in tumour development
31.	*Zingiber officinale* (Adrak)	Inhibits inflammation owing to reduce in the formation of prostaglandins and leukotrienes

PLANT TISSUE CULTURE

Plant tissue culture is defined as the sterilized and controlled cultivation of plant seeds, cells, tissues, explants, organs, or protoplasts on a chemically specified synthesized nutritional medium in sterile and controlled light, temperature, and humidity circumstances [30].

Advantages of Plant Tissue Culture for Standardization of Phytoconstituents

A biotechnological method that depends on the use of plant cell cultures is now available to reduce the unpredictability of important bioactive components as much as possible and develop product standardization. This "green" biotech technique eliminates the potential for ambient pollutants to be carried over into the final extract as a result of several traditional extraction procedures as well as tightly regulated growth conditions that result in predictable and standardized extract composition. Botanical products derived from cultivated and wild-crafted plant materials can differ considerably in the content of putatively bioactive constituents due to diverse growth conditions and plant developmental processes at the time of collection. Besides the quality and steadiness of the raw material, the subsequent handling and extraction, which can also differ enormously amongst manufacturers in various countryside, are also responsible for the final product composition. During this process, other botanical and non-botanical pollutants may be introduced into the final product. The latest green biotech technology focuses on the use of plant cell cultures to construct active metabolites that have proven to be an essential substitute method for conquering many of the disadvantages associated with standardisation, availability, and safety issues [31].

STANDARDIZATION OF NATURAL IMMUNOSTIMULANTS

A. *Tinospora Crispa*

Description

The family Menispermaceae includes the tree *Tinospora crispa* (TC) [32]. TC's antibacterial, antihyperglycemic, antiparasitic, antioxidant, cardiovascular,anti-atherosclerosis, antiproliferative, and immunomodulatory properties have been discovered [33 - 35].

Collection and Extraction

The whole plants of TC were obtained. The pulverised stems of TC were extracted for 72 hours at room temperature with 80 percent ethyl alcohol (3 x 3 litres) & then filtered using Whatman No. 1 filter paper.The extra solvent was vaporized from the filtrate using rotary evaporator at temperature between 55 & 60°C.

Standardization

The TC extract was standardized by HPLC with the following conditions:

Apparatus: Waters (USA)

Detectors: 2998 Photodiode Array Detector

Column: RP, Xbridge® C18 (5 µm, 250 mm x 4.6 mm id)

Mobile phase: Acetonitrile & water + 0.02% of trifluoroacetic acid

Method: Isocratic elution

Procedure: 10:90 acetonitrile–water (10 minutes), then gradient changed to 25:75 (25 minutes).

Flow rate: 1.2 ml/min

Wavelength: Recording of UV spectrum (DAD): 210-380 nm,

Quantification of UV traces – 254 nm

Standards: Syringin & Magnoflorine

100 mg of TCE was dissolved in 1 ml of methanol, then filtered using a 0.45 µm Millipore filter before being injected into the HPLC system. The HPLC was validated for extract standardization by analysing a set of parameters: limit of detection (LOD), limit of quantification (LOQ), linearity, and precision. By comparing their retention durations & UV spectra with that of standards run independently, the standard substances syringin & magnoflorine in TCE were detected and identified.

Immunomodulatory Assays

To study the immunostimulatory effects of TCE following assays or studies were performed in male Wistar Kyoto rats:

1. Neutrophil migration assay
2. Determination of Mac-1 expression
3. Determination of phagocytosis
4. Assay for splenic lymphocytes proliferation
5. T-lymphocyte phenotyping using flow cytometric assessment
6. Quantification of Th1/Th2 cytokines

Results

Standardization

The two marker substances, syringin & magnoflorine were the basis of standardization of TCE. The results of standardization and quantitative analysis of marker compounds are mentioned in Tables **4** and **5**., respectively.

The correlation coefficient (r^2) of 0.998 was obtained from the calibration curve plotted for the standard solution of syringin at the concentration range of 62.5-1000 µg/ml. To ensure that the results were consistent, the relative standard deviation (percent RSD) was determined.

The percent RSD values of peak area & retention time were 0.77 µg/ml & 0.85 min, respectively, for intra-assay precision, whereas the percent RSD of the mean area under peak & retention time were 7.73 µg/ml & 1.98 min, respectively, for the interday assay.

The LOD of syringin was observed to be 3.11 ng/ml & the LOQ was observed to be 9.443 ng/ml. The correlation coefficient (r^2) of 0.9978 was obtained for magnoflorine & the calibration curve was linear at the concentration range of 62.5-1000 µg/ml. The percent RSD values for intra-assay precision of peak area & retention time were 0.241 µg/ml & 0.0111 min, respectively, while for interday precision, the percent RSD values of peak area & retention time were 2.78 µg/ml & 0.583 min, respectively and thus it demonstrated the reproducibility of the results. The LOD of magnoflorine was observed to be 7.792 ng/ml & the LOQ was observed to be 23.613 ng/ml.

Table 4. Results of standardization of TCE [36].

Sr. No.	Method	Wavelength	Marker Compounds	Retention Time (minutes)	
				Standard	TCE
1)	Reversed-phase HPLC	254 nm	Syringin	6.460	6.360
			Magnoflorine	20.960	20.967

Table 5. Quantitative determination of marker compounds [36].

Sr. No.	Method	Marker Compounds	Concentration of TCE (µg/mL)
1)	HPLC	Syringin	466.92±2.23
		Magnoflorine	281.21±2.078

Immunomodulatory Assays

The extract of TC triggered cell-mediated immunity by increasing neutrophil chemotactic and phagocytic action as well as the expression of the proinflammatory integrin Mac-1.TCE increased the production of splenocytes while also increasing the production of Th1 & Th2 cytokines. According to the results of the studies, the ethanolic extract of TC appears to have powerful immunostimulatory characteristics [36].

B. *Mangifera Indica & Curcuma Domestica*

Description

In male albino ICR mice, the immunostimulatory effects of methanolic extracts of *Mangifera indica* leaves & *Curcuma domestica* rhizomes on the adaptive & innate immune systems were investigated.

Collection and Extraction

The plants of *Mangifera indica* & *Curcuma domestica* were collected & labeled as MI & CD correspondingly. A mechanical grinder was used to powder the air-dried plant materials. The dried powdered plant specimen was extracted three times using 99.5 percent methanol using the cold maceration technique. Filtration of the crude extracts was done using Whatman no. 1 filter paper. The rotary evaporation technique was used to evaporate the solvent.

Phytochemical Screening

Preliminary phytochemical analysis was used to detect several plant elements such as alkaloids, phenolics, flavonoids, steroid, saponin, and triterpenes in the methanol extracts of the plants utilising the Malaysian Herbal Monograph 2009 methodology [37].

Standardization

The HPLC analysis was performed using following circumstances:

Apparatus: Waters

Sampler: 2707 auto sampler

Detectors: 2998 photodiode array detector, 2475 multi fluorescence detector

Controller: 600 controller

Degasser: In-line degasser AF

Column: HyPURITY C18 (4.60 x 250 mm, 5μm)

Standards: MangiferinM3547 & curcumin C1386

Mobile phase:Potassium dihydrogen 0.01 molar orthophosphate solution pH 2.7 ± 0.2 (I), acetonitrile (II)

Method: Isocratic elution

Flow rate: 1 ml/min

Ratio of mobile: For MI & its reference compound- 15:85 (v/v) & for CD & its reference phase solvents compound- 40:60 (v/v) (I:II)

Detection wavelength: 254 nm

Data gathering and peak assessment were accomplished by using Empower Pro System with a modest modulation.

Parameters such as limits of quantification (LOQ), & detection (LOD), linearity, precision, were evaluated for the validation of the reversed-phase HPLC method. The LOD was calculated by measuring the standard deviation (σ) of the results of the minimum concentration in a calibration curve of six runs (n=5).The slope of the calibration curves of external standards was utilised to determine LOQ. The linearity was evaluated *via* linear calibration assessment.To calculate the correlation coefficient (r^2), calibration curves were utilised. The precision of the technique was measured using intra-assay and inter-assay validation. For mangiferin & curcumin, calibration plots were produced at concentrations of 15.625 to 1000 μg/ml & 0.3 to1mg/ml, correspondingly. The related compound graph was produced as an area *versus* concentration graph. Extract and standard substance concentrations of 10 mg/ml & 1 mg/ml, correspondingly, were separately injected three times during one day & on three different days. The RSD & slope (S) of the calibration curves were used to determine LOD & LOQ using the following formulas: LOD = 3.3 x (RSD/S) & LOQ = 10 x (RSD/S).

Immunomodulatory Assays

The immunostimulatory properties of the extracts were studied using the following tests or assays:

1. Innate immune response test

2. Adaptive immune response test

3. Test for white blood cell (WBC) count

4. Spleen index (SI) test

5. Determination of haemagglutination antibody (HA)

6. Assessment of the delayed type of hypersensitivity (DTH) response.

Results

Phytochemical Screening

The MI methanolic extract comprised steroids and phenolics (tannins), while the CD extract comprised triterpenes, phenolics (tannins), alkaloids, and flavonoids, according to the qualitative preliminary phytoconstituent analysis (Table **6**).

Table 6. Preliminary phytoconstituent analysis of the *Mangifera indica* & *Curcuma domestica* methanolic extracts [38].

Sr. No.	Phytoconstituents	*Mangifera indica*	*Curcuma domestica*
1)	Saponin	-	-
2)	Flavonoids	-	+
3)	Steroids	++	-
4)	Alkaloids	-	++
5)	Phenolics (tannin)	+	+
6)	Triterpene	-	+++

Note: Not present; +: Mildly present; ++: Moderately present; +++: Extremely present.

Standardization

The results of standardization are mentioned in Table **7**. The correlation coefficient (r^2) for the mangiferin calibration curve was 0.993, and the curve obtained by plotting was linear throughout the concentration range of 15.625 to 1000 μg/ml, whereas the correlation coefficient (r^2) for curcumin was 0.957, for the concentration range of 0.3 to 1 mg/ml of standard curcumin.

Table 7. Standardization results of MI & CD methanol extract [38].

Sr. No.	Method	Wavelength (nm)	Active Constituents	Retention Time (minutes)		Concentration Found in Extract (mg/g)
				Standard	Extract	
1)	HPLC	254	Mangiferin	2.959	2.947	172
			Curcumin	4.289	4.247	80

Immunomodulatory Assays

Mangifera indica leaves (160 mg/kg) & *Curcuma domestica* rhizomes (200 mg/kg) methanolic extracts operate as effective immunostimulatory substances by raising cell-mediated & humoral immune responses, hence improving both the adaptive & innate components of the immune system. The rhizome of *Curcuma domestica* is a more potent immunostimulant than that of the leaves of *Mangifera indica* [38].

C. *Stereospermum Suaveolens*

Description

Stereospermum suaveolens (Bignoniaceae) roots & bark are utilized to treat blood diseases, liver illnesses, inflammations, pain, fevers, and asthma, *etc* [39]. Antioxidant, hepato protective, anti- hyperglycemic, anticancer & anti-inflammatory effects of the plant have been investigated [40]. Dehydro-α-lapachone & lapachol are the major active elements of *S. suaveolens* root. In albino rats, the immunomodulatory effect of standardized root extract of *S. suaveolens* was investigated.

Collection and Extraction

S. suaveolens roots were collected. The air-dried root material (500 g) was pulverized in a grinder, & the extraction was done with ethanol (70 percent) for 15 days at 25°C using the cold maceration methodology. The crude extract was filtered, evaporated using a rotary evaporator (at 40°C), & then lyophilized. 12.38 percent (w/w) yield was attained.

Phytochemical Analysis

For the identification of different phytochemicals, a preliminary phytochemical assessment of the crude extract of *S. suaveolens* was carried out. Standard colour reaction procedures were used for the analysis [41].

Standardization

Dehydro-α-lapachone & lapachol, the major bioactive components of *S.suaveolens*root extract (SSRE), were used to standardize the extract. The HPLC instrument consisting of Luna C18 (2) 100 Å, 250 x 4.6 mm filled with 5 μm particles column was utilised for this purpose. Methanol and a 5 percent acetic acid aqueous solution (80:20 v/v) formed the mobile phase. The detection wavelength chosen was 278 nm. The maximum run time was kept at 30 minutes, with a flow rate of 1 ml/min and a consistent column temperature of 25°C. The quan titative measurements of dehydro-α- lapachone & lapachol in the extract were carried out using the relevant calibration curves.

Immunomodulatory Assays

The immunostimulatory activity of the extract was checked by following tests:

1. Total & differential leukocyte count (TLC & DLC)

2. NBT reduction test

3. Delayed type hypersensitivity (DTH) response

4. Neutrophil adhesion test

5. Carbon clearance test

Results

Phytochemical Analysis

The preliminary phytochemical examination of SSRE yielded optimistic results for the occurrence of saponins, flavonoids, carbohydrates, terpenoids, tannins, gums, steroids, & alkaloids as significant phytoconstituents.

Standardization

The results of the standardization of SSRE are mentioned in Table **8**.

Table 8. Standardization results of SSRE [42].

Sr. No.	Method	Wavelength (nm)	Active Constituents of SSRE	Retention Time (minutes)	Content Present in SSRE (%) (w/w)
1)	RP-HPLC	278	Dehydro-α-lapachone	5.52±0.04	0.043±0.003
			Lapachol	7.87±0.09	0.16±0.002

Immunomodulatory Assays

In small dose concentration, SSRE displays immunostimulatory capabilities, believing that lapachol & its derivative dehydro-α-lapachone are the major active components. In lower doses to 300 mg/kg body weight, SSRE displays non-specific immunostimulatory effect [42].

D. *Barleria Prionitis*

Description

Barleria prionitis Linn. (Family- Acanthaceae), a significant Ayurvedic medicinal plant in India, has traditionally been used to cure a range of diseases, such as nervine & skin diseases, swellings, arthritic & rheumatic disorders, gout,and moreover functions as an immunorestorative [43]. Anti-respiratory syncytial virus, anti- arthritic, hepatoprotective and anti-inflammatory properties have been described, as well as anti-hepatotoxic, anti-stress, & immunorestorative, glutathione S-transferase, acetylcholinesterase suppressive, & anti-bacterial properties are also studied [44 - 47].

Collection and Storage

The airborne portions of *Barleria prionitis* (BP), at the flowering stage, were collected. The clean, shade-dried fresh airborne portions were ground coarse to fine and sieved using mesh sieve # 20 before being kept in a sealed vessel for future use.

Extraction

The shade dried & coarse-finely ground airborne portions (1 kg) of BP were extracted sequentially utilizing petroleum ether (60-80°C) & methanol using the Soxhlet apparatus.The methanolic extract was dried using a vacuum at 50°C, and the extractive value (percent w/w) was reported to be 16.82 of the dry weight of plant matter. The methanolic extract (100 g) suspended in 200 ml of 20% v/v methanol in distilled water was segregated sequentially in a separating funnel with varying quantities of n-butanol until total separation. The n-butanol fractions were mixed & dried under vacuum to yield the iridoids fraction (IFBp). The extraction yield of IFBp in the methanolic extract from BP was reported to be 42.83 percent w/w.

Phytochemical Screening

For detection of various phytoconstituents, IFBp was analyzed by preliminary phytoconstituent analysis [48].

Standardization

The composition of IFBp was analysed using the following conditions:\

Equipment: Camag HPTLC equipment

Applicator: Linomat V specimen applicator

TLC chamber: Camag Twin - TroughTLC chamber

Scanner: Camag TLC scanner III

Software: Wincats integration software

Plates: HPTLC plates (10 × 20 cm) with an aluminium backing & a 200 nm thick layer of silica gel 60 F254

Biological markers: Major iridoids in BP: shanzhiside methyl ester & barlerin

Application rate: 1 µl/15 s

Mobile phase: Chloroform-methanol (80:20 v/v)

Radiation source: Deuterium lamp

Scanning wavelength: 240 nm

Methanol solvent was utilised to make stock solutions for the samples and reference indicators.Various concentrations (5, 10 & 15 µl) from stock solutions of methanolic extract (3 mg/ml) and IFBp (2 mg/ml) from BP were spotted in the format of bands of width 6 mm on the plate using a Linomat V specimen applicator. From stock solutions of shanzhiside methyl ester and barlerin (100 µg/ml), various volumes such as 2, 4, 6, 8, and 10 µl were spotted on TLC plates to achieve concentrations of 200, 400, 600, 800, and 1000 ng for each spot. In a Camag twin-trough TLC chamber, the chromatogram was generated up to 80 mm using chamber saturation (20 min) circumstances. TLC plates were left to dry in an air current after development with the use of an air dryer. Camag TLC scanner III was used to conduct densitometric scanning at the absorbance mode of 240 nm. The data of peak area displayed against the respective concentrations was processed using linear regression analysis.

Immunomodulatory Assays

Albino mice were used to investigate the *in-vivo* immunomodulatory actions of the iridoids fraction (IFBp) on humoral & cellular immune responses to antigenic provocation by sheep erythrocytes, & utilising neutrophil adhesion assay, phagocytic action, & cyclophosphamide-induced myelosuppression. The nitroblue tetrazolium (NBT) assay and neutrophil candidacidal test were used in the *in-vivo* experiments.

Results

Phytochemical Screening

The preliminary phytoconstituent analysis of IFBp indicated a high amount of iridoids.

Standardization

IFBp was standardised for the overall content of key ingredients before its immunomodulatory actions were assessed. The proposed HPTLC procedure is selective for identifying shanzhiside methyl ester and barlerin in methanolic extract and IFBp from BP. The results of standardization are mentioned in Table **9**. The calibration curves for shanzhiside methyl ester and barlerin were linear over range of 200-1000 ng/ml, and their regression equations (correlation coefficient) were $y = 3.9175x + 482.9$ ($r^2 = 0.9956$) and $y = 4.2297x + 301.33$ ($r^2 = 0.9932$), correspondingly, where y is the response as peak area & x is the content.

Table 9. Standardization results of *Barleria prionitis* methanol extract & iridoids fraction (IFBp) [49].

Sr. No.	Method	Wavelength (nm)	Active Constituents	Retention Factor			Content Present (% w/w)	
				Standard	Methanol Extract	IFBp	Methanol Extract	IFBp
1)	HPTLC	240	Shanzhiside methyl ester	0.30	0.31	0.29	4.91 ±0.21	21.55 ±2.40
			Barlerin	0.48	0.47	0.49	4.69 ±0.15	10.03 ±1.69

Immunomodulatory Assays

IFBp has the ability to trigger both humoral and cellular immune responses. IFBp is a powerful immunostimulant, as it activates both specific and non-specific immunological systems [49].

STANDARDIZATION OF NATURAL IMMUNOSUPPRESSANTS

A. *Phyllanthus Amarus*

Description

Phyllanthus amarus belonging to the family- Euphorbiaceae is of great importance because of its vast range of physiological functions, which include antiviral (against Hepatitis B), anti-inflammatory, antimutagenic, antimicrobial, anticarcinogenic, nephroprotective, cardioprotective, hepatoprotective, and hypoglycemic [50, 51]. *P. amarus* has a wide range of therapeutic effects thanks to its phytochemicals, which include sterols, alkaloids, flavonoids, polyphenols, ellagitannins, lignans, triterpenes, and essential oils [52].

Collection and Extraction

The whole plants of *P. amarus* were obtained. About 1 Kg of plant materials was pulverised and extracted for 72 hours in 80 percent ethanol (3 x 3 L) at room temperature before being strained through Whatman® Grade 1 filter paper. Using a rotary evaporator, the accumulated filtrate was evaporated at a temperature between 55°C and 60°C to remove the excessive solvent at reduced pressure. The quantity of extracts achieved was 108 g (10.8 percent weight/weight).

Standardization

The HPLC assessment of *P. amarus* ethanolic extract (80%) was carried out by using the following circumstances:

Column: Reverse-phase C-18 column (250 mm x 4.6 mm ID, 5 m, XBridge™)

Detector: Photodiode array (PDA) detector (Waters 2998)

Wavelengths range: 205 to 270 nm

Standard I: Corilagin, gallic acid, geraniin, ellagic acid

Mobile phase: Gradient elution using acetonitrile 99.99 percent (solvent I)

and orthophosphoric acid 0.2 percent (solvent II)

Flow rate: 0.6 ml/min

Method: 5-70 percent I (0 to 15 min),

70 to 95 percent I (15 to 30 min),

and pump I was held at 95 percent for 20 minutes.

Standard II: Lignans (phyllanthin and hypophyllanthin)

Flow rate: 0.4 ml/min

Mobile phase: Acetonitrile (I) and water (acidified using 0.1 percent orthophosphoric acid) (II) that was isocratically eluted using 5 percent II, and then elevated to 95 percent over 20 minutes and held at 95 percent for 15 minutes [54].

Using two distinct chromatographic settings, constituents of the extracts and standard substances were detected and quantified [53].

The validation of HPLC for the standardization of the extract was performed by determining linearity, precision, and limits of detection (LOD) and quantification (LOQ).

Immunomodulatory Assays

The following tests/assays were performed to check the immunosuppressive effects in Wistar-Kyoto rats of the obtained extract:

1. Cell migration assay
2. CD11b & CD18 integrin expression on leukocytes
3. Phagocytic assay
4. Antigenic stimulus
5. Assay for T & B lymphocytes proliferation
6. Flow cytometric analysis for T lymphocyte phenotyping
7. Quantification of Th1/Th2 cytokines
8. Cell viability assay

Results

Standardization

The extract of *P. amarus* revealed the presence of six main components by the chromatograms using reversed-phase HPLC, namely corilagin, gallic acid, geraniin, ellagic acid, phyllanthin and hypophyllanthin. These phenolic constituents were recognized as main peaks in the chromatograms with different retention times. The details are mentioned in Table **10**.

The standard curve plotted for reference standard of corilagin from the concentration range of 62.5 to 500 µg/ml gives a correlation coefficient (r^2) of 0.996.

For the inter-day assay, the relative standard deviations (percent RSDs) of the average area under the peak and average retention time were 1.814 percent and 0.932 percent, respectively, while the percent RSD values for intra-assay precision of peak area and retention time were 3.68 percent and 1.092 percent, respectively, confirming the results' reliability. The LOD and LOQ of corilagin were 1.863 and 5.651 ng/ml, correspondingly.

The standard curve for phyllanthin and hypophyllanthin from the concentration range of 31.25 to 250 µg/ml, was achieved with r^2 values of 0.9970 and 0.9973, correspondingly.

The reproducibility of the outcomes was illustrated, with percent RSD values of the peak area and retention time of 1.63 percent and 0.216 percent, respectively, for hypophyllanthin & 8.173 percent and 0.136 percent, respectively, for phyllanthin for the inter-day assay precision,

The reproducibility of the results was illustrated, with percent RSD values of the peak area and retention time for hypophyllanthin of 1.63 percent and 0.216 percent, respectively, and 8.173 percent and 0.136 percent, respectively, for phyllanthin for the inter-day assay precision, while the percent RSD values for intra-assay precision were 6.172 percent and 0.858 percent for the peak area and retention time, respectively, for hypophyllanthin & 7.252 percent and 0.321 percent, respectively, for phyllanthin.

The LOD and LOQ for hypophyllanthin were reported to be 2.331 and 7.0712 ng/ml, correspondingly, whereas the LOD and LOQ for phyllanthin were 5.481 and 16.621 ng/ml, respectively.

Immunomodulatory Assays

Through multiple mechanisms, the standardized ethanolic extract of *P. amarus* could inhibit the immunological response of specific and non-specific immunity in Wistar-Kyoto rats. The extract showed significant suppression of neutrophil phagocytic action by downregulating the percentage of CD11b and CD18 expression in neutrophils, as well as chemotaxis and *E. coli* phagocytosis by neutrophils. The plant extract influenced early and late events of lymphocyte stimulation in splenic lymphocytes, such as the secretion of Thl and Th2 cytokines, lymphocyte proliferation, and CD4+ and CD8+ expression. Thus, *P. amarus* has a potent immunosuppressive effect [55].

Table 10. Standardization results of *P. amarus* extract [55].

Sr. No.	Method	Wavelength (nm)	Major Constituents	Retention Time (min)	Concentration in Extract (μg/mL)
1)	RP-HPLC	205-270	Gallic acid	8.187±0.0072	181.17±0.55
			Geraniin	23.709±0.078	168.19±1.12
			Corilagin	26.519±0.370	318.14±0.46
			Phyllanthin	27.235±0.095	99.49±0.078
			Hypophyllanthin	28.081±0.117	108.11±0.48
			Ellagic acid	33.595±0.138	605.19±0.23

B. *Zingiber Zerumbet*

Description

The rhizomes of *Zingiber zerumbet* (L.) belonging to the family Zingiberaceae have been extensively used as condiments, as traditional health supplements and as a therapy to cure several forms of immunity diseases such as allergies, inflammation, asthma, rheumatoid arthritis, bacterial infections, and oedema. The natural drug has also been commonly used to treat haemorrhoids, vertigo, peptic ulcer, debility, anorexia, coughs, lesions, and injuries [56]. Antioxidant, antimicrobial, larvicidal, anti-inflammatory, immunomodulation, antihyperlipidemic, antihyperglycemic, and anthelmintic characteristics were all demonstrated in *Z. zerumbet* rhizomes [57].

Collection and Extraction

Z. zerumbet rhizomes were collected and chopped into small pieces. Further, the pieces were air-dried at room temperature below the shade and ground into a coarse powder. For the extraction of the powdered material (1.75 kg), 80 percent ethanol (3x3 L) was employed, and the extraction was carried out for three days at 25°C. The filtrates obtained were concentrated by using a rotary evaporator at 37-40°C, then lyophilized to obtain a crude *Z. zerumbet* extract (248.0 g) [58]. At 4°C, the crude extract was stored until further use.

Standardization

Reversed-phase HPLC

The HPLC assessment of *Z. zerumbet* ethanolic extract (80%) was carried out by using the following conditions:

Stock solution: 80% ethanolic extract of *Z. zerumbet* (3 mg/ml)

Reference standard: Solution of zerumbone (1 mg/ml)

Concentration range: 125 to 1000 µg/ml in a series of two-fold dilutions.

Wavelength: 250 nm

Column: Xbridge® C-18 (4.6 x 250 mm, 5 µm), and

Detector: PDA (Waters 2998).

Mobile phase: Gradient elution method,water (Solvent I),

acetonitrile (Solvent II)

Flow rate: 1.2 ml/min.

All the samples and standard solutions were sonicated for 15 minutes before filtration using a 0.45 µmMillex PTFE membrane. The extract was standardized on the grounds of the reference standard zerumbone. The diluted extract and reference standard were determined individually. The starting composition was 65 percent Solvent II & further, it was followed by elevating Solvent II to 70 percent in 10 minutes. The Solvent II concentration was gradually increased to 75 percent until 16 minutes had passed. The determination of constituents in the sample was done by comparing the retention times and UV-Vis spectra of the sample peaks with the reference peak. The standard curve for the reference standard was constructed using four concentrations of prepared standard dilution *vs.* the areas under the peaks. The standard curve equations were used to measure the components in the extract.

The International Conference on Harmonisation (ICH) guideline was implemented to validate the HPLC technique and analytical method utilized in the investigation (ICH, 2005). The validation included linearity, accuracy, precision, the limit of detection (LOD), and the limit of quantification (LOQ). The accuracy was achieved by spiking the known reference standard at a specific amount to the blank sample over nine determinations (three concentrations/three replicates). Precision was obtained from intra-assay & inter-day precisions. Intra-assay precision was obtained using the same procedure over a short period of time, while inter-day precision was obtained on various days. Using four dilutions of the reference standard (zerumbone), made in triplicate, a calibration curve was prepared by plotting respective peak areas *versus* the concentration of the standards. The linearity value was revealed by the correlation coefficient (R^2) acquired from the standard curve equation. The residual standard deviation (RSD) and slope (S) of the calibration curve were used to derive the LOD and LOQ, which were calculated using the following formulas: LOQ = 10 x (RSD/S) and LOD = 3.3 x (RSD/S).

LC-MS/MS

Ethanolic extract (80%) of *Z. zerumbet* was analyzed by LC-MS/MS for detection of bioactive and secondary metabolites by using the following conditions:

Instrument: AB Sciex 3200QTrap LC-MS/MS with

Flexar FX-15 series UHPLC

Column: Phenomenex synergy fusion column

(100 x 2.1 mm; particle size, 3 µm)

Capillary voltage: 4500 V

100-1500 m/z (full scan)and 50-1500 m/z (MS/MS scan)

Source temperature: 500°C

Eluent: Formic acid in water (0.1%) with 5-mM ammonium formate(I)

Acetonitrile with 0.1 percent formic acid and 5-mM ammonium formate(II)

The gradient programme began with 20-30 percent eluent II for 10 minutes before escalating to 40 percent eluent II for another 10 minutes. The eluent II concentration was increased to 50 percent for 10 minutes before increasing to 90 percent for the next 20 minutes. Again for 10 minutes, 90 percent eluent II was kept constant, followed by a reduction to 20 percent eluent II for the next 10 minutes. A steady flow rate of 250 µl/min was sustained during the investigation, with an injection volume of 20 µl, and negative ionization mode was employed. The observed constituent peaks were compared to a mass spectrum by using ACD Labs advanced chemometrics mass fragmentations prediction software.

Immunomodulatory Assays

The immunosuppressive activity of the standardized extract of *Zingiber zerumbet* on innate immunological responses in Wistar rats was studied by following assays:

1. Cell migration assay

2. CD11b/CD18 integrin expression assay

3. Phagocytic assay

4. ROS production assay

5. Evaluation of the levels of plasma lysozyme & ceruloplasmin

Results

RP-HPLC

In the HPLC chromatogram of ethanolic extract (80%) of *Z. zerumbet*, zerumbone was found as a prominent peak and with good concentration. Details are mentioned in Table **11**. The identity was verified by comparing the peak to the chromatogram of the reference standard, zerumbone.

The zerumbone (125-1000 µg/ml) standard curve had an R^2 value of 0.999, indicating high accuracy. The precision and repeatability of the HPLC analysis were verified using the percent RSD of intra-day and inter-day assay precision of retention times and respective peak areas Table **12**. In terms of retention time, the percent RSD for intraday and interday assay precision was 0.93 and 1.53 percent, respectively, while the percent RSD for peak area was 0.57 and 5.92 percent, respectively. The LOD of zerumbone was determined to be 0.117 µg/ml, and the LOQ was reported to be 0.355 µg/ml using this HPLC technique.

Table 11. Standardization results of *Z. zerumbet* extract [59].

Sr. No.	Method	Wavelength (nm)	Major Constituent	Retention Time (min)		Concentration in extract (mg/g)
				Standard	Extract	
1)	RP-HPLC	250	Zerumbone	9.745	9.745	242.73

LC-MS/MS

Table 12. Retention times, MS^2 fragments of tentative chemical markers in *Z.zerumbet* [59].

Sr. No.	Tentative Compounds Identified	MS^2 Fragmentation Ions	Molecular Ion Peak $(M-H)^-$	Retention Time (min)
1	Ethyl gallate	182, 169, 125, 69	197[a]	2.317
2	Gallic acid	169, 125[a], 95, 69	169	2.650
3	Catechin	271, 261, 245, 201, 125	289[a]	4.334

(Table 12) cont.....

Sr. No.	Tentative Compounds Identified	MS^2 Fragmentation Ions	Molecular Ion Peak (M-H)$^-$	Retention Time (min)
4	Kaempferol Rhamnoside	432, 327, 284[a], 256, 227, 212, 163	430	5.063
5	Kaempferol	267, 257, 229, 227, 187, 169, 143	285[a]	5.680
6	Kaempferol-3-O-(2″, 4″-diacetyl) rhamnoside isomer	516, 474, 456, 396, 285[a], 256, 228, 151	514	6.130
7	Kaempferol-3-O-(2″- or 3″-acetyl) rhamnoside isomer	474, 414, 291, 287[a], 256, 233, 228, 152	472	9.060
8	Kaempferol methylether	299, 284, 256[a], 228, 211, 183, 171, 132	298	9.331
9	Kaempferol methylether isomer	300, 256[a], 228, 212, 184, 163	298	10.848
10	Kaempferol-3-O-(3″,4″-diacetyl) rhamnoside isomer	516, 474, 456, 414, 299, 291, 287[a], 268,256, 228, 212, 152	514	12.533
11	Kaempferol-3-O-(3″,4″-diacetyl) rhamnoside isomer2	516, 474, 456, 414, 291, 286[a], 261, 256,240, 228, 212, 59	514	13.431
12	Kaempferol glucoside conjugate	556, 497, 455, 289, 284[a], 255, 227	557	16.409
13	Kaempferol glucoside conjugate	557, 498, 456, 289, 284[a], 256, 228	556	16.410
14	Desmethoxycurcumin	337, 322, 217, 202, 198, 173, 158, 134, 119[a]	337	20.510
15	Curcumin	367[a], 352, 247, 217, 202, 173, 149, 134, 119	367	20.622
16	Bisdesmethoxycurcumin	289, 187, 161, 143, 119	307[a]	21.016
17	Zerumbone	217, 201, 173, 168, 158[a], 133, 69	217	21.914
18	Curcumin isomer	354, 325, 218, 203, 173, 149, 134	369[a]	22.477

[a]Base peak.

Immunomodulatory Assays

The results of the assays demonstrate that the *Zingiber zerumbet* standardized extract has potential immunosuppressive properties [59].

C. *Momordica Charantia*

Description

The seeds of *Momordica charantia* L. containing alpha-momorcharin (α-MMC), is isolated and refined has a variety of pharmacological activities, including tumour growth suppression, antiviral activity, and immune response inhibition [60, 61]. α-MMC is a ribosome-inactivating protein (RIP) that belongs to the type I family of RIP's [62]. Alpha-MMC has been shown to have significant antitumor activity in breast cancer, melanoma, and other malignancies, making it an attractive therapeutic option for cancer therapy [63].

Collection, Extraction and Standardization

The seeds of bitter melon were obtained. The bitter gourd seeds were ground into a powder, and then extracted using a 50 mM acetate buffer solution (pH 6.3). At 2°C, 250 mM HCl was added to the crude extract to acidify it. The supernatant obtained following basic centrifugation was neutralized using 1 M sodium phosphate buffer (pH 7.0). The proteins were then precipitated using ammonium sulphate (AS). Additional purification of α-MMC was achieved by utilizing SP-Sepharose FF, Superdex 75, and MacroCap™ SP columns. The determination of alpha-MMC was accomplished using SDS-PAGE and gel filtration HPLC. The molecular weights of the unadulterated α-MMC were evaluated using matrix-assisted laser desorption ionization-time of flight mass spectrometry (MALDI-TOF-MS), and the N-terminal amino acid sequence analysis was done using electrospray ionisation quadrupole mass spectrometry (ESI-QUAD-MS). Ultimately, endotoxins were removed using Sephadex G-100 column chromatography, and the Limulus assay confirmed that the α-MMC solution was free from all the endotoxins.

Immunomodulatory Assays

The immunosuppression of α-MMC *via* the LRP1 receptor on monocytes was studied by following methods:

1. Evaluation of α-MMC induced apoptosis in THP-1, WIL2-S & H9 cells by flow cytometry.

2. Expression of cytokines in cell lysates of THP-1, WIL2-S & H9 cells.

3. Assays of western blotting for the LRP1 receptor protein from THP-1, WIL2-S & H9 cells.

4. Identification of MAPK signalling proteins.

5. LRP1 knockdown in THP-1 cells.

6. LRP1 silencing effects on cytokines & signalling proteins.

Results

Standardization

The pure α-MMC protein was chromatographically and electrophoretically homogeneous, as evidenced by a single band on the SDS-PAGE gel and a single peak eluted in the HPLC chromatogram. α-MMC was analysed by MALDI-TO--MS, and the real molecular weight of the protein was found to be 28551.6 Da Table **13**. The N-terminal 5-amino acid sequence N-Asp-Val-Ser-Phe-Arg was similar to the sequences of α-MMC published in the NCBI database. The discovered protein showed a typical mass spectrometric peak related to YLLMHLFNYDGK, which was similar to the sequence of α-MMC.

Table 13. Standardization results of α-MMC protein sample [66].

Sr. No.	Method	Test sample	Wavelength (nm)	Average molecular weight (Da)	Retention Time (min)	Area of peak obtained	Purity (%)
1)	HPLC	α-MMC protein	220	-	11.028	37116	>97
2)	MALDI-TOF-MS		-	28551.6	-	-	-

Immunomodulatory Assays

Cytotoxicity and immunomodulatory actions on macrophages/monocytes may be a significant mechanism and a leading contributor in α-MMC immunosuppression. Due to the wide distribution of the LRP1 receptor in macrophages/monocytes, α-MMC is expected to suppress the secretion of cytokines from polarized M2 macrophages in the cancer microenvironment, and α-MMC is very likely to kill M2 macrophages to suppress tumour growth and metastasis [64 - 66].

D. *Terminalia Chebula*

Description

Terminalia chebula is a common evergreen tree in India and south-east Asia (Family- Combretaceae). The fruit of *T. chebula* has been used widely as an anti-diarrheal, astringent, anti-bleeding, and antitussive agent [67]. *T. chebula* has antioxidant and cytoprotective actions in rat primary hepatocytes, liver, and kidney, as well as protective benefits against drug-induced hepatic, gastric, intestinal, and renal impairments [68, 69]. *T.chebula* has been shown to have anti-inflammatory properties in local and systemic anaphylaxis as well as LPS-activated RAW264.7 cells in recent investigations [70].

Collection, Extraction and Standardization

The exterior appearances and histological morphology of the acquired dried ripe fruits of *T. chebula* were used to identify them. The standardized extract of *T. chebula* fruits, NDI10218, was produced at Bioland Co., Ltd. The powder derived by coarse milling the fruits of *T. chebula* was extracted for 6 hours at room temperature using 50 percent ethanol. After filtration, at low pressure, the extract was evaporated and vacuum dried to powder. Standardization of NDI10218 was carried out using chebulagic acid as an indicator marker. The authentication of NDI10218 was accomplished by comparing the sample retention time to that of legitimate standards. Chebulinic acid, chebulic acid, corilagin, and punicalagin were bought from Chromadex, while gallic acid was bought from Sigma. Chebulagic acid was purified [71]. An HPLC system (Agilent 1200) with a Shiseido Capcell Pack C18 4.6 x 150 mm column was utilised for the investigation. A mobile phase of aqueous phosphoric acid (0.1 percent) and acetonitrile mixture (80:20) was utilised at a flow rate of 1 ml/min. The absorption peaks were identified at 216 nm and compared to standard marker compounds. The total chebulagic acid concentration in NDI10218 was measured to be 4.62 percent (w/w).

Immunosuppressive Effect as an Anti-arthritic Treatment

Rheumatoid arthritis (RA) is a complicated autoimmune illness that is refractory to treatment. Articular pain, polyarthritis, and joint damage are all symptoms. It is caused by a variety of pathogenic processes, such as local and systemic inflammation, humoral and cellular immunological responses, massive angiogenesis, and osteoclast and matrix metalloproteinases mediated damage of bone and cartilage [72].

As RA is an autoimmune disease, the use of immunosuppressants is one of the various ways of treatment for this disease. The anti-arthritic actions of NDI10218, a standardized ethanol extract of *T. chebula*, in mouse collagen-induced arthritis (CIA) were studied by performing the following tests:

1. Histological evaluation of the knee joints.

2. Enzyme-linked immunosorbent assay (ELISA).

3. Flow cytometry.

Results

Standardization

HPLC was used to establish the fingerprint of NDI10218, a standardized ethanol extract of *T. chebula*. On the basis of the extract's chromatogram, six primary constituent peaks were identified. The retention times for the six main component peaks detected are mentioned in Table **14**.

Table 14. Standardization results of NDI10218 obtained from *T. chebula* fruits [73].

Sr. No.	Method	Wavelength (nm)	Major Constituents	Retention Time (min)
1)	HPLC	216	Chebulic acid	5.20
			Gallic acid	8.37
			Punicalagin	27.52
			Corilagin	39.06
			Chebulagic acid	50.72
			Chebulinic acid	61.40

Immunosuppressive and Anti-arthritic Effects

NDI10218 reduced the amount of T cells and activated T cells in local lymph nodes and inhibited the migration of T cells and granulocytes to the impacted synovial joints. These findings demonstrate NDI10218's immunosuppressive activity on T cell proliferation and activation, as well as immune cells migration to the afflicted locations [73].

STANDARDIZATION OF IMMUNOMODULATING TISSUE CULTURED PLANTS

Echinacea Angustifolia

Description

Echinacea is a commonly used term for the nine species of big, daisy-like plants from the Aster family (Compositae). Aside from the conventional usage for common cold & upper respiratory tract ailments, the extracts of echinacea have demonstrated their impact on inflammation and wound healing in rats, lowering the period and/or severity of the symptoms [74 - 76].

Cell Culture Formation & Extraction

Echinacea angustifolia cell cultures were obtained from sterile root explants. After callus formation and preliminary testing, the cell culture was adjusted to proliferate in liquid suspension using Gamborg B5 culture media. Fourteen days old culture suspensions developed at 25°C, were treated for extract production using mechanical homogenization & filtering. The dissolved strained homogenate was further subjected to a chromatographic column comprising XAD4 resin for enhancing its principle active constituents. Ethanol was used to elute the compounds that remained in the column post-washing, and the eluate was taken & evaporated using an evaporator. The extremely concentrated aqueous solution was subjected to lyophilization to produce the final powder extract.

Standardization

Echinacea angustifolia cell culture extract is an amber colour powder that dissolves readily in water. The product standardization was done using organic maltodextrins and titrated in echinacoside at a concentration of 4%. The extract's HPLC analysis revealed various peaks, as follows: the primary peak corresponds to echinacoside, while smaller components like chlorogenic acid, cynarin, & 1,5-di-caffeoylquinic acid (1,5-DCQ) can be attributed to derivatives of caffeoylquinic acids.

Immunomodulatory Assays

The immunomodulatory action of the extract was studied on cell line of mouse monocyte macrophage- RAW 264.7. The following tests were performed:

1. Analysis for the presence of NO_2.

2. Cell viability study using the MTT assay [77].

Echinacea extracts have significant immunomodulatory properties, which are exerted by various constituents like polysaccharides, alkylamides & caffeic acid derivatives, according to literature. In the RAW 246.7 macrophage cell line, the capability of *Echinacea angustifolia* cell culture extract to suppress the formation of the immunomodulator/anti-inflammatory biomarker nitric oxide (NO) produced by lipopolysaccharide (LPS) was investigated Table **15**.

The major biological characteristics of a titrated extract obtained from *Echinacea angustifolia* cell cultures were revealed in the study, and the strong immunomodulating potential of echinacoside was validated in biochemical and *in-vivo* assays [31].

Table 15. Standardization results of cell culture extract of *Echinacea angustifolia* [31].

Sr. No.	Method	Major Constituents	Retention Time (min)
1)	HPLC	Chlorogenic acid	7.045
		Cynarin	7.520
		1,5-DCQ	11.598
		Echinacoside	12.921

Helicteres Angustifolia

Description

Helicteres angustifolia (Family- Sterculiaceae) is a vital medicinal plant with a wide range of unique health-enhancing properties, including anti-hyperglycemic, antioxidant, anticancer, and immunomodulatory properties due to the occurrence of the huge amount of phytoconstituents in the plant [78, 79].

Extraction of Callus Suspension Cultures

Helicteres angustifolia callus suspension cultures were cleaned and accumulated for oven drying at 60°C. The dried powders were immersed for 2 hours in an ethanol solution containing 80 percent (v/v) ethanol (500 mL) using the hot reflux extraction method. The supernatants were concentrated and lyophilized into powders using the vacuum evaporation technique, which is the callus suspension culture extract (CE). The corresponding roots were extracted by the same procedure to acquire the extract of wild roots (WE). Further, at -20°C, they were stored before analysis.

Standardization

FTIR Analysis

A FTIR spectrometer was used to examine the chemical profiling of CE in contrast to WE. The dry test specimens were pulverized into fine powder utilizing potassium bromide (KBr) and subjected under high pressure till a euphotic film formed, which was then analyzed with an FTIR spectrometer (Jasco FT/IR-300).

Phytochemical Screening

Qualitative analysis of CE and WE was performed by phytochemical screening to detect the various phytoconstituents present in the extracts Table **16**.

Table 16. Various tests for phytochemical analysis of extracts [81].

Sr. No.	Phytochemical	Test
1)	Terpenoids	Salkowski test
2)	Flavonoids	Alkaline reagent test
3)	Cardiac glycosides	Keller-Killiani test
4)	Steroids	Libermann-Burchard
5)	Phenolic compounds	Ferric chloride test
6)	Saponins	Foaming test
7)	Anthraquinone glycosides	Borntrager's test
8)	Alkaloids	Wagner's reagent
9)	Triterpenoids	Libermann-Burchard

Quantitative Analysis

The extracts were tested for quantitative assessments utilizing a UV-vis spectrophotometer (Shimazu UV-1800). The total phenolic concentration (TPC), total flavonoid concentration (TFC), total saponin concentration (TSC), & total polysaccharide concentration (TPSC) of dried materials was determined, and the TPC, TFC, TSC, and TPSC values were obtained using the following formula:

$TC_{Feedstock}(mg/g) = TC_{Extract} x$ extraction yield

TPC, TPSC, TSC, or TFC concentration in the extract from dried cultures/wild roots is $TC_{Extract}(mg/g)$, while TSC, TFC, TPC, or TPSC concentration in the dried matter of cultures/wild roots is $TC_{Feedstock}(mg/g)$.

HPLC Analysis

1 mg of extract was diluted in 1 ml of methanol & passed through 0.45 µm filter (Whatman). The nine phenolic constituents were measured utilizing an HPLC instrument having an LC-NetII/ADC system controller, UV-1570 intelligent UV/VIS detector, AS-1555-10 intelligent sampler, CO-1560 intelligent column thermostat, & PU-1580 intelligent HPLC pumps. A COSMOSIL5C18-AR-II packed column (5 µm particle size, 250 x 4.6 mm internal diameter) was used to separate the samples at 25°C. Mobile phase consisted of solvent I (methanol: acetic acid: water = 10:2:88) & solvent II (methanol: acetic acid: water = 90:3:7), with a flow rate of 1 ml/min. The volume to be injected was set at 20 microlitres. HPLC grade standards of phenolic constituents were employed as reference standards (p-coumaric acid, caffeic acid, quercetin, vanillin, rutin, gallic acid, catechol, rosmarinicacid, (-)-epicatechin). The identification was done at

wavelength of 280 nm. The individual phenolic constituents were determined by comparison of their retention times to the standards.

Immunomodulatory Assays

Immunomodulatory activities of CE were assessed on macrophages RAW 264.7 using the following assays:

1. Assay for cell proliferation.

2. Examination of nitric oxide (NO) production.

3. Assay for phagocytosis.

4. Study of protective activities on damage caused by doxorubicin (DOX).

RESULTS

Standardization

Ftir Analysis

The FTIR spectra revealed that the CE & WE have several functional groups in common from 4000-400 cm^{-1}, as depicted in the Table **17**. The findings of the FTIR spectra revealed certain similarities in the chemical characteristics of CE and WE [80].

Table 17. Results of FTIR spectra of CE & WE [81].

Sr. No.	Peak Frequency (cm^{-1})	Functional Groups Detected	Approx. Type of Substances Present in the Extracts
1)	3400	OH	Polyphenolic
2)	2920	C-H (weak stretching vibration)	-
3)	1477-1625	C=C (aromatic stretching)	-
4)	1135-1031	C-O (bending vibrations)	Glycoside & polysaccharide carbohydrates
5)	940-810 & 778.14	-	Polysaccharides

Phytochemical Screening

The qualitative assessments of CE and WE revealed similar phytoconstituent compositions, as mentioned in Table **18**, suggesting the viability of employing callus suspension cultures to synthesize saponins, terpenoids, phenolic constituents, flavonoids, & triterpenoids constituents of *H. angustifolia.*

Table 18. Results of qualitative assessment of extracts [81].

Sr. No.	Phytoconstituents	Wild Root Extract	Culture Extract
1)	Steroids	-	-
2)	Flavonoids	+	+
3)	Saponins	+	+
4)	Cardiac glycosides	-	-
5)	Triterpenoids	+	+
6)	Phenolic compounds	+	+
7)	Alkaloids	-	-
8)	Terpenoids	+	+
9)	Anthraquinone glycosides	-	-

+: Present, -: Absent.

Quantitative Analysis

In relation to the extracts, CE had less TFC, TPC, and TSC levels than WE, as mentioned in the Table **19**.

Table 19. Results of quantitative determination of the extracts & dry powders [81].

Sr. No.	Sample	Extracts				Yield (%)	Dry Powders			
		TPC (mg GAE/g)	TFC (mg RE/g)	TSC (mg OAE/g)	TPSC (mg/g)		TPC (mg GAE/g)	TFC (mg RE/g)	TSC (mg OAE/g)	TPSC (mg/g)
1)	Callus culture	72.74 ±1.13	230.13±0.83	119.70 ±10.40	56.09 ±1.94	24.40	17.75 ±0.28	56.15 ±0.20	29.21 ±2.54	13.69 ±0.47
2)	Wild roots	135.92 ±1.46	330.64 ±3.03	285.10 ±12.13	44.70 ±1.85	9.00	10.99 ±0.14	29.76 ±0.27	25.66 ±1.09	4.02 ±0.17

GAE- Gallic Acid Equivalents, RE- Rutin Equivalents, OAE- Oleanolic Acid Equivalents.

HPLC Analysis

High amount of gallic acid (10.20±0.14 µg/mg), rosmarinic acid (49.94±1.34 µg/mg) & p-coumaric acid (7.35±0.08 µg/mg) was observed in WE in the HPLC evaluation. Gallic acid (6.96±0.36 µg/mg) was the highly concentrated phenolic constituent in CE, followed by catechol, quercetin, & caffeic acid. As depicted by HPLC investigation, CE is an adequate resource of phenolic constituents of *H. angustifolia*. In comparison with WE, the levels of rosmarinic acid & p-coumaric acid in CE reduced dramatically to 0.98±0.02 and 0.62±0.02 μg/mg, as described in Table **20**. Particularly, a considerable reduction in rosmarinic acid, which had a major involvement in the reduction of TPC in CE, was discovered.

Table 20. Quantification results of phenolic constituents detected by HPLC in the extracts [81].

Sr. No.	Phenolic Constituents	Wild Root Extract (μg/mg)	Culture Extract (μg/mg)
1)	Quercetin	1.27±0.04	1.25±0.03
2)	Caffeic acid	1.04±0.01	1.02±0.02
3)	Vanillin	0.09±0.00	0.05±0.00
4)	Catechol	1.47±0.05	1.45±0.04
5)	(-)-Epicatechin	Not detected	Not detected
6)	Gallic acid	10.20±0.14	6.96±0.36
7)	p-coumaric acid	7.35±0.08	0.62±0.02
8)	Rutin	Not detected	0.98±0.01
9)	Rosmarinic acid	49.94±1.34	0.98±0.02

Immunomodulatory Assays

The results suggest that the immune response of macrophages can be stimulated by CE. Therefore, CE has the capacity to enhance immunity [81].

CONCLUDING REMARKS

Natural drugs are utilized as home therapy, over-the-counter (OTC) products, raw materials, formulations, and excipients in both developed and developing countries, and they account for a significant proportion of the worldwide drug marketplace. Natural drugs are safer and have fewer side effects. Therefore, it is important to establish optimal standardization methods in order to develop high-quality, safe, and efficacious natural products. According to WHO guidelines, standardized natural drugs will be more authentic and will make it easier to assess their quality. This can only be accomplished if the herbal products are reviewed and studied using advanced standardised techniques such as UV-visible, TLC, HPLC, GC-MS, HPTLC, spectrofluorimetric, and other procedures. The quality of a natural drug must be monitored from collection to processing to the completed packaged product in order to ensure its safety and efficacy. Many government organizations should accept a more general approach to natural drug quality by accepting the WHO recommendations and publishing monographs based on the different quality parameters listed above. This will improve the regulatory process and reduce the risk of infringement. Due to many new immune disorders and illnesses, natural medicines and their phytoconstituents with potential immunomodulatory properties are gaining popularity. Because all environmental conditions are controlled, natural pharmaceuticals developed through plant tissue culture have constant growth, improved quality, and a constant quantity of phytoconstituents. This helps to overcome the drawbacks of standardising natural drugs with polyconstituents that are present in the plants.

CONSENT FOR PUBLICATION

Not applicable.

CONFLICT OF INTEREST

The authors declare no conflict of interest, financial or otherwise.

ACKNOWLEDGEMENTS

The authors would like to acknowledge STES's Smt. Kashibai Navale College of Pharmacy, Kondhwa (Bk), Pune 411048, Maharashtra for the completion of this book chapter.

REFERENCES

[1] Bhandary MJ, Chandrashekhar KR. Glimpses of ethnic herbal medicine of coastal Karnataka. Ethnobotany 2002; 14: 1-12.

[2] World Health Organization. WHO guidelines for assessing quality of herbal medicines with reference to contaminants and residues. 2007.

[3] Ortiz MV. Alternative Medicine: Incorporation into Therapeutics Topics. Am J Pharm Educ 1998; 62: 208-12.

[4] Parasuraman S, Thing G, Dhanaraj S. Polyherbal formulation: Concept of ayurveda. Pharmacogn Rev 2014; 8(16): 73-80. [http://dx.doi.org/10.4103/0973-7847.134229] [PMID: 25125878]

[5] Ravishankar B, Shukla VJ. Indian systems of medicine: a brief profile. Afr J Tradit Complement Altern Med 2008; 4(3): 319-37. [http://dx.doi.org/10.4314/ajtcam.v4i3.31226] [PMID: 20161896]

[6] Pan SY, Litscher G, Gao SH, *et al.* Historical perspective of traditional indigenous medical practices: the current renaissance and conservation of herbal resources. Evid Based Complement Alternat Med 2014; 2014: 1-20. [http://dx.doi.org/10.1155/2014/525340] [PMID: 24872833]

[7] Ekor M. The growing use of herbal medicines: issues relating to adverse reactions and challenges in monitoring safety. Front Pharmacol 2014; 4: 177. [http://dx.doi.org/10.3389/fphar.2013.00177] [PMID: 24454289]

[8] Ahmad Khan MS, Ahmad I. Herbal Medicine. New Look to Phytomedicine [Internet]. Elsevier; 2019. p. 3–13. Available from: linkinghub.elsevier.com/retrieve/pii/B978012814619400001X

[9] Mazumder MEH, Rahman S. Pharmacological Evaluation of Bangladeshi Medicinal Plants for Antioxidant Activity. Pharm Biol 2008; 46(10-11): 704-9. [http://dx.doi.org/10.1080/13880200802215735]

[10] Kulkarni O, Mukherjee S, Bhandare R, *et al.* Evaluation of comparative free-radical quenching potential of Brahmi (*Bacopa monnieri*) and Mandookparni (*Centella asiatica*). Ayu 2011; 32(2): 258-64.
[http://dx.doi.org/10.4103/0974-8520.92549] [PMID: 22408313]

[11] Patwardhan B, Warude D, Pushpangadan P, Bhatt N. Ayurveda and traditional Chinese medicine: a comparative overview. Evid Based Complement Alternat Med 2005; 2(4): 465-73.
[http://dx.doi.org/10.1093/ecam/neh140] [PMID: 16322803]

[12] Karimi A, Majlesi M, Rafieian-Kopaei M. Herbal *versus* synthetic drugs; beliefs and facts. J Nephropharmacol 2015; 4(1): 27-30.
[PMID: 28197471]

[13] Handique PJ. A brief overview on *andrographis paniculata* (burm. F) nees., a high valued medicinal plant: boon over synthetic. Asian J Sci Technol 2010; 6: 113-8.

[14] Rao EV. Modern approaches to herbal medicine. East Pharm 2000; 43: 35-40.

[15] Folashade K O, Omoregie EH, Ochogu AP., Standardization of herbal medicines - A review. Int J Biodivers Conserv 2012; 4: 3.
[http://dx.doi.org/10.5897/IJBC11.163]

[16] Joshi VK, K O Folashade, EH Omoregie, AP Ochogu, Joshi A, Dhiman KS. The Ayurvedic Pharmacopoeia of India, development and perspectives. J Ethnopharmacol 2017; 197: 32-8.
[http://dx.doi.org/10.1016/j.jep.2016.07.030] [PMID: 27404231]

[17] Bauer R. Quality Criteria and Standardization of Phytopharmaceuticals: Can Acceptable Drug Standards Be Achieved? Drug Inf J 1998; 32(1): 101-10.
[http://dx.doi.org/10.1177/009286159803200114]

[18] Calixto JB. Efficacy, safety, quality control, marketing and regulatory guidelines for herbal medicines (phytotherapeutic agents). Braz J Med Biol Res 2000; 33(2): 179-89.
[http://dx.doi.org/10.1590/S0100-879X2000000200004] [PMID: 10657057]

[19] Wani M, Parakh P, Dehghan MH, Polshettiwar S. V.V.Chopade P, Chepurwar S. Herbal Medicine and Its Standardization. Pharm Rev 2007.

[20] Choudhary N, Sekhon BS. An overview of advances in the standardization of herbal drugs. J Pharm Educ Res 2011; 2(2): 16.

[21] Singh R, Kotecha M. A review on the Standardization of herbal medicines. Int J Pharm Sci Res 2016; 7: 97-106.

[22] Jadhav RB, Patil CR, Bhpoe S, Murumkar CV. Herbal drug standardization and quality assurance of raw materials: a rational approach. 2003.

[23] Trivedi PC, Ed. Medicinal plants: traditional knowledge. New Delhi: I.K. International Pub. House; 2006. 258 p.

[24] Sachan AK, Vishnoi G, Kumar R. Need of standardization of herbal medicines in Modern era. Int J Phytomed 2016; 8(3): 300.
[http://dx.doi.org/10.5138/09750185.1847]

[25] Mosihuzzaman M, Choudhary MI. Protocols on safety, efficacy, standardization, and documentation of herbal medicine (IUPAC Technical Report). Pure Appl Chem 2008; 80(10): 2195-230.
[http://dx.doi.org/10.1351/pac200880102195]

[26] Akerele O. WHO's traditional medicine programme: progress and perspectives. WHO Chron 1984; 38(2): 76-81.
[PMID: 6475036]

[27] Indian Herbal Trade in World Scenario - Pharmacognosy [Internet]. pharmacy180.com. [cited 2022 Jan 11]. Available from: www.pharmacy180.com/article/indian-herbal-trade-in-world-scenario-51/

[28] Doshi G, Une H, Shanbhag P. Rasayans and non-rasayans herbs: Future immunodrug - Targets. Pharmacogn Rev 2013; 7(14): 92-6. [http://dx.doi.org/10.4103/0973-7847.120506] [PMID: 24347916]

[29] Gulati K, Ray A, Debnath PK, Bhattacharya SK. Immunomodulatory Indian Medicinal Plants. J Nat Rem 2002; 2(2): 121-31. [http://dx.doi.org/10.18311/jnr/2002/142]

[30] Plant Tissue Culture - an overview | ScienceDirect Topics, Modern Applications of Plant Biotechnology in Pharmaceutical Sciences, 2015.

[31] Dal Toso R, Melandri F. Echinacea angustifolia cell culture extract. Nutrafoods 2011; 10(1): 19-24. [http://dx.doi.org/10.1007/BF03223351]

[32] Choudhary MI, Ismail M, Shaari K, *et al.* cis-Clerodane-type furanoditerpenoids from Tinospora crispa. J Nat Prod 2010; 73(4): 541-7. [http://dx.doi.org/10.1021/np900551u] [PMID: 20356064]

[33] Rungruang T, Boonmars T. *In vivo* antiparasitic activity of the Thai traditional medicine plant--Tinospora crispa--against Plasmodium yoelii. Southeast Asian J Trop Med Public Health 2009; 40(5): 898-900. [PMID: 19842370]

[34] Praman S, Mulvany MJ, Williams DE, Andersen RJ, Jansakul C. Hypotensive and cardio-chronotropic constituents of Tinospora crispa and mechanisms of action on the cardiovascular system in anesthetized rats. J Ethnopharmacol 2012; 140(1): 166-78. [http://dx.doi.org/10.1016/j.jep.2012.01.006] [PMID: 22265931]

[35] Abood WN, Fahmi I, Abdulla MA, Ismail S. Immunomodulatory effect of an isolated fraction from Tinospora crispa on intracellular expression of INF-γ, IL-6 and IL-8. BMC Complement Altern Med 2014; 14(1): 205. [http://dx.doi.org/10.1186/1472-6882-14-205] [PMID: 24969238]

[36] Ahmad W, Jantan I, Kumolosasi E, Bukhari SNA. Immunostimulatory effects of the standardized extract of Tinospora crispa on innate immune responses in Wistar Kyoto rats. Drug Des Devel Ther 2015; 9: 2961-73. [PMID: 26089645]

[37] Malaysian Herbal Monograph, Volume 2 [Internet]. [cited 2021 Dec 13]. Available from: https://www.nhbs.com/malaysian-herbal-monograph-volume-2-book

[38] Kumolosasi E, Ibrahim SNA, Ahmad Shukri SM, Ahmad W. Immunostimulant activity of standardised extracts of Mangifera indica leaf and Curcuma domestica rhizome in mice. Trop J Pharm Res 2018; 17(1): 77. [http://dx.doi.org/10.4314/tjpr.v17i1.12]

[39] Srivastava N, Khatoon S, Rawat AKS, Rai V, Mehrotra S. Chromatographic estimation of p-coumaric acid and triacontanol in an Ayurvedic root drug patala (*Stereospermum suaveolens* Roxb.). J Chromatogr Sci 2009; 47(10): 936-9. [http://dx.doi.org/10.1093/chromsci/47.10.936] [PMID: 19930809]

[40] Meena A, Yadav A, Panda P, Preet K, Rao MM. Review on Stereo spermum suaveolens DC: A Potential Herb. Drug Invention Today 2015. 2(5).

[41] Harborne JB. Phytochemical Methods. Dordrecht: Springer Netherlands; 1980 [42] Maji AK, Samanta SK, Mahapatra S, Banerji P, Banerjee D. *in-vivo* immunomodulatory activity of standardized Stereospermum suaveolens (Roxb.) DC. root extract. Orient Pharm Exp Med 2014; 14(1): 47-54.

[43] Asolkar LV, Kakkar KK, Chakre OJ. Second supplement to glossary of Indian medicinal plants with active principles: part-1 (A-K), (1965-1981). New-Dehli: Publications and information directorate 1992.

[44] Chen JL, Blanc P, Stoddart CA, *et al.* New iridoids from the medicinal plant Barleria prionitis with potent activity against respiratory syncytial virus. J Nat Prod 1998; 61(10): 1295-7. [http://dx.doi.org/10.1021/np980086y] [PMID: 9784173]

[45] Singh B, Bani S, Gupta DK, Chandan BK, Kaul A. Anti-inflammatory activity of 'TAF' an active fraction from the plant Barleria prionitis Linn. J Ethnopharmacol 2003; 85(2-3): 187-93. [http://dx.doi.org/10.1016/S0378-8741(02)00358-6] [PMID: 12639739]

[46] Singh B, Chandan BK, Prabhakar A, Taneja SC, Singh J, Qazi GN. Chemistry and hepatoprotective activity of an active fraction from Barleria prionitis Linn. in experimental animals. Phytother Res 2005; 19(5): 391-404. [http://dx.doi.org/10.1002/ptr.1509] [PMID: 16106393]

[47] Kosmulalage KS, Zahid S, Udenigwe CC, Akhtar S, Ata A, Samarasekera R. Glutathione S-Transferase, Acetylcholinesterase Inhibitory and Antibacterial Activities of Chemical Constituents of Barleria prionitis. Z Naturforsch B J Chem Sci 2007; 62(4): 580-6. [http://dx.doi.org/10.1515/znb-2007-0417]

[48] Trease and Evans' Pharmacognosy-16th Edition 2021 Dec 16. Available from: https://www.elsevier.com/books/trease-and-evans-pharmacognosy/9780702029332

[49] Ghule BV, Yeole PG. *in-vivo* and in *vivo* immunomodulatory activities of iridoids fraction from Barleria prionitis Linn. J Ethnopharmacol 2012; 141(1): 424-31. [http://dx.doi.org/10.1016/j.jep.2012.03.005] [PMID: 22440262]

[50] Foo LY. Amarulone, a Novel Cyclic Hydrolysable Tannin from *Phyllanthus amarus*. Nat Prod Lett 1993; 3(1): 45-52. [http://dx.doi.org/10.1080/10575639308043836]

[51] Shokunbi OS, Odetola AA. Gastroprotective and antioxidant activities of Phyllanthus amarus extracts on absolute ethanol-induced ulcer in albino rats. J Med Plants Res 2008; 2(10): 261-7.

[52] Patel JR, Tripathi P, Sharma V, Chauhan NS, Dixit VK. Phyllanthus amarus: Ethnomedicinal uses, phytochemistry and pharmacology: A review. J Ethnopharmacol 2011; 138(2): 286-313. [http://dx.doi.org/10.1016/j.jep.2011.09.040] [PMID: 21982793]

[53] Jantan I, Ilangkovan M, Yuandani , Mohamad HF. Correlation between the major components of Phyllanthus amarus and Phyllanthus urinaria and their inhibitory effects on phagocytic activity of human neutrophils. BMC Complement Altern Med 2014; 14(1): 429. [http://dx.doi.org/10.1186/1472-6882-14-429]

[54] Yuandani null, Ilangkovan M, Jantan I, Mohamad HF, Husain K, Abdul Razak AF. Inhibitory Effects of Standardized Extracts of Phyllanthus amarus and Phyllanthus urinaria and Their Marker Compounds on Phagocytic Activity of Human Neutrophils. Evid-Based Complement Altern Med ECAM 2013; 2013: 603634.

[55] Ilangkovan M, Jantan I, Mesaik MA, Bukhari SNA. Immunosuppressive effects of the standardized extract of Phyllanthus amarus on cellular immune responses in Wistar-Kyoto rats. Drug Des Devel Ther 2015; 9: 4917-30. [PMID: 26347462]

[56] Yob NJ, Jofrry SM, Affandi MMRMM, Teh LK, Salleh MZ, Zakaria ZA. *Zingiber zerumbet* (L.) Smith: A Review of Its Ethnomedicinal, Chemical, and Pharmacological Uses. Evid Based Complement Alternat Med 2011; 2011: 1-12. [http://dx.doi.org/10.1155/2011/543216] [PMID: 21584247]

[57] Nongalleima K, Brojendrosingh S, Swapana N, Nahakpam L, Laitonjam W. Biological and chemical properties of Zingiber zerumbet Smith: A review. Phytochem Rev 2011; 11: 113-25.

[58] Haque MA, Jantan I, Harikrishnan H. Zerumbone suppresses the activation of inflammatory mediators in LPS-stimulated U937 macrophages through MyD88-dependent NF-κB/MAPK/PI3K-Akt signaling pathways. Int Immunopharmacol 2018; 55: 312-22.

[http://dx.doi.org/10.1016/j.intimp.2018.01.001] [PMID: 29310107]

[59] Ghazalee NS, Jantan I, Arshad L, Haque MA. Immunosuppressive effects of the standardized extract of *ZINGIBER ZERUMBET* on innate immune responses in Wistar rats. Phytother Res 2019; 33(4): 929-38. [http://dx.doi.org/10.1002/ptr.6285] [PMID: 30618097]

[60] Puri M, Kaur I, Kanwar R, Gupta R, Chauhan A, Kanwar J. Ribosome inactivating proteins (RIPs) from Momordica charantia for anti viral therapy. Curr Mol Med 2009; 9(9): 1080-94. [http://dx.doi.org/10.2174/156652409789839071] [PMID: 19747115]

[61] Ng T, Wong J, Wang H. Recent progress in research on ribosome inactivating proteins. Curr Protein Pept Sci 2010; 11(1): 37-53. [http://dx.doi.org/10.2174/138920310790274662] [PMID: 20201806]

[62] Fong WP, Poon YT, Wong TM, *et al.* A highly efficient procedure for purifying the ribosome-inactivating proteins α- and β-momorcharins from Momordica charantia seeds, N-terminal sequence comparison and establishment of their N-glycosidase activity. Life Sci 1996; 59(11): 901-9. [http://dx.doi.org/10.1016/0024-3205(96)00388-8] [PMID: 8795701]

[63] Cao D, Sun Y, Wang L, *et al.* Alpha-momorcharin (α-MMC) exerts effective anti-human breast tumor activities but has a narrow therapeutic window *in vivo.* Fitoterapia 2015; 100: 139-49. [http://dx.doi.org/10.1016/j.fitote.2014.11.009] [PMID: 25447153]

[64] Jeffrey WP. Tumour-educated macrophages promote tumour progression and metastasis 2004.https://www.nature.com/articles/nrc1256

[65] Lillis AP, Van Duyn LB, Murphy-Ullrich JE, Strickland DK. LDL receptor-related protein 1: unique tissue-specific functions revealed by selective gene knockout studies. Physiol Rev 2008; 88(3): 887-918. [http://dx.doi.org/10.1152/physrev.00033.2007] [PMID: 18626063]

[66] Deng N, Li M, Shen D, *et al.* LRP1 receptor-mediated immunosuppression of α-MMC on monocytes. Int Immunopharmacol 2019; 70: 80-7. [http://dx.doi.org/10.1016/j.intimp.2019.01.036] [PMID: 30785094]

[67] Juang LJ, Sheu SJ. Chemical identification of the sources of commercial fructus chebulae. Phytochem Anal 2005; 16(4): 246-51. [http://dx.doi.org/10.1002/pca.823] [PMID: 16042149]

[68] Mahesh R, Bhuvana S, Hazeena Begum VM. Effect of *Terminalia chebula* aqueous extract on oxidative stress and antioxidant status in the liver and kidney of young and aged rats. Cell Biochem Funct 2009; 27(6): 358-63. [http://dx.doi.org/10.1002/cbf.1581] [PMID: 19548245]

[69] Reddy AG, Jyothi K, Kumar BA, Gopi KS. Acetaminophen-induced Hepato- and Nephrotoxicity and Amelioration by silymarin and Terminalia chebula in rats. Toxicol Int 2010; 17(2): 64-6. [http://dx.doi.org/10.4103/0971-6580.72672] [PMID: 21170247]

[70] Reddy DB, Reddanna P. Chebulagic acid (CA) attenuates LPS-induced inflammation by suppressing NF-κB and MAPK activation in RAW 264.7 macrophages. Biochem Biophys Res Commun 2009; 381(1): 112-7. [http://dx.doi.org/10.1016/j.bbrc.2009.02.022] [PMID: 19351605]

[71] Lee SI, Hyun PM, Kim SH, *et al.* Suppression of the onset and progression of collagen-induced arthritis by chebulagic acid screened from a natural product library. Arthritis Rheum 2005; 52(1): 345-53. [http://dx.doi.org/10.1002/art.20715] [PMID: 15641090]

[72] Smolen JS, Steiner G. Therapeutic strategies for rheumatoid arthritis. Nat Rev Drug Discov 2003; 2(6): 473-88. [http://dx.doi.org/10.1038/nrd1109] [PMID: 12776222]

[73] Seo JB, Jeong JY, Park JY, *et al.* Anti-Arthritic and Analgesic Effect of NDI10218, a Standardized

Extract of Terminalia chebula, on Arthritis and Pain Model. Biomol Ther (Seoul) 2012; 20(1): 104-12. [http://dx.doi.org/10.4062/biomolther.2012.20.1.104] [PMID: 24116282]

[74] Speroni E, Govoni P, Guizzardi S, Renzulli C, Guerra MC. Anti-inflammatory and cicatrizing activity of Echinacea pallida Nutt. root extract. J Ethnopharmacol 2002; 79(2): 265-72. [http://dx.doi.org/10.1016/S0378-8741(01)00391-9] [PMID: 11801391]

[75] Woelkart K, Linde K, Bauer R. Echinacea for preventing and treating the common cold. Planta Med 2008; 74(6): 633-7. [http://dx.doi.org/10.1055/s-2007-993766] [PMID: 18186015]

[76] Islam J, Carter R. Use of Echinacea in upper respiratory tract infection. South Med J 2005; 98(3): 311-8. [http://dx.doi.org/10.1097/01.SMJ.0000154783.93532.78] [PMID: 15813158]

[77] Kasugai S, Hasegawa N, Ogura H. A simple *in vitro* cytotoxicity test using the MTT (3-(4,5--dimethylthiazol-2-yl)-2,5-diphenyl tetrazolium bromide) colorimetric assay: analysis of eugenol toxicity on dental pulp cells (RPC-C2A). Jpn J Pharmacol 1990; 52(1): 95-100. [http://dx.doi.org/10.1016/S0021-5198(19)37772-8] [PMID: 2308240]

[78] Lin X, Huang R, Zhang S, *et al.* Methyl helicterate protects against CCl4-induced liver injury in rats by inhibiting oxidative stress, NF-κB activation, Fas/FasL pathway and cytochrome P4502E1 level. Food Chem Toxicol 2012; 50(10): 3413-20. [http://dx.doi.org/10.1016/j.fct.2012.07.053] [PMID: 22889900]

[79] Li K, Yang X, Hu X, Han C, Lei Z, Zhang Z. *in-vivo* antioxidant, immunomodulatory and anticancer activities of two fractions of aqueous extract from Helicteres angustifolia L. root. J Taiwan Inst Chem Eng 2016; 61: 75-82. [http://dx.doi.org/10.1016/j.jtice.2015.12.022]

[80] Chen N, Chen H, Li J, Sang M, Ding S, Yu H. Discrimination and similarity evaluation of tissue-cultured and wild Dendrobium species using Fourier transform infrared spectroscopy. J Mol Struct 2015; 1086: 255-65. [http://dx.doi.org/10.1016/j.molstruc.2015.01.027]

[81] Yang X, Lei Z, Yu Y, Xiao L, Cheng D, Zhang Z. Phytochemical characteristics of callus suspension culture of Helicteres angustifolia L. and its *in-vivo* antioxidant, antidiabetic and immunomodulatory activities. S Afr J Bot 2019; 121: 178-85. [http://dx.doi.org/10.1016/j.sajb.2018.11.006]

CHAPTER 5

Immunomodulators: Chemistry and Analytical Techniques

Akalya Sendrayakannan[1] and **Prashant S. Kharkar**[1,*]

[1] *Department of Food Engineering and Technology, Department of Pharmaceutical Sciences and Technology, Institute of Chemical Technology (ICT), Nathalal Parekha Marg, Matunga, Mumbai 400 019, India*

Abstract: Immunomodulators are substances that either enhance or suppress the immunity of the host. Immunomodulators have been used for ages in Ayurvedic Medicine and Traditional Chinese Medicine. In the surge of modern medicine, many chemically derived substances are used as immunomodulators. Historically, plants present a rich source of these therapeutic agents. Researchers have used these lead structures for exploring the underlying mechanisms of immunomodulation so that newer, safer agents can be designed and used clinically. Microbial sources have also been tried in search of immunomodulators. Chemically, these are a diverse group of substances that act on varied signaling pathways to cause immunomodulation. The involvement of the immune system in many diseases and disorders makes these agents essential in the treatment of these diseases, *e.g.*, cancer. This chapter discusses the chemistry of a selected few commonly known plant-derived immunomodulators along with their biological evaluation methods and provides a broad overview of their therapeutic potential with particular emphasis on the mechanism of immunomodulation.

Keywords: Adaptive Immunity, Cytokines, Emodin, Immune checkpoint inhibitors, Immunomodulators, Innate Immunity, Interleukins, Quercetin.

INTRODUCTION

Innate immunity is the first line of defense that is present in almost all vertebrates and even in the multicellular organisms; its main role being recognition of the foreign invaders such as pathogens. In most cases, the innate immune system recognizes a particular region of the pathogen known as Pathogen Associated Molecular Patterns (PAMPs) employing the so-called Pathogen Associated Receptors (PARs). The other arm of the immune system, *i.e.*, adaptive immunity,

* **Corresponding author Prashant S. Kharkar:** Department of Food Engineering and Technology, Department of Pharmaceutical Sciences and Technology, Institute of Chemical Technology (ICT), Nathalal Parekha Marg, Matunga, Mumbai 400 019, India, E-mail: ps.kharkar@ictmumbai.edu.in

Vandana S. Nikam, Sujata P. Sawarkar, Girish B. Mahajan and Supriya G. Jagtap (Eds.)

involves the generation of B and T cell receptors somatically during the B and T cell development and so are not passed on to the next generation. Hence antigenic determination cannot be made by them until they are being made to recognize them [1]. In other words, the innate immune system is more general in its capability to identify the antigens, whereas the adaptive immune system is more specific in this aspect.

The innate immune system comprises of cells such as mast cells, basophils, natural killer (NK) cells, macrophages, eosinophils, neutrophils, and dendritic cells. These cells have their way of killing and eliminating the pathogens, some of which include releasing histamines, cytokines, or chemokines, or making the cells follow the apoptotic (programmed cell death) path, by phagocytosis, or presenting the antigens to T cells. The adaptive immune system comprises of B cells, CD4+, and CD8+ cells. The B cells eliminate the pathogen mostly by the humoral immune response or by producing antibodies. The CD8+ cells recognize most of the cancerous and virus-infected cells (intracellular pathogens) and make them undergo apoptotic pathways. The CD4+ cells, which constitute Th1, Th2, Th17, and regulatory T (Treg) cells, are involved in the production of cytokines such as Interferon γ (IFN-γ), Interleukin-2 (IL-2), IL-4, IL-5, IL-13 and IL-17 [2].

The immune system is capable of recognizing self (own body cells, proteins), from non-self (antigen), which could be anything such as the viral coat, bacterial lipopolysaccharides, viral genetic material, or any substance which does not belong to the host. The problem arises if the immune system does not recognize particular antigens resulting in a particular disease (or pathological condition) or if it recognizes its own body cells that result in auto-immune disease or disorder. The latter is mostly because of the adaptive immune response since the antigen-binding site is a result of a random genetic mechanism [1]. The role of immunomodulators is essential in these cases, which helps to maintain the homeostasis of the immune system. The present chapter thoroughly discusses the chemistry of various immunomodulators derived from natural sources, followed by the analytical techniques and finally, the efficacy of immune modulation demonstrated by some of the plant-derived immunomodulators.

IMMUNOMODULATORS

Precisely, immunomodulators are substances that help to maintain the homeostasis of the immune system, *i.e.*, it could be either immunosuppressant or immunostimulant or immunoadjuvant. These agents are administered to maintain the balanced functioning of the immune system. The immunosuppressants are agents that aid in suppressing the immune system. The suppressed immune function is desirable in patients suffering from auto-immune diseases such as rheumatoid arthritis (RA), Systemic lupus erythematosus (SLE), or for suppressing the immune response in patients who have undergone organ transplant surgery to prevent graft rejection [2]. On the other hand, the immunostimulants are agents which enhance or boost the immunity of the host. Immunostimulants are mostly indicated for providing resistance to some diseases, leading to enhanced immunity without the use of vaccines [3], *e.g.*, various Immunostimulants prescribed during the COVID-19 pandemic. The immunoadjuvants are those substances which are used in a vaccine along with the antigens as carrier material. The antigen itself, in this case, would be very small and hence will not be recognizable by the host immune response. So, immunoadjuvants are used, which aid in better recognition by the immune system, leading to the profuse response by the immune system and hence, improved protection [4]. Both the Immunostimulants and immunomodulators may work *via* specific pathways or non-specifically. With respect to chemotypes, the immunomodulators could be small-molecules, proteins or peptides, carbohydrates, nucleic acids, or lipids [5]. While the field of immunomodulators is so very vast, no attempt is made to discuss all the types of immunomodulators but small-molecules, particularly those obtained from natural sources.

Commercially, many immunosuppressants are available, some of which include Rapamycin (**1**), Sirolimus, Fig. (**1**) Cyclosporin A (**2**), Cyclophosphamide (**3**), Azathioprine (**4**), and Cinanserine (**5**). Rapamycin, a macrocyclic compound produced by *Streptomyces hygroscopicus,* disrupts the T-cell growth-promoting cytokines like IL-2 or IL-4 and acts as an anti-proliferative agent. It blocks the cell cycle during the mid-to-late G1 phase, thereby arresting the G/S transition [6]. Cyclosporin A inhibits the action of calcineurin, which in turn blocks the movement of cytosolic components of the Nuclear Factor of Activated T-cell (NF-AT). Cyclophosphamide is the most widely used alkylating agent, which inhibits both the adaptive and innate immune responses. Azathioprine is an immunosuppressant that is generally used in kidney transplants, and Cinanserine is an antagonist of serotonin, which suppresses the antibodies circulating in the human body [3].

The synthetic drugs, though efficacious, come with debilitating adverse effects, including toxicity such as nephrotoxicity, neurotoxicity, and gastrointestinal toxicity, among others. Also, they act upon actively growing cells such as bone marrow cells which ultimately end up in leucopenia and thrombocytopenia [3]. Compared to synthetic drugs, natural products offer several advantages [7] due to the synergistic actions of complex molecules when used in the form of an extract or preparation. At times, pure natural products offer distinct pharmacological and therapeutic activities. The successful use of natural products as sources of new drugs has created enough research interest in the global scientific community [8].

Overall, natural product alternatives to synthetic drugs have been developed in many instances, and the immunomodulators field is no exception to that.

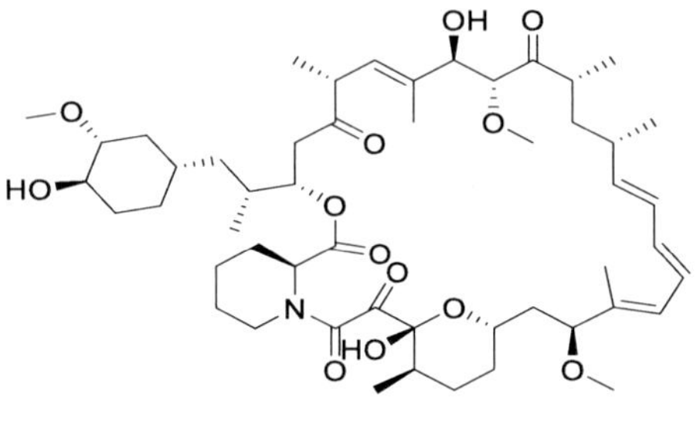

1

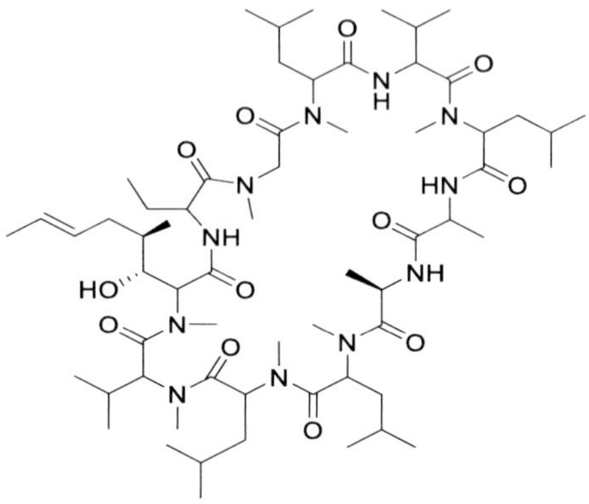

2

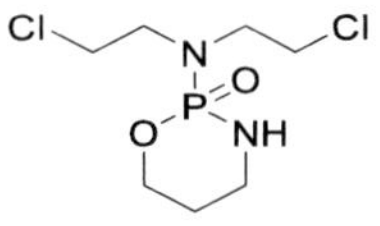

3

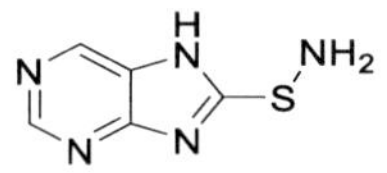

4

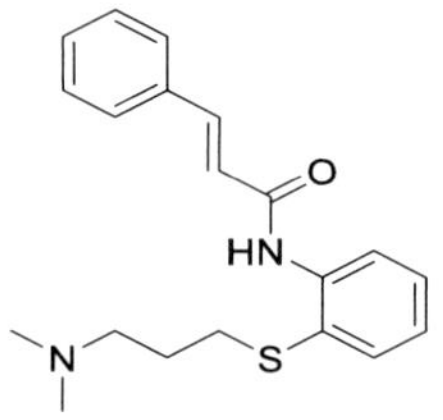

5

Fig. (1). Molecular Structures of Representative Immunosuppressant Drugs, namely Sirolimus (1), Cyclosporin A (2), Cyclophosphamide (3), Azathioprine (4), and Cinanserine (5).

Immunomodulators from Natural Sources

Countless immunomodulators have been derived from several plants, majorly from traditional systems of medicine. Exhaustive listing of these molecules is beyond the scope of this chapter. However, Table **1**. lists representative immunomodulators extracted or isolated from plants, their concentrations at which they are efficacious and their potential or definitive mode of action. They have been used most efficiently for cancer treatment, and some of the most widely used immunomodulators include resveratrol (**6**), Fig. (**2**), quercetin (**7**), emodin (**8**), and several others. Some of the immunomodulators, such as genistein (**9**), curcumin (**10**), and piperine (**11**), are used in the daily diet along with food or in food preparations. Curcuminoids (the chief compound in turmeric, *Curcuma longa*) which is available commercially in a combination of three compounds as **10**, demethoxycurcumin (**12**), and bisdemethoxycurcumin (**13**), exhibit powerful immunosuppressant activity, affecting the DCs, majorly the CD80 and CD86 (co-stimulatory molecules required for triggering T cell activation, expansion and differentiation) expressions. The structure responsible for most of the biological activity of curcumin is the methoxy phenol and methylene group. The derivative of curcumin, tetrahydrocurcumin (**14**), has a cardioprotective efficacy by modifying the structure of low-density lipoprotein (LDL) and cholesterol. Many derivatives of curcumin resulting from the chemical modifications, such as cyclocurcumin, pyrazole, and semicarbazone are efficacious as anticancer, antioxidant and anti-angiogenic agents [9]. The majority of the immunomodulators from plants are polyphenolic compounds possessing either α,β-unsaturated ketone, or conjugated alkene substructures, along with phenolic groups. These are likely to provide potent antioxidant activities, which in some way is related to their immunomodulatory potential.

Immunomodulators from fungi and mushrooms have started flourishing after the advent of microbial resistance reversal. Immunomodulators from mushrooms demonstrate immunostimulant activity on both the innate and adaptive immune systems [10, 11]. Some of them have shown a protease inhibitory activity against HIV-1 and include the compounds 3β-5α-dihydroxy-6β-methoxyergosta-7,22-diene (**15**), Ganoderic acid A-C (**16**), and Ganolucidic acid – A (**17**) extracted from the mushroom *Ganoderma lucidum*. Adenosine and iso-sinensetin are other immunomodulators extracted from the mushroom *Cordycep militaris* [13]. Protease inhibitors against viruses have been reported in fungi as well. The small organic molecules with the immunomodulatory activity have been synthesized in hyphae, and large organic molecules are extracted from fruiting bodies and fungal mycelia, which includes proteins, polysaccharides, or complex proteins and carbohydrates [14].

Table 1. Plant-based immunomodulators and their immunomodulatory effects.

S. No	Immunomodulator	Concentration Used	Plant Source	Immunomodulatory Effect	Reference
1.	Punarnavine (**18**, Lunamarine, Fig. (**3**)	40 mg/kg body weight	*Boerhaavia diffusa*	Decreased levels of cytokines like IL-6, IL-1β, and TNF-α	[13]
2.	Triphala powder	1000 mg/kg body weight	*Terminalia chebula, Terminalia belerica and Emblica officinalis*	Enhanced neutrophil function	[14]
3.	Aqueous extract	2000 mg/kg body weight	*Murraya koenigii*	Immunosuppression by reduced antibody titer	[15]
4.	Emodin (**8**, Fig. (**2**)	30 mg/kg of body weight	*Rheum palmatum*	Supressed TNF-α and NF-κB	[16]

(Table 1) cont.....

S. No	Immunomodulator	Concentration Used	Plant Source	Immunomodulatory Effect	Reference
5.	Curcumin (**10**, Fig. (**2**)	9.2 mg/kg	*Curcuma longa*	Downregulate signaling pathways of TNF-β	[17]
6.	NIM-76	120 mg/kg body weight	*Azadirachta indica*	Immune enhancement by enhancing the macrophage and lymphocyte proliferation	[18]
7.	Plant extracts	400 mg/kg body weight	*Adhatoda vasica*	Neutrophil adhesion increased and decreased hypersensitivity reaction	[19]
8.	Protein fraction	0.1 mg/ml of protein (1ml solution)	*Allium sativum*	Mannose-binding, Hemagglutination activity	[20]
9.	Aqueous extract	200 mg/kg body weight	*Ocimum basilicum*	Enhanced antibody titre values	[21]
10.	Aqueous extract of the root	-	*Heracleum maximum Bartr.*	Enhanced stimulation of IL-6 and IFNγ (in presence of priming factor)	[22]
11.	Resveratrol	15 mg/kg body weight	*Vitis vinifera*	Enhanced expression of cytokines such as IL-1α/β, IL-2, TNF-α and NF-κB	[23]

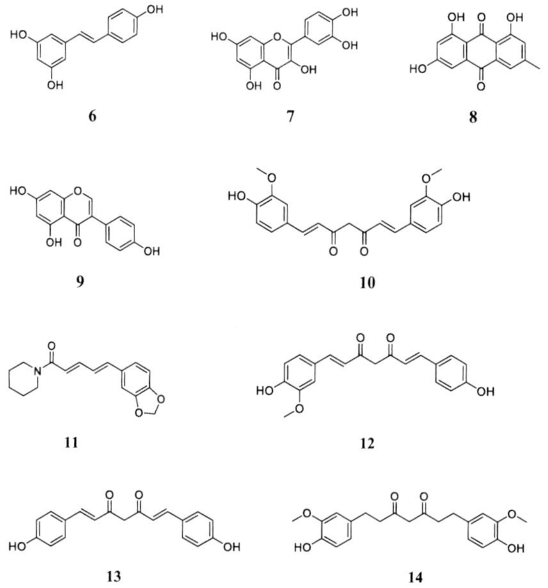

Fig. (2). Molecular Structures of Representative Immunomodulators from Plants, namely Resveratrol (6), quercetin (7), emodin (8), genistein (9), curcumin (10), piperine (11), demethoxycurcumin (12), and bisdemethoxycurcumin (13), tetrahydrocurcumin (14).

Immunostimulants are most demanding in the field of fisheries and aquaculture, and most of them include prebiotics such as malto-oligosaccharides and isomalto-oligosaccharides, β-Glucans, and galactooligosaccharides. These are provided for developing the natural immunity in the host and thereby preventing the incidences of disease [12]. The immunoadjuvants are essential agents in some vaccines, such as subunit vaccines for recognition by the host; some of them include Alum, water, and mineral oil emulsion and Freund's adjuvant (solution of antigen emulsified in mineral oil). The vaccine made from live and attenuated strains does not generally need an adjuvant, and they can stimulate immunity by themselves [4].

PHYTOCHEMICALS AS IMMUNOMODULATORS

Emodin

Emodin (**8**, (Fig. **2**), 6-methyl-1,3,8-trihydroxyanthraquinone) is an anthraquinone generally present in the rhizomes and roots of *Rheum palmatum*, *Polygonum multiflorum,* and which has its usage since ancient days as described in Traditional Chinese Medicine (TCM). Emodin has its potential efficacy in inflammation, cancer, and cardiovascular disorders. It has been used to treat various cancers, including breast, bladder, and liver. The toxicity against cancer is believed to be due to the planar and the quinoid structure. The planar structure intercalates between the DNA, which leads to the inhibition of topoisomerase II, an important enzyme required for managing DNA tangles and supercoils. The quinoid structure paves the way for forming reactive oxygen species (ROS) and hence inducing apoptosis of cancerous cells [24].

Emodin (**8**) is a powerful anticancer agent, which downregulates the androgen receptor (AR) and reduces hormone-dependent prostate cancer cell growth. Compound **8** and aloe emodin (**19**, (Fig. **3**), 1,8-dihydroxy-3-hydroxymethy-lanthra-quinone) have a stronger suppression effect on estrogen receptor alpha (ERα)-positive breast cancer cell line at the concentration $\geq$12.5 μM. Both **8** and **18** repressed the distribution of ERα protein. The mechanism by which **18** restrained ERα is by heat shock protein (HSP90)/ERα dissociation and ubiquitin-dependent degradation. Compound **8** constrained the ERα by proteasomal degradation by acting as a tyrosine kinase inhibitor. Hence, both compounds act as phytoestrogens. So far, in treating breast cancer, estrogen mimetics are used, which compensates binding of ERα-positive cells to endogenous estrogens and hence inhibit the growth of breast cancer cell lines. The synthetic mimetics of estrogens have side effects which tend to increase the risk of cancer due to unselective action [25]. Emodin has a role in regulating bladder cancer as well. Emodin does that by down-regulating Notch1 signaling, thereby acting as an anti-proliferative agent and inhibiting cell growth [26]. It limits the growth of hepatic cancerous cell lines by limiting the supply of energy to the cancerous cells, which is attributed to the inhibition of the glycolytic pathway. It has been noticed that the cells started producing ROS in larger amounts, which further leads to apoptosis due to increased damage to the mitochondria [27]. Overall, multiple pharmacological actions of **8** are responsible for its potential as an anticancer agent.

Emodin, in combination with Concanavalin A (ConA), acts as a strong anti-inflammatory and anti-proliferative agent by suppressing the level of Th1 cytokines such as IL-2, tumor necrosis factor-alpha (TNF-α), and IFN-γ, by 2.7, 3.6, and 5.0 folds, respectively and Th17 cytokines such as IL-6 and IL-17 by 1.9 and 4.7 folds, respectively. The treatment also inhibits the nuclear factor kappa B (NF-κB), thereby acting as an inhibitor of inducible nitric oxide synthase (iNOS) and hence resulting in reduced NO levels in cells. They have shown an enriched production of anti-inflammatory cytokines such as IL-4 and IL-10 by 1.5 and 4.9 folds, respectively. Hence, compound **8** works by suppressing the Th17 and enhancing the Treg cells production, which is a positive sign of suppressing the autoimmunity [28].

Emodin is an effective agent for cardiovascular disorders and complications. It acts by down-regulating the NF-κB, which results in reduced production of pro-inflammatory cytokines such as TNF-α and IL-6 [29]. The glycosylated form of emodin, E8G (emodin-8-O-glycoside), is an effective immunostimulant, which has been found to upregulate the secretion of TNF-α and IL-6, enhanced iNOS, subsequently enhanced NO in the cell and enhanced activation of NF-κB and subsequent nuclear translocation [30].

The pharmacology, toxicity and pharmacokinetics (PK) of **8** have been reviewed extensively [31], wherein it has been found to exhibit nephrotoxicity, hepatotoxicity and genotoxicity. The hepatotoxicity of emodin was proposed as a direct result of its metabolism by a variety of drug-metabolizing enzymes (DMEs) [32], which include 6-hydroxymethylemodin, (M1, Fig. **4**), 2-hydroxyemodin (M2), 5-hydroxyemodin (M3), as well as their mercapturic acid metabolites derived from glutathione conjugated counterparts. With regards to the PK, compound 8 was found to have poor intestinal absorption and rapid elimination due to phase II metabolism (glucuronidation), resulting in poor oral bioavailability.

Quercetin

Quercetin (**7**, Fig. **2**, 2-(3,4-dihydroxyphenyl)-3,5,7-trihydroxy chromen-4-one) is a flavone found in most fruits and vegetables, such as onion, apple, grapes, and nuts. Naturally, it is present as its glycoside. Once it enters the digestion cycle, it is acted by the enzymes in the mouth and converted into its aglycone form. The metabolized form of **7** has been reported in the lungs of rats and the exhaled air from the lungs of humans. Compound **7** has already been reported to be used in treating many diseases since ancient times since it is one of the major components of medicinal plant roots, stems, and bark [33].

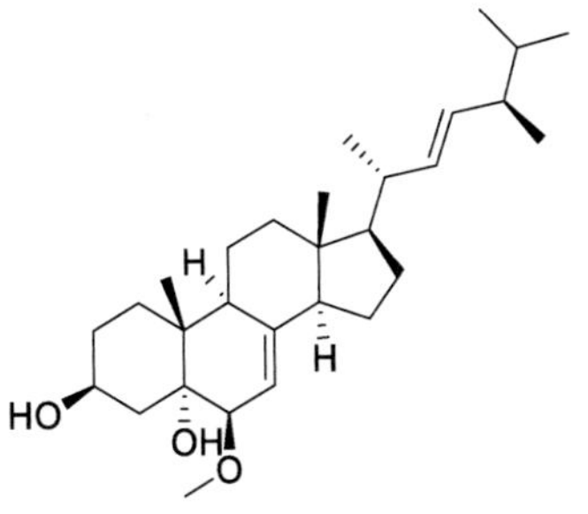

15

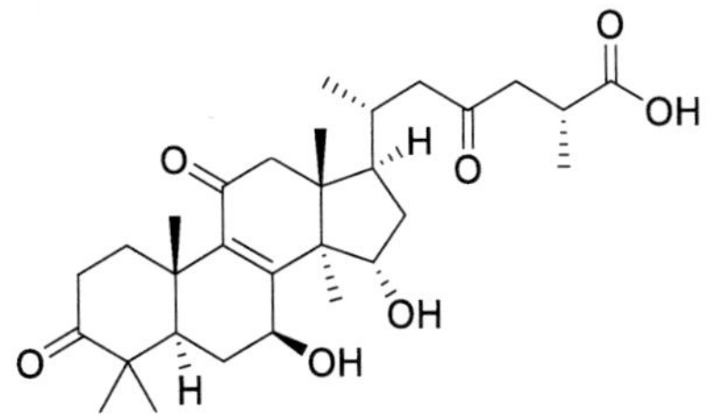

16

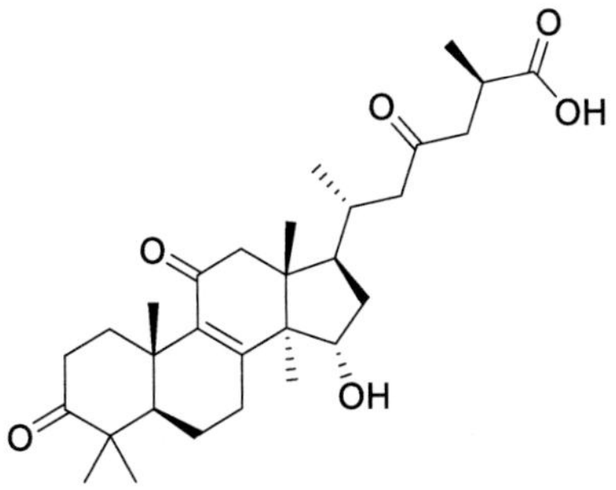

17

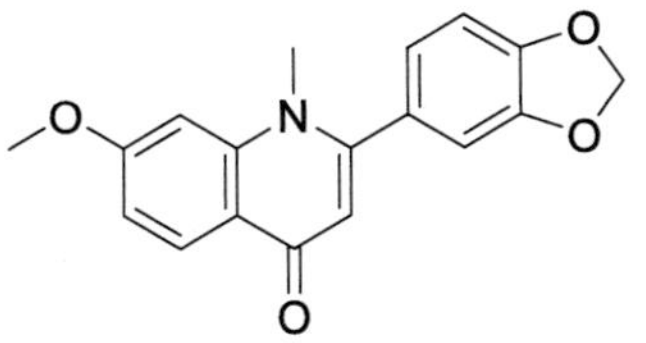

18

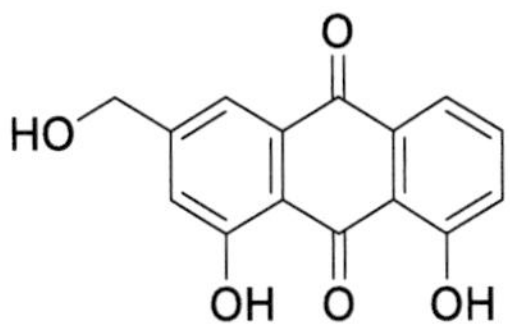

19

Fig. (3). Molecular Structures of Representative Immunomodulators from Plants, namely 3β-5α-dihydro-y-6β-methoxyergosta-7,22-diene (15), Ganoderic Acid A-C (16), and Ganolucidic Acid – A (17), Punarnavine (18) and Aloe-emodin or 8-dihydroxy-3-hydroxymethylanthra-quinone (19).

Compound **7** is a strong immunosuppressant that has a role in RA. At a concentration of 1500 mg/day along with azathioprine (100 mg/day), the levels of IL-6 and Intracellular Adhesion Molecules (ICAMs) decreased rapidly, and levels of IL-10 were subsequently increased. The levels of complement proteins such as C_3 and C_4 also decreased. The complete set of these events led to a strong anti-inflammatory effect in RA [34].

In addition, **7** has potent antiviral activity against the Influenza A virus. Upon infection by Influenza A Virus, hypersecretion of cytokines (Hypercytokinemia) has been observed, which could be fatal due to the accumulation of immune cells.

Compound **7** helps in increasing the IL-27 production while suppressing the TNF-α levels; it enhances the anti-inflammatory cytokines, and suppresses the pro-inflammatory cytokines [35]. Interestingly, **7** has been used as a strong immunomodulatory agent in asthma and asthma along with diabetes. The downstream events include constraints on the release of histamine and pro-inflammatory immune mediators such as TNF-α, IL-8, IL-1β, and IL-6 from the mast cells. Compound **7** at the concentration of 10 mg/kg reduces the number of eosinophils in the blood, Broncho Alveolar Lavage Fluid (BALF), and pulmonary parenchyma in the model treated with ovalbumin for airway inflammation. The glycosylated quercetin (Isoquercetin) has been found to be more efficient in downregulating the IL-5 in BALF [33]. In animal models with asthma and diabetes, **7** has shown a direct relationship with the dosage and mitigation of diseases. At a concentration of 30 mg/kg, it demonstrated blood glucose lowering effect in the diabetic model. The OVA challenge of both the diabetic and non-diabetic models decreased after treating them with **7** at a concentration of 30 mg/kg. However, 10 mg/kg concentration of **7** was sufficient to reduce the levels of hyperresponsivity. Compound **7** downregulated the IL-4 and upregulated the IFN-γ. It reduced the Th2 response in eosinophils of BALF and blood; hence Th1/Th2 ratio increased in the BALF and serum [36].

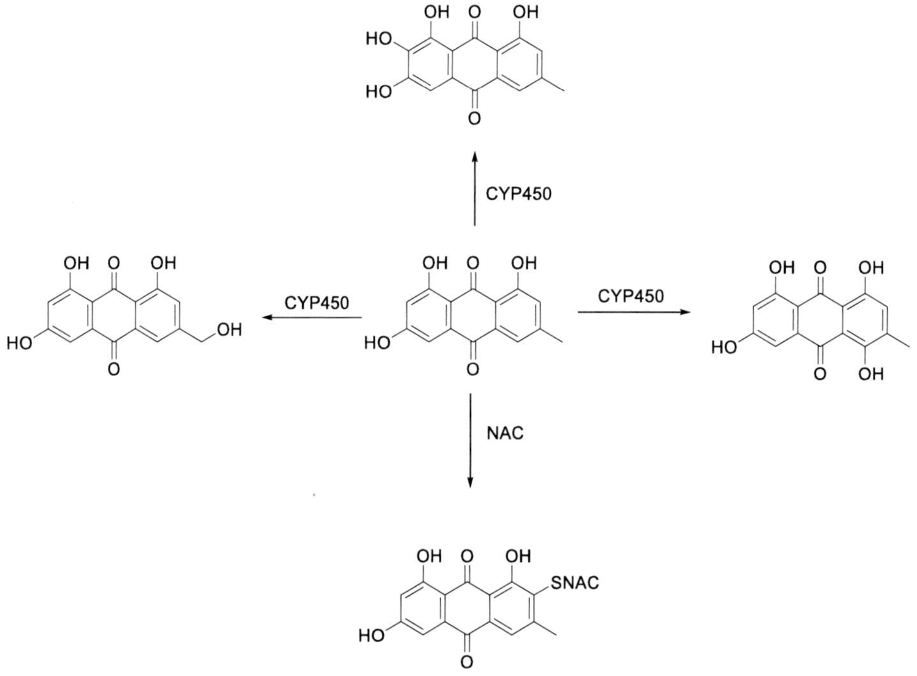

Fig. (4). Major metabolic fate of 8.

Quercetin (**7**) has the potential to revert the condition of liver cirrhosis. The anti-inflammatory and anti-necrotic effect was achieved by blocking the NF-κB activation and subsequently reducing the cytokine IL-1. The reversal of fibrosis was achieved by reduced transforming growth factor beta (TGF-β) levels [37]. The quercetin and its derivatives, Isoquercitrin q-3-O-β-D-glucopyranoside) and rutin (quercetin-3-O-rutinoside) have displayed anti-mutagenic effect. Isoquercetin displayed a very mild potentially mutagenic effect at a dose of 0.1 to 2.2 µmol per plate and rutin displayed non-mutagenic activity at the concentration of 0.1 to 1.6 µmol per plate. Quercetin at a concentration of 0.7 µmol per plate displayed the mutagenic potential. The order of increment of mutagenic potential of these compounds was rutin<isoquercetin<quercetin. The mutagenicity of these compounds depends on the presence of hydroxyl group, double bonds, and the oxo group present in these compounds [38]. In an interesting article, the effects of functional groups and sugar composition were investigated in derivatives of **7** on their free radical-scavenging properties [39]. The authors found that the isoquercetin O-gallates were far superior to **7** due to the distribution of hydroxyl substituents in the molecular structure.

The potential of **7** in COVID-19 treatment was investigated recently [40]. The authors proposed its inhibitory activity at the SARS-CoV-2 proteins, 3-chymotrypsin-like protease ($3CL_{pro}$), and papain-like protease (PL_{pro}) based on molecular modeling studies. In addition, the anti-cytokine activity was thought of advantageous for tacking the profuse cytokine storm in patients with severe disease.

Resveratrol

Resveratrol (**6**, (Fig. **2**), (*E*)-5-(4-hydroxystyryl)benzene-1,3-diol), a phytoalexin, is produced by plants belonging to the spermatophytes group such as grapes, apples, and several other fruits. A higher concentration has been reported in the skin of red grapes. It is produced in response to various stresses, including biotic (during the fungal attack) and abiotic stresses. Compound **6** exhibited a biphasic effect which indicated that at a lower dosage, it acted as an immune-enhancer, whereas, at a higher dosage, it suppressed or down-regulated the immune response. Additionally, **6** is a potent anticancer, antiviral and antioxidant compound, with strong immunomodulatory activity. Recently, its health benefits, despite being termed as a double-edged sword, have been reviewed [41].

Resveratrol (**6**) is an immune enhancer at a concentration of 30 mg/kg body weight. It has been shown to boost the immune system by increasing spleen lymphocytes and the spleen index. At a concentration of 15 mg/kg, **6** has been found to enhance the CD4+ cells and peritoneal macrophage function. The cytokines such as IL-1α/β, IL-2, TNF-α, and transcription factor NF-κB have been enhanced in a dose-dependent manner [23]. It has shown a synergistic immune enhancement effect in combination with glucans. The complex has been shown to have an improved phagocytosis activity by increased blood neutrophils and monocytes and internalization of the synthetic particles. The levels of cytokines such as IL-1, IL-6, and TNF-α were observed to increase on treatment with the complex rather than treating both of them separately. There was also a significant increase in the level of CD4 cells rather than CD8 and CD19 cells upon treatment with the complex. The complex also has shown recovery of bone marrow cells after being induced with leucopenia, which is considered as the major drawback of chemotherapy and irradiation therapy [42].

Resveratrol is an effective suppressor of the Treg cell population, which is the negative immune regulator of cancer therapy. Suppression of TGF-β is done by downregulating the CD4+/CD25+ population among the CD4+ cells and upregulating the IFN-γ of CD8+ cytotoxic T lymphocytes. Hence, resveratrol can act as a promising adjuvant for cancer immunotherapy [43]. Compound **6** exhibited a structure similar to synthetic estrogen, diethylstilbestrol. It is shown to activate estrogen-regulated genes by binding to both ERα and ERβ receptors in a dose-dependent manner. Resveratrol treatment has been shown to reduce the levels of an angiogenic factor, Vascular Endothelial Growth Factor (VEGF). It can also function similarly to Selective Estrogen Receptor Modulator (SERM), which was one of the cornerstones for treating breast cancer. But it is reported that **6** would not result in endometrial cancer, which is the drawback associated with other SERMs, such as tamoxifen [44].

Compound **6** is also a potent antiviral agent. It affects wide varieties of viruses, and it is believed that **6** affects the cellular and molecular mechanism going inside the virus rather than having a direct effect on the virus. In viruses belonging to the Herpesviridae family, **6** inhibited the viral replication by downregulating the NF-κB activation pathway. In the influenza virus, it blocked the activity of protein kinase C [45]. In the case of Middle East Respiratory Syndrome - Coronavirus (MERS-CoV), the inflammation was reduced by inhibiting the production of the pro-inflammatory cytokines and downregulating the NF-κB pathway. The antiviral activity was observed to be stimulated by promoting Sirtuin 1 (SIRT1) signals and activating apoptosis by P53 [46].

Similar to other polyphenolic immunomodulators described above, **6** undergoes metabolism mainly in the human intestine and liver, preferentially *via* glucuronidation and sulfation [47]. Metabolism of **6** by colonic microbiota is significant. The safety studies in humans have confirmed its tolerability and milder form of adverse events. At higher doses (2.5/5 g), **6** has shown mild to moderate gastrointestinal discomfort. Overall, **6** is an important phytochemical with significant immunomodulatory activities, which confirms its utility in many pathological conditions.

Genistein

Genistein (**9**, Fig. (**2**), 5,7-dihydroxy-3-(4-hydroxyphenyl)-4*H*-chromen-4-one), an isoflavone, reported to be present in soy and soy-derived products, is a powerful immune suppressor, affecting both the humoral and cell-mediated immunity. It possesses anti-inflammatory, antioxidant, and phytoestrogen activities. Genistein has a structure similar to 17β-estradiol Fig. (**5**) which binds ERβ with greater affinity than ERα; 17β-estradiol is equipotent at both the ER types. At higher concentrations, **9** demonstrated protein tyrosine kinase inhibitory activity [48].

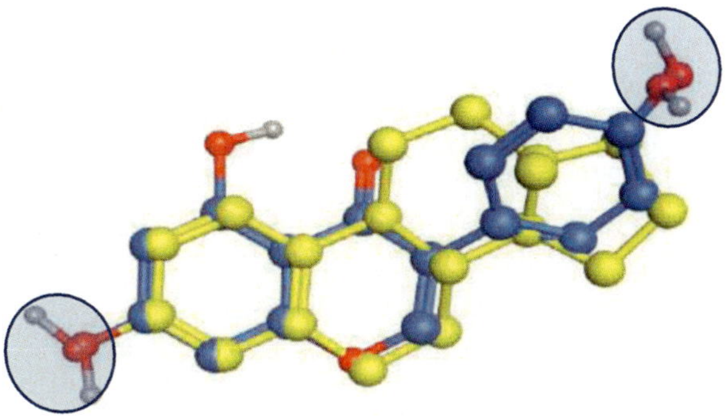

Fig. (5). Molecular Alignment of Genistein (9, blue)) with 17β-estradiol (yellow). Both Compounds are shown as Ball-and-stick Models. The Aligned -OH Groups of both Compounds are circled for clarity.

Genistein (**9**) is used for treating RA because of its strong anti-inflammatory efficacy. Treatment with **9** for two weeks in the collagen-induced rheumatoid arthritis model alleviates the inflammation of joints and the mechanism behind its action is decreased levels of inflammatory cytokines, IFN-γ and upregulation of the secretion of the cytokine IL-4. Additionally, there was a regulated expression of T-bet and GATA-3 proteins (which play an important role during the development of Th-1 and Th-2 cells). This resulted in a significantly reduced ratio of Thl to Th2, which accounts for 1:5, leading to the successful therapeutic outcome of the treatment for RA [49].

Genistein has been reported to suppress both the adaptive and humoral immune systems. It has been associated with affecting the early maturation of thymocytes and causing a decrease in both CD4+/CD8- and CD4+/CD8+ cells and finally resulting in lymphocytopenia and suppressing the immune system. Its application even has a negative effect on the thymic weight and size in a dose-dependent manner [48.50]. It has its role in epilepsy, stroke, and Alzheimer's disease. Compound **9** inhibited the JAK2/STAT3 pathway, thereby downregulating the cytokines IL-1β and TNF-α. This resulted in enhancing the expression of antioxidant proteins such as heme oxygenase-1, HO-1 and NAD(P)H:quinone dehydrogenase 1 (NQO1) and thereby downregulating the ROS release and hence reducing the oxidative damage [51].

SEARCH FOR NEWER, SAFER IMMUNOMODULATORS

Traditional Indian Medicine is full of plants and their active principles as immunomodulators. A decade-old compilation of immunomodulators in the Indian System of Medicine, *e.g.*, Ayurveda, lists common plants such as Tulsi, Kaalmegha, Kumaari, Arjuna, Naagbala, Kutki, Safed musli, Khadira, Madana and many others [52]. The bioactive compounds include glycosides, flavonoids, coumarins, sapogenins, alkaloids, and polysaccharides, along with a few minority chemical classes. Interestingly, the diversity in chemical classes in which immunomodulatory activity resides is vast. Systematic understanding of the chemical features imparting the immunomodulatory activity is lacking in the literature. There is certainly a scope on that front, which is likely to help in designing potent immunomodulators for a given disease or disorder.

The degree and target cells/organs for immunomodulatory therapies differ according to the nature of the disease/disorder. Understanding the mode and/or mechanism of immunomodulation, particularly for compounds of natural origin, clearly is critical for the optimal therapeutic outcome [53]. The recent surge in immune checkpoint inhibitors, *e.g.*, programmed death receptor 1 (PD-1) or its ligand (PD-L1) inhibitors, as anticancer agents demonstrated the usefulness of this strategy for putting brakes on cancer [54]. Few other strategies, such as cytotoxic T-cell lymphocyte-associated protein 4 (CTLA-4) inhibitors, have been used with promise for developing immunotherapeutics. The field is complex, with diverse avenues presenting daunting challenges and rewarding opportunities. The future will tell us about what's in store for us! Till then, we need to pursue the phytochemicals as leads for fine-tuning the strategies for immunomodulation within the realms of desirable safety and unavoidable adverse events.

ANALYTICAL TECHNIQUES FOR ISOLATION, PURIFICATION, QUANTIFICATION AND CHARACTERIZATION OF NATURAL IMMUNOMODULATORS

Phytoconstituents are a rich source of bioactive molecules from natural origin. They belong to different chemical classes such as flavonoids, saponins, alkaloids, tannins, terpenoids, and many others. The first step involved in the characterization of phytoconstituents is isolation and purification using appropriate method(s). The isolation of phytoconstituents from plant materials starts with usually with solvent extraction, followed by chromatographic purification, structural characterization and ultimately bioactivity screening. Extraction methods vary depending on the type of constituents that need to be extracted. Representative methods are listed in Table **2**.

Phytochemicals extraction is the first step prior to structure identification, and bioactivity evaluation. In recent years, novel extraction, isolation, and structural identification techniques and procedures have emerged, allowing for faster extraction and analysis of phytochemicals.

Elucidation of chemical structures of novel phytochemicals is the prime process for subsequent research involving structural activity relationship assessment, pharmacokinetic studies and determining the drug-likeness characteristic. As the amount of chemical constituents separated by extraction methods is negligible, their production is the next step. Hence spectral analysis is primarily employed for structural detailing [55].

A large number of advanced chromatographic and spectroscopic techniques have been employed for the detailed analysis of the immunomodulatory plant extracts, phytochemicals and formulations to ensure the quality and purity of the plant products.

Table 2. Extraction of phytoconstituents from plant.

Method	Details of the method
Solvent extraction	Appropriate solvent system selection is the key factor for successful solvent method. Using a solvent of appropriate polarity, the plant material is subjected to extraction. Solvent polarity, presence of H-bonding groups, dielectric constant, vapour pressure affect the efficiency of solvent extraction.
Immersion	Extraction of phytochemicals with appropriate solvents at room or low temperatures (<80°C). Useful for heat-sensitive compounds. It is a simple method with low efficiency.
Percolation	A percolator is used, and coarse plant material is loaded with solvents of choice. Efficient method than the immersion method.
Decoction	Plant material in the form of coarse powder or pieces is packed in an appropriate container with water, and heated to boiling for the extraction of the components of choice A useful method for volatile compounds and non-applicable for plants with a lot of starch.

(Table 2) cont.....

Method	Details of the method
Refluxing	Refluxing apparatus is used to extract plant constituents by organic solvent using heating and refluxing. Steroids, anthraquinoids, and terpenoids are extracted by this method. Constant refluxing method requires a Soxhlet extractor.
Supercritical Fluid Extraction (SCF)	Under control temperature, pressure and solvent, plant material is exposed to supercritical fluid for extraction of phytoconstituents of varying polarities, boiling points, and molecular weights.

Some of the techniques are described in Fig. (**6**) and details are below:

Chromatography

Chromatography is the most commonly used analytical technique for the separation of varied chemical constituents present in natural product extracts; their identification can also be performed by this technique. The advanced methods in this technique are:

High-Performance Liquid Chromatography (HPLC)

It is a highly efficient separation and analysis method. The principle of separation in HPLC is the same as conventional column chromatography. In the isolation, qualitative characterization, and quantification of phytochemicals, HPLC has become increasingly essential. High efficiency, high speed, and automation are all critical features of this method [55].

High-Performance Thin Layer Chromatography (HPTLC)

It is the most successful method for determining the major constituents of medicinal herbs. In comparison to TLC, the isolation and resolution are higher and the outcomes are more reliable and reproducible. By using scanning densitometry, HPTLC analysis provides the advantage of *in situ* qualitative and quantitative measurements [56]. The HPTLC can also be coupled with mass spectrometry for more efficient structural elucidation.

Droplet Counter-Current Chromatography (DCCC)

Built on the counter-current partition technique, DCCC is an advanced liquid-liquid partition chromatography. Phytoconstituents with high polarity can be separated by this method. It can be used for samples like crude extracts and gives good reproducible results [55].

High-Speed Counter-Current Chromatography (HSCCC)

It is a liquid-liquid partition chromatography. From this chromatography, the sample recovered is quantitative. It also provides good reproducibility, high purity of isolated chemicals, with a short response time. It is suitable for the separation and purification of diverse range of phytoconstituents, such as saponins, flavonoids, anthraquinoids, lignans, alkaloids, triterpenes, carbohydrates and proteins [57].

High-Performance Capillary Electrophoresis (HPCE)

It is a modern analytical technique that combines traditional electrophoresis with advanced microcolumn separation techniques. High efficiency, microamount, affordability, high automation, and extensive applications are the benefits of HPCE. It has limitations in terms of preparation ability, sensitivity, and isolation reproducibility [58].

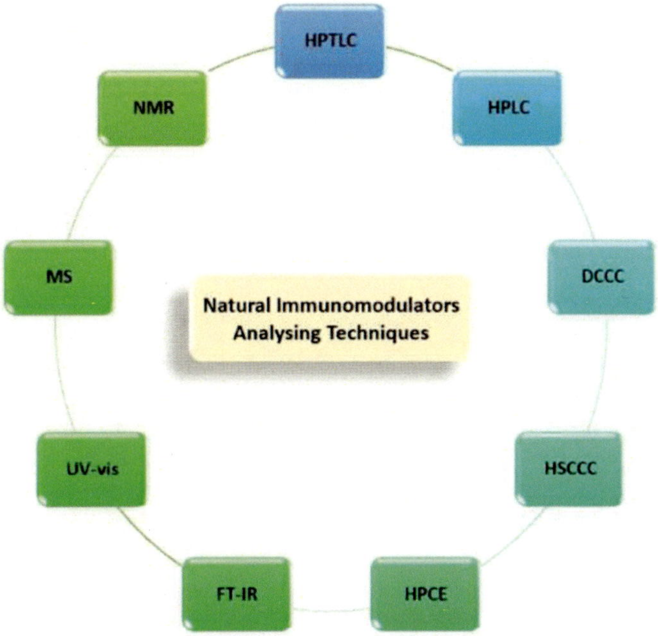

Fig. (6). Several analytical methods are used for the isolation, purification and characterization of natural immunomodulators.

Spectroscopy

Spectroscopy is majorly used for the structural identification and quantitation of phytochemicals and for checking the purity of the isolated compounds and constituents. Due to advanced techniques like Nuclear Magnetic Resonance (NMR) and Mass Spectrometry (MS), the speed and accuracy of structural determination of phytoconstituents have increased to a very high level [55]. Some of the spectroscopic methods are:

Ultraviolet/Visible (UV/Vis) Spectroscopy

It is useful for figuring out the structures of phytoconstituents with conjugated substructures. It gives information about only a part of the chemical structures. Hence, this method is used as a supplementary method to other advanced techniques [55].

Fourier-Transform Infra-Red (FT-IR) Spectroscopy

It is majorly used for the determination of functional groups and the various types of structural features, including (hetero)aromatic/(hetero)alicyclic ring substitutions. The FT-IR can be used to assess the configuration of phytochemicals under specific circumstances [55].

Mass Spectrometry (MS)

It is used to assess the molecular weights, formulae, and fragment structures of the different molecules [59]. In fact, High-Resolution Mass Spectrometry (HRMS) is an indispensable tool in the structural elucidation of novel phytochemicals and natural products.

Nuclear Magnetic Resonance (NMR) Spectroscopy

It has become the major technique to determine phytochemical structures. It can give structural details concerning the kind and number of hydrogen and carbon atoms in the molecule, as well as the modes *via* which they are coupled, the chemical environment in which they are found, arrangement, and conformation [60].

BIOACTIVITY SCREENING METHODS FOR THE IMMUNOMODULATORS

There has been the usage of both *in vivo* and *in vitro* methods for analyzing the activity of immunomodulators. One has to go for *in vivo* testing after *in vitro* evaluation. *In vitro* assays are mostly carried out in a medium containing particular cell lines, which include neutrophil adhesion test, MTT assay, Hemagglutination antibody titer, iNOS activity, inhibition of T-cell proliferation, and many more. *In vivo* studies involve either testing in an appropriate animal model representing the disease or disorder of interest; at times some chemicals are used for inducing the disease. Most of the tests to be carried out include Delayed-type hypersensitivity, Anaphylaxis, Arthritis, and many diseases of interest [19, 61]. Tables **3** and **4**. summarize the biological evaluation of immunomodulators using *in vivo* studies and *in vitro* assays.

Table 3. *In vitro* assays used for confirming the immunomodulatory activity.

S. No	Cell Lines used	Compound or Assay used	Testing Against	References
1.	HepG2 cancerous cell lines	Propidium iodide	Apoptosis analysis	[27]
		DCFH-DAP probes (2',7' Dichloro Fluorescein Diacetate)	ROS generation	
		Western blot	Immunoglobulins	
		MTT assay	Cancer cell proliferation	
2.	Splenocytes	Griess assay	Nitric oxide	[28]
		Cytometric bead assay	Cytokines	
3.	Human breast cancer cell line	Trypan blue	Cell viability	[25]
		Immunoprecipitation, Western blot, and qPCR	Detecting the ERα	
4.	*Salmonella typhimurium*	Hydrogen peroxide, tertiary butyl hydroperoxide	Mutagenicity assay	[38]

The choice of analytical method for the evaluation of immunomodulatory activity is affected by several factors such as the nature of the disease/disorder, severity, biological complexity with respect to the signaling pathways involved in the pathology of the disease/disorder, chemical nature of the putative immunomodulatory compound or preparation, and stability of the test article, to name a few. The list in Table **3** is for representation only. Few articles attempted to capture the essence of immunomodulatory analyses [62-68].

Table 4. Compounds used and disease developed for *in vivo* assays.

S. No.	The Compound used for Inducing	Disease Induced	Reference
1.	Alloxan	Diabetes	[36]
2.	Ovachallenge	Asthma	[36]
3.	Thioacetamide	Liver cirrhosis	[37]
4.	3° butyl hydroperoxide	Mutagenicity induction	[38]
5.	Collagen	Rheumatoid arthritis	[49]

CONCLUDING REMARKS

The immunomodulatory activities of natural products are of utmost importance for driving fundamental research in basic sciences and for fueling the design and discovery of novel, more potent and safer immunomodulatory compounds for various therapeutic indications in the drug discovery and development field. The major hitch is the poor or incomplete understanding of the underlying mechanism of actions of the preparations or purely natural products. A systematic understanding of the chemical features affecting the contextual immunomodulatory activity and the potential molecular targets is required for advancing the field with great speed. The advent of immune checkpoint inhibitors and their therapeutic success is definitely encouraging, but we need more such outcomes for diseases such as various difficult-to-treat cancers, RA, psoriasis, *etc.* The present book chapter is an attempt to generate interest in the reader to take up such activities and contribute to the further development of novel immunomodulators.

CONSENT FOR PUBLICATION

Not applicable.

CONFLICT OF INTEREST

The authors declare no conflict of interest, financial or otherwise.

ACKNOWLEDGEMENTS

The authors are thankful to Prof. A. B. Pandit, Vice Chancellor, Institute of Chemical Technology (ICT), Mumbai, and Prof. Shreerang V. Joshi, Head, Department of Pharmaceutical Sciences and Technology (DPST), ICT, Mumbai for arranging all the facilities required for the completion of this book chapter.

REFERENCES

[1] Medzhitov R, Janeway C Jr. Innate Immunity. N Engl J Med 2000; 343(5): 338-44. [http://dx.doi.org/10.1056/NEJM200008033430506] [PMID: 10922424]

[2] Jantan I, Ahmad W, Bukhari SNA. Plant-derived immunomodulators: an insight on their preclinical evaluation and clinical trials. Front Plant Sci 2015; 6: 655. [http://dx.doi.org/10.3389/fpls.2015.00655] [PMID: 26379683]

[3] Shukla S, Bajpai VK, Kim M. Plants as potential sources of natural immunomodulators. Rev Environ Sci Biotechnol 2014; 13(1): 17-33. [http://dx.doi.org/10.1007/s11157-012-9303-x]

[4] Nicholls EF, Madera L, Hancock REW. Immunomodulators as adjuvants for vaccines and antimicrobial therapy. Ann N Y Acad Sci 2010; 1213(1): 46-61. [http://dx.doi.org/10.1111/j.1749-6632.2010.05787.x] [PMID: 20946578]

[5] Colombani T, Haudebourg T, Decossas M, *et al.* Lipidic Aminoglycoside Derivatives: A New Class of Immunomodulators Inducing a Potent Innate Immune Stimulation. Adv Sci (Weinh) 2019; 6(16): 1900288.
[http://dx.doi.org/10.1002/advs.201900288] [PMID: 31453059]

[6] Dumont FJ, Su Q. Mechanism of action of the immunosuppressant rapamycin. Life Sci 1995; 58(5): 373-95.
[http://dx.doi.org/10.1016/0024-3205(95)02233-3] [PMID: 8594303]

[7] Karimi A, Majlesi M, Rafieian-Kopaei M. Herbal *versus* synthetic drugs; beliefs and facts. J Nephropharmacol 2015; 4(1): 27-30.
[PMID: 28197471]

[8] Newman DJ, Cragg GM. Natural Products as Sources of New Drugs from 1981 to 2014. J Nat Prod 2016; 79(3): 629-61.
[http://dx.doi.org/10.1021/acs.jnatprod.5b01055] [PMID: 26852623]

[9] Golonko A, Lewandowska H, Świsłocka R, Jasińska UT, Priebe W, Lewandowski W. Curcumin as tyrosine kinase inhibitor in cancer treatment. Eur J Med Chem 2019; 181: 111512.
[http://dx.doi.org/10.1016/j.ejmech.2019.07.015] [PMID: 31404861]

[10] El Enshasy HA, Hatti-Kaul R. Mushroom immunomodulators: unique molecules with unlimited applications. Trends Biotechnol 2013; 31(12): 668-77.
[http://dx.doi.org/10.1016/j.tibtech.2013.09.003] [PMID: 24125745]

[11] Suwannarach N, Kumla J, Sujarit K, Pattananandecha T, Saenjum C, Lumyong S. Natural bioactive compounds from fungi as potential candidates for protease inhibitors and immunomodulators to apply for coronaviruses. Molecules 2020; 25(8): 1800.
[http://dx.doi.org/10.3390/molecules25081800] [PMID: 32295300]

[12] Wu Y, Pan L, Shang QH, *et al.* Effects of isomalto-oligosaccharides as potential prebiotics on performance, immune function and gut microbiota in weaned pigs. Anim Feed Sci Technol 2017; 230: 126-35.
[http://dx.doi.org/10.1016/j.anifeedsci.2017.05.013]

[13] Manu KA, Kuttan G. Immunomodulatory activities of Punarnavine, an alkaloid from *Boerhaavia diffusa*. Immunopharmacol Immunotoxicol 2009; 31(3): 377-87.
[http://dx.doi.org/10.1080/08923970802702036] [PMID: 19555203]

[14] Srikumar R, Jeya Parthasarathy N, Sheela Devi R. Immunomodulatory activity of triphala on neutrophil functions. Biol Pharm Bull 2005; 28(8): 1398-403.
[http://dx.doi.org/10.1248/bpb.28.1398] [PMID: 16079482]

[15] Sathaye S, Amin P, Mehta V, *et al.* Immunomodulatory Activity of Aqueous Extract of *Murraya Koenigii*, L in Experimental Animals. Int J Toxicol Pharmacol Res 2011; 3(4): 7-12.

[16] Wu Y, Tu X, Lin G, *et al.* Emodin-mediated protection from acute myocardial infarction *via* inhibition of inflammation and apoptosis in local ischemic myocardium. Life Sci 2007; 81(17-18): 1332-8.
[http://dx.doi.org/10.1016/j.lfs.2007.08.040] [PMID: 17939930]

[17] Thacker PC, Karunagaran D. Curcumin and emodin down-regulate TGF-β signaling pathway in human cervical cancer cells. PLoS One 2015; 10(3): e0120045.
[http://dx.doi.org/10.1371/journal.pone.0120045] [PMID: 25786122]

[18] SaiRam M, Sharma SK, Ilavazhagan G, Kumar D, Selvamurthy W. Immunomodulatory effects of NIM-76, a volatile fraction from Neem oil. J Ethnopharmacol 1997; 55(2): 133-9.
[http://dx.doi.org/10.1016/S0378-8741(96)01487-0] [PMID: 9032626]

[19] Vinothapooshan G, Sundar K. Immunomodulatory activity of various extracts of *Adhatoda vasica Linn.* in experimental rats. Afr J Pharm Pharmacol 2011; 5(3): 306-10.
[http://dx.doi.org/10.5897/AJPP10.126]

[20] Clement F, Pramod SN, Venkatesh YP. Identity of the immunomodulatory proteins from garlic (*Allium sativum*) with the major garlic lectins or agglutinins. Int Immunopharmacol 2010; 10(3): 316-24.
[http://dx.doi.org/10.1016/j.intimp.2009.12.002] [PMID: 20004743]

[21] Jeba RC, Vaidyanathan RA, Rameshkumar G. Efficacy of *Ocimum basilicum* for immunomodulatory activity in Wistar albino rat. Int J Pharm Pharm Sci 2011; 3(4): 199-203.

[22] Webster D, Taschereau P, Lee TDG, Jurgens T. Immunostimulant properties of *Heracleum maximum Bartr.* J Ethnopharmacol 2006; 106(3): 360-3.
[http://dx.doi.org/10.1016/j.jep.2006.01.018] [PMID: 16504434]

[23] Lai X, Pei Q, Song X, *et al.* The enhancement of immune function and activation of NF-κB by resveratrol-treatment in immunosuppressive mice. Int Immunopharmacol 2016; 33: 42-7.
[http://dx.doi.org/10.1016/j.intimp.2016.01.028] [PMID: 26854575]

[24] Wen-Feng W, Feng-Sen Z, Wen-Na Z, *et al.* The synthesis, structural study and anticancer activity evaluation of emodin derivatives containing conjugative groups. Med Chem 2013; 9(4): 545-52.
[http://dx.doi.org/10.2174/1573406411309040008] [PMID: 22920154]

[25] Huang PH, Huang CY, Chen MC, *et al.* Emodin and aloe-emodin suppress breast cancer cell proliferation through ERα inhibition. Evid Based Complement Alternat Med 2013; 2013: 1-12.
[http://dx.doi.org/10.1155/2013/376123] [PMID: 23864887]

[26] Ma L, Chen K, Jiang K, *et al.* Emodin inhibits the proliferation and invasion of bladder cancer cells *via* down-regulating Notch1. Int J Clin Exp Pathol 2017; 10(9): 9452-9.
[PMID: 31966818]

[27] Xing YX, Li MH, Tao L, *et al.* Anti-cancer effects of emodin on HepG2 cells as revealed by 1H NMR based metabolic profiling. J Proteome Res 2018; 17(5): 1943-52.
[http://dx.doi.org/10.1021/acs.jproteome.8b00029] [PMID: 29676152]

[28] Sharma R, Tiku AB. Emodin inhibits splenocyte proliferation and inflammation by modulating cytokine responses in a mouse model system. J Immunotoxicol 2016; 13(1): 20-6.
[http://dx.doi.org/10.3109/1547691X.2014.995243] [PMID: 25565015]

[29] Li Q, Gao J, Pang X, Chen A, Wang Y. Molecular mechanisms of action of emodin: as an anti-cardiovascular disease drug. Front Pharmacol 2020; 11: 559607.
[http://dx.doi.org/10.3389/fphar.2020.559607] [PMID: 32973538]

[30] Lee J, Kim HJ, Nguyen TTH, *et al.* Emodin 8-O-glucoside primes macrophages more strongly than emodin aglycone *via* activation of phagocytic activity and TLR-2/MAPK/NF-κB signalling pathway. Int Immunopharmacol 2020; 88: 106936.
[http://dx.doi.org/10.1016/j.intimp.2020.106936] [PMID: 32871479]

[31] Dong X, Fu J, Yin X, *et al.* Emodin: A review of its pharmacology, toxicity and pharmacokinetics. Phytother Res 2016; 30(8): 1207-18.
[http://dx.doi.org/10.1002/ptr.5631] [PMID: 27188216]

[32] Qin B, Xu Y, Chen J, Huang W, Peng Y, Zheng J. Chemical Reactivity of Emodin and Its Oxidative Metabolites to Thiols. Chem Res Toxicol 2016; 29(12): 2114-24.
[http://dx.doi.org/10.1021/acs.chemrestox.6b00191] [PMID: 27989148]

[33] Fortunato LR, Alves CF, Teixeira MM, Rogerio AP. Quercetin: a flavonoid with the potential to treat asthma. Braz J Pharm Sci 2012; 48(4): 589-99.
[http://dx.doi.org/10.1590/S1984-82502012000400002]

[34] Al-Rekabi MD, Ali SH, Al-Basaisi H, Hashim F, Hussein AH, Abbas HK. Immunomodulatory effects of quercetin in patient with active rheumatoid arthritis. Br J Med Health Res 2015; 2(6): 23-34.

[35] Mehrbod P, Abdalla MA, Fotouhi F, *et al.* Immunomodulatory properties of quercetin-3-O-α-L-rhamnopyranoside from *Rapanea melanophloeos* against influenza a virus. BMC Complement

Altern Med 2018; 18(1): 184.
[http://dx.doi.org/10.1186/s12906-018-2246-1] [PMID: 29903008]

[36] Ravikumar N, Kavitha CN. Immunomodulatory effect of Quercetin on dysregulated Th1/Th2 cytokine balance in mice with both type 1 diabetes and allergic asthma. J Appl Pharm Sci 2020; 10(3): 80-7. [http://dx.doi.org/10.7324/JAPS.2020.103010]

[37] Casas-Grajales S, Vázquez-Flores LF, Ramos-Tovar E, *et al.* Quercetin reverses experimental cirrhosis by immunomodulation of the proinflammatory and profibrotic processes. Fundam Clin Pharmacol 2017; 31(6): 610-24.
[http://dx.doi.org/10.1111/fcp.12315] [PMID: 28802065]

[38] Valentová K, Šíma P, Rybková Z, Křížan J, Malachová K, Křen V. (Anti)mutagenic and immunomodulatory properties of quercetin glycosides. J Sci Food Agric 2016; 96(5): 1492-9. [http://dx.doi.org/10.1002/jsfa.7251] [PMID: 25960089]

[39] Kato K, Ninomiya M, Tanaka K, Koketsu M. Rffects of functional groups and sugar composition of quercetin derivatives on their radical scavenging properties. J Nat Prod 2016; 79(7): 1808-14. [http://dx.doi.org/10.1021/acs.jnatprod.6b00274] [PMID: 27314621]

[40] Derosa G, Maffioli P, D'Angelo A, Di Pierro F. A role for quercetin in coronavirus disease 2019 (COVID□19). Phytother Res 2021; 35(3): 1230-6.
[http://dx.doi.org/10.1002/ptr.6887] [PMID: 33034398]

[41] Salehi B, Mishra A, Nigam M, *et al.* Resveratrol: a double-edged sword in health benefits. Biomedicines 2018; 6(3): 91.
[http://dx.doi.org/10.3390/biomedicines6030091] [PMID: 30205595]

[42] Vetvicka V, Volny T, Saraswat-Ohri S, Vashishta A, Vancikova Z, Vetvickova J. Glucan and resveratrol complex--possible synergistic effects on immune system. Biomedical Papers of the Medical Faculty of Palacky University in Olomouc 2007; 151: 1.

[43] Yang Y, Paik JH, Cho D, Cho JA, Kim CW. Resveratrol induces the suppression of tumor-derived CD4+CD25+ regulatory T cells. Int Immunopharmacol 2008; 8(4): 542-7.
[http://dx.doi.org/10.1016/j.intimp.2007.12.006] [PMID: 18328445]

[44] Garvin S, Öllinger K, Dabrosin C. Resveratrol induces apoptosis and inhibits angiogenesis in human breast cancer xenografts *in vivo.* Cancer Lett 2006; 231(1): 113-22.
[http://dx.doi.org/10.1016/j.canlet.2005.01.031] [PMID: 16356836]

[45] Campagna M, Rivas C. Antiviral activity of resveratrol. Biochem Soc Trans 2010; 38(1): 50-3. [http://dx.doi.org/10.1042/BST0380050] [PMID: 20074034]

[46] Ramdani LH, Bachari K. Potential therapeutic effects of Resveratrol against SARS-CoV-2. Acta Virol 2020; 64(3): 276-80.
[http://dx.doi.org/10.4149/av_2020_309] [PMID: 32985211]

[47] Sergides C, Chirilă M, Silvestro L, Pitta D, Pittas A. Bioavailability and safety study of resveratrol 500 mg tablets in healthy male and female volunteers. Exp Ther Med 2016; 11(1): 164-70. [http://dx.doi.org/10.3892/etm.2015.2895] [PMID: 26889234]

[48] Cooke PS, Selvaraj V, Yellayi S. Genistein, estrogen receptors, and the acquired immune response. J Nutr 2006; 136(3): 704-8.
[http://dx.doi.org/10.1093/jn/136.3.704] [PMID: 16484547]

[49] Wang J, Zhang Q, Jin S, He D, Zhao S, Liu S. Genistein modulate immune responses in collagen-induced rheumatoid arthritis model. Maturitas 2008; 59(4): 405-12.
[http://dx.doi.org/10.1016/j.maturitas.2008.04.003] [PMID: 18499367]

[50] Yellayi S, Zakroczymski MA, Selvaraj V, *et al.* The phytoestrogen genistein suppresses cell-mediated immunity in mice. J Endocrinol 2003; 176(2): 267-74.
[http://dx.doi.org/10.1677/joe.0.1760267] [PMID: 12553875]

[51] Hu QP, Huang XY, Feng W, *et al.* Genistein protects epilepsy-induced brain injury through regulating the JAK2/STAT3 and keap1/nrf2 signaling pathways in the developing rats. Eur J Pharmacol 2021. 912: 174620.

[52] Kumar D, Arya V, Kaur R, Bhat ZA, Gupta VK, Kumar V. A review of immunomodulators in the Indian traditional health care system. J Microbiol Immunol Infect 2012; 45(3): 165-84. [http://dx.doi.org/10.1016/j.jmii.2011.09.030] [PMID: 22154993]

[53] Chun-Chu , Abd Rahman MB, Alitheen NB, *et al.* Evaluation of immunomodulatory effect: Selection of the correct targets for immunostimulation study. Am J Immunol 2011; 7(2): 17-23. [http://dx.doi.org/10.3844/ajisp.2011.17.23]

[54] Alsaab HO, Sau S, Alzhrani R, *et al.* PD-1 and PD-L1 checkpoint signaling inhibition for cancer immunotherapy: mechanism, combinations, and clinical outcome. Front Pharmacol 2017; 8: 561. [http://dx.doi.org/10.3389/fphar.2017.00561] [PMID: 28878676]

[55] Feng W, Li M, Hao Z, Zhang J. Analytical Methods of Isolation and Identification [Internet]. Phytochemicals in Human Health. IntechOpen 2019. [cited 2022 Jun 1]. Available from: https://www.intechopen.com/chapters/undefined/state.item.id

[56] OneroofTechnologies. HPTLC Laboratory | HPTLC Testing Labs | HPTLC Analysis in Mumbai [Internet]. HPTLC Laboratory | HPTLC Testing Labs | HPTLC Analysis in Mumbai. [cited 2022 Jun 1]. Available from: https://anchrom.in/

[57] Gu M, Ouyang F, Su Z. Comparison of high-speed counter-current chromatography and high-performance liquid chromatography on fingerprinting of Chinese traditional medicine. J Chromatogr A 2004; 1022(1-2): 139-44. [http://dx.doi.org/10.1016/j.chroma.2003.09.038] [PMID: 14753780]

[58] Horie H, Kohata K. Analysis of tea components by high-performance liquid chromatography and high-performance capillary electrophoresis. J Chromatogr A 2000; 881(1-2): 425-38. [http://dx.doi.org/10.1016/S0021-9673(99)01345-X] [PMID: 10905725]

[59] Kumar K, Siva B, Rama Rao N, Suresh Babu K. Rapid identification of limonoids from Cipadessa baccifera and Xylocarpus granatum using ESI-Q-ToF-MS/MS and their structure-fragmentation study. J Pharm Biomed Anal 2018; 152: 224-33. [http://dx.doi.org/10.1016/j.jpba.2017.12.050] [PMID: 29427881]

[60] Monakhova YB, Kuballa T, Lachenmeier DW. Chemometric methods in NMR spectroscopic analysis of food products. J Anal Chem 2013; 68(9): 755-66. [http://dx.doi.org/10.1134/S1061934813090098]

[61] Nair A, Chattopadhyay D, Saha B. Plant-derived immunomodulators. New Look to Phytomedicine 2019; 435-99. [http://dx.doi.org/10.1016/b978-0-12-814619-4.00018-5]

[62] Bilitewski U. Determination of immunomodulatory effects: focus on functional analysis of phagocytes as representatives of the innate immune system. Anal Bioanal Chem 2008; 391(5): 1545-54. [http://dx.doi.org/10.1007/s00216-008-2089-6] [PMID: 18427788]

[63] Zimmermann P, Ziesenitz VC, Curtis N, Ritz N. The Immunomodulatory Effects of Macrolides—A Systematic Review of the Underlying Mechanisms. Front Immunol 2018; 9: 302. [http://dx.doi.org/10.3389/fimmu.2018.00302] [PMID: 29593707]

[64] Yuliastri WO, Diantini A, Ghozali M, Sahidin I, Isrul M. Immunomodulatory activity and phytochemical analysis of *Hibiscus sabdariffa* L. flower fractions. J Appl Pharm Sci 2021; 11(11): 131-40. [http://dx.doi.org/10.7324/JAPS.2021.1101117]

CHAPTER 6

Bioassays and Other Methods for Immunomodulators in Preclinical and Clinical Setting

Priyanka P. Nigade[1], **Pranjali S. Dhamane**[2] and **Vandana S. Nikam**[1,*]

[1] *Department of Pharmacology, STES's Smt. Kashibai Navale College of Pharmacy, Kondhwa, S. P. Pune University, Pune, Maharashtra, India*

[2] *M. Pharm Pharmacology, STES's, Smt. Kashibai Navale College of Pharmacy, Kondhwa (Bk), Pune-411048, Maharashtra, India*

Abstract: The availability of appropriate animal models is essential for effective translation of immunomodulatory research into clinical settings. Bioassays and other methods for immunomodulators in the preclinical and clinical setting are being used to assess the quality and quantification of the immune response, find the best suitable route of administration and formulation method, protect the transmission of infection, and assess the safety and toxicity of immunomodulators. Identifying the appropriate animal model has become very important, since each model has its own pro's and cons. The scope of this chapter is to outline the assaying of immunomodulatory activity, the approaches and the experimental strategies. This chapter discusses various *in-vitro* models such as cell lines, assays and murine models, which are being used for quantification of the immune response, assessment of overall immune functions, immunosuppressive activity, screening of anti-allergic drugs and agents used in the treatment of various autoimmune disorders and transplant-related and autoimmune diseases. The most important questions that we should keep in mind while choosing a suitable animal model are, selection of suitable species, physiological relevance of model, immunological functions to be evaluated, and its practical implications.

Keywords: Adaptive Immunity, Immune System, Immunomodulation, Innate Immunity.

INTRODUCTION

Scientist Edward Jenner, who performed the first 'vaccination' against smallpox in 1796, brought the concept of Immunomodulation. Further, various efforts were undertaken to modify the immune system to combat both external and internal pathogen attacks, with the intention of improving disease resistance. With this

* **Corresponding author Vandana S. Nikam:** Department of Pharmacology, STES's Smt. Kashibai Navale college of Pharmacy, Kondhwa, S. P. Pune University, Pune, Maharashtra, India; E-mail: vandananikam@sinhgad.edu

goal, the immune response can be modified by applying immunosuppression, immunestimulation, and immunerestoration [1 - 3]. Immuno-stimulatory adjuvants are required in vaccines to activate the innate immune system and generate specific adaptive immunological responses. Immunoadjuvants increase the amount of antibody generated while decreasing the amount of antigen required for injection and, as a result, the frequency of injection. Examples of best-known types of immunoadjuvants are Toll-like receptor agonists (TLR), inorganic immunoadjuvants, plant-derived immunoadjuvants, exosomes, and endogenous proteins. However, their short response rates and undesirable effects limit their use. As a result, there is a continued demand for immunoadjuvants with enhanced efficacy and lower toxicity, as well as improved bioactivity and bioavailability [4, 5]. Also, many novel multifunctional adjuvants are being developed with the modified delivery system. Nanoparticle-based immunoadjuvant [4] and the incorporation of multifunctional immunoadjuvants into pDNA/mRNA vaccines [6] are two of the most promising. Immunostimulants are appealing compounds that trigger the immune system for disease prevention and improve natural resistance to numerous viral and bacterial infections. Immunostimulants act in specific and non-specific ways in the body, causing the production of specific antibodies and cytokines, which can be used to treat infectious disorders and diseases with suppressed immunity like malignancies, AIDS, SARS, *etc* [7, 8]. Immunosuppressive drugs are used to treat severe hypersensitivity immune reactions, transplant-related and autoimmune diseases caused by autoreactive B lymphocytes or T lymphocytes (CD4+ or CD8+ cells) [9, 10].

ASSOCIATION OF INNATE IMMUNITY AND ADAPTIVE IMMUNITY AND THEIR MEASUREMENTS

Innate immunity is the first-line immune system with no memory generates fast and blunt, non-specific responses to infection and tissue injury in response to the signals from germline-coded proteins termed Pattern Recognition Receptors (PRRs). PRRs have evolved to recognize molecular patterns shared by numerous pathogen classes called Pathogen-Associated Molecular Patterns (PAMPs) or Damage-Associated Molecular Patterns (DAMPs). To activate the adaptive immune system, dendritic cells, macrophages, mast cells, neutrophils, basophils and eosinophils directly interact with other cells or release cytokines and other compounds such as reactive oxygen species, nitric oxide, and lipid inflammatory mediators which are involved in the inflammatory response. Other lymphocytes without antigen specificity, such as gamma-delta T cells and Natural Killer (NK) cells, are considered innate cells with some resemblance to effector lymphocytes [11, 12]. Dendritic cells (DC) are important agents between innate and adaptive immunity by triggering primary immune responses. DC, as a component of the innate immune system, organises and transports information from the outside world to the adaptive immune system [13].

Adaptive immunity generates an antigen-specific, flexible response and has immunologic memory. So, it permits vertebrates to thrive in an environment where they are constantly exposed to infections. This system relies on the clonal selection and expansion of lymphocytes *via* antigen (T cell and B cell) receptors. Antigen receptors are clonal receptors that have been genetically altered to bind to antigens expressed in Major Histocompatibility Complex (MHC) molecules on antigen-presenting cells [14].

Although the innate and adaptive immune systems are opposite, independent systems of the host response, they work together see Fig. (**1**). The innate system acts as the first line of defense against pathogens, thus activating antigen-specific cells. These antigen-specific cells further help in recognizing and responding to microorganisms. As a result, coordination between innate and adaptive immune responses is important, even though they operate *via* different mechanisms.

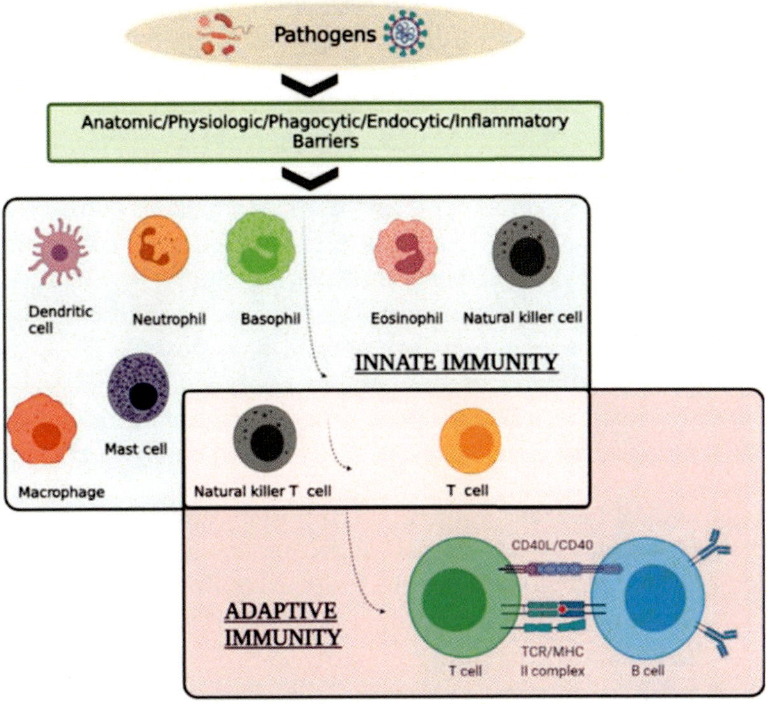

Fig. (1). Association between innate immunity and adaptive immunity.

Screening of Immunomodulators

Immune system modulation has emerged as a rapidly expanding new milestone not only in drug discovery but also in recent applications such as enhancement of disease resistance, boosting of vaccination immunity, prevention from various infections, malignancies, stress-related diseases, autoimmune diseases, and disorders such as HIV, SARS-CoV-2, and their complications. Immunomodulators are becoming increasingly popular as people know the importance of a fit immune system in illness prevention and recovery. This necessitates further research in order to design molecules that can increase immunity in a constantly changing environment. Traditional and new immunomodulators such as adjuvants, cytokines, hormones, glucocorticoids, host defense peptides, microbial products, toll-like receptors, synthetic compounds, probiotics, nutrients, vitamins, minerals, herbs, panchgavya (cow therapy), polysaccharides, helminths, vaccines, and others are capable of modifying immune responses [2]. Thus, immunomodulatory medicines, which are not routinely used to treat life-threatening illnesses, may require a larger safety factor in order to avoid major side effects or cytotoxicity. Various pre-clinical experiments employing laboratory animals and isolated human cells will thus continue to be an important part of the drug development process for the foreseeable future.

The discovery of new drugs that show activity against a protein or cell process implicated in causing a pathological state is part of the preclinical phase. This phase also includes additional studies to examine the compound's potency and selectivity against its target, as well as the mechanism of action if it is unclear. Compounds that successfully pass these efficacy and safety tests then enter into the clinical stage of drug discovery and development. In the second step, the compounds are evaluated in humans for further safety and efficacy analysis. If successful, the outcome of this effort will be the approval of a new, safe, and effective immunomodulator for one of the many diseases that impair human health. Thus, during the evaluation of a novel immunomodulator, one should design a screening approach to integrate several assays into an efficient workflow.

Also, for the sake of simplicity, the most important questions that should keep in mind while choosing a suitable animal model like the selection of suitable species, immunological functions to be evaluated along with practical implications of the model [15].

The scope of this chapter is to outline the assaying of immunomodulatory activity, the approaches and the experimental strategies. For testing immunomodulatory activity, a wide range of *in vitro* and *in vivo* methods are available.

Animal Models used for Immunomodulatory Studies

Experimental animals are often considered one of the most effective models for testing immunomodulators. Rat species (*e.g.*, albino wistar, sprague-dawley), C57 BL/6J mice, BALB/c mice, transgenic OT mice, Swiss albino mice, Dunkin-Hartley guinea pigs, and fish (*e.g.*, Cyprinus carpio) are among species employed in immunomodulatory experiments [16].

PRECLINICAL EVALUATION FOR IMMUNOMODULATORS CELL CULTURE

For cell culture assays, cells are handled in a Class II biosafety cabinet, and all treatment and stimulation steps are carried out in sterile conditions. Complete T cell media is used for all cultures, and cells are incubated at 37°C with 5% CO_2 [17]. Common cell lines used for screening immunomodulators are presented in Table **1**.

Table 1. Cell lines used for evaluation of immunomodulators [18, 19].

Cell Lines	Features
Monocyte/macrophage RAW264.7	These cells are obtained from BALB/c mice and used to examine cellular responses.
Bone marrow-derived macrophages (BMDM)	Derived from mice bone marrow as it provides a large number of macrophages for studying host-pathogen interactions.
Single-cell splenocyte suspension	Removed spleens are processed into single-cell splenocyte suspensions and are used in graft ***Vs.*** host diseases.
ConA-stimulated splenocytes	T cell differentiation is assessed using these cell lines.
LPS-stimulated splenocytes	Bacterial lipopolysaccharide (LPS) causes stimulation of B cells and macrophage also induces B cell proliferation and differentiation.
K562 cell line	Stimulation of NK cells activity against cancerous (*K562 cell line*) and non-cancerous cells.
J 779 macrophage cell line	Used for evaluation of cytotoxicity, phagocytosis, and oxidant burst.

IN VITRO METHODS FOR IMMUNOMODULATORS EVALUATION

Common *in vitro* methods used for screening immunomodulators are presented in Table **2**.

Table 2. *In vitro* methods for immunomodulators evaluation.

Sr. No.	*In Vitro* Methods	Application
1.	Inhibition of histamine release from mast cells	Testing of immunological factors
2.	Mitogen-induced lymphocyte proliferation	Assessment of non-specific cellular immunity
3.	Inhibition of T cell proliferation	Mainly used in the evaluation of immunosuppressants
4.	Phagocytosis evaluation 4.1 Chemiluminescence in macrophages 4.2 Polymorphonuclear (PMN) leucocyte's function test	It can be used to measure phagocytic activity. Phagocytes play a significant role in innate immunity and contribute to adaptive immunity, as well as tissue remodelling and tissue homeostasis, due to their versatility and diversity.
5.	PFC (plaque forming cell) assay	Assessment of the ability to develop a humoral immune response
6.	Inhibition of dihydro-orotate dehydrogenase	Evaluation of therapeutics used in autoimmune disorders, immunosuppression, and cancer
7.	Cell viability Assay MTT	MTT assay is used to detect cell not viability and growth, as well as cell proliferation in response to growth factors, cytokines, and cytotoxicity. It is also used to investigate cell activation.
8.	Cytokine ELISA Assay	Quantification of cytokines
9.	Nitrite Measurement	Quantification of nitric oxide (immunomodulator) in biological fluids
10.	NBT reduction assay	Assessment of phagocytic oxidase activity
11.	Myeloperoxidase Activity Assay	Determination of neutrophil activation levels
12.	Hydrogen Peroxide production	Determination of macrophages activation
13.	Vacuole Formation Assay	Determination of macrophages activation
14.	Spreading Index	Determination of macrophages activation

(Table 2) cont.....

Sr. No.	*In Vitro* Methods	Application
15.	Flow Cytometry-Based Immune Assessment:	
	a) Assay for evaluation of Natural Killer (NK) Cell Activity	It can be used to test NK cell cytotoxicity and thereby quantify immunological function.
	b) Direct and indirect allo-recognition assay	It permits risk assessment and mechanistic understanding of graft rejection by measuring the subject's immune reactivity against allo-antigens presented in the transplanted tissue.
	c) Lymphocyte proliferation assay (LPA)	Assessment of T-cell function
	d) Granulocyte/monocyte oxidative burst assay	Assessment of granulocyte/monocyte immune competency, phagocytosis and oxidative burst activity
	e) Intracellular cytokine staining (ICS) of antiviral lymphocytes	Evaluation of cell degranulation, cytokine production by T cells and NK cells stimulation.

Inhibition of Histamine Release from Mast Cells [20 - 22]

Hypersensitivity reactions can be induced either immunologically or non-immunologically. Immunologically induced hypersensitivity is allergic reactions to natural or synthetic compounds mediated by IgE and non-immunologically induced, such as activation of mediator release from cells *via* direct contact without induction or mediation of immune responses. Mast cells release some mediators that cause hypersensitive reactions. Histamine is a key mediator of allergic reactions found in mast cells. Mast cells release histamine in response to allergens or the calcium ionophore 48/80. The o-phthalaldehyde reaction can be used to assess histamine levels. Histamine concentration can be determined by a fluorescence detector (using 350 and 450 nm, the excitation and emission wavelengths, respectively). Percent histamine release can be calculated by the following formula:

$$\frac{\text{Sample histamine release - Spontaneous histamine release}}{\text{100\% histamine release - Spontaneous histamine release}} \times 100$$

Disodium cromoglycate has been reported to inhibit histamine release and mast cell degranulation in rats. Few non-steroid anti-inflammatory drugs, such as indomethacin, flufenamate and meclofenamate, suppress the release of histamine from rat peritoneal mast cells induced by pharmacological or immunological stimulation *in vitro*. Natural chymase inhibitors like secretory leukocyte protease inhibitor (SLPI) and alpha (1)-antitrypsin have also been reported to inhibit histamine release.

Mitogen-Induced Lymphocyte Proliferation /T Cell Proliferation Assay [17, 20, 23, 24]

T cell proliferation assay is also known as T cell transformation test. T cells are stimulated *in vitro* by a specific material known as mitogens, and cell metabolism and morphology are constantly changed to increase protein and nucleic acid synthesis in 24 to 48h, resulting in a series of changes in proliferation, cytoplasm expansion, vacuoles, nuclear chromatin lose, and so on. Therefore, lymphocytes will differentiate into lymphoblasts. As a result, lymphocyte proliferation is also known as lymphocyte transformation, and it can influence the responsiveness and function of lymphocytes.

Polyclonal mitogens increase lymphocyte proliferation *in vitro* using non-antigenic stimuli. Because many of them are nearly exclusive activators of T or B cells, they are used to create model systems for studying the roles of T and B cells in the immune system. Plant lectins, concanavalin A (Con A) and phytohemagglutinin (PHA) are common T lymphocyte mitogens. Both activate T lymphocytes and cause them to produce numerous lymphokines, but the population of their target cells and their reliance on accessory cells for mitogenic activity expression differ. Whereas, bacterial lipopolysaccharide (LPS) is a well-known mitogen of murine B lymphocytes. LPS directly activate B lymphocytes and differentiates them into immunoglobulin-secreting cells. While pokeweed *mitogen* (PWM) activates both T and B cells. Tuberculin, staphylococcal toxin, tetanus toxoid, streptococcal kinase, tumour antigen, and allogeneic tissue antigen stimulate T cell proliferation using antigenic stimuli. These different stimulants can be employed in the screening of immunomodulators using total peripheral blood lymphocyte population or with individual lymphocyte sub-population, including B-lymphocytes, T4 and T8 lymphocytes or with target cells such as murine splenocytes. The rate of proliferation of lymphocyte fraction under the influence of mitogens is measured by the determination of the rate of incorporation of 3H-thymidine into the DNA of lymphocytes. In the procedure, lymphocyte fraction is adjusted to a cell density of 105 cells per millimeter, to which mitogens are added for pre-stimulation along with the test substance. After 70-88 hours of incubation, 3H-thymidine is added, and incubation is continued for further 18 hours. The incorporated 3H-thymidine is quantitated by a scintillation counter.

Inhibition of T Cell Proliferation [20]

The activation and/or proliferation of clonal T cell populations are required for the onset of an antigen-specific immune response. Thus, inhibiting T cell activation is a highly effective method of inhibiting certain immunological responses. T cell activation can be suppressed by a variety of immunosuppressive drugs. After purification of peripheral blood leukocytes and T cells, *in vitro* inhibition can be assessed by various assays such as Mixed lymphocyte reaction, Lymphocyte stimulation and proliferation, ELISA assays, IL-2R assays *etc.* After stimulation with antiCD3 or anti-CD28, dose-response curves of inhibition of one-way mixed lymphocyte reaction and IL-2 in the supernatant are established.

Phagocytosis Evaluation

Chemiluminescence in Macrophages [20]

The stimulation of macrophages by antigen, complement, phorbol esters, and other oxygen metabolites results in the production of O_2 and other oxygen metabolites. *In vivo*, superoxide ions and other highly reactive oxygen metabolites serve as the foundation for an effective microbicidal system. However, tissue damage frequently occurs when these radicals are produced in reaction to self-antigens. Inhibiting this mechanism can be used to assess the immunomodulating effects of substances. The oxygen metabolites can create light-emitting reactions (chemiluminescence), which can be measured when amplified with appropriate indicators, such as cyclic hydrazide luminol or lucigenin and zymosan. The luminescence is measured by a luminometer. The maximum count time for the positive control is recorded. The ratio of counts per 10 s for all groups is calculated at that time and compared to the positive control counts per 10 s, and the % change is calculated. This test can be performed with macrophages, monocytes or Kupffer cells from the liver.

Polymorphonuclear (PMN) Leucocyte's Function Test using Candida Albicans Spores [25, 26]

Polymorphonuclear leukocytes (PMNs) are a type of white blood cells that include neutrophils, eosinophils, basophils, and mast cells found abundantly in circulating blood, providing the first line of defense. Phagocytosis and elimination of invading microbes is a major function of the polymorphonuclear leukocyte (PMN). In the procedure, The PMN cells in combination with Candida albicans should be cultured for one hour at 37°C in a 5% CO_2 environment with the test compound. (Cell density adjusted to 1X10 6 cells/ml for both). After incubation, fix the smear with methanol, stain with Giemsa and study under 100 X 'oil immersion objective' to determine the phagocytic activity of PMN cells.

Phagocytic index, as the ratio of the number of *Candida albicans* ingested to the total number of neutrophils and the percentage of PMN cells involved in phagocytosis, can be calculated.

PMN function can also be assessed using some other *in vitro* procedures such as quantitative nitro blue tetrazolium reduction, chemiluminescence and iodination.

PFC (Plaque Forming Cell) Assay [27]

The development of humoral immune response in the human body is assessed by PFC assay. The specific antigen used for this purpose is sheep red blood cells (SRBC). Following exposure to SRBCs or other T-cell-dependent antigens, the development of an antigen-specific antibody response necessitates the collaboration and interaction of numerous immune cell types, including antigen-presenting cells (*e.g.*, macrophages, T cells, and B cells). Thus, there are several points in the process where changes in the function of certain cells might affect B cells' ability to make antigen-specific antibodies. Because of this complicated cell interaction, it was revealed that quantifying the plaque-forming cell (PFC) response (*i.e.*, the specific antibody-forming cell SRBC response) was one of the best predictors of immunotoxicity in mice. Immunocompetent cells from lymphoid organs, especially the spleen, are used in the PFC response to SRBC. Furthermore, T cell-independent antigens can be employed in the PFC assay to identify the major immune cell type (s) targeted by a certain drug. These antigens do not require T cells to stimulate antibody production by B cells. Regardless of the antigen, the PFC assay is based on SRBC, which comprises consists of the antigen or conjugated hapten for the specific antibody generated by B cells. The plaque count corresponds with the density of antibody-producing cells. The ELISPOT assay is a modification of the PFC assay that enables the measurement of antibody-forming cells (AFCs) that generate antibodies of different isotypes such as immunoglobulins IgM, IgG, IgE, or IgA. The methodology of the ELISPOT assay is identical to that of the ELISA.

Inhibition of Dihydro-Orotate Dehydrogenase [20]

Dihydro-orotate dehydrogenase catalyzes the rate-limiting step in the biosynthesis of pyrimidines. Small molecule dihydro-orotate dehydrogenase inhibitors are an appealing therapeutic agent for autoimmune disorders, immunosuppression, and cancer because rapidly multiplying human T cells have an exceptional requirement for *de novo* pyrimidine production. The immunosuppressive substance leflunomide and its active metabolites are thought to work by inhibiting the enzyme dihydroorotate dehydrogenase.

The inhibitory potency of the agents can be determined by the initial velocity of the dihydro-orotate dehydrogenase reaction which is measured at saturating substrate concentrations, 1 mM dihydro-orotate and 100 M QD, and varying concentrations of the drugs (1 nM through100 μM). The initial velocity is calculated by using the following equation:

$$v = V / \{1 + [I]/IC50\}.$$

[I] is the inhibitory concentration in order to find the concentration causing 50% inhibition of the enzyme activity (IC50).

MTT Assay & Cyclic Voltammetry for Cell Viability and Proliferation

The MTT assay measures the function of cells, proliferation, and cytotoxicity by measuring cellular metabolic activity. This colorimetric assay converts yellow tetrazolium compound (3-(4,5-dimethylthiazol-2-yl)-2,5-diphenyltetrazolium bromide or MTT) into violet formazan crystals using metabolically active cells. In live cells, the NAD(P)H-dependent oxidoreductase enzyme reduces MTT to formazan. Then formazan particles that are insoluble are dissolved in a solubilization solution, and the resultant-colored solution is then measured with a multi-well spectrophotometer at 500-600 nm. The darker solution indicates that cells are more viable and metabolically active. This non-radioactive, colorimetric assay system based on MTT was originally developed by Mosmann and has since been improved by a number of other researchers [28, 29].

Electrochemical methods such as cyclic voltammetry test is an efficient analytical method that can provide a simple platform for the electrochemical research of lymphocyte proliferation and viability, where proliferation in cell cultures and whole blood can be evaluated electrochemically using cyclic voltammetry. In Compared to the colorimetric (MTT) assay, cyclic voltammetry provided the best association with cell count data throughout a range of 1200–300,000 cells/well of a microplate. Aside from the advantages of a short assay duration that is 4 hours and speed, the possibility to use fresh blood without further processing would result in more precise results because cells would be monitored in an intact environment [30].

Cytokine ELISA and Biological Assay [31]

Cytokine ELISA and biological assays are used for the quantification of cytokines such as TNF-, IL-1, IL-6, and IFN- in cell supernatants. Cytokines have been linked with a variety of diseases, such as cancer and neurodegenerative illnesses, in addition to immunological and inflammatory responses. The accurate determination of cytokines in biological fluids such as plasma, serum, and tissue culture samples allow researchers to completely comprehend the mechanisms behind the disease in physiological contexts.

Nitrite Determination using Colorimetric Griess Reaction Assay [32]

Nitric oxide is a crucial biomolecule that controls cellular signalling. It performs a variety of biological functions, such as immunomodulation, inflammatory processes, microbes' elimination, and cancer cell elimination. When activated by cytokines and microbial antigens, macrophages completely eradicate a wide range of microbes or parasites, as well as tumor cells, by releasing a wide range of effectors, including NO. Nitrite acquired in macrophage culture supernatant is calculated as an indicator of NO production using the colorimetric Griess reaction assay technique, which is one of the most popular and simplest methods for detecting nitrite concentration. The components of Griess reagent include Sulphanilamide in phosphoric acid and naphthylethylenediamine dihydrochloride suspended in water. This reagent combines with nitrite in samples to produce a purple azo product which is measured at an absorbance of 540 nm.

Additional well-known methods such as fluorescent assays, chemiluminescence assay, and electrochemical detection also can be applied for the determination of nitrate concentration.

Nitro-blue tetrazolium (NBT) Reduction Assay [33]

This test is used for the identification of bacterial infection and examination of phagocytic abnormalities. Typically, macrophage phagocytosis is accompanied by a burst of oxidative metabolism, allowing the formation of oxygen species that convert yellow NBT to dark blue formazan, which can be identified using NBT dye reduction. The greater the reduction in the NBT assay, the greater the activity of the oxidase enzyme, demonstrating the activation of phagocytes in proportion to the foreign particles ingested.

Myeloperoxidase Activity Assay [33]

Myeloperoxidase (MPO) is a heme-containing peroxidase predominantly found in neutrophils and, to a lesser extent, monocytes. Therefore, MPO activity test can be used to determine neutrophil activation. MPO catalyses the production of reactive oxygen species, such as hypochlorous acid, including hydrogen peroxide and halides (HOCl). HOCl is a crucial part of the host's defense response against invading microorganisms. If the stimulation index of myeloperoxidase increases after exposure to varying concentrations of the test substance, it suggests that the cells' defense potential against pathogenic organisms has improved.

A Flow Cytometry-Based Assay for Natural Killer Cell Activity Evaluation

Natural killer (NK) cells are defence cells from innate immune system that have been proven to have a role in early viral infection management and immuno-surveillance in humans and animals. Also, these cells have been discovered as important makers of cytokines such as interferon (IFN-), tumour necrosis factor (TNF), and interleukin IL-10 under various physiological and diseased conditions. NK cell cytotoxicity is a common and significant biomarker of immune function that has been shown to be reduced in people with primary immunodeficiency, late-stage HIV-infected patients, and women who are pregnant.

Flow cytometric tests avoid the issues associated with the use of radioactivity (as in the chromium release assay) and are faster and easier to standardise, also required less time. Firstly, DiO (Dioctadecyloxacarbocyanine Perchlorate), a green lipophilic fluorescent dye, is incorporated into the membrane surface of target cells grown in culture. Flow cytometry can easily distinguish target cells from effector cells using this dye. Furthermore, by introducing propidium iodide (PI), the PI-induced nuclear DNA intercalation might be used to identify dead cells. Because PI fluoresces in the orange-red spectrum, the dual-fluorescence analysis might correctly measure the fraction of target cells destroyed by effector NK cells [34].

IN VIVO METHODS FOR IMMUNOMODULATORS EVALUATION

Common *in vivo* methods used for screening immunomodulators are presented in Table **3**.

Table 3. ***In vivo*** **methods for immunomodulators evaluation.**

Sr. No.	*In Vivo* Methods	Application
1.	Assessment of cellular immunity 1.1 Carbon-clearance test 1.2 Neutrophil adhesion test	Assessment of cellular immunity and phagocytic index
2.	Hypersensitivity reaction (Arthus type immediate hypersensitivity and delayed hypersensitivity)	Measurement of cellular immune response
3.	Reversed passive arthus reaction	Evaluation of anti-inflammatory drugs
4.	Assessment of Humoral immunity 4.1 Hemagglutination antibody titer test 4.2 Mice lethality test	Assessment of Humoral immune response
5.	Calculation of immune organ index in mice	Measurement of innate and adaptive immune response and thus overall immunity
6.	Calculation of serum hemolysin level in mice	Measurement of humoral immune function

(Table 3) cont.....

Sr. No.	*In Vivo* Methods	Application
7.	Systemic anaphylaxis in mice	Examination of activities of IgG, IgE antibodies
8.	Passive cutaneous anaphylaxis	Examination of the activities of IgE antibody
9.	Adjuvant arthritis in rats	Evaluation of anti-inflammatory and immunosuppressive activity
10.	Collagen type II-induced arthritis in rats	Evaluation of anti-inflammatory and immunosuppressive activity
11.	Experimental autoimmune thyroiditis	Best model for Hashimoto's thyroiditis
12.	Spontaneous autoimmune disease in animals	Screening of agents used in the treatment of various autoimmune disorders
13.	Anti-anaphylactic activity (Schultz-Dale reaction)	Screening of anti-allergic medicines
14.	Proteoglycan-induced progressive polyarthritis in mice	Screening of anti-polyarthritis agents
15.	Coxsackievirus B3-induced myocarditis	Evaluation of immunosuppressive activity
16.	Experimental allergic encephalomyelitis	Evaluation of immunosuppressive activity
17.	Prevention of experimentally induced myasthenia gravis in rats	Screening of drugs used in myasthenia gravis
18.	Inhibition of allogeneic transplant rejection	Evaluation of immunosuppressive activity
19.	Influence on systemic lupus erythematosus (SLE)-like disorder in MRL/lpr mice	Evaluation of immunosuppressive activity
20.	Glomerulonephritis induced by anti-basement membrane antibody in rats	Evaluation of immunosuppressive activity
21.	Acute graft *versus* host disease (GvHD) in rats	Best model for GvHD

Assessment of Cellular Immunity

Carbon-Clearance Test for Determination of Macrophage Phagocytic Index [35]

Phagocytosis is performed by phagocytic cells in which foreign particles, microorganisms, and apoptotic cells are ingested and eliminated. Among the *in vivo* test, the carbon-clearance method is used to determine the phagocytic activity of macrophages. Enhanced phagocytic activity of macrophages is assessed by the rate of elimination of exogenously administered antigen particles. Particles used in this test vary greatly from Indian ink (carbon particles with a diameter of about 250A^0, coated with gelatin), polystyrene latex particles, an emulsion of lipid droplets, to aggregated bovine serum albumin. The test system involves the feeding of test drug to the animal orally or i.p. for a particular period of treatment followed by injection of Indian ink intravenously. Blood sample were drawn from the retro-orbital plexuses at periodic intervals. The carbon clearance, also known as the phagocytic index (K), is the rate of carbon elimination from the blood, which is determined spectrophotometrically and calculated using an equation:

Phagocytic index = [body weight/ (liver weight + spleen weight)] ×[(lgOD2-lgOD10)/(t10-t2)]1/3. OD2=the absorbance of 2 min after injection of Indian ink, OD10=the absorbance of 10 min after injection of Indian ink. t10=10 min, t2=2min.

Neutrophil Adhesion Test [36]

Animals should be provided the test drug orally prior to the 14-day experiment. Animals should be given the test drug orally prior to the 14-day experiment. Blood samples are collected from ventricular puncture on day 14 at the end of treatment and examined for total leucocyte counts (TLC) and differential leukocyte counts (DLC). Following the initial counts, blood samples are incubated for 15 minutes at 37°C with 80 mg/ml nylon fibres. The incubated samples are analyzed again for TLC and DLC to determine the neutrophil index of blood samples. The product of TLC and percent neutrophil is being used to calculate the neutrophil index (NI) of a blood sample. The following formula is used to calculate the % neutrophil adhesion.

Neutrophil adhesion = (NIu − Nit) × 100/ NIu

(Where, NIu is neutrophil index of untreated blood sample; Nit, neutrophil index of a treated blood sample)

Neutrophil index (NI) = TLC × % neutrophil

Hypersensitivity Reaction [16]

Hypersensitivity resulting from the antigen-antibody complex is termed as Arthus type immediate hypersensitivity, and that resulting from T lymphocyte termed as a delayed-type hypersensitivity reaction. Both types of hypersensitivities can be estimated by footpad test using sheep erythrocytes (SRBC). In this test, hypersensitivity is induced by injecting SRBC suspension in animals into the right hind paw on day zero. On day 5, the thickness of the paw is measured, and the same amount of SRBCs suspension is re-administered to the animals in the left hind paw. Paw thickness is assessed after an interval of 24, 48, 72, and 96 hours of challenge. A blood sample is collected from the retro-orbital route after 96 hours for analysis of WBC and total platelets. DTH response is measured by the change in paw thickness after being challenged by SRBC.

Reversed Passive Arthus (RPA) Reaction [37]

Reversed passive Arthus reaction is an outstanding *in vivo* model investigated as a screening test for immune complex-mediated acute inflammation in the tissue. In the RPA reaction, an excess of Ab is being injected into the skin of animals that have been previously administered with a sufficient amount of Ag by the i.v route. So, the resulting inflammatory response is characterized by perivascular IC deposition in the dermis along with edema, neutrophilia, bleeding, and tissue necrosis. The development of inflammatory tissue injury using RPA reaction has been reported in animals like rabbits, guinea pigs, and rats. So, these animal experimentations indicate that complement activation by ICs is the most crucial step and also a requirement for neutrophils and mast cells to develop inflammatory events. Recent research, however, suggests that IC-mediated inflammatory response in the RPA reaction can be stimulated by Fc gamma receptor-triggered pathways.

Assessment of Humoral Immune Immunity [38]

Hemagglutination Antibody Titer Test

The humoral response can be demonstrated by antibody molecules, which are produced by B lymphocytes and plasma cells. The hemagglutination reaction is used to assess humoral immunity, and it is investigated by injecting sheep erythrocytes (SRBCs). Hemagglutination is an agglutination process in which antibodies bind to Red Blood Cells (RBCs). RBCs act as an antigen and, due to their abundance, make excellent targets. It is a widely used assay for measuring antibody titers in serum, viral quantification, and blood grouping. Agglutination is the result of an antigen-antibody response. The reciprocal of the highest dilution, which is capable of causing visible agglutination, is known as the relative strength of an antibody titer. The antibody titer can be used to track variations in the number of antibodies produced throughout an immunological response. The antibody titer is selected in such a way that it shows highest serum dilution along with visible hemagglutination.

Mice Lethality Test

Animals are pre-treated with test compounds for three weeks in mice lethality test. On day 7 and day 17, animals are immunized with a 'hemorrhagic septicemia vaccine'. On the 21st day, 0.2 ml of Pasteurella multocida culture containing 107 cells per ml is injected into the animals subcutaneously. For the next three days (72 hours), animals are kept under observation, and the percentage mortality is calculated by using the following formula.

% mortality = Number of animal dead X 100 /Total number of animals.

Determination of Immune Organ Index in Mice [35, 39]

The immune system organs and tissues are categorized into the primary lymphoid organs (*e.g.* bone marrow and thymus) and secondary lymphoid organs (*e.g.*, spleen, lymph node and epithelial and mucosa-associated lymphoid tissues). Primary lymphoid organs are the site for the production of cells of the innate and adaptive immune system. Secondary lymphoid tissues act as the anatomic site for the adaptive immune response. Therefore, spleen and thymus organ indexes represent the overall immune function of the body.

The obtained organ index values are compared to those of the control groups. Increased readings suggest an increase in immune cell proliferation in the respective organ and can reflect, an increase in the immune response. During the determination of immune organ index in mice, animals are weighed and sacrificed by cervical dislocation on the 7th day of treatment. Then thymus and spleen are removed and weighed. The formula for calculating thymus and spleen indices is,

Thymus or spleen index (mg/g) = Weight of thymus or spleen/Body weight.

Determination of Serum Hemolysin Level in Mice [35]

Good indication of humoral immunity is serum hemolysin antibody and B-lymphocytes release it in response to a diversity of antigens. As a result, in reaction to SRBC, the level of serum hemolysin in mice is measured. Serum hemolysin levels that are significantly higher suggest that the test drug improves humoral immune function through increasing serum hemolysin levels.

Systemic Anaphylaxis in Mice [40, 41]

A severe, systemic hypersensitivity reaction is called anaphylaxis. It manifests quickly and is marked by life-threatening respiratory, breathing, and/or circulatory difficulties, as well as skin and mucosal abnormalities. Various effector molecules and receptors thought to contribute to systemic anaphylaxis, such as IgE and IgG antibodies, Fc-gamma receptors, IgE receptor (Fc epsilon RI), anaphylatoxins, Mast cells, Basophils, Monocytes/macrophages, Neutrophils, Platelets, Histamine, Platelet-Activating Factor (PAF), Cysteinyl leukotrienes (CysLTs) *etc.* Mouse models of systemic anaphylaxis are a device to study the functioning of the mast cell elucidating anaphylaxis pathomechanisms, and discovering and characterizing potential treatments for anaphylaxis. Various conventions and agreements for systemic anaphylaxis mouse models have been reported in the literature. The experimental allergens, route and mechanism of sensitization, and challenges are the primary distinctions between these models. So, mouse models indicated and 2 important pathways of systemic anaphylaxis.

Passive sensitization, which injects antigen-specific IgE antibody 24 hours before dealing with an antigen, directs to the classical pathway mediated by IgE, Fc epsilon RI, mast cells, histamine, and platelet-activating factor (PAF). On the contrary, Active sensitization is performed by sensitization with antigen 18–21 days prior to challenge, leading to an alternative pathway mediated by IgG, Fc gamma receptors, macrophages, and PAF.

Numerous manual mice models of anaphylaxis have been discovered to scrutinize the activities of human antibodies, Fc receptors, and effector cells in anaphylaxis. Transgenic mice are created that express human FcRI instead of mouse protein (hFcRITg mice), and the expression profile of the hFcRI transgene is extremely identical as compared to that detected in humans. Immunodeficient NOD-scid gamma (NSG) mice engrafted with human stem cells and knock-*in* mice are examples of the novel strains used to generate 'humanized' models of anaphylaxis. These types of anaphylaxis reactions can cause partial inhibition using a PAF receptor antagonist, histamine receptor 1 antagonist and Anti-IgG/Anti-IgE antibody.

Adjuvant Arthritis in Rats [42]

Adjuvant arthritis (AA) is a form of (sub)chronic arthritis that resembles human rheumatoid arthritis in many ways. Rat strains have a different and modifying genetic predisposition to AA, On the other hand, mice are usually resistant. Although few strains of rats can be promoted with oil adjuvant when mycobacteria are not present AA is effortlessly induced with mycobacteria suspended in oil. T cell–mediated autoimmune arthritis is a disorder that is basically used to examine immunological features in human rheumatoid arthritis (RA) and other arthritic or inflammatory disorders. It is also utilized as a technique for the development and testing of anti-inflammatory medicines.

Lewis rats are commonly used to induce AA. Adjuvant arthritis is promoted in Lewis rats using ground, heat-killed Mycobacterium tuberculosis H37Ra suspended in incomplete Freund's adjuvant in the traditional manner. During the critical period (days 10 to 35 post immunization), disease development is monitored daily using one or more techniques for assessment of motility and study of skin redness and swelling at the site of ankle and wrist joints and small interphalangeal joints.

Collagen Type II Induced Arthritis in Rats [43]

Collagen-induced arthritis (CIA) is one of the typically used RA animal models. Class II major histocompatibility complex (MHC) molecules regulate CIA genetically. CIA is very useful technique for deciphering the mechanisms underlying immune responses to an auto antigen that may have a role in human disease. Many strains of rats can be easily immunized with heterogonous or homologous native type II collagen emulsified in incomplete Freund's adjuvant to cause collagen arthritis. Sensitized spleen and lymph node cells, as well as IgG antibodies to type II collagen, can passively transfer this illness, which is characterized by the development of both cellular and humoral immune responses to type II collagen. These data support the theory that collagen arthritis is caused by immunologic hypersensitivity to type II collagen. According to a recent study, rats with adjuvant arthritis have both humoral and cellular sensitivity to homologous type II collagen. When CII is injected into the dermis, antigen-presenting cells instantly capture it (APCs). T and B lymphocytes that are antigen-specific and auto-reactive are activated in disease. T cells and T cell-derived cytokines enhance macrophage, osteoclast, and fibroblast development and activation, resulting in severe erosive arthritis.

Experimental Autoimmune Thyroiditis [44]

The mouse model of experimental autoimmune thyroiditis (EAT) is a magnificent model for Hashimoto's thyroiditis (HT). It is invaded by thyroglobulin (Tg) and recently, thyroperoxidase which are known thyroid autoantigens shared by mice and humans, and because of which numerous conserved thyroiditogenic epitopes have been detected. A homologous antigen, mouse thyroglobulin (MTg), is used because it has maximum distinct epitope(s) and generates more severe and long-lasting thyroid inflammation than heterologous mammalian Tg. Bacterial lipopolysaccharide (LPS) and supplemented complete Freund's adjuvant are two popularly utilised adjuvants to promote induction of experimental autoimmune thyroiditis with mouse thyroglobulin. The susceptibility of mouse strains is determined by genes in the major histocompatibility complex (MHC) class II. EAT is assessed using appropriate assay variables such as thyroid histology and *in vitro* proliferative response. Thyroid histology distinguishes susceptible from resistant strains and demonstrates the amount of mononuclear cell invasion and death. EAT is a T cell-mediated illness, and the *in vitro* proliferative response to MTg correlates well with EAT susceptibility. The ELISA test is used to assess the quantity of antibodies to MTg, and the T cell proliferation assay utilization can be done to test the antigenicity of synthetic peptides produced from MTg or heterologous Tg.

SPONTANEOUS AUTOIMMUNE DISEASE IN ANIMALS [20]

Several inbred animal strains have been found to have spontaneous autoimmune disorders listed in Table **4**.

Table 4. Animal models used for spontaneous autoimmune diseases.

Animal Model	Features
New Zealand black mouse (NZB mouse)	The NZB mouse develops autoimmune hemolytic anemia, splenomegaly, glomerulonephritis, lymphoproliferative diseases, and peptic ulcers.
New Zealand black/white F1 (B/W) mouse	The nephritis in these animals is approximate to that observed in people with systemic lupus erythematosus.
Immunodeficient alymphoplasia mice	Suggested as a voluntary method for Sjogren's syndrome (immune disorder characterized by dry mouth and eyes). Mice with alymphoplasia have structural deficiencies in their lymphoid organs and are more susceptible to viral infections.
Palmerston North autoimmune mouse	Recommended as a model for otic capsule osteogenesis and otosclerosis because it exhibits both spontaneous systemic autoimmune illness and otic capsule bone production.
Motheaten mice and viable motheaten	These mice develop the systemic autoimmune and inflammatory disease as they represent a single recessive mutation which is associated with systemic immune abnormalities.
Non-obese diabetic mouse (NOD mouse)	The inbred NOD mouse observed as a righteous model for type I diabetes mellitus and autoimmune thyroiditis.
Bio-breeding rat (BB rat)	Suggested as an effective model for type I diabetes mellitus (IDDM)
Obese strain chicken (OS chicken)	Well-reported model for an organ-specific, autoimmune disease, *e.g.*, spontaneous autoimmune thyroiditis. UCD-200 chicken model can produce an inherited inflammatory, fibrotic disease which is approximate to that observed in human progressive systemic sclerosis

Anti-anaphylactic Activity (Schultz-Dale Reaction) [45]

This immunopharmacological technique can be used to demonstrate immediate-type hypersensitivity in actively or passively sensitised tissues, as well as to examine the nature of the major pharmacological mediators implicated in a given tissue and for screening of anti-anaphylactic (anti-allergic) medicines. In this test, Guinea pigs (300–350 g) are used, and they are sensitized by alum-precipitated egg albumin. After three weeks, the animals are sacrificed, and the ileum is isolated. The ileum's contractility is assessed by adding BaCl2 solution and recording contractions. According to modified methods, the histamine release in the lung and trachea can be assessed.

Proteoglycan-Induced Progressive Polyarthritis in Mice [46]

By injecting human cartilage proteoglycan into BALB/c (H-2d) mice, proteoglycan-induced arthritis (PGIA) can be seen with remissions and exacerbations. The development of symmetrical synovitis, marginal erosions, polarised pannus formation, and synovial infiltration comprised of lymphocytes, plasma cells, and histiocytes are all convincing histological characteristics that resemble rheumatoid arthritis. PG injections are given at weekly intervals for a total of four injections. Arthritis appears on day 11 and peaks between 2 and 4 weeks after the last PG injection. Serum samples were obtained by a retroorbital puncture after the treatment period to determine antibodies to proteoglycans. After that, certain organs of the animals, such as limbs, tails, and lumbar spines, are isolated, decalcified, and stored in paraffin for histological study. Non-parametric statistics are applied for comparison of mean values of inter malleoli diameter and antibody titres of treated and control animals.

Coxsackievirus B3-Induced Myocarditis [47]

In the Coxsackievirus B3-induced myocarditis model, mice are used. This model is mainly used for the evaluation of immunosuppressive drugs. It shows signs of cardiac injury similar to what is seen in humans. CVB3 (coxsackievirus B3) is the most well-studied human pathogen of viral myocarditis. The pathogenesis of viral myocarditis is a multistage process that begins with cardiomyocyte infection, progresses through immune system activation, and ends with myocardial fibrosis and left ventricular failure. Pappritz K *et al.* reported both immunomodulatory effects of opioids in the experimental CVB3-induced myocarditis model.

Experimental Allergic Encephalomyelitis [20]

Delayed hypersensitivity in nerve tissue causes experimental allergic encephalomyelitis, an immunologic illness. In many ways, the model is similar to autoimmune diseases seen in humans, particularly demyelinating diseases. The approach is used to assess the immunosuppressive effects of the compound.

Prevention of Experimentally Induced Myasthenia Gravis in Rats [20]

Myasthenia gravis is an autoimmune illness characterized by skeletal muscle weakening. The patient usually has drooping eyes, a blank expression on his or her face, and weak, halting speech. Pathogenesis of this disease is characterized by the generation of autoantibodies against the nicotinic acetylcholine receptor. These autoantibodies are further responsible for the gradual degradation of receptors that are present in skeletal muscles that receive nerve impulses and produce muscular contractions. This causes muscle weakness, and as a result, muscles fail to respond to nerve signals. Injecting rats with AChR which are derived from different species or recombinant subunits of the AChR can elicit experimental myasthenia gravis (EMG) where symptoms and detectable anti-receptor antibodies of myasthenia gravis are found in animals. The two subunits are potential targets of pathogenic autoantibodies because they show crosslinking, complement-mediated lysis and inhibition of acetylcholine binding to the receptor. Although the course of the disease varies, the majority of animals possess at least a weakness and fatigability in their leg gripping. The condition causes aberrant gait in the animals, eventually resulting in their inability to move or even balance themselves. Female AO strain rats, aged 6–10 weeks, are generally used for this experiment. The rats in the study are divided into three groups:

1. Treatment group (animals immunised with acetylcholine receptor)

2. Non-treated group (animals are immunised with AChR); and

3. Control group (animals are nonimmunised)

Drug is administered by oral route on a daily basis. Treatment starts on the day of immunization, and the final dose is given on the day of sacrifice. Antibodies to the anti-AChR protein are evaluated using an ELISA method.

Inhibition of Allogeneic Transplant Rejection [20]

When allogeneic organs are transplanted into recipients, the transplants are rejected. Immunosuppressive drugs can reduce or delay this effect. In animal studies, various organs such as skin sections, heart, small intestine, and cornea are employed for allogeneic transplantation. A strong allogeneic system or a major histocompatibility complex variant strain combination can be used to assess immunosuppressive activity.

In a xenotransplantation model of mouse-to-rat skin grafts, Lewis rats served as recipients while Balb/c mice served as donors. Rat tail skin (donor) is sliced into 0.5 to 1.0 cm square pieces and transplanted into recipient rats' tails. Once the skin graft becomes turns red-brown and hard, it is described as rejection. Then titers of xeno-specific IgM and IgG antibodies are measured. Flow cytometry is used to examine the samples.

Influence on SLE-like Disorder in MRL/lpr Mice [48, 49]

The autoimmune MRL Mpf lprflpr (MRL/lpr) mice species develop a systemic lupus erythematosus (SLE)-like disorder. SLE-like disorder affects a number of organs, including skin, kidneys, heart, lungs, and joints. In addition to peripheral organ dysfunction, neuropsychiatric symptoms, such as headaches, cognitive dysfunction, and psychiatric disorders, are common in SLE patients. Particularly, the affective disorder is reported in 40-70% patients. Excessive T-lymphocyte proliferation, the production of antibodies against particular types of self-antigens, and immune-mediated disease are all symptoms of this condition. Autoantibodies directed against nuclear antigens, notably double-stranded DNA (dsDNA), are the most common autoantibodies generated during this disease. These autoantibodies form complexes with their antigens and deposit in small blood vessels with complement, resulting in extensive vasculitis. As these immune complex deposits first in the renal glomeruli, they cause glomerulonephritis and renal failure. Examples of drugs that have been screened using this model are immunosuppressive agents such as cyclophosphamide, steroids, leflunomide, cyclosporin A, azathioprine and prednisolone. After the treatment period, the survival rate and disease index in animals are calculated. For the calculation of the disease index, various clinical parameters are taken into consideration (*e.g.*, Inflammation, lesion, and/or granuloma formation in the skin). The score for the clinical index is assigned according to symptoms severity, and the average score of the treatment group is calculated and compared with the control group.

CONCLUSION

The immune system has been classified into two functional defensive structures: innate and adaptive immunity. Immune system modulation has emerged as a rapidly expanding new milestone not only in drug discovery but also in recent applications such as enhancement of disease resistance, boosting of vaccination immunity, prevention from various infections, malignancies, stress-related diseases, autoimmune diseases, and disorders such as HIV, SARS-CoV-2, and their complications. An immunomodulator is a biological or synthetic substance that can stimulate, suppress or modulate any constituent of the immune system, including both adaptive and innate arms of the immune system, combat both external and internal pathogen attacks, with the intention of improving disease resistance. The complexity and depth of the immune system make it difficult to reach the girth of the system and identify the precise target and screening model for modulation. Thus, during the evaluation of a novel immunomodulator, one should design a screening approach to integrate several assays into an efficient workflow. Also, for the sake of simplicity, the most important questions should be kept in mind while choosing a suitable animal model, such as the selection of suitable species, immunological functions to be evaluated, and the practical implications of the model.

Therefore, the accurate selection of screening model by considering the complexity of the disease and its pathological mechanism revives the hope of scientists to unravel the potential of natural or synthetic immunomodulators in the service of human health.

CONSENT FOR PUBLICATION

Not applicable.

CONFLICT OF INTEREST

The author declares no conflict of interest, financial or otherwise.

ACKNOWLEDGEMENTS

The authors of this chapter would like to acknowledge STES's Smt. Kashibai Navale College of Pharmacy, Kondhwa, Pune 411048, Maharashtra, India

REFERENCES

[1] Aridoğan BC. Immunomodulatory Effects of Phytocompounds. Mod Phytomedicine Turn Med Plants into Drugs. 2006; 341-56. [http://dx.doi.org/10.1002/9783527609987.ch16]

[2] Dhama K, Saminathan M, Jacob SS, *et al.* Effect of immunomodulation and immunomodulatory agents on health with some bioactive principles, modes of action and potent biomedical applications. Vol. 11. Int J Pharmacol 2015; 11(4): 253-90. [http://dx.doi.org/10.3923/ijp.2015.253.290]

[3] Kumar D, Arya V, Kaur R, Bhat ZA, Gupta VK, Kumar V. A review of immunomodulators in the Indian traditional health care system. J Microbiol Immunol Infect 2012; 45(3): 165-84. [http://dx.doi.org/10.1016/j.jmii.2011.09.030] [PMID: 22154993]

[4] Banstola A, Jeong JH, Yook S. Immunoadjuvants for cancer immunotherapy: A review of recent developments. Acta Biomater 2020; 114(August): 16-30. [http://dx.doi.org/10.1016/j.actbio.2020.07.063] [PMID: 32777293]

[5] Crowe JE. Prevention of fetal and early life infections through maternal-neonatal immunization 2011; 1212-30. [http://dx.doi.org/10.1016/B978-1-4160-6400-8.00038-9]

[6] Abbasi S, Uchida S. Multifunctional immunoadjuvants for use in minimalist nucleic acid vaccines. Pharmaceutics 2021; 13(5): 644. [http://dx.doi.org/10.3390/pharmaceutics13050644] [PMID: 34062771]

[7] Shahbazi S, Bolhassani A. Immunostimulants: Types and Functions. J Med Microbiol Infect Dis 2016; 4(3): 45-51.

[8] Petrunov B, Nenkov P, Shekerdjiisky R. The role of immunostimulants in immunotherapy and immunoprophylaxis. Biotechnol Biotechnol Equip 2007; 21(4): 454-62. [http://dx.doi.org/10.1080/13102818.2007.10817494]

[9] Rathee P, Chaudhary H, Rathee S, Rathee D., Immunosuppressants : A Review. Pharm Innovat J 2014; 1 (12).

[10] Felippe MJB. Felippe MJB. Immunotherapy. Second Edition. Elsevier Inc. 2013; 584-97.

[11] Clark R, Kupper T. Old meets new: the interaction between innate and adaptive immunity. J Invest Dermatol 2005; 125(4): 629-37.

[http://dx.doi.org/10.1111/j.0022-202X.2005.23856.x] [PMID: 16185260]

[12] Černý J, Stříž I. Adaptive innate immunity or innate adaptive immunity? Clin Sci (Lond) 2019; 133(14): 1549-65.
[http://dx.doi.org/10.1042/CS20180548] [PMID: 31315948]

[13] Palucka K, Banchereau J. Dendritic cells: a link between innate and adaptive immunity. J Clin Immunol 1999; 19(1): 12-25.
[http://dx.doi.org/10.1023/A:1020558317162] [PMID: 10080101]

[14] Marshall JS, Warrington R, Watson W, Kim HL. An introduction to immunology and immunopathology. Allergy Asthma Clin Immunol 2018; 14(S2) (Suppl. 2): 49.
[http://dx.doi.org/10.1186/s13223-018-0278-1] [PMID: 30263032]

[15] House R V. Preclinical evaluation of immunomodulation. 2000; 246-50.

[16] Ganeshpurkar A, Saluja AK. Experimental animal models used for evaluation of potential immunomodulators: A mini review. Bull Fac Pharm Cairo Univ 2017; 55(2): 211-6.
[http://dx.doi.org/10.1016/j.bfopcu.2017.08.002]

[17] Patel V. A screening strategy to identify novel immunomodulators. 2019.

[18] Heukels P, Hulst JAC, Van , *et al.* Fibrocytes are increased in lung and peripheral blood of patients with idiopathic pulmonary fibrosis. Respir Res 2018; 19(1): 90.
[http://dx.doi.org/10.1186/s12931-018-0798-8]

[19] UCLA Health. Flow Cytometry Based Immune Assessment - Pathology at UCLA, Los Angeles, California (CA).

[20] Dayan AD. Drug Discovery and Evaluation edited by HG Vogel and WH Vogel. 1998.
[http://dx.doi.org/10.1191/096032798678907883]

[21] Lewis GP, Whittle BJR. The inhibition of histamine release from rat peritoneal mast cells by non-steroid anti-inflammatory drugs and its reversal by calcium. Br J Pharmacol 1977; 61(2): 229-35.
[http://dx.doi.org/10.1111/j.1476-5381.1977.tb08409.x] [PMID: 72577]

[22] He SH, Xie H, Zhang XJ, Wang XJ. Inhibition of histamine release from human mast cells by natural chymase inhibitors. Acta Pharmacol Sin 2004; 25(6): 822-6.
[PMID: 15169639]

[23] Nakamura A, Nagai K, Suzuki S, Ando K, Tamura G. A novel method of screening for immunomodulating substances, establishment of an assay system and its application to culture broths of microorganisms. J Antibiot (Tokyo) 1986; 39(8): 1148-54.
[http://dx.doi.org/10.7164/antibiotics.39.1148] [PMID: 3759665]

[24] The Introduction of T Cell Proliferation Assay - Creative Biolabs Blog.

[25] Gabhe SY, Tatke PA, Khan TA. Evaluation of the immunomodulatory activity of the methanol extract of *Ficus benghalensis* roots in rats. Indian J Pharmacol 2006; 38(4): 271-5.
[http://dx.doi.org/10.4103/0253-7613.27024]

[26] Roth JA, Kaeberle ML. Evaluation of bovine polymorphonuclear leukocyte function. Vet Immunol Immunopathol 1981; 2(2): 157-74.
[http://dx.doi.org/10.1016/0165-2427(81)90047-7] [PMID: 7344267]

[27] Ladics GS. Plaque-Forming Cell Assays. Encycl Immunotoxicol 2016; 698-702.
[http://dx.doi.org/10.1007/978-3-642-54596-2_1171]

[28] Doskocil I, Havlik J, Verlotta R, *et al. In vitro* immunomodulatory activity, cytotoxicity and chemistry of some central European polypores. Pharm Biol 2016; 54(11): 2369-76.
[http://dx.doi.org/10.3109/13880209.2016.1156708] [PMID: 26984176]

[29] Aro AO, Dzoyem JP, Goddard A, Fonteh P, Kayoka-Kabongo PN, McGaw LJ. *In vitro* Antimycobacterial, Apoptosis-Inducing Potential, and Immunomodulatory Activity of Some

Rubiaceae Species. Front Pharmacol 2019; 10(March): 185.
[http://dx.doi.org/10.3389/fphar.2019.00185] [PMID: 30890938]

[30] Nikbakht M, Pakbin B, Nikbakht Brujeni G. Evaluation of a new lymphocyte proliferation assay based on cyclic voltammetry; an alternative method. Sci Rep 2019; 9(1): 4503.
[http://dx.doi.org/10.1038/s41598-019-41171-8] [PMID: 30872745]

[31] Arteaga Figueroa L, Barbosa Navarro L, Patiño Vera M, Petricevich VL. Preliminary studies of the immunomodulator effect of the bougainvillea xbuttiana extract in a mouse model. Evid Based Complement Alternat Med 2015; 2015; 479412.
[http://dx.doi.org/10.1155/2015/479412]

[32] Chen W gui, Sun J, Shen W wei, Yang S zhen, Zhang Y, Hu X, *et al.* Sema4D expression and secretion are increased by HIF-1α and inhibit osteogenesis in bone metastases of lung cancer. Clin Exp Metastasis. 2019; 36(1): 39-56.

[33] Kasa P, Tippana A, Usha R. Evaluation of *In vitro* Immunomodulatory effects of Soyabean (Glycine max. L) Extracts on mouse immune system. Int J Pharm Sci Res 2015; 9951-5.
[http://dx.doi.org/10.1007/s10585-018]

[34] Valiathan R, Lewis JE, Melillo AB, Leonard S, Ali KH, Asthana D. Evaluation of a flow cytometry-based assay for natural killer cell activity in clinical settings. Scand J Immunol 2012; 75(4): 455-62.
[http://dx.doi.org/10.1111/j.1365-3083.2011.02667.x] [PMID: 22150284]

[35] Guo Z, Xu HY, Xu L, Wang SS, Zhang XM. *In vivo* and *In vitro* immunomodulatory and anti-inflammatory effects of total flavonoids of astragalus. Afr J Tradit Complement Altern Med 2016; 13(4): 60-73.
[http://dx.doi.org/10.21010/ajtcam.v13i4.10] [PMID: 28852721]

[36] Nfambi J, Bbosa GS, Sembajwe LF, Gakunga J, Kasolo JN. Immunomodulatory activity of methanolic leaf extract of Moringa oleifera in Wistar albino rats. J Basic Clin Physiol Pharmacol 2015; 26(6): 603-11.
[http://dx.doi.org/10.1515/jbcpp-2014-0104] [PMID: 26103628]

[37] Szalai AJ, Digerness SB, Agrawal A, *et al.* The Arthus reaction in rodents: species-specific requirement of complement. J Immunol 2000; 164(1): 463-8.
[http://dx.doi.org/10.4049/jimmunol.164.1.463] [PMID: 10605043]

[38] Zahoor B, Javeed A, Naeem ur Rehman, Tokhi A, Ahmed Z, Esmaeilpour K *et al.*, Evaluation of Cellular and Humoral Immune Responses of Piroxicam in Murine Model. Ann Pharmacol Pharm 2020; 5(3).

[39] Rao DS. Overview and Compartmentalization of the Immune System. In book: Hematology 2018. pp.199-209
[http://dx.doi.org/10.1016/B978-0-323-35762-3.00019-6]

[40] Reber LL, Hernandez JD, Galli SJ. The pathophysiology of anaphylaxis. J Allergy Clin Immunol 2017; 140(2): 335-48.
[http://dx.doi.org/10.1016/j.jaci.2017.06.003] [PMID: 28780941]

[41] Doyle E, Trosien J, Metz M. Protocols for the induction and evaluation of systemic anaphylaxis in mice. Methods Mol Biol 2013; 1032: 133-8.
[http://dx.doi.org/10.1007/978-1-62703-496-8_10] [PMID: 23943449]

[42] van Eden W, Wagenaar-Hilbers JPA, Wauben MHM. Adjuvant Arthritis in the Rat. Curr Protoc Immunol 1996; 19(1): 1-8.
[http://dx.doi.org/10.1002/0471142735.im1504s19] [PMID: 18432736]

[43] Pandey S. Various techniques for the evaluation of anti arthritic activity in animal models. J Adv Pharm Technol Res 2010; 1(2): 164-71.
[PMID: 22247842]

[44] Creemers BYP, Rose NR, Kong AYM. Experimental autoimmune thyroiditis. *In vitro* cytotoxic

effects of T lymphocytes on thyroid monolayers J Exp Med 1983; 559-71.

[45] Chand N, Eyre P. The Schultz-Dale reaction: A review. Agents Actions 1978; 8(3): 171-84. [http://dx.doi.org/10.1007/BF01966600] [PMID: 352112]

[46] K. D. M. Rajesh Rajaiah, Animal Models, in Rheumatoid Arthritis, M. H. W. Marc C. Hochberg, Alan J. Silman, Josef S. Smolen, Michael E. Weinblatt, Ed. 2009, pp. 218–224.

[47] Pappritz K, Savvatis K, Miteva K, *et al.* Immunomodulation by adoptive regulatory T-cell transfer improves Coxsackievirus B3-induced myocarditis. FASEB J 2018; 32(11): 6066-78. [http://dx.doi.org/10.1096/fj.201701408R] [PMID: 29863913]

[48] Bartlett RR, Raiss RX, Popovic S. Development of auto immunity in MRL/ipr mice and the effects of drugs on this murine disease. Scand J Rheumatol 1988; 17(sup75): 290-9. [http://dx.doi.org/10.3109/03009748809096781]

[49] Gulinello M, Putterman C. The MRL/lpr mouse strain as a model for neuropsychiatric systemic lupus erythematosus. J Biomed Biotechnol 2011; 2011; 207504. [http://dx.doi.org/10.1155/2011/207504]

CHAPTER 7

Natural Immunomodulators in Cancer Therapy

Chaitrali Shevkar[1] and **Abhijeet S. Kate**[1,*]

[1] *Department of Natural Products, National Institute of Pharmaceutical Education and Research, Ahmedabad, Gujarat, India*

Abstract: Cancer is a complex disease, ranking among the top causes of mortality worldwide. There are numerous therapies available however, they are showing limited success in a complete cure. The advanced treatment regime includes immunotherapy that improves the body's natural defences. The approved immunotherapies are imiquimod (Zyclara®), lenalidomide (Revlimid®) pomalidomide (Pomalyst®), and thalidomide (Thalomid®). However, these therapies have severe side effects like nausea, high blood pressure, blood clot, severe allergies, *etc.* Hence, natural products with immunomodulatory properties are being widely used as adjuvant therapy in cancer treatment. Plant secondary metabolites, such as curcumin, resveratrol, zerumbone, quercetin, genistein and betulinic acid, which are used as a member of the cancer medications and possess immunomodulatory potential, have been described in this chapter. We have discussed the mode of action, *in vitro*, *in vivo*, formulation studies and plant source of these natural immunomodulators. This chapter also discusses the current state of these pure compounds in context to their development as anticancer treatments in the future.

Keywords: Anticancer, Antitumor, Curcumin, Cytotoxicity, Immunotherapy, Natural Immunomodulators, Quercetin and Betulinic Acid, Resveratrol.

INTRODUCTION

Cancer imposes the largest worldwide healthcare burden as it is the second prominent cause of death globally, accounting for approximately 9.6 million deaths in 2018 [1 - 3]. At present, chemotherapy, endocrine treatment, targeted cure, radiation, surgery and immunomodulation are used for the management of cancer [4]. Multiple genetic and epigenetic factors influence cancer cell sensitivity leading to drug resistance in cancer which has posed a huge challenge in cancer therapeutics [5]. High doses of a drug, rapid metabolism, higher elimination rate, lower bioavailability, adverse effects, and toxicity to normal cells are the drawbacks associated with the existing chemotherapeutics [6]. There are numero-

* **Corresponding author Abhijeet S. Kate:** Department of Natural Products, National Institute of Pharmaceutical Education and Research, Ahmedabad, Gujarat, 382355 India; E-mails: kate.abhi.s@gmail.com; abhijeetk@niperahm.ac.in

Vandana S. Nikam, Sujata P. Sawarkar, Girish B. Mahajan and Supriya G. Jagtap (Eds.)

us adverse effects of radiation therapy as well like cardiovascular disease, dermatitis, pneumonitis, and sexual dysfunction [7]. Immunotherapy is a clinically validated emerging treatment for the management of broad cancer types [8]. Tumour's immune resistance mechanisms, such as specific immune responses mediating collateral tissue damage and immune-inhibitory pathways, can be effectively targeted against cancer [9].

The immunomodulatory checkpoints like cytotoxic T lymphocyte antigen 4, CD25+ (Interleukin-2 receptor alpha chain), CD4+ (cluster of differentiation 4), foxp3-expressing Tregs (suppressor T Cells), Interleukin-2 (IL-2) and Interleukin-15 (IL-15) are used as tools to enhance the effects of immunotherapeutic. Inhibiting pro-inflammatory cytokines like Interleukin-6 (IL-6), which activate the signal transducer and activator of transcription 3 (STAT3) and NF-κβ (nuclear factor kappa light chain enhancer of activated B cells) pathways, prevents the upregulation of anti-apoptotic peptides like Bcl-2 (B-cell lymphoma 2) [10, 11]. Macrophages infiltrating the tumour microenvironment prompt the immune response to counter the tumour by increasing reactive nitrogen and reactive oxygen species, leading to DNA impairment and tumour destruction [12]. Monoclonal antibodies in unmodified form or modified with add-on toxins and radionuclides are extensively used as magic bullets to treat cancer as an immunotherapeutic [13]. However, these monoclonal antibodies have limitations in cost, production and purification, risk of virus association, *etc* [14]. Currently, lenalidomide (Revlimid®), pomalidomide (Pomalyst®), Imiquimod (Zyclara®), and thalidomide (Thalomid®) are among the authorised immunotherapies against cancer. Lenalidomide and pomalidomide are the synthetic analogues of thalidomide used against several haematological malignancies and regulates various aspects of the immune system, including cytokine production, T cell co-stimulatory activity, and Natural Killer cell cytotoxicity [15, 16]. However, these therapies have severe side effects like severe allergies, nausea, high blood pressure and blood clot [17].

For ages, nature-based treatment systems, such as Ayurveda, Unani, Siddha, and Traditional Chinese Medicine have used immunomodulation for healing [18, 19]. Several plants like *Withania somnifera*, *Paris polyphylla*, *Astragalus melanophrurius*, *Astragalus oleifolius*, *Ocimum sanctum*, *Panax ginseng*, *Alternanthera tenella*, *Terminalia arjuna*, *Tinospora cordifolia*, *etc.* have been used as immunomodulatory agents [20]. These plants, in the form of various ayurvedic formulations such as Rasayanas, are known to inhibit tumour development in mice by improving natural killer (NK) cell activity while enhancing the production of Granulocyte-macrophage colony-stimulating factor (GM-CSF), Interferon gamma (INF-γ), and IL-2 [19]. A formulation of *Withania somnifera* containing a 1:1 ratio of alcoholic extract of roots and leaves showed enhanced Type 1 T helper (Th1) expression in tumour-bearing mice, repressing the expression of STAT3. This formulation has also shown increased (cluster of differentiation 8) CD8+ and CD4+ T cell proliferation which is useful in inhibiting cancer growth [21]. Numerous *in-vitro* (human lung cancer cell lines- A549, H1264, H1299, Calu-6) and *in-vivo* studies of *Panax ginseng* against lung cancer have been reported indicating its multiple molecular targets of immunomodulation [22]. A nano-particle of *Panax ginseng* using silver has shown cytotoxicity against the A549 cell line (IC_{50} value 20 μg/mL) by inducing apoptosis *via* the p38 mitogen-activated protein kinase (MAPK)/p53 pathway [23].

These studies indicate that plant secondary metabolites have the potential to modulate the immune system through multitargeted pathways and produce the desired pharmacological action, which is also applicable to treating cancer. This hypothesis has been proved for a few Natural Products such as curcumin, resveratrol, quercetin, genistein, betulinic acid, and zerumbone Fig (**1**). [24]. This chapter examines numerous secondary metabolites showing anti-cancer activities through immunomodulation Table **1**, and the established natural products have been described to the greatest extent possible.

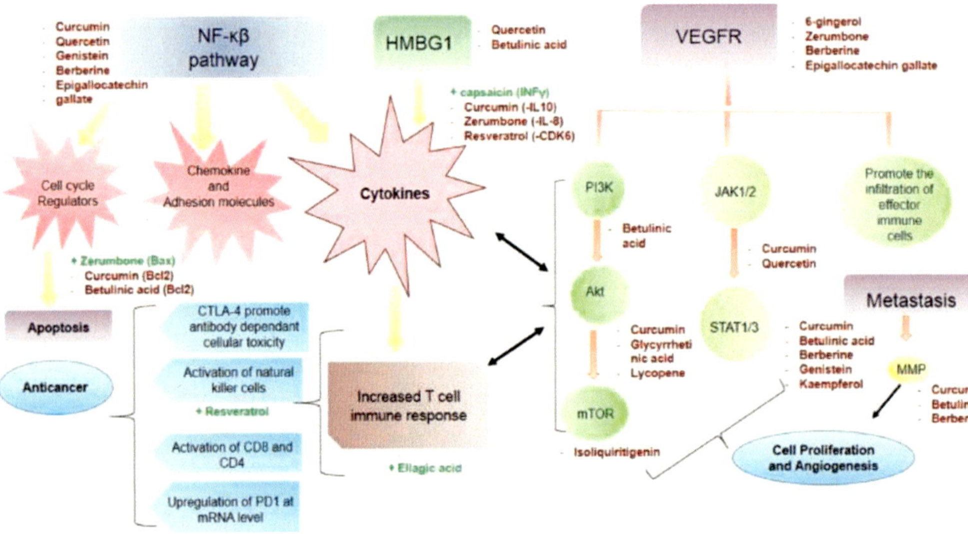

Fig. (1). Anticancer activity of selected natural products *via* immunomodulation (-ve sign indicates inhibition and +ve sign indicates activation).

Table 1. List of Natural Products with their plant source having anticancer activity *via* immunomodulation.

Sr. No.	Compound	Plant Sources	References
1	Curcumin	*Curcuma longa*	[25]
2	Resveratrol	*Fallopia japonica*	[26]
3	6-gingerol	*Zingiber officinalis*	[27]
4	*Gallic acid*	*Vaccinium angustifolium, Juglans nigra*	[28, 29]
5	Ellagic acid	Fragaria x ananassa	[30]
6	Capsaicin	*Capsicum annuum* and other *Capsicum* sp.	[31]
7	Magnoflorine	*Magnolia grandiflora, Magnolia officinalis*	[32]
8	Berberine	*Coptis chinensis*	[33]
9	Pseudocoptisine	*Corydalis turtschaninovii Besser*	[34]
10	Piperine	*Piper longum* Linn	[35]
11	Colchicine	*Colchicum autumnale*	[36]
12	Quercetin	*Citrus, Vaccinium spp.*	[37]
13	Kaempferol	*Aloe vera, Ginkgo biloba L., Hypericum perforatum L.,*	[38]
14	Rutin	*Ruta graveolens*	[39]
15	Epigallocatechin-3-gallate	*Camellia sinensis* L.	[40]
16	Genistein	*Vicia faba*	[41]
17	Puerarin	*Pueraria lobata*	[42]
18	Luteolin	*Lonicera Japonica*	[43]
19	Apigenin	*Portulaca oleracea, Mentha longifolia, Cynodon dactylon, Salvia officinalis* L.	[44]
20	Daidzein	*Pueraria lobata, Pueraria mirifica*	[45]
21	Chrysin	*Picea crassifolia*	[46]
22	Baicalein	*Scutellaria altissima* L.	[47]
23	Shikonin	*Lithospermum erythrorhyzon*	[48]
24	Apocynin	*Picrorhiza kurroa*	[49]
25	Andrographolide	*Andrographis paniculata*	[50]
26	Betulin	*Aldus subcordata* L., *Plumeria obtusa*	[51]
27	Zerumbone	*Zingiber zerumbet*	[52]
28	β-carotene	*Daucus carota, Spinacia oleracea*	[53]
29	Lycopene	*Lycopersicon esculentum, Citrullus lanatus*	[54]

(Table 1) cont.....

Sr. No.	Compound	Plant Sources	References
30	Astaxanthin	*Euphausia pacifica, Haematococcus pluvialis, Pandalus borealis*	[55]
31	Genipin	*Gardenia jasminoides*	[56]
32	Ginsan	*Panax ginseng*	[57]
33	Oleanolic acid	*Luffa cylindrica, Phytolacca americana*	[58]
34	Madecassoside	*Centella asiatica*	[59]
35	11-keto-*β*-boswellic acid	*Boswellia carteri*	[60]

Curcumin

Curcumin Fig. (**2**), a phenolic pigment, is obtained as a major constituent from the bulbs of *Curcuma longa* and is traditionally well known for its wound-healing properties [61]. Curcumin shows anticancer activity through a variety of immunogenic routes, including suppression of transcription factors, such as NF-κB, STAT, and Activator protein 1 (AP-1), as well as downregulation of antiapoptotic proteins (Bcl-2 and Bcl-Xl) and metastasis protein (MMP2) Fig.(**1**). [62]. This compound has shown cytotoxicity when tested *in-vitro* against colon cancer cell line (HCT116) with IC_{50} of 10.2 μM [63]. Further, the efficacy of curcumin has been established by *in-vivo* studies using a cancer mouse model developed in which swiss albino mice were inoculated with Ehrlich's ascites carcinoma (EAC), a murine mammary carcinoma cell line to induce cancer. Here, curcumin was given to the treated group with a dose of 50 mg/kg body weight for every alternate day for a week. It was observed that EAC cells grew up to 390 million in untreated mice, but the number of EAC cells was reduced to 20 million in curcumin-treated mice. This reduction in tumour size was due to enhanced immune response of T cells and suppression of anti-inflammatory cytokines such as TGF-β, IL10, and IL-4 in tumour-bearing hosts [64].

Drug likeliness of curcumin is largely restricted due to its poor bioavailability. Hence, the formulation of liposome-encapsulated curcumin has been developed, which inhibited head and neck squamous cell carcinoma by reducing the expression of Bcl-2, Bcl-xL, cyclin D1, matrix metalloproteinase-9, cyclooxygenase-2, Myeloid cell leukemia-1 (Mcl-1L), and Mcl-1S. In this study, liposomal curcumin was administered at 50 mg/kg dose four times per week through tail vein injection for 26 days. The results showed reduced tumour weight (33.09 mg) as compared to the control animals (89.36mg) [65]. This molecule has been extensively studied and 33 clinical trials were conducted in the previous decade. These studies indicated the potential of curcumin as an anti-cancer agent showing significant improvement in tumour markers and other parameters associated with several cancers along with symptomatic relief [66]. Along with the positive therapeutic results, it has several challenges like adverse effects (hyperplasia, anaemia, ulcers and inflammation), bioavailability, and metabolism [67]. Efforts are needed to resolve these challenges and maximise the benefits of curcumin against cancer.

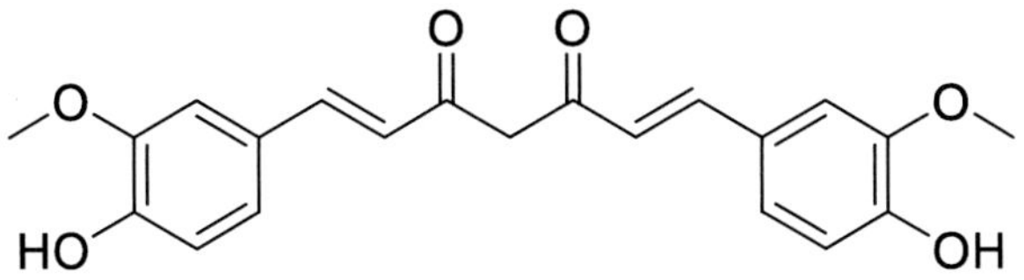

Fig. (2). Chemical structure of Curcumin.

Resveratrol

Resveratrol can be found in a variety of grapes, cherries, berries, and peanuts [68]. Resveratrol Fig.(**3**) has been traditionally used for antioxidant, anticarcinogenic, antiviral, neuroprotective, and anti-inflammatory properties [69]. It enhances tumour cell elimination by promoting the formation of natural killer cells, natural killer group 2D, and T-lymphocytes [70]. This compound inhibits A549 cells (human lung cancer) *in-vitro* with IC_{50} value 8.9±1.3 μM along with *in-vivo* in a dose dependant manner. An *in vivo* study was carried out on a nude mice model developed by implanting A549 cells. In this study, the tumour size was reduced in dose-dependent manner when resveratrol was administered intravenously at different doses like 15, 30, and 60 mg/kg [71]. Resveratrol promotes cell cycle arrest at the G1/S phase when tested against HCT116 and Caco-2 human colon cancer cells showing IC_{50} values of 120 and 170 μM, respectively. It increases the amounts of apoptotic proteins caspase 7 and caspase 9 and reduces the levels of CDK6, CDK4, cyclin D1, and P21 [72].

This compound has shown a synergistic effect with doxorubicin by increasing its inhibitory action by 2.5 folds against breast cancer cell lines, namely MCF-7 and MDA-MB-231, by downregulating the expression of NF-κB and Cyclo oxygenase -2 (COX-2) [73]. TriCurin, a formulation including curcumin, resveratrol, and epicatechin gallate, lowers the tumour growth of a head and neck squamous cell cancer cell line by 85 percent by increasing p53 levels [74]. Despite all this excellent efficacy, resveratrol's clinical development has been hindered due to its poor physicochemical qualities resulting in limited success in developing therapeutic formulations utilising traditional drug delivery systems. Several nano-formulations have been developed in an attempt to overcome their physicochemical limitations, however, each one of them has its own set of benefits and challenges [75]. One such formulation is the dual encapsulation of resveratrol with cyclodextrin complex made in liposomal formulations. This resveratrol formulation showed better efficacy, enhanced solubility and stability as compared with the compound alone (Concentration of resveratrol =50 μM) [76, 77]. Such kind of efforts is further required for the clinical translation of this molecule.

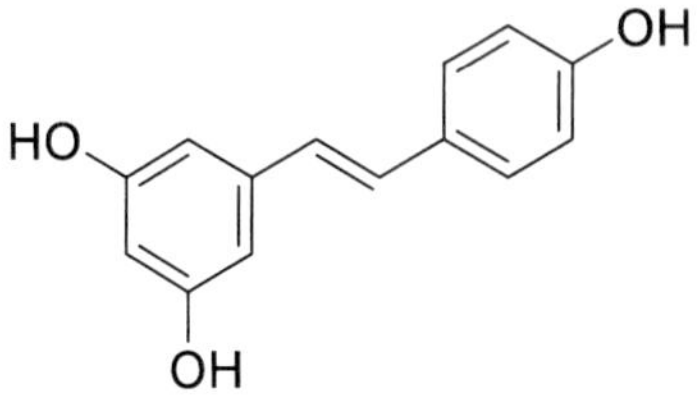

Fig. (3). Chemical structure of Resveratrol.

Quercetin

Quercetin is biosynthesised *via* phenylalanine and possesses radical scavenging activity due to the presence of a phenolic hydroxyl group at the 3rd position of the B ring Fig. (**4**) [78]. It is present abundantly in fruits like berries, apples and several other vegetables. Quercetin acts on the high-mobility group box protein 1 (HMGB1) pathway, thymic stromal lymphopoietin (TSLP) activation, and the Janus kinase (JAK)-STAT signalling pathway to have a multitargeted anticancer impact Fig. (**1**) [79]. Inducible nitric acid synthase (iNOS), proinflammatory cytokines, p21 CDK, and NF-κB activation are getting inhibited by quercetin, causing the cell cycle to stall in the G1/S phase [80, 81]. *in-vitro* anticancer activity of quercetin was evaluated against 9 cancer cell lines such as CT-26, LNCaP, PC12, MCF-7, MOLT-4, U266B1, Raji, and CHO by using MTT assay. It showed potent activity against MOLT-4 (acute lymphoblastic leukemia), Raji (human lymphoid), and U266B1 (human myeloma) cell line with an IC_{50} value of 2.91±0.54, 3.52±0.46, and 6.13±0.73 μM respectively. *In-vivo* tumour reduction in quercetin-treated mice was observed in MCF-7 and CT-26 tumour bearing mice at different doses (50, 100 and 200 mg/kg; i.p.) [82]. Similar *in-vivo* studies were conducted on the HepG2-induced mice model, which was treated with quercetin 10 mg/kg dose administered intraperitoneally for 7 days. The results of this study showed significant tumour volume reduction up to 600 mm^3 in the treated group as compared to 1400 mm^3 in the control group at the end of 21 days as compared to the control group along with suppression of cyclin D1 [83].

Similar to other natural products, quercetin needs further aid in enhancing its pharmacokinetic properties like aqueous solubility and oral bioavailability. Efforts are being made by formulating various nano-based formulations like ligand-conjugated biodegradable quercetin nanoparticles, liposomal copper (II) quercetin, polymeric micelles, *etc* [84, 85]. One such nano-self-emulsifying formulation has been developed and showed anticancer activity at an IC_{50} value of 21.62 µg/ml after 24 hrs, which was better than only quercetin, which was 69.90 µg/ml against the MCF-7 cell line. The formulation was also tested on female Sprague Dawley rats induced with 7,12-dimethylbenz-α anthracene (DMBA) tumours, and it effectively reduced the tumour volume up to 355 mm^3 compared to quercetin alone, which could reduce the tumour volume up to 530 mm^3 [86]. These investigations show that quercetin has the potential to become an anticancer drug but the rigorous studies in the abovementioned directions.

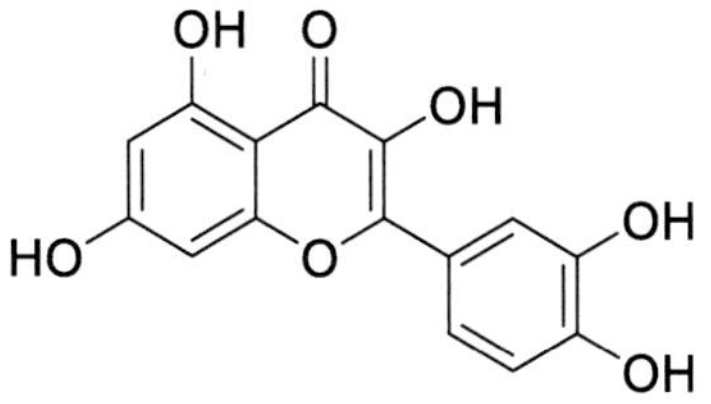

Fig. (4). Chemical structure of Quercetin.

Genistein

Genistein, an isoflavone that is majorly found in soybeans, lupin, fava beans, and other plants [87, 88]. Asian people routinely consume soya products and an epidemiological study carried out on a large population (metadata) indicated a reduced risk of breast cancer in Asian women. This study report revealed that the higher consumption of soy products shows the protective effects against cancer mainly due to its major secondary metabolite genistein Fig. (**5**) [89]. The immunomodulatory activity of genistein produces an anticancer effect by inhibiting the transcriptional factors like NF-κB, Akt, STAT3 and STAT5 along with downregulation of apoptotic and metastatic proteins like Bcl-2, Bcl-Xl and MMP-9, MMP2 respectively [90]. Genistein inhibits human prostate cancer cell line PCa by arresting the cell cycle at the G2/M phase in a dose dependant manner with an IC_{50} value of 25 µM after 72 hrs of treatment [91]. The anti-cancer activity of genistein was evaluated by *in-vivo* histological study in which the model having hepatocellular carcinoma was developed using male Wistar rats induced with N-nitrosodiethylamine along with phenobarbital. The group in which genistein was administered at 15 mg/Kg, as a suspension in olive oil for 15 days, showed increased Caspase-3 activity, DNA fragmentation (indicating apoptosis), and a significant reduction in proliferating cell nuclear antigen in the HCC-bearing rats [92].

A phase 2 trial for genistein against prostate cancer was conducted in a randomised way on 54 patients. A soy-rich diet equivalent to 30 mg of genistein was given to patients and showed a 7.8% reduction of serum prostate-specific antigen levels. This study showed good anticancer efficacy with a mild side effect. However, few patients showed cardiac adverse events [93]. Phase 1 and 2 pilot studies indicated a synergistic effect of genistein along with FOLFOX-Bevacizumab. Here, genistein (60mg) was administered orally for 7 days after every 2 weeks and showed significant improvement against metastatic colorectal cancer (mCRC). These clinical trials suggest the anticancer potential of genistein, although both studies showed mild and rare cardiac adverse events [94]. Hence, a thorough assessment of genistein for its cardiac effects and other toxicities should be established before further development.

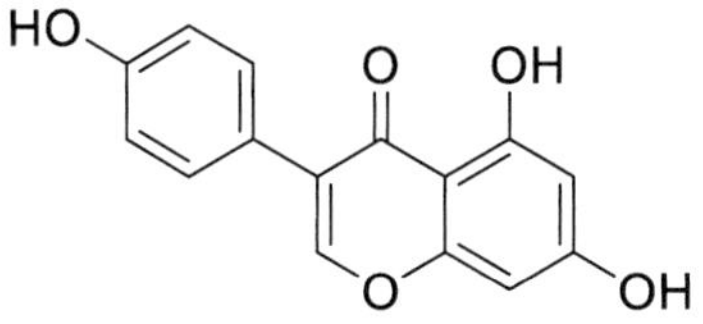

Fig. (5). Chemical structure of Genistein.

Betulinic Acid

Betulinic acid Fig. (**6**) is a leading analogue of betulin which is a prominent pentacyclic triterpene present in the bark of birch trees (*Betula*) along with various other plants like *Syzygium farmosanum*, *Ancistrocladus heyneaus*, *Tetracera bolivia*na, and *Tryphyllum peltatum* [95]. *Betulinic acid* has a wide spectrum of pharmacological activities like anti-HIV, antioxidant, anti-inflammatory, anticancer, *etc* [96]. Betulinic acid Betulinic acid downregulates phosphatidylinositol 3-kinase (PI3K) subunit, STAT3, Bcl-2,which subsequently suppresses Akt phosphorylation at Thr308 and Ser473 [97]. Thus, betulinic acid exhibits anticancer action by interacting with various molecular targets. Betulinic acid shows *in-vitro* anticancer activity against cell line VA-13 (human lung cancer), and HepG2 (human liver cancer) with an IC_{50} value of 11.6 and 21 µM, respectively [98].

In human prostate cancer cells (PC3), betulinic acid suppresses the production of NF-κB, resulting in a decrease in IKK activity and phosphorylation of IκBa. After 24 hrs treatment, betulinic acid resulted in a dose-dependent loss in cell viability in PC-3 cells, at doses of 1–40 µM (IC_{50}:10 µM) [99]. Betulinic acid showed anticancer activity with an IC_{50} value of 29.55 µM against the MCF-7 cell line. It was further evaluated *in-vivo* on female balb/c athymic nude mice transplanted with human breast cancer cells (MCF-7) and showed a 77% reduction in tumour size as compared to control at 100mg/kg of betulinic acid i.p. concentration at 37 days [100]. Modifications at the C-3 position of betulinic acid were done to form di-hydro betulinic acid derivatives to improvise the ADME (absorption, distribution, metabolism and elimination) profile of betulinic acid. The derivatives 2-4-difluoro-benzoyloxy, 2-4-difluoro-benzylidene-amino, benzoyl-hydrazono showed improved metabolic stability while all the derivatives showed poor aqueous solubility, low-moderate permeability and high plasma binding [101].

To address the solubility and absorption issues of betulinic acid, several liposomal-based formulations have been developed [102, 103]. Polyethylene glycol-modified liposomes of betulinic acid have been devised such that the hydrophobic betulinic acid remains enclosed within the lipid bilayer with coating of hydrophilic polyethylene glycol layer. This formulation showed a two-fold increase in the tumour growth inhibition *in-vivo* owing to the slow release of betulinic acid, optimised particle size (leading to accumulation at tumour site), lowered opsonisation due to brush-like configuration of liposomes [104].

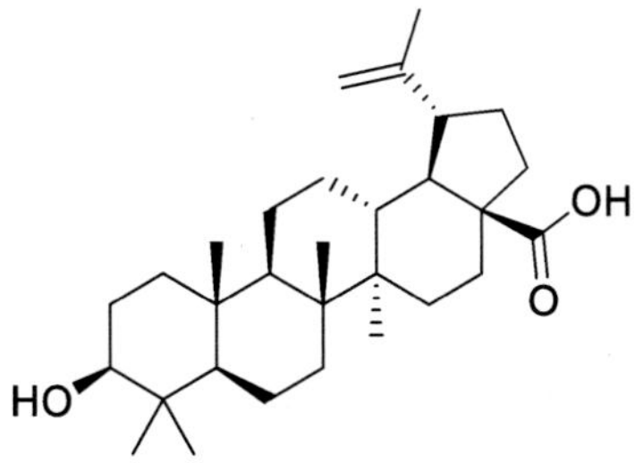

Fig. (6). Chemical structure of Betulinic acid.

Zerumbone

Zerumbone is a cyclic eleven-membered sesquiterpene that is obtained from rhizomes of bitter ginger, *Zingiber zerumbet* (L.) Smith Fig. (**7**) [105]. Zerumbone shows potent anticancer activity against human breast cancer cell line MCF-7 with an IC_{50} value of 2.9 ± 0.8 μM. It has also shown remarkable anticancer activity against the HepG2 cell line (IC_{50} value - 15.80 μM) through triggering the apoptotic process by upregulation of Bax protein [106]. Zerumbone halts the cell cycle at the G2/M phase by downregulating NF-κB activity, further reducing MMP-3, COX-2 and IL-8 expression [107]. In a terminal deoxynucleotidyl transferase-mediated dUTP nick-end labeling (TUNEL) assay, zerumbone was administered at 7.5 and 15.7 mg/kg body weight to immunodeficient female mice in that tumour was induced with MDA-MB231-luc-D3H1 cells. The results revealed a statistically significant increase in the number of apoptotic bodies after zerumbone treatment [108]. Further, clinical development of zerumbone is limited due to its low water solubility, poor absorption, or concomitant low bioavailability. A comprehensive report on formulation development to overcome the biopharmaceutical barriers of zerumbone has been published by Kesharwani, S. S., & Bhat, G. J [109]. According to this report, 7 formulations have been developed based on nanotechnology against different cancer forms.

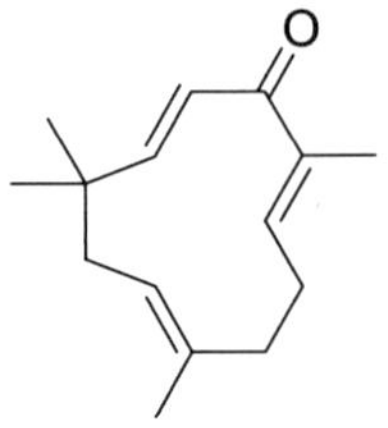

Fig. (7). Chemical structure of Zerumbone.

Berberine

Berberine Fig. (**8**), also known as umbellatine, is a yellow-coloured isoquinoline quaternary alkaloid first isolated from *Xanthoxylon cava* and also present in other medicinal plants like *Berberis vulgaris* L. *Phellondendron amurense*, *Phellondendron chinense schneid, Berberis aristata*, *Hydrastis canadensis*, *Coptis rhizome*, *Coptis chinensis*, *Coptis japonica* [110, 111]. It has been used traditionally in Ayurvedic and Chinese medicine for its antimicrobial and antiprotozoal properties [112]. A spectrum of targets is reported for berberine as it acts against cancer by downregulation of COX-2, NF-κB, STAT3, Bcl-2, Bcl-xL, and MMP [113]. Berberine shows *in-vitro* anticancer activity against gastric cancer cell lines MKN45 and SGC7901 with an IC_{50} value of 20.4 μM and 36.9 μM, respectively [114].

Berberine reverses the doxorubicin resistance by suppressing the autophagy-associated protein LC3II, resulting in a cellular build-up of p62, and reduced cell proliferation [115]. Berberine oral gavage with 50, 100, or 200 mg /kg body weight was administered to 6-7 weeks old female athymic immunodeficient mice to evaluate its antitumor effect. The results showed a 62% tumour volume reduction at the dose of 200mg/kg body weight along with a significant reduction in anti-apoptotic proteins Bcl-2 and Bcl-xL [116]. Several structural modifications at C-8, C-9, and C-13 positions have been carried out to boost the efficiency of berberine. According to the primary structure-activity relationship, 13-alkyl berberine derivatives had much stronger anti-tumour activities as compared to shorter alkyl chain lengths [117]. However, poor absorption, quick metabolism, and removal of berberine have been identified as major hurdles in the further drug development process [118]. Various new delivery techniques, including nano-sized dosage forms, liposomes, and phospholipid complexes, show promising possibilities and should be investigated further to improve bioavailability [119, 120].

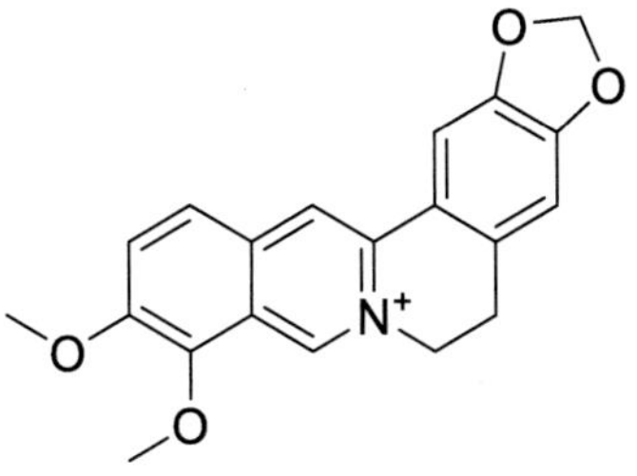

Fig. (8). Chemical structure of berberine.

Epigallocatechin Gallate

Epigallocatechin gallate (EGCG) is a major active constituent of the polyphenolic fraction of *Camellia sinensis* and *Camellia assamica* (green tea) Fig. (**9**) [121]. Its antioxidant property has been well established [122]. The reactive oxygen species produced by epigallocatechin gallate inhibits (IkappaB kinase) IKKβ, which further leads to NF-κB blockage [123]. In addition, EGCG downregulates COX-2, apoptotic proteins, VEGF and STAT1, leading to anticancer activity [124]. The prolonged use of chemotherapy generally leads to a lowered response of tumour cells towards the drugs. EGCG has shown increased sensitivity of anticancer drug like 5-Fluorouracil when delivered together. In this study, EGCG (50 μM) increased the sensitisation of 5-Fluorouracil by 8 (IC_{50} value 5 ± 0.36 μM) and 14 (IC_{50} value 11 ± 0.96 μM) times against HCT-116 and DLD1 colorectal cancer cell lines [125]. An *in vivo* study was carried out to check the efficacy of EGCG, and a prostate cancer model was induced in six-week-old male athymic mice by injecting 15μL of BCaPM-T10 cells (100,000). 0.06% EGCG in water was administered and tumour size was monitored. The results showed 50% reduction in tumour growth after 1 month of epigallocatechin gallate treatment [126].

Due to its low stability and restricted penetration, EGCG has a low oral bioavailability [127]. The bioavailability of EGCG is highly altered with different food intake patterns [128]. Efforts to increase the bioavailability of EGCG by making nutritional modifications have been reported by Andreu Fernandez, V., and the team. In this trial, healthy men (5) and women (5) volunteers were administered Teavigo® (green tea extract) alone, Teavigo® with a standard breakfast, and lastly FontUp® (Teavigo® commercially prepared with fats, carbohydrates, proteins, vitamins, and minerals) with the washup period of seven days. This study showed that after fasting overnight, using a green tea extract enhanced with EGCG (Teavigo®, 94 percent EGCG) leads to the maximum exposure to EGCG in both men and women (AUC0–360 and Cmax). Furthermore, Teavigo® reduced epigallocatechin gallate bioavailability when consumed with a Mediterranean diet breakfast [129]. Further approaches like synergistic effects with curcumin, synthetic analogues and formulation development are being utilised to elevate the efficiency and pharmacokinetics of epigallocatechin gallate [130, 131].

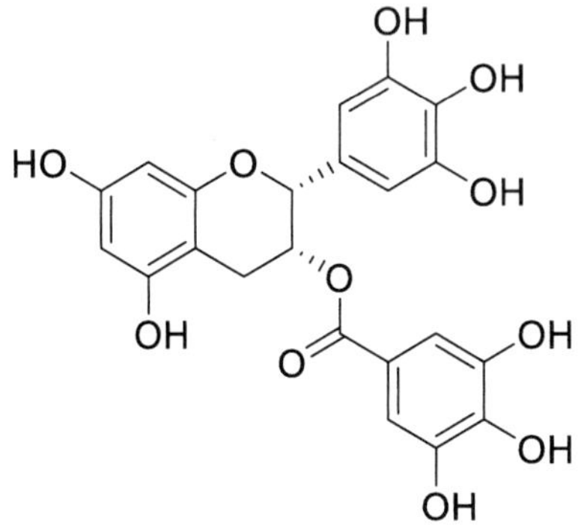

Fig. (9). Chemical structure of epigallocatechin gallate.

Miscellaneous

Alkaloids are secondary metabolites widely distributed in various natural sources like plants, insects, marine life, *etc.*, and have immense structural and pharmacological diversity [132]. Capsaicin Fig. (**10**) is an alkaloid commonly found in genus Capsicum [31]. Capsaicin exhibits an anticancer effect by stimulating immunogenic cell death by stimulating the secretion of interferon gamma (IFN-γ) [133]. It degrades tumour-specific T-cells and alters the tumour microenvironment, resulting in anti-tumour activity [134]. Capsaicin-loaded solid nanoparticles have been formulated to improvise their solubility. The formulation showed anticancer activity against human liver cancer cell lines (HepG2) with an IC_{50} value of 21.36 μg × ml^{-1} *in-vitro* [135]. Magnoflorine Fig. (**10**) is another alkaloid, which exhibits anticancer activity through immunomodulation. It is present in plants like *Magnolia grandiflora* L., *Magnolia officinalis* Rehder & E.H. Wilson, *Tinospora crispa*, *etc* [136]. In a cell viability study, magnoflorine was examined using the tumour cell lines like U251, HEPG2, and Hela and the compound showed anticancer activity against HEPG2 and U251 with IC_{50} 0.4 and 7 μg $mL^{-1,}$ respectively, while it had shown no effect on the Hela cancer cell [137]. Magnoflorine increases the sensitivity of cisplatin and suppresses the expression of HMGB1 (high-mobility group protein-1) a proinflammatory cytokine, and also inhibits NF-κB in osteosarcoma cells [138].

A phenolic secondary metabolite, 6-gingerol Fig. (**10**) from *Zingiber officinale* [139], has the ability to slow down the metastasis of renal cell carcinoma by reducing MMP2, slugs, and vimentin protein levels [140]. The anti-metastasis effect of 6-gingerol was observed on lung B16F10 melanoma by inhibiting vascular endothelial growth factor (VEGF) induced angiogenesis and COX-2 [141]. Gallic acid Fig. (**10**) a phenolic compound, found in pomegranate, tea leaves, bearberry, pomegranate, gallnuts, witch hazel, sumac [142], exhibits the tumour suppressive effect by binding to epidermal growth factor receptor and triggering the activation of p53 in non-small cell lung cancer [143]. Ellagic acid Fig. (**10**) present in berries, fruits and nuts [144], also shows antitumor activity by inducing T-cell activation *via* blocking programmed cell death protein 1 and programmed death ligand 1 [145].

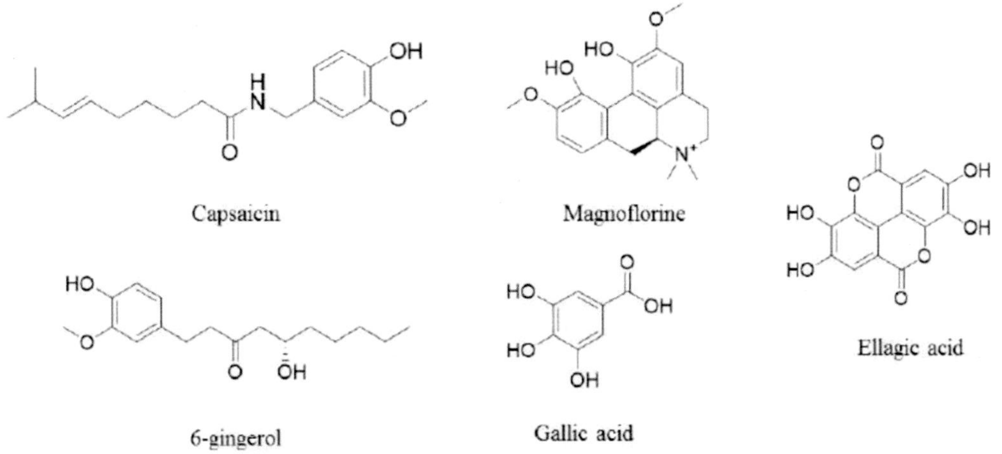

Fig. (10). Chemical structures of miscellaneous compounds having anticancer activity *via* immunomodulation.

Flavonoids are polyphenolic plant secondary metabolites with significant structural diversity and biological activities like antioxidant, anti-inflammatory, antimutagenic *etc* [146]. The biosynthesis of flavonoids occurs *via* the phenylpropanoid pathway, which is initiated by 4-coumaryl CoA [147]. Isoliquiritigenin Fig. (**11**) obtained from the roots of *Glycyrrhiza glabra* L., inhibits the growth of DU145 and LNCaP prostate cancer cell lines with the IC_{50} value of 11 μM and 13 μM respectively by increasing the expression of GADD153 (growth arrest and DNA damage-inducible gene 153) leading to S and G2/M phase arrest of the cell cycle [148]. Tangeretin Fig. (**11**) widely distributed in citrus fruits, is a polymethoxylated anti-cancer activity in several cancer cells like breast, ovary, colorectal *etc.* It inhibits cell proliferation *via* modulation of Notch, mTOR, and MAPK signalling pathways [149]. Apigenin (4′, 5, 7-trihydroxyflavone) Fig. (**11**) occurs in various common fruits and vegetables that show anticancer activity by various mechanisms like apoptosis, autophagy, immunomodulation, cell cycle arrest, and inhibition of invasion. Reduction of

Janus kinase/signal transducers and activators of transcription (JAK/STAT) occurs in the immunomodulation mechanism, leading to its anticancer effect [150]. Kaempferol Fig. (**11**), a dietary flavonoid, is present in various fruits and vegetables. It acts *via* inhibition of serine/threonine-protein kinase (MAPK and RSK2) and decreased expression of JAK3, IL8, STAT6 and NF-κB to exhibit an anti-cancer effect [151]. Rutin Fig. (**11**), also known as rutoside, is mostly present in Eucalyptus, buckwheat and Japanese pagoda trees [152]. A detailed review of rutin and how it modulates various intracellular signalling pathways, as verified by *in-vitro* and *in-vivo* research shows that rutin acts through JAK/STAT and EGFR signalling pathways to inhibit cell proliferation [153].

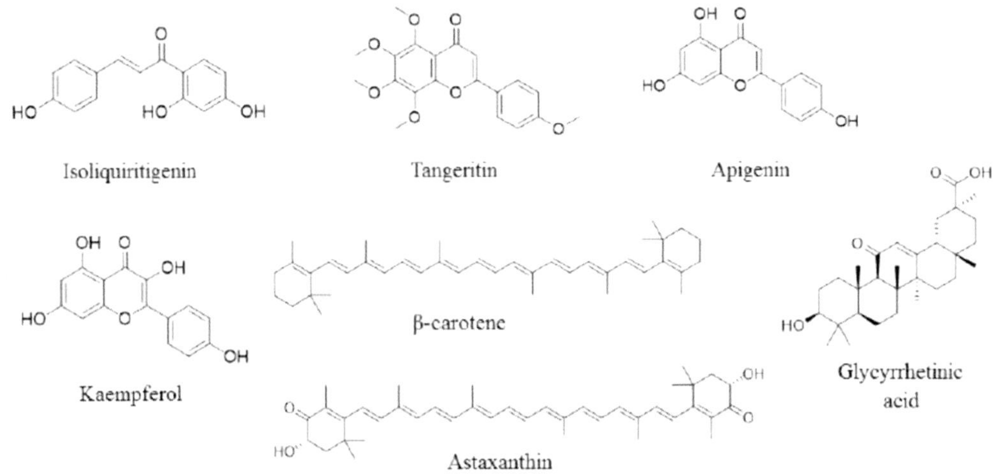

Fig. (11). Chemical structures of miscellaneous compounds having anticancer activity *via* immunomodulation.

Kekule is credited with coining the name "terpen" to characterise $C_{10}H_{18}$ hydrocarbons found in turpentine (German, "Terpentin") oil that has now taken on a generic meaning and is used to refer to isoprene-based secondary metabolites [154]. Glycyrrhetinic acid (Fig. **11**), a triterpenoid is obtained from *Glycyrrhiza glabra* L. roots [37]. Glycyrrhetinic acid-conjugated allicin-loaded gelatin nanoparticles have been formulated against hepatic cancer (HepG2 cell line) and showed an IC_{50} value of 5.046 μM [155] Glycyrrhetinic acid inactivates the AkT pathway, downregulating NF-κB against the prostate cancer cell line LNCaP [156]. β-carotene, a vitamin A pre-cursor, is available in various fruits and vegetables [157]. It slows the growth rate of prostate cancer cell lines PC-3, DU145, and LNCaP [158]. Tomatoes, olives, watermelon, pink guava, papaya, and rosehip contain lycopene [159]. Lycopene Fig. (**11**) shows anticancer activity against the human colon cancer cell line HT-29 with an IC_{50} value of 10 μM by suppressing the Akt pathway and expression of cyclin D1 [160]. Astaxanthin (3,

3′-dihydroxy-β, β′-carotene-4, 4′-dione) Fig. (**11**) occurs naturally in various species of algae, salmon, yeast, shrimp, krill, crayfish, and trout [161]. *In-vitro* anticancer studies of astaxanthin were conducted on various cell lines like VMM917, MCF7, A549, HepG2, and WiDr. Results revealed that astaxanthin had selective activity against lung and colon cancer cell lines that are A549 and WiDr, with an IC_{50} value of 61 μM and 75μM, respectively [162].

CONCLUDING REMARKS

Cancer treatment is driven by two important paradigms: modifications of oncogenes and immune-oncology. The management of tumour heterogeneity and increasing drug resistance are the major setbacks for current chemotherapeutics. Immune checkpoint inhibitors allow for increased longevity benefits but are restricted by less validated markers to optimise the therapy. The discovery of emerging immune checkpoints in the tumour microenvironment has helped to strategize the key immunomodulators for cancer treatment. The use of natural products for anticancer activity is emerging due to the better understanding between immunology and oncology. In this chapter, the authors have highlighted the leading natural compounds that have immunomodulatory benefits against various cancer types. Molecules like curcumin, resveratrol, quercetin, betulinic acid, and zerumbone have been well studied for their anticancer potential and show multitargeted action for tumour destruction. Curcumin, genistein, and betulinic acid have been further evaluated in various clinical trials. The solubility and other pharmacokinetic parameters of these molecules need further improvisation to translate them into potential anticancer drugs. Few molecules, such as resveratrol, zerumbone and capsaicin, have shown anticancer potential in their *in-vitro* and *in-vivo* studies, but further research into their structure-activity relationship and formulation development studies are needed to improve their pharmacokinetics and toxicity profile for better drug likeliness. Natural immunomodulators, as a result, appear to be a potential field of research for advanced cancer therapy in the ensuing years.

CONSENT FOR PUBLICATION

Not applicable.

CONFLICT OF INTEREST

The authors declare no conflict of interest, financial or otherwise.

ACKNOWLEDGEMENTS

We acknowledge the Department of Pharmaceuticals, Ministry of Chemicals and Fertilizers, Government of India and National Institute of Pharmaceutical Education and Research (NIPER), Ahmedabad, for providing continuous support and facilities.

REFERENCES

[1] Mattiuzzi C, Lippi G. Current cancer epidemiology. J Epidemiol Glob Health 2019; 9(4): 217-22. [http://dx.doi.org/10.2991/jegh.k.191008.001] [PMID: 31854162]

[2] Nikolaou M, Pavlopoulou A, Georgakilas AG, Kyrodimos E. The challenge of drug resistance in cancer treatment: a current overview. Clin Exp Metastasis 2018; 35(4): 309-18. [http://dx.doi.org/10.1007/s10585-018-9903-0] [PMID: 29799080]

[3] https://www.who.int/health-topics/cancer

[4] Wang X, Zhang H, Chen X. Drug resistance and combating drug resistance in cancer. Cancer Drug Resist 2019; 2(2): 141-60. [http://dx.doi.org/10.20517/cdr.2019.10] [PMID: 34322663]

[5] Roberti A, Sala DL, Cinti C. Multiple genetic and epigenetic interacting mechanisms contribute to clonally selection of drug-resistant tumors: Current views and new therapeutic prospective. J Cell Physiol 2006; 207(3): 571-81. [http://dx.doi.org/10.1002/jcp.20515] [PMID: 16250021]

[6] Nurgali K, Jagoe RT, Abalo R. Adverse effects of cancer chemotherapy: Anything new to improve tolerance and reduce sequelae? Front Pharmacol 2018; 9: 245. [http://dx.doi.org/10.3389/fphar.2018.00245] [PMID: 29623040]

[7] Berkey FJ. Managing the adverse effects of radiation therapy. Am Fam Physician 2010; 82(4): 381-388, 394. [PMID: 20704169]

[8] Farkona S, Diamandis EP, Blasutig IM. Cancer immunotherapy: the beginning of the end of cancer? BMC Med 2016; 14(1): 73. [http://dx.doi.org/10.1186/s12916-016-0623-5] [PMID: 27151159]

[9] Pardoll DM. The blockade of immune checkpoints in cancer immunotherapy. Nat Rev Cancer 2012; 12(4): 252-64. [http://dx.doi.org/10.1038/nrc3239] [PMID: 22437870]

[10] Waldmann TA. Effective cancer therapy through immunomodulation. Annu Rev Med 2006; 57(1): 65-81. [http://dx.doi.org/10.1146/annurev.med.56.082103.104549] [PMID: 16409137]

[11] Lee JY, Lee HT, Shin W, *et al.* Structural basis of checkpoint blockade by monoclonal antibodies in cancer immunotherapy. Nat Commun 2016; 7(1): 13354. [http://dx.doi.org/10.1038/ncomms13354] [PMID: 27796306]

[12] Ma Y, Shurin GV, Peiyuan Z, Shurin MR. Dendritic cells in the cancer microenvironment. J Cancer 2013; 4(1): 36-44. [http://dx.doi.org/10.7150/jca.5046] [PMID: 23386903]

[13] Brodsky FM. Monoclonal antibodies as magic bullets. Pharm Res 1988; 5(1): 1-9. [http://dx.doi.org/10.1023/A:1015860525341] [PMID: 3072552]

[14] Coulson, A., Levy, A. and Gossell-Williams, M. Monoclonal antibodies in cancer therapy: mechanisms, successes and limitations. West Indian Med J 2014; 63(6), p.650.

[http://dx.doi.org/10.7727/wimj.2013.241]

[15] Brennan FR, Morton LD, Spindeldreher S, *et al.* Safety and immunotoxicity assessment of immunomodulatory monoclonal antibodies. MAbs 2010; 2(3): 233-55. [http://dx.doi.org/10.4161/mabs.2.3.11782] [PMID: 20421713]

[16] Jan M, Sperling AS, Ebert BL. Cancer therapies based on targeted protein degradation — lessons learned with lenalidomide. Nat Rev Clin Oncol 2021; 18(7): 401-17. [http://dx.doi.org/10.1038/s41571-021-00479-z] [PMID: 33654306]

[17] Kotla V, Goel S, Nischal S, *et al.* Mechanism of action of lenalidomide in hematological malignancies. J Hematol Oncol 2009; 2(1): 36. [http://dx.doi.org/10.1186/1756-8722-2-36] [PMID: 19674465]

[18] Vallet S, Palumbo A, Raje N, Boccadoro M, Anderson KC. Thalidomide and lenalidomide: Mechanism-based potential drug combinations. Leuk Lymphoma 2008; 49(7): 1238-45. [http://dx.doi.org/10.1080/10428190802005191] [PMID: 18452080]

[19] Arivarasan VK. Shree Devi MS. *in-vitro* Immunomodulatory activity and Thrombolytic potential of Kabasura Kudineer (KSK), an official Siddha polyherbal formulation. *S.S.* RN 2020; 2(3): 1-21. [http://dx.doi.org/10.2139/ssrn.3670659]

[20] Diwanay S, Chitre D, Patwardhan B. Immunoprotection by botanical drugs in cancer chemotherapy. J Ethnopharmacol 2004; 90(1): 49-55. [http://dx.doi.org/10.1016/j.jep.2003.09.023] [PMID: 14698508]

[21] Alamgir M, Uddin SJ. Recent advances on the ethnomedicinal plants as immunomodulatory agents. Ethnomedicine: a source of complementary therapeutics 2010; 37(661): 2.

[22] Malik F, Kumar A, Bhushan S, *et al.* Immune modulation and apoptosis induction: Two sides of antitumoural activity of a standardised herbal formulation of Withania somnifera. Eur J Cancer 2009; 45(8): 1494-509. [http://dx.doi.org/10.1016/j.ejca.2009.01.034] [PMID: 19269163]

[23] Kim S, Kim N, Jeong J, *et al.* Anti-Cancer Effect of Panax Ginseng and Its Metabolites: From Traditional Medicine to Modern Drug Discovery. Processes (Basel) 2021; 9(8): 1344. [http://dx.doi.org/10.3390/pr9081344]

[24] Castro-Aceituno V, Ahn S, Simu SY, *et al.* Anticancer activity of silver nanoparticles from Panax ginseng fresh leaves in human cancer cells. Biomed Pharmacother 2016; 84: 158-65. [http://dx.doi.org/10.1016/j.biopha.2016.09.016] [PMID: 27643558]

[25] Abood WN. Immunomodulatory and natural immunomodulators. J Allergy Inflamm 2017; 1: 101.

[26] Paulucci VP, Couto RO, Teixeira CCC, Freitas LAP. Optimization of the extraction of curcumin from Curcuma longa rhizomes. Rev Bras Farmacogn 2013; 23(1): 94-100. [http://dx.doi.org/10.1590/S0102-695X2012005000117]

[27] Chen H, Deng Q, Ji X, Zhou X, Kelly G, Zhang J. Glucose oxidase-assisted extraction of resveratrol from Japanese knotweed (Fallopia japonica). New J Chem 2016; 40(9): 8131-40. [http://dx.doi.org/10.1039/C6NJ01294A]

[28] Wohlmuth H, Leach DN, Smith MK, Myers SP. Gingerol content of diploid and tetraploid clones of ginger (Zingiber officinale Roscoe). J Agric Food Chem 2005; 53(14): 5772-8. [http://dx.doi.org/10.1021/jf050435b] [PMID: 15998147]

[29] Martin LJ, Matar C. Increase of antioxidant capacity of the lowbush blueberry (Vaccinium angustifolium) during fermentation by a novel bacterium from the fruit microflora. J Sci Food Agric 2005; 85(9): 1477-84. [http://dx.doi.org/10.1002/jsfa.2142]

[30] Mahoney N, Molyneux RJ. Phytochemical inhibition of aflatoxigenicity in Aspergillus flavus by constituents of walnut (Juglans regia). J Agric Food Chem 2004; 52(7): 1882-9.

[http://dx.doi.org/10.1021/jf030812p] [PMID: 15053524]

[31] da Silva Pinto M, Lajolo FM, Genovese MI. Bioactive compounds and quantification of total ellagic acid in strawberries (Fragaria x ananassa Duch.). Food Chem 2008; 107(4): 1629-35. [http://dx.doi.org/10.1016/j.foodchem.2007.10.038]

[32] Sanatombi K, Sharma GJ. Capsaicin content and pungency of different Capsicum spp. cultivars. Not Bot Horti Agrobot Cluj-Napoca 2008; 36(2): 89-90.

[33] Farag MA, Al-Mahdy DA. Comparative study of the chemical composition and biological activities of *Magnolia grandiflora* and *Magnolia virginiana* flower essential oils. Nat Prod Res 2013; 27(12): 1091-7. [http://dx.doi.org/10.1080/14786419.2012.696256] [PMID: 22690913]

[34] Yan D, Jin C, Xiao XH, Dong XP. Antimicrobial properties of berberines alkaloids in Coptis chinensis Franch by microcalorimetry. J Biochem Biophys Methods 2008; 70(6): 845-9. [http://dx.doi.org/10.1016/j.jbbm.2007.07.009] [PMID: 17804078]

[35] Tao Y, Huang S, Yan J, Cai B. Establishment of a rapid and sensitive UPLC-MS/MS method for pharmacokinetic determination of nine alkaloids of crude and processed Corydalis turtschaninovii Besser aqueous extracts in rat plasma. J Chromatogr B Analyt Technol Biomed Life Sci 2019; 1124: 218-25. [http://dx.doi.org/10.1016/j.jchromb.2019.06.018] [PMID: 31233942]

[36] Sunila ES, Kuttan G. Immunomodulatory and antitumor activity of Piper longum Linn. and piperine. J Ethnopharmacol 2004; 90(2-3): 339-46. [http://dx.doi.org/10.1016/j.jep.2003.10.016] [PMID: 15013199]

[37] Sapra S, Bhalla Y, Nandani , *et al.* Colchicine and its various physicochemical and biological aspects. Med Chem Res 2013; 22(2): 531-47. [http://dx.doi.org/10.1007/s00044-012-0077-z]

[38] Batiha GES, Beshbishy AM, Ikram M, *et al.* The pharmacological activity, biochemical properties, and pharmacokinetics of the major natural polyphenolic flavonoid: quercetin. Foods 2020; 9(3): 374. [http://dx.doi.org/10.3390/foods9030374] [PMID: 32210182]

[39] Devi KP, Malar DS, Nabavi SF, *et al.* Kaempferol and inflammation: From chemistry to medicine. Pharmacol Res 2015; 99: 1-10. [http://dx.doi.org/10.1016/j.phrs.2015.05.002] [PMID: 25982933]

[40] Parray SA, Bhat JU, Ahmad G, Jahan N, Sofi G. Iqbal SMF. Ruta graveolens: from traditional system of medicine to modern pharmacology: an overview. Am J Pharm Tech Res 2012; 2(2): 239-52.

[41] Sharangi AB. Medicinal and therapeutic potentialities of tea (*Camellia sinensis* L.) – A review. Food Res Int 2009; 42(5-6): 529-35. [http://dx.doi.org/10.1016/j.foodres.2009.01.007]

[42] Kaufman PB, Duke JA, Brielmann H, Boik J, Hoyt JE. A comparative survey of leguminous plants as sources of the isoflavones, genistein and daidzein: implications for human nutrition and health. J Altern Complement Med 1997; 3(1): 7-12. [http://dx.doi.org/10.1089/acm.1997.3.7] [PMID: 9395689]

[43] Liu X, Mei Z, Qian J, Zeng Y, Wang M. Puerarin partly counteracts the inflammatory response after cerebral ischemia/reperfusion *via* activating the cholinergic anti-inflammatory pathway. Neural Regen Res 2013; 8(34): 3203-15. [PMID: 25206641]

[44] Ziyan L, Yongmei Z, Nan Z, Ning T, Baolin L. Evaluation of the anti-inflammatory activity of luteolin in experimental animal models. Planta Med 2007; 73(3): 221-6. [http://dx.doi.org/10.1055/s-2007-967122] [PMID: 17354164]

[45] Nicholas C, Batra S, Vargo MA, *et al.* Apigenin blocks lipopolysaccharide-induced lethality *in vivo* and proinflammatory cytokines expression by inactivating NF-kappaB through the suppression of p65

phosphorylation. J Immunol 2007; 179(10): 7121-7.
[http://dx.doi.org/10.4049/jimmunol.179.10.7121] [PMID: 17982104]

[46] Hämäläinen M, Nieminen R, Vuorela P, Heinonen M, Moilanen E. Anti-inflammatory effects of flavonoids: genistein, kaempferol, quercetin, and daidzein inhibit STAT-1 and NF-kappaB activations, whereas flavone, isorhamnetin, naringenin, and pelargonidin inhibit only NF-kappaB activation along with their inhibitory effect on iNOS expression and NO production in activated macrophages. Mediators Inflamm 2007; 2007(3): 45673.
[PMID: 18274639]

[47] Bae Y, Lee S, Kim SH. Chrysin suppresses mast cell-mediated allergic inflammation: Involvement of calcium, caspase-1 and nuclear factor-κB. Toxicol Appl Pharmacol 2011; 254(1): 56-64.
[http://dx.doi.org/10.1016/j.taap.2011.04.008] [PMID: 21515303]

[48] Chandrashekar N, Selvamani A, Subramanian R, Pandi A, Thiruvengadam D. Baicalein inhibits pulmonary carcinogenesis-associated inflammation and interferes with COX-2, MMP-2 and MMP-9 expressions *in-vivo*. Toxicol Appl Pharmacol 2012; 261(1): 10-21.
[http://dx.doi.org/10.1016/j.taap.2012.02.004] [PMID: 22369883]

[49] Andújar I, Recio MC, Bacelli T, Giner RM, Ríos JL. Shikonin reduces oedema induced by phorbol ester by interfering with IκBα degradation thus inhibiting translocation of NF-κB to the nucleus. Br J Pharmacol 2010; 160(2): 376-88.
[http://dx.doi.org/10.1111/j.1476-5381.2010.00696.x] [PMID: 20423347]

[50] Stefanska J, Pawliczak R. Apocynin: molecular aptitudes. Mediators Inflamm 2008; 2008(11): 106507.
[PMID: 19096513]

[51] Ajaya Kumar R, Sridevi K, Vijaya Kumar N, Nanduri S, Rajagopal S. Anticancer and immunostimulatory compounds from Andrographis paniculata. J Ethnopharmacol 2004; 92(2-3): 291-5.
[http://dx.doi.org/10.1016/j.jep.2004.03.004] [PMID: 15138014]

[52] Tolstikov GA, Flekhter OB, Shultz EE, Baltina LA, Tolstikov AG. Betulin and its derivatives. Chemistry and biological activity. Chem Sustain Dev 2005; 13(1): 1-29.

[53] Singh YP, Girisa S, Banik K, *et al.* Potential application of zerumbone in the prevention and therapy of chronic human diseases. J Funct Foods 2019; 53: 248-58.
[http://dx.doi.org/10.1016/j.jff.2018.12.020]

[54] Bogacz-Radomska L, Harasym J. β-Carotene—properties and production methods. Food Quality and Safety 2018; 2(2): 69-74.
[http://dx.doi.org/10.1093/fqsafe/fyy004]

[55] Suwanaruang T. Analyzing lycopene content in fruits. Agric Agric Sci Procedia 2016; 11: 46-8.
[http://dx.doi.org/10.1016/j.aaspro.2016.12.008]

[56] Dave D, Liu Y, Pohling J, Trenholm S, Murphy W. Astaxanthin recovery from Atlantic shrimp (Pandalus borealis) processing materials. Bioresour Technol Rep 2020; 11: 100535.
[http://dx.doi.org/10.1016/j.biteb.2020.100535]

[57] Lee SW, Lim JM, Bhoo SH, Paik YS, Hahn TR. Colorimetric determination of amino acids using genipin from Gardenia jasminoides. Anal Chim Acta 2003; 480(2): 267-74.
[http://dx.doi.org/10.1016/S0003-2670(03)00023-0]

[58] Song JY, Han SK, Son EH, Pyo SN, Yun YS, Yi SY. Induction of secretory and tumoricidal activities in peritoneal macrophages by ginsan. Int Immunopharmacol 2002; 2(7): 857-65.
[http://dx.doi.org/10.1016/S1567-5769(01)00211-9] [PMID: 12188027]

[59] Brinker AM, Ma J, Lipsky PE, Raskin I. Medicinal chemistry and pharmacology of genus Tripterygium (Celastraceae). Phytochemistry 2007; 68(6): 732-66.
[http://dx.doi.org/10.1016/j.phytochem.2006.11.029] [PMID: 17250858]

[60] Li H, Gong X, Zhang L, *et al.* Madecassoside attenuates inflammatory response on collagen-induced arthritis in DBA/1 mice. Phytomedicine 2009; 16(6-7): 538-46. [http://dx.doi.org/10.1016/j.phymed.2008.11.002] [PMID: 19135346]

[61] Ammon H. Boswellic acids in chronic inflammatory diseases. Planta Med 2006; 72(12): 1100-16. [http://dx.doi.org/10.1055/s-2006-947227] [PMID: 17024588]

[62] Cundell D, Wilkinson F. D.; Wilkinson, F. Curcumin: powerful immunomodulator from turmeric. Curr Immunol Rev 2014; 10(2): 122-32. [http://dx.doi.org/10.2174/1573395510666141029233003]

[63] Gautam SC, Gao X, Dulchavsky S. Gautam, S.C.; Gao, X.; Dulchavsky, S. Immunomodulation by curcumin. The Molecular Targets and Therapeutic Uses of Curcumin in Health and Disease 2007; 321-41.

[64] Tamvakopoulos C, Dimas K, Sofianos ZD, *et al.* Metabolism and anticancer activity of the curcumin analogue, dimethoxycurcumin. Clin Cancer Res 2007; 13(4): 1269-77. [http://dx.doi.org/10.1158/1078-0432.CCR-06-1839] [PMID: 17317839]

[65] Bhattacharyya S, Md Sakib Hossain D, Mohanty S, *et al.* Curcumin reverses T cell-mediated adaptive immune dysfunctions in tumor-bearing hosts. Cell Mol Immunol 2010; 7(4): 306-15. [http://dx.doi.org/10.1038/cmi.2010.11] [PMID: 20305684]

[66] Wang D, Veena MS, Stevenson K, *et al.* Liposome-encapsulated curcumin suppresses growth of head and neck squamous cell carcinoma *in vitro* and in xenografts through the inhibition of nuclear factor kappaB by an AKT-independent pathway. Clin Cancer Res 2008; 14(19): 6228-36. [http://dx.doi.org/10.1158/1078-0432.CCR-07-5177] [PMID: 18829502]

[67] Salehi B, Stojanović-Radić Z, Matejić J, *et al.* The therapeutic potential of curcumin: A review of clinical trials. Eur J Med Chem 2019; 163: 527-45. [http://dx.doi.org/10.1016/j.ejmech.2018.12.016] [PMID: 30553144]

[68] Kumar G, Mittal S, Sak K, Tuli HS. Molecular mechanisms underlying chemopreventive potential of curcumin: Current challenges and future perspectives. Life Sci 2016; 148: 313-28. [http://dx.doi.org/10.1016/j.lfs.2016.02.022] [PMID: 26876915]

[69] Dhingra AK, Rathi V, Chopra B. Resveratrol. In naturally occurring chemicals against Alzheimer's disease. 2021; 33-47. [http://dx.doi.org/10.1016/B978-0-12-819212-2.00037-2]

[70] Salehi B, Mishra A, Nigam M, *et al.* Resveratrol: A double-edged sword in health benefits. Biomedicines 2018; 6(3): 91. [http://dx.doi.org/10.3390/biomedicines6030091] [PMID: 30205595]

[71] Trung LQ, An DTT. Is resveratrol a cancer immunomodulatory molecule? Front Pharmacol 2018; 9: 1255. [http://dx.doi.org/10.3389/fphar.2018.01255] [PMID: 30459616]

[72] Yin HT, Tian QZ, Guan L, Zhou Y, Huang XE, Zhang H. *in vitro* and *in vivo* evaluation of the antitumor efficiency of resveratrol against lung cancer. Asian Pac J Cancer Prev 2013; 14(3): 1703-6. [http://dx.doi.org/10.7314/APJCP.2013.14.3.1703] [PMID: 23679260]

[73] Rai G, Mishra S, Suman S, Shukla Y. Resveratrol improves the anticancer effects of doxorubicin *in vitro* and *in vivo* models: A mechanistic insight. Phytomedicine 2016; 23(3): 233-42. [http://dx.doi.org/10.1016/j.phymed.2015.12.020] [PMID: 26969377]

[74] Liu B, Zhou Z, Zhou W, *et al.* Resveratrol inhibits proliferation in human colorectal carcinoma cells by inducing G1/S-phase cell cycle arrest and apoptosis through caspase/cyclin-CDK pathways. Mol Med Rep 2014; 10(4): 1697-702. [http://dx.doi.org/10.3892/mmr.2014.2406] [PMID: 25050564]

[75] Piao L, Mukherjee S, Chang Q, *et al.* TriCurin, a novel formulation of curcumin, epicatechin gallate,

and resveratrol, inhibits the tumorigenicity of human papillomavirus-positive head and neck squamous cell carcinoma. Oncotarget 2017; 8(36): 60025-35.
[http://dx.doi.org/10.18632/oncotarget.10620] [PMID: 28947951]

[76] Summerlin N, Soo E, Thakur S, Qu Z, Jambhrunkar S, Popat A. Resveratrol nanoformulations: Challenges and opportunities. Int J Pharm 2015; 479(2): 282-90.
[http://dx.doi.org/10.1016/j.ijpharm.2015.01.003] [PMID: 25572692]

[77] Soo E, Thakur S, Qu Z, Jambhrunkar S, Parekh HS, Popat A. Enhancing delivery and cytotoxicity of resveratrol through a dual nanoencapsulation approach. J Colloid Interface Sci 2016; 462: 368-74.
[http://dx.doi.org/10.1016/j.jcis.2015.10.022] [PMID: 26479200]

[78] Patil BS, Jayaprakasha GK, Chidambara Murthy KN, Vikram A. Bioactive compounds: historical perspectives, opportunities, and challenges. J Agric Food Chem 2009; 57(18): 8142-60.
[http://dx.doi.org/10.1021/jf9000132] [PMID: 19719126]

[79] Khan F, Niaz K, Maqbool F, *et al.* Molecular targets underlying the anticancer effects of quercetin: an update. Nutrients 2016; 8(9): 529.
[http://dx.doi.org/10.3390/nu8090529] [PMID: 27589790]

[80] Murakami A, Ashida H, Terao J. Multitargeted cancer prevention by quercetin. Cancer Lett 2008; 269(2): 315-25.
[http://dx.doi.org/10.1016/j.canlet.2008.03.046] [PMID: 18467024]

[81] Jeong JH, An JY, Kwon YT, Rhee JG, Lee YJ. Effects of low dose quercetin: Cancer cell-specific inhibition of cell cycle progression. J Cell Biochem 2009; 106(1): 73-82.
[http://dx.doi.org/10.1002/jcb.21977] [PMID: 19009557]

[82] Hashemzaei M, Far AD, Yari A, *et al.* Anticancer and apoptosis-inducing effects of quercetin *in vitro* and *in vivo*. Oncol Rep 2017; 38(2): 819-28.
[http://dx.doi.org/10.3892/or.2017.5766] [PMID: 28677813]

[83] Zhou J, Fang L, Liao J, *et al.* Investigation of the anti-cancer effect of quercetin on HepG2 cells *in vivo*. PLoS One 2017; 12(3): e0172838.
[http://dx.doi.org/10.1371/journal.pone.0172838] [PMID: 28264020]

[84] Lozano O, Lázaro-Alfaro A, Silva-Platas C, *et al.* Nanoencapsulated quercetin improves cardioprotection during hypoxia-reoxygenation injury through preservation of mitochondrial function. Oxid Med Cell Longev 2019; 2019(1): 1-14.
[http://dx.doi.org/10.1155/2019/7683051] [PMID: 31341535]

[85] Kumar P, Sharma G, Kumar R, *et al.* Promises of a biocompatible nanocarrier in improved brain delivery of quercetin: Biochemical, pharmacokinetic and biodistribution evidences. Int J Pharm 2016; 515(1-2): 307-14.
[http://dx.doi.org/10.1016/j.ijpharm.2016.10.024] [PMID: 27756627]

[86] Jain AK, Thanki K, Jain S. Novel self-nanoemulsifying formulation of quercetin: Implications of pro-oxidant activity on the anticancer efficacy. Nanomedicine 2014; 10(5): e959-69.
[http://dx.doi.org/10.1016/j.nano.2013.12.010] [PMID: 24407148]

[87] Gaur A, Bhatia A. Genistein: A multipurpose isoflavone. Int J Green Pharm 2009; 3(3): 176-83.
[http://dx.doi.org/10.4103/0973-8258.56270]

[88] https://go.drugbank.com/drugs/DB01645

[89] Spagnuolo C, Russo GL, Orhan IE, *et al.* Genistein and cancer: current status, challenges, and future directions. Adv Nutr 2015; 6(4): 408-19.
[http://dx.doi.org/10.3945/an.114.008052] [PMID: 26178025]

[90] Banerjee S, Li Y, Wang Z, Sarkar FH. Multi-targeted therapy of cancer by genistein. Cancer Lett 2008; 269(2): 226-42.
[http://dx.doi.org/10.1016/j.canlet.2008.03.052] [PMID: 18492603]

[91] Davis JN, Singh B, Bhuiyan M, Sarkar FH. Genistein-induced upregulation of p21 WAF1, downregulation of cyclin B, and induction of apoptosis in prostate cancer cells. Nutr Cancer 1998; 4(1): 12-8.

[92] Chodon D, Banu SM, Padmavathi R, Sakthisekaran D. Inhibition of cell proliferation and induction of apoptosis by genistein in experimental hepatocellular carcinoma. Mol Cell Biochem 2007; 297(1-2): 73-80.
[http://dx.doi.org/10.1007/s11010-006-9324-2] [PMID: 17006617]

[93] Lazarevic B, Boezelijn G, Diep LM, *et al.* Efficacy and safety of short-term genistein intervention in patients with localized prostate cancer prior to radical prostatectomy: a randomized, placebo-controlled, double-blind Phase 2 clinical trial. Nutr Cancer 2011; 63(6): 889-98.
[http://dx.doi.org/10.1080/01635581.2011.582221] [PMID: 21714686]

[94] Pintova S, Dharmupari S, Moshier E, Zubizarreta N, Ang C, Holcombe RF. Genistein combined with FOLFOX or FOLFOX–Bevacizumab for the treatment of metastatic colorectal cancer: phase I/II pilot study. Cancer Chemother Pharmacol 2019; 84(3): 591-8.
[http://dx.doi.org/10.1007/s00280-019-03886-3] [PMID: 31203390]

[95] Hordyjewska A, Ostapiuk A, Horecka A, Kurzepa J. Betulin and betulinic acid: triterpenoids derivatives with a powerful biological potential. Phytochem Rev 2019; 18(3): 929-51.
[http://dx.doi.org/10.1007/s11101-019-09623-1]

[96] Amiri S, Dastghaib S, Ahmadi M, *et al.* Betulin and its derivatives as novel compounds with different pharmacological effects. Biotechnol Adv 2020; 38: 107409.
[http://dx.doi.org/10.1016/j.biotechadv.2019.06.008] [PMID: 31220568]

[97] Xu T, Pang Q, Wang Y, Yan X. Betulinic acid induces apoptosis by regulating PI3K/Akt signaling and mitochondrial pathways in human cervical cancer cells. Int J Mol Med 2017; 40(6): 1669-78.
[http://dx.doi.org/10.3892/ijmm.2017.3163] [PMID: 29039440]

[98] Fu L, Zhang S, Li N, *et al.* Three new triterpenes from Nerium oleander and biological activity of the isolated compounds. J Nat Prod 2005; 68(2): 198-206.
[http://dx.doi.org/10.1021/np040072u] [PMID: 15730243]

[99] Rabi T, Shukla S, Gupta S. Betulinic Acid Suppresses Constitutive and TNFα-induced NF-κB Activation and Induces Apoptosis in Human Prostate Carcinoma PC-3 Cells. Mol Carcinog 2008; 47(12): 964–973.

[100] Damle AA, Pawar YP, Narkar AA. Anticancer activity of betulinic acid on MCF-7 tumors in nude mice. Indian J Exp Biol 2013; 51(7): 485-91.
[PMID: 23898546]

[101] Rajendran P, Jaggi M, Singh MK, Mukherjee R, Burman AC. Pharmacological evaluation of C-3 modified Betulinic acid derivatives with potent anticancer activity. Invest New Drugs 2008; 26(1): 25-34.
[http://dx.doi.org/10.1007/s10637-007-9081-4] [PMID: 17851638]

[102] Dehelean CA, Feflea S, Ganta S, Amiji M. Anti-angiogenic effects of betulinic acid administered in nanoemulsion formulation using chorioallantoic membrane assay. J Biomed Nanotechnol 2011; 7(2): 317-24.
[http://dx.doi.org/10.1166/jbn.2011.1297] [PMID: 21702370]

[103] Mullauer FB, van Bloois L, Daalhuisen JB, *et al.* Betulinic acid delivered in liposomes reduces growth of human lung and colon cancers in mice without causing systemic toxicity. Anticancer Drugs 2011; 22(3): 223-33.
[http://dx.doi.org/10.1097/CAD.0b013e3283421035] [PMID: 21263311]

[104] Liu Y, Gao D, Zhang X, *et al.* Antitumor drug effect of betulinic acid mediated by polyethylene glycol modified liposomes. Mater Sci Eng C 2016; 64: 124-32.
[http://dx.doi.org/10.1016/j.msec.2016.03.080] [PMID: 27127036]

[105] da Silva TM, Pinheiro CD, Orlandi PP, Pinheiro CC, Pontes GS. Zerumbone from Zingiber zerumbet (L.) smith: a potential prophylactic and therapeutic agent against the cariogenic bacterium Streptococcus mutans. BMC Complement Altern Med 2018; 18(1): 1-9.
[PMID: 29295712]

[106] Girisa S, Shabnam B, Monisha J, *et al.* Potential of zerumbone as an anti-cancer agent. Molecules 2019; 24(4): 734.
[http://dx.doi.org/10.3390/molecules24040734] [PMID: 30781671]

[107] Sharifah Sakinah SA, Tri Handayani S, Azimahtol Hawariah LP. Zerumbone induced apoptosis in liver cancer cells *via* modulation of Bax/Bcl-2 ratio. Cancer Cell Int 2007; 7(1): 4.
[http://dx.doi.org/10.1186/1475-2867-7-4] [PMID: 17407577]

[108] Sehrawat A, Arlotti JA, Murakami A, Singh SV. Zerumbone causes Bax- and Bak-mediated apoptosis in human breast cancer cells and inhibits orthotopic xenograft growth *in vivo*. Breast Cancer Res Treat 2012; 136(2): 429-41.
[http://dx.doi.org/10.1007/s10549-012-2280-5] [PMID: 23053663]

[109] Kesharwani SS, Bhat GJ. Formulation and Nanotechnology-Based Approaches for Solubility and Bioavailability Enhancement of Zerumbone. Medicina (Kaunas) 2020; 56(11): 557.
[http://dx.doi.org/10.3390/medicina56110557] [PMID: 33114101]

[110] Hahn FE, Ciak J. Berberine. In Mechanism of Action of Antimicrobial and Antitumor Agents. Antibiot 1975.III 1975, 577-584.

[111] Imanshahidi M, Hosseinzadeh H. Pharmacological and therapeutic effects of Berberis vulgaris and its active constituent, berberine. Phytother Res 2008; 22(8): 999-1012.
[http://dx.doi.org/10.1002/ptr.2399] [PMID: 18618524]

[112] Vuddanda PR, Chakraborty S, Singh S. Berberine: a potential phytochemical with multispectrum therapeutic activities. Expert Opin Investig Drugs 2010; 19(10): 1297-307.
[http://dx.doi.org/10.1517/13543784.2010.517745] [PMID: 20836620]

[113] Guamán Ortiz L, Lombardi P, Tillhon M, Scovassi A. Berberine, an epiphany against cancer. Molecules 2014; 19(8): 12349-67.
[http://dx.doi.org/10.3390/molecules190812349] [PMID: 25153862]

[114] Wang J, Yang S, Cai X, *et al.* Berberine inhibits EGFR signaling and enhances the antitumor effects of EGFR inhibitors in gastric cancer. Oncotarget 2016; 7(46): 76076-86.
[http://dx.doi.org/10.18632/oncotarget.12589] [PMID: 27738318]

[115] Wang Y, Liu Y, Du X, Ma H, Yao J. Berberine reverses doxorubicin resistance by inhibiting autophagy through the PTEN/Akt/mTOR signaling pathway in breast cancer. OncoTargets Ther 2020; 13: 1909-19.
[http://dx.doi.org/10.2147/OTT.S241632] [PMID: 32184626]

[116] Katiyar SK, Meeran SM, Katiyar N, Akhtar S. p53 cooperates berberine-induced growth inhibition and apoptosis of non-small cell human lung cancer cells *in vitro* and tumor xenograft growth *in vivo*. Mol Carcinog 2009; 48(1): 24-37.
[http://dx.doi.org/10.1002/mc.20453] [PMID: 18459128]

[117] Zou K, Li Z, Zhang Y, *et al.* Advances in the study of berberine and its derivatives: a focus on anti-inflammatory and anti-tumor effects in the digestive system. Acta Pharmacol Sin 2017; 38(2): 157-67.
[http://dx.doi.org/10.1038/aps.2016.125] [PMID: 27917872]

[118] Chitlange S. Bioavailability of berberine: challenges and solutions. *İstanbul*. J Pharm (Cairo) 2021; 51(1): 141-53.

[119] Azadi R, Musavi SE, Motekef N, Rezayat SM, Jafari M. Preparation and Characterization of Berberine loaded Micelle Formulations with Approach to Oral Drug Delivery. Trends Pharmacol Sci 2020; 6(4): 255-62.

[120] Xue M, Yang M, Zhang W, *et al.* Characterization, pharmacokinetics, and hypoglycemic effect of berberine loaded solid lipid nanoparticles. Int J Nanomedicine 2013; 8: 4677-87. [http://dx.doi.org/10.2147/IJN.S51262] [PMID: 24353417]

[121] Bartosikova L, Necas J. Epigallocatechin gallate: a review. Vet Med (Praha) 2018; 63(10): 443-67. [http://dx.doi.org/10.17221/31/2018-VETMED]

[122] Xu YQ, Gao Y, Granato D. Effects of epigallocatechin gallate, epigallocatechin and epicatechin gallate on the chemical and cell-based antioxidant activity, sensory properties, and cytotoxicity of a catechin-free model beverage. Food Chem 2021; 339: 128060. [http://dx.doi.org/10.1016/j.foodchem.2020.128060] [PMID: 32950901]

[123] Muraoka K, Shimizu K, Sun X, *et al.* Flavonoids exert diverse inhibitory effects on the activation of nf-κb. Transplant Proc 2002; 34(4): 1335-40. [http://dx.doi.org/10.1016/S0041-1345(02)02795-1] [PMID: 12072354]

[124] Hong MH, Kim MH, Chang HJ, *et al.* (−)-Epigallocatechin-3-gallate inhibits monocyte chemotactic protein-1 expression in endothelial cells *via* blocking NF-κB signaling. Life Sci 2007; 80(21): 1957-65. [http://dx.doi.org/10.1016/j.lfs.2007.02.024] [PMID: 17379255]

[125] La X, Zhang L, Li Z, Li H, Yang Y. (−)-Epigallocatechin Gallate (EGCG) enhances the sensitivity of colorectal cancer cells to 5-FU by inhibiting GRP78/NF-κB/miR-155-5p/MDR1 pathway. J Agric Food Chem 2019; 67(9): 2510-8. [http://dx.doi.org/10.1021/acs.jafc.8b06665] [PMID: 30741544]

[126] Moses MA, Henry EC, Ricke WA, Gasiewicz TA. The heat shock protein 90 inhibitor, (---epigallocatechin gallate, has anticancer activity in a novel human prostate cancer progression model. Cancer Prev Res (Phila) 2015; 8(3): 249-57. [http://dx.doi.org/10.1158/1940-6207.CAPR-14-0224] [PMID: 25604133]

[127] Mazyed EA, Helal DA, Elkhoudary MM, Abd Elhameed AG, Yasser M. Formulation and Optimization of Nanospanlastics for Improving the Bioavailability of Green Tea Epigallocatechin Gallate. Pharmaceuticals (Basel) 2021; 14(1): 68. [http://dx.doi.org/10.3390/ph14010068] [PMID: 33467631]

[128] Kim HS, Quon MJ, Kim JA. New insights into the mechanisms of polyphenols beyond antioxidant properties; lessons from the green tea polyphenol, epigallocatechin 3-gallate. Redox boil. 2014; 2: 187-95.

[129] Andreu Fernández V, Almeida Toledano L, Pizarro Lozano N, *et al.* Bioavailability of epigallocatechin gallate administered with different nutritional strategies in healthy volunteers. Antioxidants 2020; 9(5): 440. [http://dx.doi.org/10.3390/antiox9050440] [PMID: 32438698]

[130] Manikandan R, Beulaja M, Arulvasu C, *et al.* Synergistic anticancer activity of curcumin and catechin: An *in vitro* study using human cancer cell lines. Microsc Res Tech 2012; 75(2): 112-6. [http://dx.doi.org/10.1002/jemt.21032] [PMID: 21780253]

[131] Granja A, Pinheiro M, Reis S. Epigallocatechin gallate nanodelivery systems for cancer therapy. Nutrients 2016; 8(5): 307. [http://dx.doi.org/10.3390/nu8050307] [PMID: 27213442]

[132] Roberts MF. Alkaloids: biochemistry, ecology, and medicinal applications. Spr Sci Busin Media 2013; 2(1): 1-45.

[133] Jin T, Wu H, Wang Y, Peng H. Capsaicin induces immunogenic cell death in human osteosarcoma cells. Exp Ther Med 2016; 12(2): 765-70. [http://dx.doi.org/10.3892/etm.2016.3368] [PMID: 27446273]

[134] Ghosh AK, Basu S. Tumor macrophages as a target for Capsaicin mediated immunotherapy. Cancer Lett 2012; 324(1): 91-7.

[http://dx.doi.org/10.1016/j.canlet.2012.05.002] [PMID: 22579786]

[135] Kunjiappan S, Sankaranarayanan M, Karan Kumar B, *et al.* Capsaicin-loaded solid lipid nanoparticles: design, biodistribution, *in silico* modeling and *in vitro* cytotoxicity evaluation. Nanotechnology 2021; 32(9): 095101.
[http://dx.doi.org/10.1088/1361-6528/abc57e] [PMID: 33113518]

[136] Xu T, Kuang T, Du H, *et al.* Magnoflorine: A review of its pharmacology, pharmacokinetics and toxicity. Pharmacol Res 2020; 152: 104632.
[http://dx.doi.org/10.1016/j.phrs.2020.104632] [PMID: 31911246]

[137] Mohamed SM, Hassan EM, Ibrahim NA. Cytotoxic and antiviral activities of aporphine alkaloids of *Magnolia grandiflora* L. Nat Prod Res 2010; 24(15): 1395-402.
[http://dx.doi.org/10.1080/14786410902906959] [PMID: 19764006]

[138] Okon E, Luszczki JJ, Kukula-Koch W, *et al.* Synergistic or additive pharmacological interactions between magnoflorine and cisplatin in human cancer cells of different histological origin. Int J Mol Sci 2020; 21(8): 2848.
[http://dx.doi.org/10.3390/ijms21082848] [PMID: 32325867]

[139] Mao QQ, Xu XY, Cao SY, *et al.* Bioactive compounds and bioactivities of ginger (Zingiber officinale Roscoe). Foods 2019; 8(6): 185.
[http://dx.doi.org/10.3390/foods8060185] [PMID: 31151279]

[140] Xu S, Zhang H, Liu T, *et al.* 6□Gingerol suppresses tumor cell metastasis by increasing YAP ^{ser127} phosphorylation in renal cell carcinoma. J Biochem Mol Toxicol 2021; 35(1): e22609.
[http://dx.doi.org/10.1002/jbt.22609] [PMID: 32926756]

[141] Kim EC, Min JK, Kim TY, *et al.* [6]-Gingerol, a pungent ingredient of ginger, inhibits angiogenesis *in vitro* and *in vivo*. Biochem Biophys Res Commun 2005; 335(2): 300-8.
[http://dx.doi.org/10.1016/j.bbrc.2005.07.076] [PMID: 16081047]

[142] Goldberg I, Rokem JS. Organic and fatty acid production. Encyclopedia of microbiology. 2009; 3: 441-2.

[143] Kang DY, Sp N, Jo ES, *et al.* The inhibitory mechanisms of tumor PD-L1 expression by natural bioactive gallic acid in non-small-cell lung cancer (NSCLC) cells. Cancers (Basel) 2020; 12(3): 727.
[http://dx.doi.org/10.3390/cancers12030727] [PMID: 32204508]

[144] Muthukumaran S, Tranchant C, Shi J, Ye X, Xue SJ. Ellagic acid in strawberry (Fragaria spp.): Biological, technological, stability, and human health aspects. Food Quality and Safety 2017; 1(4): 227-52.
[http://dx.doi.org/10.1093/fqsafe/fyx023]

[145] Ri MH, Ma J, Jin X. Development of natural products for anti-PD-1/PD-L1 immunotherapy against cancer. J Ethnopharmacol 2021; 281(1): 114370.
[http://dx.doi.org/10.1016/j.jep.2021.114370] [PMID: 34214644]

[146] Panche AN, Diwan AD, Chandra SR. Flavonoids: an overview. J Nutr Sci 2016; 5: e47.
[http://dx.doi.org/10.1017/jns.2016.41] [PMID: 28620474]

[147] Falcone Ferreyra ML, Rius SP, Casati P. Flavonoids: biosynthesis, biological functions, and biotechnological applications. Front Plant Sci 2012; 3: 222.
[http://dx.doi.org/10.3389/fpls.2012.00222] [PMID: 23060891]

[148] Kanazawa M, Satomi Y, Mizutani Y, *et al.* Isoliquiritigenin inhibits the growth of prostate cancer. Eur Urol 2003; 43(5): 580-6.
[http://dx.doi.org/10.1016/S0302-2838(03)00090-3] [PMID: 12706007]

[149] Raza W, Luqman S, Meena A. Prospects of tangeretin as a modulator of cancer targets/pathways. Pharmacol Res 2020; 161(2): 105202.
[http://dx.doi.org/10.1016/j.phrs.2020.105202] [PMID: 32942013]

[150] Yan X, Qi M, Li P, Zhan Y, Shao H. Apigenin in cancer therapy: anti-cancer effects and mechanisms of action. Cell Biosci 2017; 7(1): 50.
[http://dx.doi.org/10.1186/s13578-017-0179-x] [PMID: 29034071]

[151] Chen AY, Chen YC. A review of the dietary flavonoid, kaempferol on human health and cancer chemoprevention. Food Chem 2013; 138(4): 2099-107.
[http://dx.doi.org/10.1016/j.foodchem.2012.11.139] [PMID: 23497863]

[152] Al-Dhabi NA, Arasu MV, Park CH, Park SU. An up-to-date review of rutin and its biological and pharmacological activities. EXCLI J 2015; 14: 59-63.
[PMID: 26535031]

[153] Perk AA, Shatynska-Mytsyk I, Gerçek YC, *et al.* Rutin mediated targeting of signaling machinery in cancer cells. Cancer Cell Int 2014; 14(1): 124.
[http://dx.doi.org/10.1186/s12935-014-0124-6] [PMID: 25493075]

[154] Dev S. Terpenoids Natural products of woody plants 1989; 691-807.

[155] Ossama M, Hathout RM, Attia DA, Mortada ND. Enhanced allicin cytotoxicity on HEPG-2 cells using glycyrrhetinic acid surface-decorated gelatin nanoparticles. ACS Omega 2019; 4(6): 11293-300.
[http://dx.doi.org/10.1021/acsomega.9b01580] [PMID: 31460232]

[156] Jayasooriya RGPT, Dilshara MG, Park SR, *et al.* 18β-Glycyrrhetinic acid suppresses TNF-α induced matrix metalloproteinase-9 and vascular endothelial growth factor by suppressing the Akt-dependent NF-κB pathway. Toxicol. *in vitro* 2014; 28(5): 751-8.
[http://dx.doi.org/10.1016/j.tiv.2014.02.015] [PMID: 24613819]

[157] Ullah N, Khan A, Khan FA, *et al.* Composition and isolation of beta carotene from different vegetables and their effect on human serum retinal level. Middle East J Sci Res 2011; 9(4): 496-502.

[158] Williams AW, Boileau TWM, Zhou JR, Clinton SK, Erdman JW Jr. β-carotene modulates human prostate cancer cell growth and may undergo intracellular metabolism to retinol. J Nutr 2000; 130(4): 728-32.
[http://dx.doi.org/10.1093/jn/130.4.728] [PMID: 10736321]

[159] Caseiro M, Ascenso A, Costa A, Creagh-Flynn J, Johnson M, Simões S. Lycopene in human health. Lebensm Wiss Technol 2020; 127: 109323.
[http://dx.doi.org/10.1016/j.lwt.2020.109323]

[160] Tang FY, Shih CJ, Cheng LH, Ho HJ, Chen HJ. Lycopene inhibits growth of human colon cancer cells *via* suppression of the Akt signaling pathway. Mol Nutr Food Res 2008; 52(6): 646-54.
[http://dx.doi.org/10.1002/mnfr.200700272] [PMID: 18537129]

[161] Ambati R, Phang SM, Ravi S, Aswathanarayana R. Astaxanthin: sources, extraction, stability, biological activities and its commercial applications--a review. Mar Drugs 2014; 12(1): 128-52.
[http://dx.doi.org/10.3390/md12010128] [PMID: 24402174]

[162] Demir S, Demir EA, Aliyaziciglu Y. Selective Cytotoxic Effect of Astaxanthin on Human Lung and Colon Cancer Cells. J Agric Nat 2020; 23(6): 1489-94.

CHAPTER 8

Natural Immunomodulators for Infections and Other Diseases

Aaliya Liyakath Ali[1], **Namrata Nailwal**[1], **Sujata Sawarkar**[2] and **Gaurav Doshi**[1,*]

[1] *Department of Pharmacology, SVKM'S Dr. Bhanuben Nanavati College of Pharmacy, Mithibai Campus, Vile Parle (W), Mumbai-400056, India*

[2] *Department of Pharmaceutics, SVKM'S Dr. Bhanuben Nanavati College of Pharmacy, Mithibai Campus, Vile Parle (W), Mumbai-400056, India*

Abstract: Infection is one of the most common occurring issues in an individual. Diseases caused by infections hamper the immune system of an individual. To modulate the immune system, immunomodulatory drugs work by either stimulating or suppressing the immune system. Several drugs like levamisole and azathioprine are available in the market today to overcome various infections. But an alternative is required to overcome the drug resistance and other side effects associated with these available drugs. To tackle these problems, many plant-based immunomodulators are being explored and have proven to be beneficial against these infections. This chapter focuses on the mechanism of action and application of natural immunomodulators like Curcumin, Resveratrol, and Genistein on various infections. The primary goal of this chapter is to understand the role of natural immunomodulators in the body for various infections and related disease conditions. With the help of findings, one can conclude that all-natural immunomodulators have areas that need attention, including their therapeutic risk-benefit ratio and their target binding affinity for various infections. However, further investigations into these drugs are necessary for a clear understanding to maximize their clinical applications

Keywords: Natural Immunomodulators, Antimicrobial, Antibacterial, Antiviral, Antiparasitic, Ayurveda, Curcumin, Genistein, Immunosuppressants, Immunostimulants, Infection, Resveratrol.

INTRODUCTION

An immune response is the ability of the human body to be shielded, protecting itself against various harmful agents [1]. Immunomodulators are drugs that modify the response of the immune system either by stimulating or suppressing

* **Corresponding author Gaurav Doshi:** Department of Pharmacology, SVKM'S Dr. Bhanuben Nanavati College of Pharmacy, Mithibai Campus, Vile Parle (W), Mumbai-400056, India; E-mail: gaurav.pharmacology@gmail.com

Vandana S. Nikam, Sujata P. Sawarkar, Girish B. Mahajan and Supriya G. Jagtap (Eds.)

the release and production of antibodies in human serum. They are used to restore the level of the immune response [2]. A well-balanced immune system enhances defence mechanisms against various infections, hypersensitivity reactions, and autoimmune diseases. Immunomodulators are used in treating chronic infections, cancer, and organ transplantation [3]. There is a rise in the emergence of novel immunomodulators as the understanding of autoimmune diseases increases globally [4, 5]. Immunostimulants act by showing prophylactic action in normal individuals by activating the primary immune responses [6]. These agents are used in the treatment of inflammation and cancer by enhancing the body's defence mechanism. T and B lymphocytes act as primary targets for immune-stimulating agents. Immunostimulants act by affecting cytokines and specifically inhibiting or enhancing populations of immune cells like lymphocytes, neutrophils, macrophages, NK cells, and cytotoxic T lymphocytes [7].

Immunosuppression mainly decreases the body's resistance to fight against infections [8]. These agents have been clinically used to treat graft rejections and autoimmune diseases and hence are termed antirejection agents [9]. They are the most widely used drug in the treatment of inflammatory bowel disease (IBD) like Crohn's disease [3]. Drugs such as prasterone and hydroxychloroquine are immunomodulators, used to manage immunological conditions like rheumatoid arthritis and systemic lupus erythematosus [10]. The present immunomodulant therapy consists of drugs that have a specific mode of action and give rise to various side effects. Some of the side effects caused by these immunomodulators are pulmonary toxicity, myelosuppression, and hypertension [11]. These adverse effects can often lead to being the cause of death in immunocompromised patients [12]. Cyclosporine is an immunosuppressant that causes adverse effects like hyperkalemia, convulsion and hepatitis when given orally or intravenously. It is not recommended during pregnancy. Other alternatives like tacrolimus and mycophenolate are used instead of cyclosporine, however, they increase the risk of diabetes [13 - 15]. Immunomodulators also manifest oral adverse effects like Sjogren's syndrome and oral lichen planus [16 - 18]. Immunostimulants are a class of immunomodulators that enhance body's resistance against infections, while immunosuppressants are agents that inhibit or suppress the active immune system. Natural immunomodulators have the potential to fight off infections caused by microorganisms like bacteria, viruses, and fungi.

INFECTIOUS DISEASES

Infection is a bodily condition produced by the introduction of one or multiple pathogens like bacteria, fungi, and viruses. The severity of infection can range from mild to severe and sometimes may be fatal. There are four major agents responsible for infections: Bacteria, fungi, viruses, and parasites, as depicted in Table **1**.

Table 1. Various infectious agents and diseases caused by them.

Sr. No.	Type of Infective Agent	Name	Disease	Reference
1	Bacteria	*Bacillus anthracis*	Anthrax	[19]
2	Bacteria	*Mycobacterium tuberculosis*	Tuberculosis	[20]
3	Bacteria	*Vibrio cholerae*	Cholera	[21]
4	Fungi	*Pneumocystis*	Pneumonia	[22]
5	Fungi	*Candida species*	Mucocutaneous infections	[23]
6	Virus	*Human immunodeficiency virus*	Acquired Immuno Deficiency Syndrome (AIDS)	[24]
7	Virus	*Severe acute respiratory syndrome coronavirus 2 (SARS-CoV-2) virus*	Covid-19	[25]
8	Virus	*Poliovirus*	Poliomyelitis	[26]
9	Virus	*Hepatitis virus*	Hepatitis	[27]
10	Parasite	*Plasmodium species*	Malaria	[28]
12	Parasite	*Wuchereria bancrofti*	Filariasis	[29]

Antibiotics are active drugs that are used to treat various infections. Antibiotics either destroy or prevent the multiplication of microbes, which allows the immune system to clear infections. Antibiotic resistance, these days, is limiting the efficacy of many of these drugs. Using an antibiotic is advised even after no more symptoms are seen to heal the infection and prevent the growth of resistant microbes. Antibiotic development presently focuses on targets that are critical for bacterial metabolism; however, studies into how bacterial species communicate with one another could lead to the creation of newer medications that reduce resistance. Antibiotics are not effective against infectious diseases caused by viruses like influenza; instead, antiviral drugs are used for viral infections. These drugs elicit their therapeutic effect either by limiting or hampering the multiplication capacity of the virus or by increasing the immunological response of the body to the infection. Antiviral drugs are divided into various categories, each of these is used to treat different types of viral infections, including influenza, HIV, herpes, and hepatitis B. Viruses, similar to bacteria, evolve throughout time and become resistant to antiviral medications [30]. Several studies have looked at the current state of immunomodulatory techniques for infection prevention in neonatal immunological deficiencies and recent breakthroughs in the developing field of immunotherapies to increase immune functions and antimicrobial defences in neonates [31]. The innate immune system, formerly thought to be primitive, is now being revealed to be extremely sophisticated, controlled, and intricately linked with the acquired immune system and the neurological system. Understanding the exact regulatory mechanisms and active molecules of the innate immune system might lead to discovery of medicines that are effective against a wider range of fatal pathogens. Understanding how the natural microbiota communicates with the immune system of the body and how the immune system recognizes infections might lead to development of medicines that assist the natural microbiota in outcompete bacterial pathogens [32].

Due to the growing number of infections emerging each day, it has become burdensome to treat them with antibiotics as they have become less effective. New drug resistance mechanisms are emerging and spreading globally, leading to difficulty treating infections, causing longer stays in hospitals, and increasing medical costs and mortality rates. There is an important and urgent need to come up with an alternative to treat infectious diseases.

Natural immunomodulators can help treat these infections by various mechanisms. Natural immunomodulators like curcumin, piperine, quercetin, resveratrol, and artemisinin are plant-derived biochemicals that have the potential to modulate the human immune system [33]. Berberine and Piperine, belonging to the chemical class of alkaloids, have proven to down-regulate the production and release of interleukin-2 (IL-2), interleukin-4 (IL-4) and reduce the level of pro-inflammatory cytokines like interleukin-1β (IL-1β) and interleukin-6 (IL-6) [34, 35]. Switching to natural immunomodulators will resolve the problem of antimicrobial drug resistance and also result in lesser side effects, unlike synthetic immunomodulators [36].

This chapter focuses on the mechanism of action and applications of natural immunomodulators in treating various infectious diseases. Indigenous medicines have seen an increase in clinical usage in the past few years, owing to their lack of significant adverse effects and higher efficacy. Furthermore, the continual rise in antibiotic-resistant bacteria, as well as several adverse effects induced by synthetic medicines, has motivated researchers to explore herbal immunomodulators to treat a variety of illnesses. Herbal medicines are believed to boost the natural resistance of the body to combat infection, and their immunomodulatory properties have been documented in a variety of plants [37]. Immunomodulatory action has been reported for a variety of Indian medicinal herbs and different 'Rasayanas'. The Rasayana category of medicines is said to enhance health, immunity, and lifespan. According to Ayurveda, these Rasayanas strengthen all body tissues, reduce aging, improve intelligence, and prevent sickness [37 - 39]. Herbal medicines have long been a staple of pharmacological therapy, and they are now being explored for synergistic combinations.

Natural immunomodulators are broadly classified into two categories based on their mechanism of action, they are immunostimulants and immunosuppressants. They have the potential to generate an immune response or defend against infections. Immunomodulatory action of these natural immunomodulators occurs mainly *via* stimulation of phagocytotic pathways, activation of macrophages, and increment in the count of immunity mediators, total white cells and natural killer cells [33]. Naturally obtained compounds showing potential as an immunomodulator are briefly described further.

Curcumin

Curcumin contains a diarylheptanoid chemical structure found in *Curcuma longa* and its relatedrhizome species. Curcumin's medicinal properties have been recognized for ages. Curcumin has been shown to have anti-cancer, antioxidant, anti-angiogenic, anti-proliferative, and other biological and pharmacological effects. Curcumin is a chemical that has been researched widely for its immunomodulatory effects. Curcumin inhibited NO generation, cyclooxygenase-2 (COX-2), nuclear factor-kappa B (NFkB), inducible nitric oxide synthase (iNOS), and lipoxygenase in NK cells and TNFα-activated macrophages, reducing the inflammatory reactions [40, 41]. Curcumin reduced the production of pro-inflammatory cytokines TNF-α, IL-1, IL-6, and IL-12 in macrophages and dendritic cells [42, 43].

Antibacterial Activity

Studies show that curcumin exerts a potential antibacterial effect against both methicillin-sensitive *Staphylococcus aureus* (MSSA) and methicillin-resistant *Staphylococcus aureus* (MRSA) [44, 45]. When coupled with antibiotics like ampicillin, ciprofloxacin, norfloxacin, gentamicin, and amikacin, curcumin has a significant synergistic antibacterial action against *Staphylococcus aureus* [44]. Curcumin inhibits the development of highly pathogenic bacteria, such as *Enterococcus faecalis*, *Pseudomonas aeruginosa*, *Escherichia coli*, and *Klebsiella pneumonia* [45].

Antifungal Activity

[1,7-Bis(3,4,5- trimethoxy phenyl)-1,6-heptadiene-3,5-dione (L1) and 1,7-di(--anthracenyl)-1,6-heptadiene-3,5 dione was synthesised and evaluated for antifungal efficacy against *Aspergillus, penicillium*, and *Alternaria spp*. These two derivatives had a possible inhibitory impact on the development of the cultures examined, with L1 having a little advantage over the other derivative [46]. Curcumin, along with a significant inhibitory effect on *Candida albicans* [47], can also reduce *Candida albicans* resistance to fluconazole when used together [48].

Argyreia Speciosa

Argyreia speciosa is a species of Argyreia belonging to the family of Convolvulaceae. It is frequently utilized in Ayurveda, India's old traditional medical system, since it has a variety of therapeutic qualities. It is a woody climber that may be cultivated throughout India, including Assam, West Bengal, Bihar, Orissa, and South India [49]. The fatty oil extracted from the seeds of *Argyreia speciosa* was reported to contain palmitic, oleic, stearic, behenic, linoleic, and linolenic acid glycosides.N-triacontanol, sitosterol, p-hydroxycinnamoyl octadecanolate, and caffeic acid have been found in the fruits of *Argyreia speciosa* [50]. It has been observed that a 95 percent ethanolic extract of *A. speciosa* dried root can stimulate cellular and humoral immunity [51].

Antibacterial Activity

The leave's alcoholic extract had antibacterial action against *Staphylococcus aureus* but not against *Escherichia coli*. Both bacteria were unaffected by the aqueous extract [52]. *In vitro* antibacterial activity against *Klebsiella species*, *Escherichia coli*, *Pseudomonas aeruginosa*, *Bacillus anthracis*, *Salmonella typhi*, *Salmonella paratyphi*, *Shigella boydii*, *Shigella flexneri*, *Streptococcus haemolyticus*, and *Bacillus subtilis* was discovered in the seed oil [53].

Antifungal Activity

Aspergillus flavus, *Colletotrichum capsici*, *Cryptococcus neoformans*, *Alternaria solani*, *Helminthosporium sp.*, *Colletotrichum dematium*, *Aspergillus niger*, *A. sydowi*, and *Fusarium oxysporum* were all shown to have antifungal action in the seed oil. *Penicillium sp.* was discovered to be oil-resistant [53]. Antifungal activity of hexadecanyl p-hydroxycinnamate and scopoletin extracted from the root was evaluated against *Fusarium fusiformis*, *Fusarium semitectum*, and *Alternaria alternative* [54].

Antiviral Activity

In CAM (chorioallantoic membranes) cultures, the extract of the plant and fruits exhibited interferon-like antiviral activity against the vaccinia virus, but no action against Ranikhet sickness virus [55].

Antiparasitic Activity

The impact of aqueous and alcoholic extracts of *A. speciosa* leaves on the spontaneous movements of the adult worm and a nerve/muscle preparation of *Setariacervi*, a bovine filarial worm, as well as the survival of microfilariae *in vitro*, was investigated. The nerve/muscle preparation was completely paralyzed with the aqueous extract at a dosage of 25 g/ml, but the alcoholic extract needed only 50 ng/ml [56].

Mangifera Indica

For thousands of years, *Mangifera indica* (MI), commonly known as mango, has been an important plant in Ayurveda and other traditional medicinal systems. Mangoes are members of the genus Mangifera, which includes around 30 tropical fruiting trees in the Anacardiaceae flowering plant family. As a polyphenol antioxidant and glucosyl xanthone, mangiferin has potent antioxidant, anti-lipid peroxidation, immunomodulation, cardiotonic, hypotensive, wound healing, antidegenerative, and antidiabetic properties. It is native to tropical Asia and has grown for over 4000 years in the Indian subcontinent, which has now naturalized in most tropical nations. Roots, bark, leaves, fruits, seeds, flowers, and kernels are among the parts utilized for medicinal purposes.

Antiviral Activity

Mangiferin's effect on Herpes simplex virus type 2 (HSV-2) was investigated *in vitro*; mangiferin does not directly inactivate HSV-2, but it does suppress the late events in HSV-2 replication. *In vitro*, mangiferin inhibited HSV-1 viral multiplication in cells and counteracted the cytopathic effects of HIV [57 - 59].

Antiparasitic Activity

Mangiferin, at a dose level of 100 mg/kg, shows an equivalent inhibitory effect on *Cryptosporidium parvum* in a neonatal mouse model to the same dose (100 mg/kg) of paromomycin [60].

Antibacterial And Antifungal Activities

Mangiferin showed effectiveness against seven bacterial species, including *Bacillus pumilus*, *Bacillus cereus*, *Staphylococcus aureus*, *Staphylococcus citreus*, *Escherichia coli*, *Salmonella agona*, and *Klebsiella pneumoniae*, as well as one yeast (*Saccharomyces cerevisiae*) and four fungi, in an *in vitro* agar diffusion technique (*Thermoascus aurantiacus*, *Trichoderma reesei*, *Aspergillus flavus*, and *A. fumigatus*) [61].

Tinospora Sinensis

Tinospora sinensis, also known as Tinospora malabarica belongs to the Menispermaceae family of Menispermaceae and is found almost everywhere in India and Southeast Asia. This plant's stem has long been used to treat debility, dyspepsia, fever, inflammation, syphilis, ulcer, bronchial diseases, jaundice, urinary illness, skin diseases, and liver diseases [62], and it's also recognized for its adaptogenic and immunomodulatory characteristics. The anti-inflammatory, anti-diabetic, hepatoprotective, immunomodulatory, and adaptogenic properties of this species' aqueous and alcoholic extracts have been observed [63].

Antimicrobial Activity

Tinospora sinensis's ethanolic leaf extract exhibited antibacterial efficacy against *Candida albicans*, *Pseudomonas aeruginosa*, and *Aspergillus niger*. Antimicrobial activity of ethanolic stem and flower extract was found against the gram-positive bacterium *Staphylococcus aureus* and the fungus strain *Aspergillus niger*. The presence of alkaloids may account for the antibacterial action. Extracts, which include ethanolic, methanolic, and chloroform extracts, except aqueous extract, inhibited fungal growth as well as the development of gram-negative and gram-positive bacteria *in vitro* [64].

Antiviral Activity

Due to the presence of several bioactive chemicals such as alkaloids, diterpenoid lactones, glycosides, and steroids, *T. sinensis* is known to have immunomodulatory and immune-stimulating characteristics [65]. The crude extract contains anti-HIV potential and inhibits HIV reverse transcriptase activity, according to studies [66].

Trigonella Foenum-gracium

Trigonella foenum-graecum, belonging to the Fabaceae family, often known as fenugreek, has been used for its therapeutic qualities in Mediterranean and Asian civilizations for ages. Many traditional systems, including Ayurvedic medicine, utilize the seed and leaf of this plant to cure diabetes [67].

Antifungal Activity

The antifungal potential of aqueous extracts from various plant parts of fenugreek leaves and stems, roots, ground and non-ground seeds in petroleum ether, ethyl acetate, and methanol fractions of the aerial parts against fungal strains such as *Botrytis cinerea*, *Fusarium graminearum*, *Alternaria species*, *Pythium aphanidermatum*, and *Rhizoctonia solani* is established. The antifungal potential of the fenugreek plant was found in all sections of the plant, with the degree of the impact varying depending on the fungus species and plant parts. The antifungal activity of the methanol extract is the most potent, completely inhibiting the development of *R. solani* and *Alternaria species* [68].

Antibacterial Activity

Several studies have shown that Trigonella extracts are efficient against *Helicobacter pylori* [69 - 71]. One study which used honey samples with the best antibacterial activity against *Pseudomonas aeruginosa*, *Escherichia coli*, and *Staphylococcus aureus* revealed the highest levels of pollen from Trigonella, among other plants [72].

Antiparasitic Activity

The methanol soluble fraction of Trigonella extract has nematocidal activity and induced considerable mortality of *Meloidogyne javanica* larvae (>92%), indicating that it may be utilized to combat nematodes [73].

Platycodon Grandiflorum

In China, Japan, and Korea, *Platycodon grandiflorum* (PG) roots which belong to the Campanulaceae family, have long been used as herbal medicine and food to cure a variety of lung illnesses and respiratory problems [74]. Many chemical components have been discovered in PG, including saponins, polysaccharides, flavonoids, phenolic acids, fatty acids, and sterols. Furthermore, PG has anti-diabetic, anti-cancer, anti-inflammatory, immunomodulatory, and anti-allergic properties [75 - 80].

Antimicrobial Activity

The antimicrobial activities of PG extracts were investigated against bacteria that cause bronchitis (such as *Mycobacterium sp.*, *Staphylococcus aureus*, *Klebsiella pneumoniae*, *Corynebacterium diphtheriae*, and *Streptococcus pyogenes*) and bacteria that cause food poisoning (*i.e.*, *Escherichia coli* and *Bacillus cereus*) [81].

Antiviral Activity

PG root extract and/or PG saponin components were used to produce a pharmaceutical formulation. This medication proved effective as an antiviral drug in the treatment and prevention of hepatitis C. Because the components of this invention are non-toxic to humans and prevent the growth of the hepatitis C virus, it can be utilized as a hepatitis C preventative or therapeutic agent [82].

Resveratrol

Resveratrol which is chemically known as (5-[(E)-2-(4-hydroxyphenyl) ethenyl] benzene-1, 3-diol), is a derivative of stilbene and phytoalexin. It is abundantly found in dietary supplements and plant sources, including grapevines, red wine, and peanuts. Resveratrol was found to exert a variety of pharmacological activities such as antimicrobial, chemo preventive, anticancer, anti-inflammatory, and antioxidant properties. The inflammatory molecules are strongly inhibited by resveratrol. Resveratrol inhibits NF-β in PMA, LPS, or TNFα-mediated macrophages, and dendritic cells, among other immunomodulatory actions. Resveratrol reduced NF- β activation by blocking Iβ kinase [83 - 85]. The production of IL-12, IL-6, IL-1, TNF-α, and IFNα by splenic macrophages and lymphocytes, was also suppressed by resveratrol [86].

Antibacterial Activity

Resveratrol presented antibacterial activity against all tested Gram-positive bacteria like *Bacillus cereus*, *Staphylococcus aureus* MSSA *Staphylococcus aureus* MRSA *Staphylococcus aureus* and *Enterococcus faecalis*. It also shows antimicrobial activity against Gram-negative bacteria like *Escherichia coli*, *Klebsiella pneumonia,* and *Salmonella typhimurium* [87].

Antifungal Activity

Resveratrol has inhibitory action at a dose level of 25– 50 g/mL against the fungal dermatophytes *Trichophyton mentagrophytes*, *Trichophyton tonsurans*, *Trichophyton rubrum*, *Epidermophyton floccosum*, and *Microsporumgypseum* [88]. The inhibitory activity for *Candida albicans*, *Saccharomyces cerevisiae*, and *Trichosporonbeigelii* is 10–20 g/mL [89].

Antiparasitic Activity

Resveratrol showed strong antiparasitic activity against *Trypanosoma cruzi*, *Setariacervi*, and *Leishmania amazonensis* [90 - 92].

Antiviral Activity

Resveratrol has been demonstrated to have a strong antiviral potential in both human and animal viral infections. Blockage of viral protein synthesis, suppression of different transcription and signaling pathways, and inhibition of viral-associated gene expressions were shown to be the major antiviral strategies.

Resveratrol showed significant suppression in viral infections like the influenza virus, respiratory syncytial virus [93 - 97], varicella-zoster virus [98], Epstein-

Barr virus [99, 100], herpes simplex virus [101 - 104], human immunodeficiency virus [105, 106], African swine fever virus, enterovirus, human metapneumonia virus, and duck enteritis virus.

Epigallocatechin-3-Gallate

Epigallocatechin-3- gallate (EGCG), chemically [(2R,3R)-5,7-dihydroxy-2-(3,4, 5-trihydroxyphenyl)-3,4-dihydro-2H-chromen-3-yl]3,4,5-trihydroxybenzoate], is among the most active and abundantly present polyphenols in green tea *Camellia sinensis* from Theaceae family. Its chemo preventive, anti-angiogenic, anti-invasive, anti-proliferative, anti-inflammatory and anti-oxidant properties *in vitro* and *in vivo* have been widely described [107, 108].

Antibacterial Activity

Epicatechin gallate (ECG) and epigallocatechin gallate (EGCG) are two catechins that have very potent antibacterial properties and are more efficient against Gram-positive bacteria than Gram-negative bacteria [109]. These polyphenolic compounds have a broad antibacterial spectrum and inhibit various pathogenic bacteria like *Bacillus cereus*, *Campylobacter species.*, *Clostridium perfringens*, *Escherichia coli*, *Helicobacter pylori*, *Legionella pneumophila*, *Mycobacterium tuberculosis*, *Mycoplasma pneumonia*, *Proteus vulgaris*, *Pseudomonas aeruginosa*, *Salmonella spp.*, *Serratia marcescens*, *Staphylococcus species.*, oral pathogenic *Streptococci species* [110].

Antiviral Activity

EGCG inhibits adenovirus [111], bovine coronavirus, and bovine rotavirus [112]. EGCG also inhibited the expression of Epstein-Barr Virus lytic proteins [113]. Catechins also showed antiherpetic activity against HSV [114]. ECGC prevents infection by the influenza virus by binding to the viral hemagglutinin [115].

Antifungal Activity

EGCG exhibited variable time and concentration-dependent fungicidal activities against several fungi like *Candida Albicans* and Trichophyton [116].

Antiparasitic Activity

The most common flavonoid component of green tea, epigallocatechin 3-O-gallate (EGCG), has been shown to have an action against several Leishmania species, including visceral leishmaniasis species *L. Infantum* [117].

Genistein

Genistein, also known as 4,5,7-trihydroxyisoflavone, is a phytoestrogen found in soy and soy-derived products. It has been found that genistein has the potential for induction of apoptosis, and cell cycle arrest, as well as anti-angiogenic, antimetastatic, and anti-inflammatory effects. The tyrosine kinase inhibitor genistein is well-known. Soy, which originated in Asia, is a legume with grains that grow in pods. Only the berries are used in food, while other parts of the plant, especially the root, are used in industry and medicine. It contains important amino acids as well as proteins, lipids, carbohydrates, mineral salts, enzymes, lecithin, and vitamins A, B1, B2, C, D, and E, which account for about 40% of the total. Soybean crops, which were first planted in eastern China, have expanded fast across the world, owing to the excellent nutritious content of the grains [118].

Antibacterial Activity

Genistein reduced the growth of *S. Aureus* and *B. Anthracis in vitro* [19]. It inhibits the *in vitro* invasion of many bacterial species, including *Yersinia enterocolitica* [120], enteropathogenic *E.coli* [121], *Mycobacterium avium* [122], *S. aureus* [123, 124], *Listeria monocytogenes* [125], and *Fonsecaeapedrosi* [126].

Antiviral Activity

Genistein shows antiviral activity against several herpes viruses, including HSV-1, cytomegalovirus, and bovine herpesvirus-1, as well as non-herpesviruses, which include SV40, human papillomavirus, porcine reproductive and respiratory syndrome virus, African swine fever virus, and human immunodeficiency virus [127 - 135].

Antiparasitic Activity

In vitro treatment of cestodes and trematodes with genistein results in worm immobilization and flaccid paralysis in a dose-dependent manner, suggesting that genistein works predominantly on the flatworm's tegument, where it interacts with enzymes and produces permanent changes in structure [136].

Quercetin

The flavonol quercetin, whose chemical name is 2-(3,4-dihydroxyphenyl)-3,-,7-trihydroxychromen-4-one, belongs to the polyphenol family, which includes widely distributed secondary plant metabolites. Tea, capers, red onions, broccoli, berries, grapevines, and apples are just a few of the foods that contain quercetin. Anti-mutagenic, anti-oxidative, anti-inflammatory, anticancer, neuroprotective, antihypertensive, and blood glucose-lowering properties have been discovered in quercetin [137]. Quercetin scavenges nitrogen and reactive oxygen species (ROS), targets well-known pro-inflammatory signal transduction pathways like MAPK, NF-β, and STAT1, and suppresses viral multiplication as well as target cell infectivity [138].

Antibacterial Activity

Quercetin has shown significant bacteriostatic activity against *Salmonella enterica* serotype *Typhimurium*, *Pseudomonas aeruginosa*, *Pseudomonas fluorescens*, *Helicobacter pylori*, *Staphylococcus epidermidis*, *S. aureus*, *Yersinia enterocolitica*, *Micrococcus luteus*, *Campylobacter jejuni*, and *Escherichia coli* [139]. Derivatives of quercetin showed potent antibacterial activity with 100% inhibition of *Listeria monocytogenes*, *Pseudomonas aeruginosa*, and *Aeromonas hydrophila* [140].

Antifungal Activity

Quercetin showed the strongest antifungal activities against *Candida albicans*, *Cryptococcus neoformans*, and *Aspergillus niger* [141].

Antiparasitic Activity

Several studies show that quercetin can inhibit the growth of many protozoan parasites, including Toxoplasma, Babesia, Theileria, Trypanosoma, and Leishmania. In *in vitro* and *in vivo*, quercetin has been shown to suppress the growth of *Trypanosoma brucei rhodesiense*, *T. brucei*, *Trypanosoma cruzi*, and *Leishmania donovani* parasites [142].

Antiviral Activity

The effectiveness of quercetin against the human T-lymphotropic virus 1 (HTLV-1) and the Japanese encephalitis virus (JEV) produced by Japanese encephalitis, a mosquito-borne illness, has been established [143, 144]. By inhibiting the action of the nonstructural protein 3 protease, quercetin has been shown to inhibit the dengue virus type 2 and the hepatitis C virus [145, 146].

Colchicine

Colchicine, a tropolone derivative (N-[(7S)-1,2, 3,10-tetramethoxy-9-oxo-6,7-dihydro-5H-benzo(a)heptalen-7] -ylacetamide), is the primary alkaloid of *Colchicum autumnale* (family: Colchicaceae), often known as autumn crocus. For ages, preparations from this plant have been used to treat gout problems. Colchicine has been recognized by the US Food and Drug Administration for the management and cure of familial Mediterranean fever and acute gout flares [147].

Antibacterial Activity

Colchicine has some antibacterial action on *S. aureus*, *G. tetragenus*, *B. subtilis*, *M. phlei*, *C. hofmanni*, *S. typhi*, *S. Paratyphi*, *S. flexneri*, *E.coli*, *V. cholera*, and *K. Pneumonia* [148].

Antiviral Activity

Colchicine has been shown to inhibit virus replication in viruses such as dengue and Zika viruses by inhibiting microtubule polymerization [149]; blocks transport and reduces replication of the recombinant demyelinating strain of the mouse hepatitis virus, and inhibits respiratory syncytial virus (RSV) infection in neonatal rats by regulating antioxidative enzymes [150]. Furthermore, colchicine and colchicine derivatives have been shown to affect HIV viral load [151].

Capsaicin

Capsaicin (E)-N-[(4-hydroxy-3-methoxyphenyl) methyl]-8-methylnon-6-enamide, has been used as a counter-irritant and topical rubefacient in traditional medicine to treat joint and muscular discomfort. It was discovered that capsaicin inhibited the NF-β pathway, iNOS production, and COX-2 activity in macrophages in a TRPV1-independent manner [152].

Antibacterial Activity

Capsaicin and its derivatives have been found to have both direct and indirect antibacterial actions, depending on a variety of parameters, including bacterial species and strains. A capsaicin derivative was discovered to be an efficient *E. coli* inhibitor [153]. Capsaicin only mildly inhibited the development of several strains of *C. violaceum*, *S. marcescens*, and *P. aeruginosa* [154]. Only four of the Gram-positive bacterial strains studied exhibited considerable sensitivity to capsaicin or its derivatives: *S. aureus*, *B. subtilis*, *S. mutans*, and *P. Larva* [155 - 157].

Andrographolide

Andrographolide is a diterpenoid lactone discovered in *Andrographis paniculate*. Andrographolide has been shown to have a wide range of biological actions. *In vitro*, andrographolide has been shown to exhibit several immunomodulatory effects, including the decrease of IL-12, TNF-α, PGE2, NO, COX-2, and iNOS in microglia and macrophages. Andrographolide inhibited the generation of NK cells, IFN-α, IL-2, and TNF-α, among other factors [158].

Antibacterial Activity

Andrographolide was found to be a quorum-sensing inhibitor of *Pseudomonas aeruginosa*. Antimicrobial activity was found against *Bacillus subtilis*, *Staphylococcus aureus*, *Escherichia coli*, *Pseudomonas aeruginosa*, and *Candida albicans* using a synergistic combination of andrographolide and arabinogalactan proteins [159].

Antiviral Activity

A derivative of andrographolide inhibited the herpes simplex virus type 1 (HSV-1) infection at the post-entry step [160].

Antiparasitic Activity

In vitro, andrographolide combined with curcumin has antiplasmodial action against *Plasmodium falciparum* erythrocytic stages and *Plasmodium berghei* erythrocytic stages [161 - 163]. Based on the results of docking studies, andrographolide may be a protease inhibitor against malaria parasites [164].

Tripterugium Wilfordii

Tripterygium wilfordii Hook F (TwHF) is a wood vine plant that is widely used in traditional Chinese medicine in southern China. TwHF has been used to treat rheumatoid arthritis, Systemic lupus erythematosus, nephritis, autoimmune disorders, and allergic Skin diseases because of its immunoregulatory, anti-inflammatory, anti-tumor, anti-fertility, antibacterial, and other pharmacological characteristics [165 - 167]. TwHF's primary active components are tripodine, triptonide, triptolide (TPT), and tripdiolide (TPO).

Antibacterial Activity

Ethanolic extract of *Tripterygium wilfordii* showed effective antimicrobial activity against *Staphylococcus aureus*, methicillin-resistant *Staphylococcus aureus (MRSA),* and *Candida albicans* [168].

Acorus Calamus

Acorus calamus belonging to the Araceae family is also known as sweet flag or calamus. It is a semiaquatic, perennial, aromatic herb with creeping rhizomes. The plant is found in the northern temperate and subtropical regions of Asia, North America, and Europe. Neurological conditions and respiratory conditions like asthma, fever, cough, epilepsy, depression, bronchitis, sedative, and circulatory disorders have all been treated with the plant. Rheumatism, fever, and swollen joints are treated with rhizome paste. Rhizome has a strong effect on the central nervous system, improving grasping capacity, memory, cognition, and speaking, as well as correcting emotional, mood, and personality disorders. The Rhizome also has aphrodisiac properties and is used as an aphrodisiac [169].

Antibacterial Activity

Acorus calamus L. has a wide range of biological activity, including antibacterial properties. The ethanol extract of *A. calamus* L. rhizome has been shown to have antibacterial action against *E. coli*, *Staphylococcus aureus*, and *Candida albicans* [170]. The ethanol and methanol extracts of the Rhizome of the *Acorus Calamus* can inhibit *E. coli*, *S. epidermidis*, and *S. aureus* from proliferating. It was discovered that the ethanol extract of *A. calamus* contains phenylpropanoids, monoterpenes, sesquiterpenes, and asarone, which exhibit antimicrobial activity [171]. Essential oils isolated from *A. calamus* rhizome potentially inhibited the growth of *S. aureus* and *E. coli* and *Candida albicans* [172].

Antifungal Activity

A. calamus L. also shows antifungal activity against *Fusarium oxysporum* f. sp. *lycopersici* [173]. The essential oil showed antifungal activity against *Aspergillus oryzae*, *A. nidulans*, *A. jumigatis*, *P. aculeatum*, *Phomopsis destuctum*, *P. digitatum*, *P . italicum*, *Diplodianatalensis*, *Alternaria tenuis*, *C. albicans*, *Epidermophyton cresens*, and *Microsporum gypseum* [174, 175]. The alcohol extract possesses antifungal activity against *Aspergillus niger*, *Penicillium selenium*, and *Saccharomyces* [176]. The fungitoxicity data of the oil with those of its major constituent's β -asarone, asaraldehyde, acoradin against *Helminthosporiumoryzae* indicated that β -asarone was the most active. β -Asarone present was primarily responsible for its fungitoxicity [177].

Antiviral Activity

It was found that the alcohol extract of the Rhizome showed potent antiviral activity against Herpes simplex virus HSV-1 and HSV-2 at a concentration well below the cytotoxic concentration. β-asarone possesses strong inhibitory activity against the replication of both virus types [178].

Antiparasitic Activity

The alcoholic extract was reported to show *in vitro* anthelmintic activity against human *Ascaris lumbricoides*. The essential oil inhibited the amplitude of rhythmic contractions of *Ascaris lumbricoides* within 5 minutes of exposure. In one study, the essential oil showed nematicidal activity against *Meloidogyne incognita* [179].

The essential oil shows insecticidal activity against houseflies *Musca domestica*. The oil inhibits the interstitial cell activity of instar larvae of *Dysdercuskoenigii*. β -asarone, with its antigonadal function, represented a new type of antigonadal agent that might afford a newer and safer approach toward insect control [180].

Emblica Officinalis

Emblica Officinalis (EO), belonging to the Euphorbiaceae family, often known as "Indian gooseberry" or "Amla," is one of the most important therapeutic herbs in Indian traditional medicine [181 - 184]. EO is a tropical and subtropical plant native to India, but it is now found in Sri Lanka, Uzbekistan, Southeast Asia, and China [185]. In traditional medicine, EO has a wide range of health benefits, including liver tonic, diuretic, laxative, aiding digestion, antipyretic, hair tonic, anti-ulcer, and treating common colds and fevers [186 - 189]. It can also be used to improve memory, reduce cholesterol, neutralize snake venom, cure viral illnesses, and act as an immunomodulator [190]. Polyphenols, ellagic acid, chebulinic acid, gallic acid, chebulagic acid, apigenin, quercetin, corilagin, and luteolin are among the bioactive components found in the Amla fruit [182, 183, 191].

Antibacterial Activity

The major phytoconstituents of EO, gallic and tannic acid, have significant antibacterial properties [186]. When evaluated for *E.coli*, *K. pneumoniae*, *S. aureus*, *B. cereus*, *V. cholerae*, and *C. albicans* [192], EO extracts showed a high zone of inhibition (ZOI). Antimicrobial efficacy for Gram-positive, Gram-negative, and fungal organisms indicates the use of *P. emblica* fruit as a treatment for a variety of microbial diseases [193]. Gram-positive bacteria are more resistant to EO than Gram-negative bacteria, which might be related to variations in the cell wall structure and composition [194].In comparison to the standards, the methanolic extract of EO showed considerable antibacterial activity. In comparison to the standards, the methanolic extract of EO showed considerable antibacterial activity. Antibacterial activity was also observed in ethyl acetate and aqueous extracts of EO. Against *E.coli* and *Staphylococcus aureus*, a methanolic extract of EO provided the largest inhibitory zone [195].

Antifungal Activity

Aqueous extracts of EO were found to have antifungal action against eight *Aspergillus species,* namely *Aspergillus candidus*, *Aspergillus columnaris*, *Aspergillus flavipes*, *Aspergillus flavus*, *Aspergillus fumigatus*, *Aspergillus niger*, *Aspergillus ochraceus*, and *Aspergillus tamari*. Methanol extract of EO exhibited superior antifungal activity compared to the other solvents like petroleum ether, chloroform, benzene, and ethanol [196]. Emblica extracts in ethanol and acetone showed considerable suppression of *F. equiseti* and *C. albicans*, with Griseofulvin as the standard antifungal agent [197].

Antiviral Activity

Phyllaemblicin B isolated from plant roots was shown to be effective against Coxsackie virus, while phenolic content was found to be beneficial against HSV 1 and 2 [198 - 200]. P. emblica's 1, 2, 4, 6-tetra-O-galloyl-D-glucose has antiviral efficacy against HSV *in vitro*. EO's polyphenolic component may have anti-HSV effects by inactivating extracellular viral particles and interfering with viral production in host cells, making it a possible treatment option for HSV [200]. Influenza A is inhibited by pentagalloylglucose as its viral replication is inhibited by preventing virus adsorption and reducing virus release [201].

Evolvulus Alsinoides

In India, *Evolvulus alsinoides* is a prominent and essential medicinal plant. *Evolvulus alsinoides* have therapeutic properties in all of its plant parts. Ayurvedic medicine makes extensive use of this herb. It may be seen growing in open, grassy areas over nearly all of India and subtropical regions across the world. *E. alsinoides* L. is mostly utilized in East Asian traditional medicine. In Ayurveda, the herb is utilized as a brain tonic to treat neurodegenerative disorders, asthma, and dementia. The plant's roots and stem extract are used to cure dysentery and depression in Sri Lanka. Respiratory and mental problems are treated with leaves [202].

Antibacterial Activity

Gram-negative bacteria like *Bacillus cereus* and *Staphylococcus aureus* were more resistant to all plant extracts than gram-positive bacteria like *Bacillus subtilis, E. coli* & *P. aeruginosa*. The plant root extract showed maximum antibacterial activity against various microorganisms [203].

Antifungal Activity

Aspergillus flavus and *Aspergillus niger* are greatly inhibited by ethanolic extracts of the plant [204].

CONCLUSION

Immunomodulators are either natural or synthetic substances that can suppress, stimulate, or modulate the immune system, including both adaptive and innate immunity. The rising frequency of infectious diseases, along with the undesirable effects of synthetic immunomodulators, has resulted in the search for natural immunomodulators. Herbal medicine presents a fresh target for drug discovery methodologies and medication development for researchers. Herbal immune drugs may offer an opportunity to explore a wide range of synergistic chemical moieties when used in combination, operate on various molecular targets and broaden the therapeutic range. Traditional knowledge and methods combined with practical experience help to create a safer and more cost-effective platform for the development of novel scaffolds and immune drugs. In this chapter, we have summarised the importance of medicinal plants as producers of immunomodulatory molecules with a wide range of chemistry with potential applications in animal and human health.

CONSENT FOR PUBLICATION

Not applicable.

CONFLICT OF INTEREST

The authors declare no conflict of interest, financial or otherwise.

ACKNOWLEDGEMENTS

The authors of this chapter would like to acknowledge SVKM's Dr. Bhanuben Nanavati College of Pharmacy, V.M. Road, Vile Parle (W), Mumbai-400056.

REFERENCES

[1] AA, Sabir S, Jan A. Physiology, Immune Response. StatPearls. 2020. Sep 27. Available from: https://www.ncbi.nlm.nih.gov/books/NBK539801/ (accessed on 7 october 2021).

[2] Bascones-Martinez A, Mattila R, Gomez-Font R, Meurman JH. Immunomodulatory drugs: Oral and systemic adverse effects. Med Oral Patol Oral Cir Bucal 2014; 19(1): e24-31. [http://dx.doi.org/10.4317/medoral.19087] [PMID: 23986016]

[3] Preiss JC, Zeitz M. Use of methotrexate in patients with inflammatory bowel diseases. Clin Exp Rheumatol 2010; 28(5) (Suppl. 61): S151-5. [PMID: 21044450]

[4] Ben-Efraim S. Immunomodulating anticancer alkylating drugs: targets and mechanisms of activity. Curr Drug Targets 2001; 2(2): 197-212. [http://dx.doi.org/10.2174/1389450013348597] [PMID: 11469719]

[5] Naga PN, Rajeshwari P. An overview on immunomodulators. Int J Curr Pharmaceutical & Clinical Research 2014; 4(2): 108-14.

[6] Wagner H. Search for plant derived natural products with immunostimulatory activity: recent advances. Pure Appl Chem 1990; 62(7): 1217-22. [http://dx.doi.org/10.1351/pac199062071217]

[7] Lee SJ, Chinen J, Kavanaugh A. Immunomodulator therapy: Monoclonal antibodies, fusion proteins, cytokines, and immunoglobulins. J Allergy Clin Immunol 2010; 125(2) (Suppl. 2): S314-23. [http://dx.doi.org/10.1016/j.jaci.2009.08.018] [PMID: 20036416]

[8] Makare N, Bodhankar S, Rangari V. Immunomodulatory activity of alcoholic extract of Mangifera indica L. in mice. J Ethnopharmacol 2001; 78(2-3): 133-7. [http://dx.doi.org/10.1016/S0378-8741(01)00326-9] [PMID: 11694357]

[9] Yatim KM, Lakkis FG. A brief journey through the immune system. Clin J Am Soc Nephrol 2015; 10(7): 1274-81. [http://dx.doi.org/10.2215/CJN.10031014] [PMID: 25845377]

[10] Durcan L, Petri M. Immunomodulators in SLE: Clinical evidence and immunologic actions. J Autoimmun 2016; 74: 73-84. [http://dx.doi.org/10.1016/j.jaut.2016.06.010] [PMID: 27371107]

[11] Kremer JM, Alarcón GS, Lightfoot RW Jr, *et al.* Methotrexate for rheumatoid arthritis. Arthritis & Rheumatism. Official J Am College Rheumatol 1994; 37(3): 316-28.

[12] Schonder KS, Mazariegos GV, Weber RJ. Adverse effects of immunosuppression in pediatric solid organ transplantation. Paediatr Drugs 2010; 12(1): 35-49. [http://dx.doi.org/10.2165/11316180-000000000-00000] [PMID: 20034340]

[13] Bradford K, Shih DQ. Optimizing 6-mercaptopurine and azathioprine therapy in the management of inflammatory bowel disease. World J Gastroenterol 2011; 17(37): 4166-73. [http://dx.doi.org/10.3748/wjg.v17.i37.4166] [PMID: 22072847]

[14] Toscano E, Cotta J, Robles M, Lucena MI, Andrade RJ. Toxicidad hepática inducida por los nuevos fármacos inmunosupresores. Gastroenterol Hepatol 2010; 33(1): 54-65. [http://dx.doi.org/10.1016/j.gastrohep.2009.07.003] [PMID: 19889479]

[15] Prokai A, Fekete A, Pásti K, *et al.* The importance of different immunosuppressive regimens in the development of posttransplant diabetes mellitus. Pediatr Diabetes 2012; 13(1): 81-91. [http://dx.doi.org/10.1111/j.1399-5448.2011.00782.x] [PMID: 21595806]

[16] Ng WF, Bowman SJ. Biological therapies in primary Sjögren's syndrome. Expert Opin Biol Ther 2011; 11(7): 921-36. [http://dx.doi.org/10.1517/14712598.2011.574120] [PMID: 21457124]

[17] Leverenz DL, St Clair EW. Recent advances in the search for a targeted immunomodulatory therapy for primary Sjögren's syndrome. F1000 Res 2019; 8: 8. [http://dx.doi.org/10.12688/f1000research.19842.1] [PMID: 31508200]

[18] López-Jornet P, Camacho-Alonso F, Salazar-Sanchez N. Topical tacrolimus and pimecrolimus in the treatment of oral lichen planus: an update. J Oral Pathol Med 2010; 39(3): 201-5. [http://dx.doi.org/10.1111/j.1600-0714.2009.00830.x] [PMID: 19943858]

[19] Chambers J, Yarrarapu SN, Mathai JK. Anthrax Infection. StatPearls 2021. https://www.ncbi.nlm.nih.gov/books/NBK535379/

[20] Pai M. Tuberculosis: the story after the Primer. Nat Rev Dis Primers 2020; 6(1): 29. [http://dx.doi.org/10.1038/s41572-020-0161-5] [PMID: 32327661]

[21] Fanous M, King KC. Cholera. StatPearls 2021. https://www.ncbi.nlm.nih.gov/books/NBK470232/

[22] Jain V, Vashisht R, Yilmaz G, Bhardwaj A. Pneumonia Pathology. StatPearls. 2021. https://www.ncbi.nlm.nih. gov/books/NBK526116/

[23] Kühbacher A, Burger-Kentischer A, Rupp S. Interaction of Candida species with the skin. Microorganisms 2017; 5(2): 32. [http://dx.doi.org/10.3390/microorganisms5020032] [PMID: 28590443]

[24] Waymack JR, Sundareshan V. Acquired immune deficiency syndrome (AIDS). Treasure Island (FL). 2020 Jan. Available from: https://pubmed.ncbi.nlm.nih.gov/30725978/ (accessed on 26 october 2021).

[25] Cascella M, Rajnik M, Aleem A, Dulebohn S, Di Napoli R. Features, evaluation, and treatment of coronavirus (COVID-19). StatPearls. 2021 Apr 20. Available from: https:

//www.ncbi.nlm.nih.gov/books/NBK554776/ (accessed on 26 october 2021).

[26] Wolbert JG, Higginbotham K. Poliomyelitis (Polio). StatPearls. 2020. Available from: https://www.ncbi.nlm.nih.gov/books/NBK558944/ (accessed on 7 october 2021).

[27] Zarrin A, Akhondi H. Viral Hepatitis. StatPearls. 2021 Apr 7. Available from: https://www.ncbi.nlm.nih.gov/books/NBK556029/ (accessed on 7 october 2021).

[28] Buck E, Finnigan NA. Malaria. StatPearls. 2021 Apr 11. Available from: https://www.ncbi.nlm.nih.gov/books/NBK551711/ (accessed on 7 october 2021).

[29] Newman TE, Juergens AL. Filariasis. StatPearls. 2020 Aug 11. Available from: https://www.ncbi.nlm.nih.gov/books/NBK556012/ (accessed on 7 october 2021).

[30] Drexler M. How Infection Works. What You Need to Know About Infectious Disease. 2010.

[31] Futata EA, Fusaro AE, de Brito CA, Sato MN. The neonatal immune system: immunomodulation of infections in early life. Expert Rev Anti Infect Ther 2012; 10(3): 289-98. [http://dx.doi.org/10.1586/eri.12.9] [PMID: 22397563]

[32] National Research Council Treating infectious diseases in a microbial world: report of two workshops on novel antimicrobial therapeutics. 2006.

[33] Jantan I, Ahmad W, Bukhari SNA. Plant-derived immunomodulators: an insight on their preclinical evaluation and clinical trials. Front Plant Sci 2015; 6: 655. [http://dx.doi.org/10.3389/fpls.2015.00655] [PMID: 26379683]

[34] Lin WC, Lin JY. Berberine down-regulates the Th1/Th2 cytokine gene expression ratio in mouse primary splenocytes in the absence or presence of lipopolysaccharide in a preventive manner. Int Immunopharmacol 2011; 11(12): 1984-90. [http://dx.doi.org/10.1016/j.intimp.2011.08.008] [PMID: 21867779]

[35] Vaibhav K, Shrivastava P, Javed H, *et al.* Piperine suppresses cerebral ischemia–reperfusion-induced inflammation through the repression of COX-2, NOS-2, and NF-κB in middle cerebral artery occlusion rat model. Mol Cell Biochem 2012; 367(1-2): 73-84. [http://dx.doi.org/10.1007/s11010-012-1321-z] [PMID: 22669728]

[36] Kimura Y, Tsukada J, Tomoda T, *et al.* Clinical and immunologic evaluation of dendritic cell-based immunotherapy in combination with gemcitabine and/or S-1 in patients with advanced pancreatic carcinoma. Pancreas 2012; 41(2): 195-205. [http://dx.doi.org/10.1097/MPA.0b013e31822398c6] [PMID: 21792083]

[37] Patwardhan B, Kalbag D, Patki PS, Nagsampagi BA. Search of immunomodulatory agents: a review. Indian drugs. 1990; 28(2): 56-63.

[38] Puri A, Saxena R, Saxena RP, Saxena KC, Srivastava V, Tandon JS. Immunostimulant activity of Nyctanthes arbor-tristis L. J Ethnopharmacol 1994; 42(1): 31-7. [http://dx.doi.org/10.1016/0378-8741(94)90020-5] [PMID: 8046941]

[39] Ziauddin M, Phansalkar N, Patki P, Diwanay S, Patwardhan B. Studies on the immunomodulatory effects of Ashwagandha. J Ethnopharmacol 1996; 50(2): 69-76. [http://dx.doi.org/10.1016/0378-8741(95)01318-0] [PMID: 8866726]

[40] Bhaumik S, Jyothi MD, Khar A. Differential modulation of nitric oxide production by curcumin in host macrophages and NK cells. FEBS Lett 2000; 483(1): 78-82. https://www.sciencedirect.com/science/article/pii/S0014579300020895 [http://dx.doi.org/10.1016/S0014-5793(00)02089-5] [PMID: 11033360]

[41] Surh YJ, Chun KS, Cha HH, *et al.* Molecular mechanisms underlying chemopreventive activities of anti-inflammatory phytochemicals: down-regulation of COX-2 and iNOS through suppression of NF-κB activation. Mutat Res 2001; 480-481: 243-68. [http://dx.doi.org/10.1016/S0027-5107(01)00183-X] [PMID: 11506818]

[42] Gao X, Kuo J, Jiang H, *et al.* Immunomodulatory activity of curcumin: suppression of lymphocyte

proliferation, development of cell-mediated cytotoxicity, and cytokine production *in vitro*. Biochem Pharmacol 2004; 68(1): 51-61.
[http://dx.doi.org/10.1016/j.bcp.2004.03.015] [PMID: 15183117]

[43] Kim GY, Kim KH, Lee SH, *et al.* Curcumin inhibits immunostimulatory function of dendritic cells: MAPKs and translocation of NF-κ B as potential targets. J Immunol 2005; 174(12): 8116-24.
[http://dx.doi.org/10.4049/jimmunol.174.12.8116] [PMID: 15944320]

[44] Mun SH, Joung DK, Kim YS, *et al.* Synergistic antibacterial effect of curcumin against methicillin-resistant *Staphylococcus aureus*. Phytomedicine 2013; 20(8-9): 714-8.
[http://dx.doi.org/10.1016/j.phymed.2013.02.006] [PMID: 23537748]

[45] Gunes H, Gulen D, Mutlu R, Gumus A, Tas T, Topkaya AE. Antibacterial effects of curcumin. Toxicol Ind Health 2016; 32(2): 246-50.
[http://dx.doi.org/10.1177/0748233713498458] [PMID: 24097361]

[46] Thomachan S, Sindhu S, John VD. Synthesis, characterization, antibacterial, antifungal and cytotoxic activity of curcuminoid analogues with trisubstituted phenyl and anthracenyl ring and their zinc (II), copper (II) and vanadyl (IV) chelates. Int J Pharmac Chem 2016; 6: 78-86.

[47] Dovigo LN, Pavarina AC, Ribeiro APD, *et al.* Investigation of the photodynamic effects of curcumin against Candida albicans. Photochem Photobiol 2011; 87(4): 895-903.
[http://dx.doi.org/10.1111/j.1751-1097.2011.00937.x] [PMID: 21517888]

[48] Garcia-Gomes AS, Curvelo JAR, Soares RMA, Ferreira-Pereira A. Curcumin acts synergistically with fluconazole to sensitize a clinical isolate of *Candida albicans* showing a MDR phenotype. Med Mycol 2012; 50(1): 26-32.
[http://dx.doi.org/10.3109/13693786.2011.578156] [PMID: 21539505]

[49] Krishnamurthi A. The Wealth of India: Raw Materials: Vol. VIII. Ph-Re. 1969. Available from: https://www.cabdirect.org/cabdirect/abstract/19710305452 (accessed on 7 october 2021).

[50] Purushothaman KK, Sarada A, Loganathan D. Phytochemical study of Argyreia speciosa (Vridhadaru). Bull Med Ethnobot Res 1982; 3: 250-3.

[51] Gokhale AB, Damre AS, Saraf MN. Investigations into the immunomodulatory activity of Argyreia speciosa. J Ethnopharmacol 2003; 84(1): 109-14.
[http://dx.doi.org/10.1016/S0378-8741(02)00168-X] [PMID: 12499085]

[52] George M, Pandalai KM. Investigations on Plant Antibiotics. Part IV. Further Search for Antibiotic Substances in Indian Medicinal Plants. Indian J Med Res 1949; 37(2): 169-81. Corpus ID: 90081337.

[53] Mishra SH, Chaturvedi SC. Antibacterial and antifungal activity of the oil and unsaponifiable matter of Argyreia speciosa sweet. Indian Drugs and Pharmaceuticals 1978; 13: 29-31.

[54] Shukla YN, Srivastava A, Kumar S, Kumar S. Phytotoxic and antimicrobial constituents of Argyreia speciosa and Oenothera biennis. J Ethnopharmacol 1999; 67(2): 241-5.
[http://dx.doi.org/10.1016/S0378-8741(99)00017-3] [PMID: 10619391]

[55] Babbar OP, Joshi MN, Madan AR. Evaluation of plants for antiviral activity. Indian J Med Res. 1982 Dec 1;76(S): 54-65.

[56] Parveen N, Khan NU, Singhal KC. Antifilarial activity of Argyria speciosa against Setaria cervi *in vitro*. Phytother Res 1990; 4(4): 162-4.
[http://dx.doi.org/10.1002/ptr.2650040409]

[57] Zhu XM, Song JX, Huang ZZ, Wu YM, Yu MJ. [Antiviral activity of mangiferin against herpes simplex virus type 2 in vitro]. Chung Kuo Yao Li Hsueh Pao 1993; 14(5): 452-4.
[PMID: 8010041]

[58] Zheng MS, Lu ZY. Antiviral effect of mangiferin and isomangiferin on herpes simplex virus. Chin Med J (Engl) 1990; 103(2): 160-5.
[PMID: 2167819]

[59] Guha S, Ghosal S, Chattopadhyay U. Antitumor, immunomodulatory and anti-HIV effect of mangiferin, a naturally occurring glucosylxanthone. Chemotherapy 1996; 42(6): 443-51. [http://dx.doi.org/10.1159/000239478] [PMID: 8957579]

[60] Perrucci S, Fichi G, Buggiani C, Rossi G, Flamini G. Efficacy of mangiferin against Cryptosporidium parvum in a neonatal mouse model. Parasitol Res 2006; 99(2): 184-8. [http://dx.doi.org/10.1007/s00436-006-0165-4] [PMID: 16547730]

[61] Stoilova I, Gargova S, Stoyanova A, Ho I. Antimicrobial and antioxidant activity of the polyphenol mangiferin. Herba Pol 2005; 1(51).

[62] Akhtar MS, Iqbal Z, Khan MN, Lateef M. Anthelmintic activity of medicinal plants with particular reference to their use in animals in the Indo–Pakistan subcontinent. Small Rumin Res 2000; 38(2): 99-107. [http://dx.doi.org/10.1016/S0921-4488(00)00163-2] [PMID: 10760446]

[63] Kirtikar KR, Basu BD. Indian medicinal plants. Dehradun. International book distributors. 1987; 2.

[64] Devi MA, Prasad BD, Rambabu B. Study of antimicrobial properties of Tinospora sinensisby agar well diffusion method. Scandinavian J Pharm Sci Res 2014; 1(1): 1-5.

[65] Thawani VR, Varadpande UK, Sontakke SD, Singh RP, Khiyani RK, Kalikar MV. Immunomodulatory effect of *Tinospora cordifolia* extract in human immuno-deficiency virus positive patients. Indian J Pharmacol 2008; 40(3): 107-10. [http://dx.doi.org/10.4103/0253-7613.42302] [PMID: 20040936]

[66] Estari M, Venkanna L, Reddy AS. *In vitro* anti-HIV activity of crude extracts from Tinospora cordifolia. BMC Infect Dis 2012; 12(S1): P10. [http://dx.doi.org/10.1186/1471-2334-12-S1-P10]

[67] Nahas R, Moher M. Complementary and alternative medicine for the treatment of type 2 diabetes. Can Fam Physician 2009; 55(6): 591-6. [PMID: 19509199]

[68] Haouala R, Hawala S, El-Ayeb A, Khanfir R, Boughanmi N. Aqueous and organic extracts of Trigonella foenum-graecum L. inhibit the mycelia growth of fungi. J Environ Sci (China) 2008; 20(12): 1453-7. [http://dx.doi.org/10.1016/S1001-0742(08)62548-6] [PMID: 19209631]

[69] O'Mahony R, Al-Khtheeri H, Bogahawata A, *et al.* Bactericidal and anti-adhesive properties of culinary and medicinal plants against Helicobacter pylori: P477. Clinical Microbiology & Infection Supplement 2005; (Apr): 11.

[70] Randhir R, Shetty K. Improved α-amylase and Helicobacter pylori inhibition by fenugreek extracts derived *via* solid-state bioconversion using Rhizopus oligosporus. Asia Pac J Clin Nutr 2007; 16(3): 382-92. [PMID: 17704018]

[71] Randhir R, Lin Y, Shetty K. Phenolics, their antioxidant and antimicrobial activity in dark germinated fenugreek sprouts in response to peptide and phytochemical elicitors. Asia Pac J Clin Nutr 2004; 13(3): 295-307. [PMID: 15331344]

[72] Mercan N, Guvensen A, Celik A, Katircioglu H. Antimicrobial activity and pollen composition of honey samples collected from different provinces in Turkey. Nat Prod Res 2007; 21(3): 187-95. [http://dx.doi.org/10.1080/14786410600906277] [PMID: 17365707]

[73] Zia T, Hasnain SN, Hasan SK. Evaluation of the oral hypoglycaemic effect of Trigonella foenum-graecum L. (methi) in normal mice. J Ethnopharmacol 2001; 75(2-3): 191-5. [http://dx.doi.org/10.1016/S0378-8741(01)00186-6] [PMID: 11297850]

[74] Li W, Liu Y, Wang Z, *et al.* Platycodin D isolated from the aerial parts of Platycodon grandiflorum

protects alcohol-induced liver injury in mice. Food Funct 2015; 6(5): 1418-27. [http://dx.doi.org/10.1039/C5FO00094G] [PMID: 25927324]

[75] Zhang L, Wang Y, Yang D, *et al.* Platycodon grandiflorus – An Ethnopharmacological, phytochemical and pharmacological review. J Ethnopharmacol 2015; 164: 147-61. [http://dx.doi.org/10.1016/j.jep.2015.01.052] [PMID: 25666431]

[76] Han LK, Zheng YN, Xu BJ, Okuda H, Kimura Y. Saponins from platycodi radix ameliorate high fat diet-induced obesity in mice. J Nutr 2002; 132(8): 2241-5. [http://dx.doi.org/10.1093/jn/132.8.2241] [PMID: 12163669]

[77] Chun J, Joo EJ, Kang M, Kim YS. Platycodin D induces anoikis and caspase-mediated apoptosis *via* p38 MAPK in AGS human gastric cancer cells. J Cell Biochem 2013; 114(2): 456-70. [http://dx.doi.org/10.1002/jcb.24386] [PMID: 22961809]

[78] Wang C, Schuller Levis GB, Lee EB, *et al.* Platycodin D and D3 isolated from the root of Platycodon grandiflorum modulate the production of nitric oxide and secretion of TNF-α in activated RAW 264.7 cells. Int Immunopharmacol 2004; 4(8): 1039-49. [http://dx.doi.org/10.1016/j.intimp.2004.04.005] [PMID: 15222978]

[79] Xie Y, Sun HX, Li D, Platycodin D. Platycodin d improves the immunogenicity of newcastle disease virus-based recombinant avian influenza vaccine in mice. Chem Biodivers 2010; 7(3): 677-89. [http://dx.doi.org/10.1002/cbdv.200900183] [PMID: 20232336]

[80] Han EH, Park JH, Kim JY, Chung YC, Jeong HG. Inhibitory mechanism of saponins derived from roots of Platycodon grandiflorum on anaphylactic reaction and IgE-mediated allergic response in mast cells. Food Chem Toxicol 2009; 47(6): 1069-75. [http://dx.doi.org/10.1016/j.fct.2009.01.041] [PMID: 19425227]

[81] Lee SJ, Bang WS, Hong JY, Kwon OJ, Shin SR, Yoon KY. Antioxidant and antimicrobial activities of black Doraji (Platycodon grandiflorum). Hanguk Sikpum Jeojang Yutong Hakoeji 2013; 20(4): 510-7. [http://dx.doi.org/10.11002/kjfp.2013.20.4.510]

[82] Kim J, Lee S, Lim J, Park S. Kim J, Lee S, Lim J, Park S.. Pharmaceutical composition for preventing or treating Hepatitis C, comprising the roots extract of Platycodon grandiflorum or Platycodon grandiflorum saponin. WO patent 085091 2010.

[83] Holmes-McNary M, Baldwin AS Jr. Chemopreventive properties of trans-resveratrol are associated with inhibition of activation of the IkappaB kinase. Cancer Res 2000; 60(13): 3477-83. [PMID: 10910059]

[84] Manna SK, Mukhopadhyay A, Aggarwal BB. Resveratrol suppresses TNF-induced activation of nuclear transcription factors NF-κ B, activator protein-1, and apoptosis: potential role of reactive oxygen intermediates and lipid peroxidation. J Immunol 2000; 164(12): 6509-19. [http://dx.doi.org/10.4049/jimmunol.164.12.6509] [PMID: 10843709]

[85] Gao X, Xu YX, Janakiraman N, Chapman RA, Gautam SC. Immunomodulatory activity of resveratrol: suppression of lymphocyte proliferation, development of cell-mediated cytotoxicity, and cytokine production. Biochem Pharmacol 2001; 62(9): 1299-308. [http://dx.doi.org/10.1016/S0006-2952(01)00775-4] [PMID: 11705464]

[86] Kowalski J, Samojedny A, Paul M, Pietsz G, Wilczok T. Effect of apigenin, kaempferol and resveratrol on the expression of interleukin-1beta and tumor necrosis factor-alpha genes in J774. 2 macrophages. Pharmacological reports: PR. 2005; 57(3): 390-4.

[87] Paulo L, Ferreira S, Gallardo E, Queiroz JA, Domingues F. Antimicrobial activity and effects of resveratrol on human pathogenic bacteria. World J Microbiol Biotechnol 2010; 26(8): 1533-8. [http://dx.doi.org/10.1007/s11274-010-0325-7]

[88] Chan MMY. Antimicrobial effect of resveratrol on dermatophytes and bacterial pathogens of the skin. Biochem Pharmacol 2002; 63(2): 99-104. [http://dx.doi.org/10.1016/S0006-2952(01)00886-3] [PMID: 11841782]

[89] Jung HJ, Hwang IA, Sung WS, *et al.* Fungicidal effect of resveratrol on human infectious fungi. Arch Pharm Res 2005; 28(5): 557-60.
[http://dx.doi.org/10.1007/BF02977758] [PMID: 15974442]

[90] Salehi B, Mishra A, Nigam M, *et al.* Resveratrol: A double-edged sword in health benefits. Biomedicines 2018; 6(3): 91.
[http://dx.doi.org/10.3390/biomedicines6030091] [PMID: 30205595]

[91] Passos CLA, Ferreira C, Soares DC, Saraiva EM. Leishmanicidal effect of synthetic trans-resveratrol analogs. PLoS One 2015; 10(10): e0141778.
[http://dx.doi.org/10.1371/journal.pone.0141778] [PMID: 26517558]

[92] Mukherjee N, Parida PK, Santra A, *et al.* Oxidative stress plays major role in mediating apoptosis in filarial nematode Setaria cervi in the presence of trans-stilbene derivatives. Free Radic Biol Med 2016; 93: 130-44.
[http://dx.doi.org/10.1016/j.freeradbiomed.2016.01.027] [PMID: 26849945]

[93] Cheng K, Wu Z, Gao B, Xu J. Analysis of influence of baicalin joint resveratrol retention enema on the TNF-α, SIgA, IL-2, IFN-γ of rats with respiratory syncytial virus infection. Cell Biochem Biophys 2014; 70(2): 1305-9.
[http://dx.doi.org/10.1007/s12013-014-0055-9] [PMID: 24938899]

[94] Liu T, Zang N, Zhou N, *et al.* Resveratrol inhibits the TRIF-dependent pathway by upregulating sterile alpha and armadillo motif protein, contributing to anti-inflammatory effects after respiratory syncytial virus infection. J Virol 2014; 88(8): 4229-36.
[http://dx.doi.org/10.1128/JVI.03637-13] [PMID: 24478430]

[95] Xie X, Zang N, Li S, *et al.* Resveratrol Inhibits respiratory syncytial virus-induced IL-6 production, decreases viral replication, and downregulates TRIF expression in airway epithelial cells. Inflammation 2012; 35(4): 1392-401.
[http://dx.doi.org/10.1007/s10753-012-9452-7] [PMID: 22391746]

[96] Zang N, Li S, Li W, *et al.* Resveratrol suppresses persistent airway inflammation and hyperresponsivess might partially *via* nerve growth factor in respiratory syncytial virus-infected mice. Int Immunopharmacol 2015; 28(1): 121-8.
[http://dx.doi.org/10.1016/j.intimp.2015.05.031] [PMID: 26044349]

[97] Zang N, Xie X, Deng Y, *et al.* Resveratrol-mediated gamma interferon reduction prevents airway inflammation and airway hyperresponsiveness in respiratory syncytial virus-infected immunocompromised mice. J Virol 2011; 85(24): 13061-8.
[http://dx.doi.org/10.1128/JVI.05869-11] [PMID: 21937650]

[98] Docherty JJ, Sweet TJ, Bailey E, Faith SA, Booth T. Resveratrol inhibition of varicella-zoster virus replication *in vitro.* Antiviral Res 2006; 72(3): 171-7.
[http://dx.doi.org/10.1016/j.antiviral.2006.07.004] [PMID: 16899306]

[99] Espinoza JL, Takami A, Trung LQ, Kato S, Nakao S. Resveratrol prevents EBV transformation and inhibits the outgrowth of EBV-immortalized human B cells. PLoS One 2012; 7(12): e51306.
[http://dx.doi.org/10.1371/journal.pone.0051306] [PMID: 23251493]

[100] Yiu CY, Chen SY, Chang LK, Chiu YF, Lin TP. Inhibitory effects of resveratrol on the Epstein-Barr virus lytic cycle. Molecules 2010; 15(10): 7115-24.
[http://dx.doi.org/10.3390/molecules15107115] [PMID: 20948499]

[101] Chen X, Qiao H, Liu T, *et al.* Inhibition of herpes simplex virus infection by oligomeric stilbenoids through ROS generation. Antiviral Res 2012; 95(1): 30-6.
[http://dx.doi.org/10.1016/j.antiviral.2012.05.001] [PMID: 22584350]

[102] Docherty J, Fu M, Hah J, Sweet T, Faith S, Booth T. Effect of resveratrol on herpes simplex virus vaginal infection in the mouse. Antiviral Res 2005; 67(3): 155-62.
[http://dx.doi.org/10.1016/j.antiviral.2005.06.008] [PMID: 16125258]

[103] Docherty JJ, Fu MMH, Stiffler BS, Limperos RJ, Pokabla CM, DeLucia AL. Resveratrol inhibition of herpes simplex virus replication. Antiviral Res 1999; 43(3): 145-55. [http://dx.doi.org/10.1016/S0166-3542(99)00042-X] [PMID: 10551373]

[104] Docherty J, Smith J, Fu M, Stoner T, Booth T. Effect of topically applied resveratrol on cutaneous herpes simplex virus infections in hairless mice. Antiviral Res 2004; 61(1): 19-26. [http://dx.doi.org/10.1016/j.antiviral.2003.07.001] [PMID: 14670590]

[105] Clouser CL, Chauhan J, Bess MA, *et al.* Anti-HIV-1 activity of resveratrol derivatives and synergistic inhibition of HIV-1 by the combination of resveratrol and decitabine. Bioorg Med Chem Lett 2012; 22(21): 6642-6. [http://dx.doi.org/10.1016/j.bmcl.2012.08.108] [PMID: 23010273]

[106] Heredia A, Davis C, Amin MN, *et al.* Targeting host nucleotide biosynthesis with resveratrol inhibits emtricitabine-resistant HIV-1. AIDS 2014; 28(3): 317-23. [http://dx.doi.org/10.1097/QAD.0000000000000168] [PMID: 24326355]

[107] Singh BN, Shankar S, Srivastava RK. Green tea catechin, epigallocatechin-3-gallate (EGCG): Mechanisms, perspectives and clinical applications. Biochem Pharmacol 2011; 82(12): 1807-21. [http://dx.doi.org/10.1016/j.bcp.2011.07.093] [PMID: 21827739]

[108] Yang H, Landis-Piwowar K, Chan TH, Dou QP. Green tea polyphenols as proteasome inhibitors: implication in chemoprevention. Curr Cancer Drug Targets 2011; 11(3): 296-306. [http://dx.doi.org/10.2174/156800911794519743] [PMID: 21247384]

[109] Mabe K, Yamada M, Oguni I, Takahashi T. *In vitro* and *in vivo* activities of tea catechins against Helicobacter pylori. Antimicrob Agents Chemother 1999; 43(7): 1788-91. [http://dx.doi.org/10.1128/AAC.43.7.1788] [PMID: 10390246]

[110] Friedman M. Overview of antibacterial, antitoxin, antiviral, and antifungal activities of tea flavonoids and teas. Mol Nutr Food Res 2007; 51(1): 116-34. [http://dx.doi.org/10.1002/mnfr.200600173] [PMID: 17195249]

[111] Weber JM, Ruzindana-Umunyana A, Imbeault L, Sircar S. Inhibition of adenovirus infection and adenain by green tea catechins. Antiviral Res 2003; 58(2): 167-73. [http://dx.doi.org/10.1016/S0166-3542(02)00212-7] [PMID: 12742577]

[112] Clark KJ, Grant PG, Sarr AB, *et al.* An *in vitro* study of theaflavins extracted from black tea to neutralize bovine rotavirus and bovine coronavirus infections. Vet Microbiol 1998; 63(2-4): 147-57. [http://dx.doi.org/10.1016/S0378-1135(98)00242-9] [PMID: 9850995]

[113] Chang LK, Wei TT, Chiu YF, *et al.* Inhibition of Epstein–Barr virus lytic cycle by (−)-epigallocatechin gallate. Biochem Biophys Res Commun 2003; 301(4): 1062-8. [http://dx.doi.org/10.1016/S0006-291X(03)00067-6] [PMID: 12589821]

[114] Savi LA, Barardi CRM, Simões CMO. Evaluation of antiherpetic activity and genotoxic effects of tea catechin derivatives. J Agric Food Chem 2006; 54(7): 2552-7. [http://dx.doi.org/10.1021/jf052940e] [PMID: 16569042]

[115] Nakayama M, Suzuki K, Toda M, Okubo S, Hara Y, Shimamura T. Inhibition of the infectivity of influenza virus by tea polyphenols. Antiviral Res 1993; 21(4): 289-99. [http://dx.doi.org/10.1016/0166-3542(93)90008-7] [PMID: 8215301]

[116] Okubo S, Toda M, Hara Y, Shimamura T. Antifungal and fungicidal activities of tea extract and catechin against Trichophyton. Jpn J Bacteriol 1991; 46(2): 509-14. [http://dx.doi.org/10.3412/jsb.46.509] [PMID: 2062004]

[117] Inacio JDF, Fonseca MS, Almeida-Amaral EE. (−)-Epigallocatechin 3-O-gallate as a new approach for the treatment of visceral Leishmaniasis. J Nat Prod 2019; 82(9): 2664-7. [http://dx.doi.org/10.1021/acs.jnatprod.9b00632] [PMID: 31503486]

[118] Dixon R, Ferreira D. Dixon RA, Ferreira D. Genistein. Phytochemistry. 2002 Jun 1 2002; 60(3): 205-

11.

[119] Hong H, Landauer MR, Foriska MA, Ledney GD. Antibacterial activity of the soy isoflavone genistein. J Basic Microbiol 2006; 46(4): 329-35. [http://dx.doi.org/10.1002/jobm.200510073] [PMID: 16847837]

[120] Rosenshine I, Duronio V, Finlay BB. Tyrosine protein kinase inhibitors block invasin-promoted bacterial uptake by epithelial cells. Infect Immun 1992; 60(6): 2211-7. [http://dx.doi.org/10.1128/iai.60.6.2211-2217.1992] [PMID: 1587588]

[121] Crane JK, Majumdar S, Pickhardt DF III. Host cell death due to enteropathogenic Escherichia coli has features of apoptosis. Infect Immun 1999; 67(5): 2575-84. [http://dx.doi.org/10.1128/IAI.67.5.2575-2584.1999] [PMID: 10225923]

[122] Bermudez LE, Young LS. Factors affecting invasion of HT-29 and HEp-2 epithelial cells by organisms of the Mycobacterium avium complex. Infect Immun 1994; 62(5): 2021-6. [http://dx.doi.org/10.1128/iai.62.5.2021-2026.1994] [PMID: 8168968]

[123] Jett BD, Gilmore MS. Internalization of Staphylococcus aureus by human corneal epithelial cells: role of bacterial fibronectin-binding protein and host cell factors. Infect Immun 2002; 70(8): 4697-700. [http://dx.doi.org/10.1128/IAI.70.8.4697-4700.2002] [PMID: 12117986]

[124] Lammers A, Nuijten PJM, Kruijt E, *et al.* Cell tropism of Staphylococcus aureus in bovine mammary gland cell cultures. Vet Microbiol 1999; 67(2): 77-89. [http://dx.doi.org/10.1016/S0378-1135(99)00018-8] [PMID: 10414363]

[125] Tang P, Sutherland CL, Gold MR, Finlay BB. Listeria monocytogenes invasion of epithelial cells requires the MEK-1/ERK-2 mitogen-activated protein kinase pathway. Infect Immun 1998; 66(3): 1106-12. [http://dx.doi.org/10.1128/IAI.66.3.1106-1112.1998] [PMID: 9488402]

[126] Limongi CL, De Souza W, Rozental S. Protein kinase antagonists inhibit invasion of mammalian cells by Fonsecaea pedrosoi. J Med Microbiol 2003; 52(3): 201-9. [http://dx.doi.org/10.1099/jmm.0.04945-0] [PMID: 12621084]

[127] Akula SM, Hurley DJ, Wixon RL, Wang C, Chase CCL. Effect of genistein on replication of bovine herpesvirus type 1. Am J Vet Res 2002; 63(8): 1124-8. [http://dx.doi.org/10.2460/ajvr.2002.63.1124] [PMID: 12171165]

[128] Lyu SY, Rhim JY, Park WB. Antiherpetic activities of flavonoids against herpes simplex virus type 1 (HSV-1) and type 2 (HSV-2) *in vitro.* Arch Pharm Res 2005; 28(11): 1293-301. [http://dx.doi.org/10.1007/BF02978215] [PMID: 16350858]

[129] Evers DL, Chao CF, Wang X, Zhang Z, Huong SM, Huang ES. Human cytomegalovirus-inhibitory flavonoids: Studies on antiviral activity and mechanism of action. Antiviral Res 2005; 68(3): 124-34. [http://dx.doi.org/10.1016/j.antiviral.2005.08.002] [PMID: 16188329]

[130] Stantchev TS, Markovic I, Telford WG, Clouse KA, Broder CC. The tyrosine kinase inhibitor genistein blocks HIV-1 infection in primary human macrophages. Virus Res 2007; 123(2): 178-89. [http://dx.doi.org/10.1016/j.virusres.2006.09.004] [PMID: 17030448]

[131] Arabyan E, Hakobyan A, Kotsinyan A, *et al.* Genistein inhibits African swine fever virus replication *in vitro* by disrupting viral DNA synthesis. Antiviral Res 2018; 156: 128-37. [http://dx.doi.org/10.1016/j.antiviral.2018.06.014] [PMID: 29940214]

[132] Yura Y, Yoshida H, Sato M. Inhibition of herpes simplex virus replication by genistein, an inhibitor of protein-tyrosine kinase. Arch Virol 1993; 132(3-4): 451-61. [http://dx.doi.org/10.1007/BF01309554] [PMID: 8397505]

[133] Hirasawa K, Kim A, Han HS, Han J, Jun HS, Yoon JW. Effect of p38 mitogen-activated protein kinase on the replication of encephalomyocarditis virus. J Virol 2003; 77(10): 5649-56. [http://dx.doi.org/10.1128/JVI.77.10.5649-5656.2003] [PMID: 12719557]

[134] Vela EM, Bowick GC, Herzog NK, Aronson JF. Genistein treatment of cells inhibits arenavirus infection. Antiviral Res 2008; 77(2): 153-6.
[http://dx.doi.org/10.1016/j.antiviral.2007.09.005] [PMID: 17961732]

[135] Vella C, Festenstein H. Coxsackievirus B4 infection of the mouse pancreas: the role of natural killer cells in the control of virus replication and resistance to infection. J Gen Virol 1992; 73(6): 1379-86.
[http://dx.doi.org/10.1099/0022-1317-73-6-1379] [PMID: 1607859]

[136] Tandon V, Pal P, Roy B, Rao HSP, Reddy KS. *In vitro* anthelmintic activity of root-tuber extract of Flemingia vestita, an indigenous plant in Shillong, India. Parasitol Res 1997; 83(5): 492-8.
[http://dx.doi.org/10.1007/s004360050286] [PMID: 9197399]

[137] Middleton E Jr, Kandaswami C, Theoharides TC. The effects of plant flavonoids on mammalian cells: implications for inflammation, heart disease, and cancer. Pharmacol Rev 2000; 52(4): 673-751.
[PMID: 11121513]

[138] Boots AW, Haenen GRMM, Bast A. Health effects of quercetin: From antioxidant to nutraceutical. Eur J Pharmacol 2008; 585(2-3): 325-37.
[http://dx.doi.org/10.1016/j.ejphar.2008.03.008] [PMID: 18417116]

[139] Wang S, Yao J, Zhou B, *et al.* Bacteriostatic effect of quercetin as an antibiotic alternative *in vivo* and its antibacterial mechanism *in vitro*. J Food Prot 2018; 81(1): 68-78.
[http://dx.doi.org/10.4315/0362-028X.JFP-17-214] [PMID: 29271686]

[140] Osonga FJ, Akgul A, Miller RM, *et al.* Antimicrobial activity of a new class of phosphorylated and modified flavonoids. ACS Omega 2019; 4(7): 12865-71.
[http://dx.doi.org/10.1021/acsomega.9b00077] [PMID: 31460413]

[141] Abd-Allah WE, Awad HM, AbdelMohsen MM. HPLC analysis of quercetin and antimicrobial activity of comparative methanol extracts of Shinus molle L. Int J Curr Microbiol Appl Sci 2015; 4: 550-8.

[142] Tasdemir D, Kaiser M, Brun R, *et al.* Antitrypanosomal and antileishmanial activities of flavonoids and their analogues: *in vitro, in vivo*, structure-activity relationship, and quantitative structure-activity relationship studies. Antimicrob Agents Chemother 2006; 50(4): 1352-64.
[http://dx.doi.org/10.1128/AAC.50.4.1352-1364.2006] [PMID: 16569852]

[143] Coelho-dos-Reis JGA, Gomes OA, Bortolini DE, *et al.* Evaluation of the effects of Quercetin and Kaempherol on the surface of MT-2 cells visualized by atomic force microscopy. J Virol Methods 2011; 174(1-2): 47-52.
[http://dx.doi.org/10.1016/j.jviromet.2011.03.019] [PMID: 21507333]

[144] Johari J, Kianmehr A, Mustafa M, Abubakar S, Zandi K. Antiviral activity of baicalein and quercetin against the Japanese encephalitis virus. Int J Mol Sci 2012; 13(12): 16785-95.
[http://dx.doi.org/10.3390/ijms131216785] [PMID: 23222683]

[145] Zandi K, Teoh BT, Sam SS, Wong PF, Mustafa MR, AbuBakar S. Antiviral activity of four types of bioflavonoid against dengue virus type-2. Virol J 2011; 8(1): 560.
[http://dx.doi.org/10.1186/1743-422X-8-560] [PMID: 22201648]

[146] Bachmetov L, Gal-Tanamy M, Shapira A, *et al.* Suppression of hepatitis C virus by the flavonoid quercetin is mediated by inhibition of NS3 protease activity. J Viral Hepat 2012; 19(2): e81-8.
[http://dx.doi.org/10.1111/j.1365-2893.2011.01507.x] [PMID: 22239530]

[147] Sadiq NM, Robinson KJ, Terrell JM. Colchicine. StatPearls [Internet]. 2020 Jan. (accessed on 26 october 2021).

[148] Gohar MA, Makkawi M. The antibacterial action of colchicine and colchicine. J Pharm Pharmacol 1951; 3(7): 415-9.
[PMID: 14851212]

[149] Richter M, Boldescu V, Graf D, *et al.* Synthesis, Biological Evaluation, and Molecular Docking of Combretastatin and Colchicine Derivatives and their hCE1-Activated Prodrugs as Antiviral Agents.

ChemMedChem 2019; 14(4): 469-83.
[http://dx.doi.org/10.1002/cmdc.201800641] [PMID: 30605241]

[150] Biswas K, Das Sarma J. Effect of microtubule disruption on neuronal spread and replication of demyelinating and nondemyelinating strains of mouse hepatitis virus *in vitro*. J Virol 2014; 88(5): 3043-7.
[http://dx.doi.org/10.1128/JVI.02545-13] [PMID: 24352473]

[151] Worachartcheewan A, Songtawee N, Siriwong S, Prachayasittikul S, Nantasenamat C, Prachayasittikul V. Rational design of colchicine derivatives as anti-HIV agents *via* QSAR and molecular docking. Med Chem 2019; 15(4): 328-40.
[http://dx.doi.org/10.2174/1573406414666180924163756] [PMID: 30251609]

[152] Kim CS, Kawada T, Kim BS, *et al.* Capsaicin exhibits anti-inflammatory property by inhibiting IkB-a degradation in LPS-stimulated peritoneal macrophages. Cell Signal 2003; 15(3): 299-306.
[http://dx.doi.org/10.1016/S0898-6568(02)00086-4] [PMID: 12531428]

[153] Wang X, Yu L, Li F, Zhang G, Zhou W, Jiang X. Synthesis of amide derivatives containing capsaicin and their antioxidant and antibacterial activities. J Food Biochem 2019; 43(12): e13061.
[http://dx.doi.org/10.1111/jfbc.13061] [PMID: 31612542]

[154] Rivera MLC, Hassimotto NMA, Bueris V, Sircili MP, Almeida FA, Pinto UM. Effect of Capsicum frutescens extract, capsaicin, and luteolin on quorum sensing regulated phenotypes. J Food Sci 2019; 84(6): 1477-86.
[http://dx.doi.org/10.1111/1750-3841.14648] [PMID: 31132155]

[155] Santos MMP, Vieira-da-Motta O, Vieira IJC, *et al.* Antibacterial activity of Capsicum annuum extract and synthetic capsaicinoid derivatives against Streptococcus mutans. J Nat Med 2012; 66(2): 354-6.
[http://dx.doi.org/10.1007/s11418-011-0579-x] [PMID: 21858615]

[156] Molina-Torres J, García-Chávez A, Ramírez-Chávez E. Antimicrobial properties of alkamides present in flavouring plants traditionally used in Mesoamerica: affinin and capsaicin. J Ethnopharmacol 1999; 64(3): 241-8.
[http://dx.doi.org/10.1016/S0378-8741(98)00134-2] [PMID: 10363839]

[157] Flesar J, Havlik J, Kloucek P, *et al. In vitro* growth-inhibitory effect of plant-derived extracts and compounds against Paenibacillus larvae and their acute oral toxicity to adult honey bees. Vet Microbiol 2010; 145(1-2): 129-33.
[http://dx.doi.org/10.1016/j.vetmic.2010.03.018] [PMID: 20409652]

[158] Maiti K, Gantait A, Kakali M, Saha BP, Mukherjee PK. Therapeutic potentials of andrographolide from Andrographis paniculata: a review. J Nat Rem 2006; 6(1): 1-3.

[159] Singha PK, Roy S, Dey S. Antimicrobial activity of Andrographis paniculata. Fitoterapia 2003; 74(7-8): 692-4.
[http://dx.doi.org/10.1016/S0367-326X(03)00159-X] [PMID: 14630176]

[160] Kongyingyoes B, Priengprom T, Pientong C, Aromdee C, Suebsasana S, Ekalaksananan T. 3,19-isopropylideneandrographolide suppresses early gene expression of drug-resistant and wild type herpes simplex viruses. Antiviral Res 2016; 132: 281-6.
[http://dx.doi.org/10.1016/j.antiviral.2016.07.012] [PMID: 27424493]

[161] Mishra K, Dash AP, Dey N. Andrographolide: a novel antimalarial diterpene lactone compound from Andrographis paniculata and its interaction with curcumin and artesunate. J Trop Med 2011; 2011: 1-6.
[http://dx.doi.org/10.1155/2011/579518] [PMID: 21760808]

[162] Widyawaruyanti A, Asrory M, Ekasari W, *et al. In vivo* antimalarial activity of Andrographis paniculata tablets. Procedia Chem 2014; 13: 101-4.
[http://dx.doi.org/10.1016/j.proche.2014.12.012]

[163] Zaid OI, Abd Majid R, Sabariah MN, *et al.* Andrographolide effect on both Plasmodium falciparum

infected and non infected RBCs membranes. Asian Pac J Trop Med 2015; 8(7): 507-12. [http://dx.doi.org/10.1016/j.apjtm.2015.06.007] [PMID: 26276279]

[164] Megantara S, Levita J, Ibrahim S. *In Silico* Study of Andrographolide as Protease Inhibitors for Antimalarial Drug Discovery. Proceeding of 3rd International Conference on Computation for Science and Technology 2015. Jan 10 (pp. 36-39). [http://dx.doi.org/10.2991/iccst-15.2015.8]

[165] Wang X, Zu Y, Huang L, *et al.* Treatment of rheumatoid arthritis with combination of methotrexate and Tripterygium wilfordii: A meta-analysis. Life Sci 2017; 171: 45-50. [http://dx.doi.org/10.1016/j.lfs.2017.01.004] [PMID: 28088452]

[166] Patavino T, Brady DM. Natural medicine and nutritional therapy as an alternative treatment in systemic lupus erythematosus. Altern Med Rev 2001; 6(5): 460-71. [PMID: 11703166]

[167] Mao SJ, Huang XM. Tripterygium wilfordii Hook F is efficacious in the treatment of Henoch-Schönlein purpura nephritis in children. World J Pediatr 2016; 12(3): 375-6. [http://dx.doi.org/10.1007/s12519-016-0032-z] [PMID: 27351576]

[168] Alam ST, Hwang H, Son JD, *et al.* Natural photosensitizers from Tripterygium wilfordii and their antimicrobial photodynamic therapeutic effects in a Caenorhabditis elegans model. J Photochem Photobiol B 2021; 218: 112184. [http://dx.doi.org/10.1016/j.jphotobiol.2021.112184] [PMID: 33848804]

[169] Sharma V, Singh I, Chaudhary P. *Acorus calamus* (The Healing Plant): a review on its medicinal potential, micropropagation and conservation. Nat Prod Res 2014; 28(18): 1454-66. [http://dx.doi.org/10.1080/14786419.2014.915827] [PMID: 24824923]

[170] Susanah RW, Retno K, Dira SI. Total phenolic and flavonoid contents and antimicrobial activity of Acorus calamus L. rhizome ethanol extract. Res J Chem Environ 2018; 22: 65-70.

[171] Rahamoz-Haghighi S, Asadi MH, Riahi-Madvar A, Baghizadeh A. Antibacterial effect of Acorus calamus extractions against gram positive and negative bacteria. Ethno-Pharmaceutical products 2014; 1(1): 1-7.

[172] Rita W, Suirta I, Prisanti P, Utami P. Antibacterial activity of jeringau rhizome essential oil (Acorus calamus Linn.) against Escherichia coli and Staphylococcus aureus bacteria. Cakra Kim 2017; 5(2): 130-6.

[173] Rawal P, Adhikari RS, Danu K, Tiwari A. Antifungal activity of Acorus calamus against Fusarium oxysporum f. sp. Lycopersii. Int J Curr Microbiol Appl Sci 2015; 4(11): 710-5.

[174] Alankararao GS, Rajendra Prasad Y. Antimicrobial property of Acorus calamus Linn: *in vitro* studies. Indian perfumer. 1981. Available from: https://agris.fao.org/agris-search/search.do?recordID=US201302005358 (accessed on 7 october 2021).

[175] Kapil VB, Sinha AK, Sinha GK. Antibacterial and antifungal study of some essential oils and their constituents from the plants of Kumaon and its Tarai tract. Bull Med Ethnobot Res 1983; 4: 124-9.

[176] Vashi IG, Patel HC. chemical-constituents and antimicrobial activity of acorus-calamus linn. Comp Physiol Ecol 1987; 12(1): 49-51.

[177] Saxena DB, Tomar SS, Singh RP. Fungitoxicity of chemical components and some derivatives from Anethum sowa and Acorus calamus. Indian Perfumer 1990; 34(3): 199-203.

[178] Badam L. Badam L. *In vitro* Studies on the Effects of Acorus calamus Extract and Beta-Asarone on Herpes Viruses. Deerghayu international. 1995; 11: 16-8.

[179] Singh RP, Tomar SS, Devakumar C, Goswami BK, Saxena DB. Nematicidal efficacy of some essential oils against Meloidogyne incognita. Indian Perfumer 1991; 35(1): 35-7.

[180] Saxena BP, Koul O, Tikku K, Atal CK. A new insect chemosterilant isolated from Acorus calamus L. Nature 1977; 270(5637): 512-3.

[http://dx.doi.org/10.1038/270512a0]

[181] Vasant BS, Bhaskarrao DA, Bhanudas SR. Emblica officinalis-the wonder of ayurvedic medicine. World J Pharma Sci 2013; 3(1): 285-306.

[182] Variya BC, Bakrania AK, Patel SS. Emblica officinalis (Amla): A review for its phytochemistry, ethnomedicinal uses and medicinal potentials with respect to molecular mechanisms. Pharmacol Res 2016; 111: 180-200.
[http://dx.doi.org/10.1016/j.phrs.2016.06.013] [PMID: 27320046]

[183] Yadav SS, Singh MK, Singh PK, Kumar V. Traditional knowledge to clinical trials: A review on therapeutic actions of Emblica officinalis. Biomed Pharmacother 2017; 93: 1292-302.
[http://dx.doi.org/10.1016/j.biopha.2017.07.065] [PMID: 28747010]

[184] Lanka S. A review on pharmacological, medicinal and ethnobotanical important plant: Phyllanthus emblicalinn. (syn. Emblica officinalis). World J Pharm Res 2018; 7(04): 380-96.

[185] Baliga MS, Dsouza JJ. Amla (Emblica officinalis Gaertn), a wonder berry in the treatment and prevention of cancer. Eur J Cancer Prev 2011; 20(3): 225-39.
[http://dx.doi.org/10.1097/CEJ.0b013e32834473f4] [PMID: 21317655]

[186] Patil SG, Deshmukh AA, Padol AR, Kale DB. *In vitro* antibacterial activity of Emblica officinalis fruit extract by tube Dilution Method. Int J Toxicol Appl Pharmacol 2012; 2(4): 49-51.

[187] Kulkarni KV, Ghurghure SM. Indian gooseberry (Emblica officinalis): Complete pharmacognosy review. Int J Chem Stud 2018; 2(2): 5-11.

[188] Kumar KS, Bhowmik D, Dutta A, *et al.* Recent trends in potential traditional Indian herbs Emblica officinalis and its medicinal importance. J Pharmacogn Phytochem 2012; 1(1): 18-28.

[189] Baby B, Antony P, Vijayan R. Antioxidant and anticancer properties of berries. Crit Rev Food Sci Nutr 2018; 58(15): 2491-507.
[http://dx.doi.org/10.1080/10408398.2017.1329198] [PMID: 28609132]

[190] Jain R, Pandey R, Mahant RN, Rathore DS. A review on medicinal importance of Emblica officinalis. Int J Pharm Sci Res 2015; 6(1): 72-84. [IJPSR].

[191] Patel JR, Tripathi P, Sharma V, Chauhan NS, Dixit VK. Phyllanthus amarus: Ethnomedicinal uses, phytochemistry and pharmacology: A review. J Ethnopharmacol 2011; 138(2): 286-313.
[http://dx.doi.org/10.1016/j.jep.2011.09.040] [PMID: 21982793]

[192] Siraj MB, Khan AA, Jahangir U. Therapeutic Potential of Evolvulus alsinoides. J Drug Delivery and Therapeutics. 2019 Aug 15;9(4-s):696-701.

[193] D Ojha, C Maity, PD Mohapatra, A Samanta. *In vitro* antimicrobial potentialities of different solvent extracts of ethnomedicinal plants against clinically isolated. J Phytol 2010; 2(4): 57-64.

[194] Hossen SM, Sarkar R, Mahmud S, Aziz NA. Medicinal potential of Phyllanthus emblica (Linn.) fruits extracts: biological and pharmacological activities. J Pharm Res Int 2014; 1486-99.

[195] Dharajiya D, Patel P. in NM-CT, 2015 undefined. Antibacterial activity of Emblica officinalis (Gaertn.) fruits and Vitex negundo (L.) leaves. Available from: https://www.indianjournals.com/ijor.aspx? target=ijor: ctbp& volume=9& issue=4&article=007 (accessed on 7 october 2021)

[196] Vijayalakshmi S, Arunkumar V, Anju D, Gunasundari P, Moorthy P, Chandrasekharan AK. Comparative antimicrobial activities of Emblica officinalis and Ocimum sanctum. Anc Sci Life 2007; 27(2): 1-6.
[PMID: 22557261]

[197] Satish S, Mohana DC, Ranhavendra MP, Raveesha KA. Antifungal activity of some plant extracts against important seed borne pathogens of Aspergillus sp. Agric Technol Thail 2007; 3(1): 109-19.

[198] Hossain MM, Mazumder K, Hossen SM, Tanmy TT, Rashid MJ. *In vitro* studies on antibacterial and antifungal activities of Emblica officinalis. Int J Pharm Sci Res 2012; 3(4): 1124-7.

[199] Liu Q, Wang YF, Chen RJ, *et al.* Anti-coxsackie virus B3 norsesquiterpenoids from the roots of Phyllanthus emblica. J Nat Prod 2009; 72(5): 969-72. [http://dx.doi.org/10.1021/np800792d] [PMID: 19374435]

[200] Wang YF, Wang XY, Ren Z, *et al.* Phyllaemblicin B inhibits Coxsackie virus B3 induced apoptosis and myocarditis. Antiviral Res 2009; 84(2): 150-8. [http://dx.doi.org/10.1016/j.antiviral.2009.08.004] [PMID: 19699238]

[201] Xiang Y, Pei Y, Qu C, *et al. In vitro* anti-herpes simplex virus activity of 1,2,4,6-tetra-O-galloy--β-D-glucose from *Phyllanthus emblica* L. (Euphorbiaceae). Phytother Res 2011; 25(7): 975-82. [http://dx.doi.org/10.1002/ptr.3368] [PMID: 21213355]

[202] Liu G, Xiong S, Xiang YF, *et al.* Antiviral activity and possible mechanisms of action of pentagalloylglucose (PGG) against influenza A virus. Arch Virol 2011; 156(8): 1359-69. [http://dx.doi.org/10.1007/s00705-011-0989-9] [PMID: 21479599]

[203] Saranya B, Sarathadevi D, Somasundaram SS. Investigation of antibacterial activities of Evolvulus alsinoides (L.) against clinical pathogens. Int J Curr Microbiol Appl Sci 2015; 4: 491-7.

[204] Priya T. Antimicrobial Activity of Evovulus Alisinoids (L) Extract with Different Organic Solvents in Pathogenic Bacteria and Fungal Species. Available from: https://papers.ssrn.com/sol3/papers.cfm?abstract_id=3090982 (accessed on 7 october 2021).

CHAPTER 9

Delivery of Immunomodulators: Challenges and Novel Approaches

Mansi Damani[1], **Prabha Singh**[1] and **Sujata Sawarkar**[1,*]

[1] *Department of Pharmaceutics, SVKM's Dr. Bhanuben Nanavati College of Pharmacy, University of Mumbai, India*

Abstract: Immunomodulators can be either synthetic in origin or naturally obtained. Natural plant-based compounds can influence the immune system by either affecting antibody secretion to control the infection or affecting the functions of immune cells, thus contributing to maintaining immune homeostasis. Phytochemicals in plants, such as polysaccharides, lactones, flavonoids, alkaloids, diterpenoids and glycosides, have been reported to possess immunomodulating properties. However, there are many challenges limiting the clinical use of natural immunomodulators. In this chapter, we have discussed in detail standardization, formulation development, route of administration and regulatory concerns of natural immunomodulators. In order to overcome these challenges and ensure that natural immunomodulators reach the target site at therapeutic concentrations, different polymer and lipid-based nanocarrier delivery systems have been developed. These nanocarriers by virtue of their size, can easily penetrate and reach the target site and deliver the drugs. Many nanocarriers like liposomes, niosomes, nanoparticles, microemulsions, phytosomes and other vesicular systems designed for natural immunomodulators are discussed in this chapter.

Keywords: Drug Delivery Challenges, Drug Delivery Systems, Immunomodulators, Immunostimulants, Immunosuppressants, Immunoadjuvants, Nanocarriers, Natural Products, Phytoconstituents.

INTRODUCTION

Immunity is the ability of the body to combat a wide array of potential pathogens, resist diseases and prevent any organ or tissue damage. It comprises of series of balanced complex, multicellular and physiologic mechanisms that enable the host body to differentiate between self and foreign entity and eliminate it [1, 2]. Vertebrates have an extremely complex and advanced immune system, which is capable of producing a large variety of cells to arrest the growth of various microbes and the development of subsequent infections. The immune system is

* **Corresponding author Sujata Sawarkar:** Department of Pharmaceutics, SVKM's Dr. Bhanuben Nanavati College of Pharmacy, University of Mumbai, India; E-mail: sujata.sawarkar@bncp.ac.in

Vandana S. Nikam, Sujata P. Sawarkar, Girish B. Mahajan and Supriya G. Jagtap (Eds.)

not confined to any particular organ or tissue; rather, it is active for the entire body of the host. The immune system is simply a collaborative amalgamation between cells and proteins that work systemically to provide protection against infection or any foreign entity [3].

The development process of all immune cells originates from hemopoietic stem cells in the bone marrow. These cells either migrate to the thymus and differentiate into mature T-lymphocytes (T-cells) or remain in the bone marrow to differentiate and mature into B- lymphocytes (B-cells). B-cells differentiate into plasma cells, eventually producing immunoglobulins or antibodies. In a mature state, B-cells are generally found in bone marrow, spleen, intestine, lymph nodes and bloodstream. On interaction with a foreign entity or an antigen, B-cells mature into plasma cells and produce highly specialized serum protein molecules to destroy antigens; B-cells also mature as memory cells to ensure a quick response to the same antigen if the infection is encountered again. After leaving the thymus, T-cells populate either in the spleen, bone marrow, lymph nodes or blood and further mature into cytotoxic T-cells and helper T-cells for exhibiting cell-mediated immune response. T-cells have antigen-specific molecules that help them recognize and eliminate specific antigens. Helper T cells assist B-cells to produce antibodies and assist killer T-cells in their attack on foreign entities [4].

Immunity is categorized as active immunity and passive immunity. When immunity is achieved by exposure to a disease organism triggering the host immune system, it is an active type of immunity. This type of immunity is long-lasting and involves memory B-cells. Natural active immunity is achieved when the body is exposed to an infection or by introducing killed or attenuated forms of the disease pathogens through vaccination, called induced active immunity. Passive immunity is acquired when antibodies are directly provided to an individual without involvement or activation of the immune system. Natural passive immunity is attained from the mother to her child by the passage of antibodies either through the placenta or through breast milk. Passive immunity is transient in nature and lasts only for a few weeks to months but provides immediate protection in contrast to active immunity, which develops after a longer period of time, however, it is long-lasting [5, 6].

Over the past few decades, the health industry and biomedical research have collectively emphasized the importance and maintenance of the healthy immune system for prevention against various infections and rapid recovery from diseases. Ironically, immunity is not always as beneficial to the host body, especially when it causes tissue damage, hypersensitivity and or leads to other autoimmune diseases. In such cases, it becomes necessary to modulate immunity by suppressing it in order to treat autoimmune diseases or prevent graft rejection. On the other hand, in infectious and by enhancing immunity to fight off infections. Over the years, research has led to the development of a group of molecules that can target the immune system [7, 8].

NATURAL IMMUNOMODULATORS

Synthetic and chemical immunomodulating drugs have been used to treat cancer, graft rejections and other autoimmune disorders for years. For example, cyclophosphamide is a widely used alkylating agent that acts as an immunosuppressor against animal and human malignancies. It has the tendency to inhibit both humoral and cell-mediated immune responses. Cyclophosphamide, however, is associated with renal toxicity and renal failure. Synthetic immunomodulators are often associated with nephrotoxicity, hypertension, hepatotoxicity, hirsutism, gastrointestinal toxicity (nausea, vomiting, diarrhea, anorexia and abdominal pain), neurotoxicities such as headache, insomnia, pain, cardiovascular toxicity and metabolic toxicity like hyperkalemia, hypomagnesemia, hyperglycemia *etc.* Drugs like azathioprine used as a disease-modifying anti-rheumatic drug (DMARD) also affect rapidly growing cells, including bone marrow and gastrointestinal cells resulting in thrombocytopenia, leucopenia and gastrointestinal toxicity. Anti-thymocyte globulin, synthetically prepared polyclonal IgG component from the serum of various animals used in the treatment of renal allograft rejection causes serum sickness and nephritis. Some of the chemical immunomodulators also cause fever, leucopenia, thrombocytopenia, skin rashes and infertility due to the destruction of testicular and ovarian cells [9].

Clinical drawbacks and limitations of synthetic immunomodulators have led to increased interest in the study of natural and plant-based immunomodulators. Studies have indicated that many natural products have the ability to repair impaired immune systems either by activating the components of innate immunity, such as stimulation of macrophages and lymphocytes, or by modulating the cytokine profile and stimulating the process of apoptosis, thus reducing the incidence of infections. Natural immunomodulators can help potentiate humoral immunity (HI) or cell-mediated immunity (CMI) by causing a significant increase in serum immunoglobulin (Ig) levels and other mediators of CMI in various body fluids. Natural products also cause a significant increase in the populations of mature T cells, interleukins, tumor necrosis factor-alpha (TNF-α), interferons, *etc.* Natural immunostimulants can also activate humoral as well as cell-mediated immune response against tumors facilitating recognition and destruction of the tumor, and enhancing the ability of the host to tolerate damage caused by toxic chemicals [1].

There are many plants that are reported to have immunomodulating activities [9 - 13]. Various phytoconstituents isolated from plants belonging to chemical classes of alkaloids, flavones, saponins, glycosides, stilbenes, terpenoids, flavanols *etc.*, have shown immunomodulatory activity Table **1**. Similarly, various extracts of plant parts have also shown immunomodulatory activity Table **2**.

Table 1. Plants with immunomodulatory activities [12, 14].

Sr No.	Article-title	Phytoconstituent	Activity
		ALKALOIDS	
1.	*Piper longum Linn*	Piperine	Immunostimulant
2.	*Coptis chinensis* *Berberis vulgaris* *Tinospora Cordilfolia*	Berberine	Immunostimulant, Immunosupressant
3.	*Chelidonium majus L.*	Chelerythrine	Immunosupression
4.	*Corydalis turtschaninovii*	Pseudocoptisine	Immunostimulant
5.	*Sinomenium acutum*	Sinomenine	Immunosuppression
6.	*Sophora alopecuroides L.*	Sophocarpine	Immunostimulant
7.	*Leonurus japonica*	Leonurine	Immunostimulant
8.	*Lycoris radiate*	Lycorine	Immunosuppression
9.	*Stephania tetrandra*	Tetrandrine	Immunostimulant
1.	*Capsicum species*	Colchicine	Immunostimulant
11.	*Achillea millefolium C.*	Trigonelline	Immunostimulant
12.	*Pilocarpus microphyllus*	Pilocarpine	Immunostimulant
		FLAVANOIDS (CHALCONE, ISOFLAVONES, FLAVONES, FLAVANOLS)	
13.	*Semecarpus anacardium,*	Butein	Immunosuppressant
14.	*Humulus lupulus*	Xanthohumol, Dihydroxanthohumol	Immunostimulant
15.	*Mallotus, Philippinensis*	MallotophilippenS	Immunostimulant
16.	*Glycyrrhiza inflate*	Licochalcone E	Immunosuppressant
17.	*Ruta graveolens*	Rutin	Immunosuppressant
18.	*Camellia sinensis*	Epigallocatechin-3- gallate	Immunostimulant
19.	*Pueraria mirifica, Pueraria lobate*	Diadzein	Immunostimulant
20.	*Glycine max, Glycine soja*	Genistein	Immunosuppressant
21.	*Helichrysum italicum*	Arzanol	Immunostimulant
22.	*Myrtus communi*	Myrtucommulone	Immunostimulant

(Table 1) cont.....

Sr No.	Article-title	Phytoconstituent	Activity
23.	*Soinacia oleracea, Phaseolus vulgaris*	Kaempferol	Immunosuppressant
24.	*Citrus limon, Citrus sinensis*	Quercetin	Immunosuppressant
25.	*Lonicera Japonica*	Luteolin	Immunosuppressant
26.	*Cynodon dactylon*	Apigenin	Immunostimulant
27.	*Picea crassifolia*	Chrysin	Immunosuppressant
28.	*Scutellariae altissima*	Baicalein	Immunosuppressant
29.	*Scutellariae baicalensis*	Oroxylin A	Immunosuppressant
30.	*Artemisia princeps*	Eupafolin	Immunosuppressant
TERPENOIDS			
31.	*Zingiber zerumbet*	Zerumbone	Immunosuppressant
32.	*Andrographis paniculata*	Andrographolide	Immunosuppressant
33.	*Panax ginseng*	Ginsan	Immunostimulant
34.	*Phytolacca Americana*	Oleanolic acid	Immunosuppressant
35.	*Luffa cylindrical*	Echinocystic acid	Immunosuppressant
36.	*Centella asiatica*	*Asiaticoside,*	Immunosuppressant
37.	*Tripterygium wilfordii*	Triptolide, celastrol	Immunosuppressant
38.	*Rabdosia rubescens*	Oridonin	Immunosuppressant
SAPONINS			
39.	*Glycyrrhiza glabra*	Glycrhhizin, glycyrhrritic acid	Immunosuppressant
40.	*Bupleurum falcatum*	Saikosaponin-a and d	Immunosuppressant
COUMARINS			
41.	*Cnidium monnieri* (Fructus Cnidii)	Osthole	Immunosuppressant
42.	*Newbouldia laevis*	2-Acetylfuro-1,4-naphtoquinone	Immunosuppressant
43.	*Mammea americana*	Coumarin A	Immunosuppressant
POLYPHENOLS			
44.	*Curcuma longa*	Curcumin	Immunosuppressant
45.	*Dumortiera angust*	Manchartin C	Immunosuppressant
46.	*Arctostaphylos uva-ursi, vitis vinifera*	Gallic acid	Immunosuppressant
47.	*Morus alba, Arachis hypogea*	Resveratrol	Immunostimulant
48.	*Zingiber officinalis*	6-Gingerol	Immunosuppressant
49.	*Fallopia japonica*	Piceatannol	Immunosuppressant

(Table 1) cont.....

Sr No.	Article-title	Phytoconstituent	Activity
		QUINONES	
50.	*Nigella sativa L.*	Thymoquinone	Immunostimulant
51.	*Polygonum amplexicaule*	Emodin	Immunostimulant
52.	*Lithospermum erythrorhyzon*	Shikonin	Immunostimulant
		CAROTENOIDS	
53.	*Citrus sinensis, Daucus carota*	β-Carotene	Immunostimulant
54.	*Citrullus lanatus, Solanum lycopersicum*	Lycopene	Immunostimulant

Table 2. Plants extracts with immunomodulatory activity.

Sr. No.	Plant (Family)	Part	Extract	References
		IMMUNOSTIMULANT ACTIVITY		
1.	Root of *Withania Somnifera* (Solanaceae)	Root	-	[6]
2.	*Morus Alba* (Moraceae)	Plant	Methanolic	[6]
3.	*Picrorhiza Scrophulariiflora* (Plantaginaceae)	-	Methanolic, Diethylether,ethyl acetate, aqueous	[3, 6]
4.	Seeds of *Plantago asiatica* L. (Plantaginaceae)	Seeds	-	[6]
5.	*Panax ginseng* (Araliaceace)	Roots	Aqueous-Ethanolic	[6]
6.	Seeds of *Caesalpinia bonducella* (Fabaceae)	Seeds	Ethanolic	[6]
7.	Leaves of *Cynodon dactylon* (Poaceae)	Leaves	Aqueous	[6]
8.	Fruits of *Schisandra arisanensis* (Schisandraceae)	Fruits	Acetone	[6]
9.	Whole plant of *Toxicodendron pubescens* (Anacardiaceae)	Whole	Aqueous, methanolic	[6]
10.	Stem of *Tinospora cordifolia* (Menispermaceae)	Stem	Aqueous	[3, 6]
11.	Leaves of *Ocimum sanctum* (Labiateae)	Leaves	Aqueous	[3]
12.	Whole plant of *Achillea millefolium* C. (Compositae)	Whole plant	Alcoholic	[3]
13.	Leaves of *Andrographis paniculata* Nees (Acanthaceae)	Leaves	Alcoholic	[3]
14.	Leaves of *Murraya Koenigii* L. (Rutaceace)	Leaves	Methanolic	[3]

(Table 2) cont.....

Sr. No.	Plant (Family)	Part	Extract	References
15.	Fruits of *Lagenaria siceraria* Mol. (Cucurbitaceae)	Fruits	Ethanolic	[3]
16.	Roots of *Asparagus racemosus* (Liliaceae)	Root	Aqueous	[3]
17.	Whole plant of *Ganoderma lucidum* (Polyporaceae)	Whole plant	Aqueous,ethanolic	[3]
18.	Flowers of *Couroupita guianensis* Aubl. (Lecythidaceae)	Flowers	Aqueous, methanolic	[3]
19.	Heartwood of *Acacia catechu* (Leguminosae)	Heartwood	Aqueous	[3]
20.	Flower of *Hibiscus rosa sinensis* Linn. (Malvaceae)	Flower	Hydroalcoholic	[3]
21.	Leaves of *Urena lobate* Linn (Malvaceae)	Leaves	Methanolic	[3]
22.	Fruit peel of *Citrus natsudaidai Hayata* (Rutaceae)	Fruit peel	Oil	[3]
23.	Whole plant of *Cleome gynandra* Linn. (Capperdiceae)	Whole plant	Aqueous, ethanolic	[3]
24.	Fruits of *Randia dumetorum* Lamk. (Rubiaceae)	Fruits	Chlorofom, petroleumether, methanolic	[3]
25.	Bark of *Terminalia arjuna* Roxb. (Combretaceae)	Bark	Aqueous, alcoholic	[3]
26.	Stem and bark of *Bauhinia variegate* Linn. (Caesalpiniaceae)	Stem, bark	Ethanolic	[3]
27.	Leaves of *Gymnema sylvestre* (Asclepiadaceae)	Leaves	Aqueous	[3]
28.	Aerial parts of *Cordia superba* Cham. (Boraginaceae)	Aerial parts	Methanolic	[3]
29.	Fruits of *Heracleum persicum* (Apiaceae)	Fruits	Aqueous	[3]
30.	Leaves of *Moringa Oliefera* (Moringaceae)	Leaves	Alcoholic	[15]
31.	Rhizome of *Zingiber officinale* (Zingiberaceae)	Rhizome	Aqueous, alcoholic	[16]
32.	Seeds of *Argyreia speciosa* Convolvulaceae	Seeds	Distilled water and ethanolic	[9]
33.	Seeds of *Centrosema pubescens* Fabaceae	Seeds	Chloroform	[9]
34.	Whole plant of *Isatis cappadoica* Brassicaceae	Whole plant	Ethanolic	[9]
35.	Stem bark of *Mangifera indica* Anacardiaceae	Stem bark	Alcoholic	[9]
36.	Seeds of *Nigella sativa* Ranunculaceae	Seeds	Ethanolic	[9]

(Table 2) cont.....

Sr. No.	Plant (Family)	Part	Extract	References
37.	Whole plant of *Trigonella foenum* graecum Leguminosae	Whole plant	Aqueous	[9]
IMMUNOSUPPRESSIVE ACTIVITY				
32.	Whole plant of *Artemisia argyi* (Asteraceae)	Whole plant	Ethyl acetate extract	[17]
33.	Seeds of *Moringa olifera* (Moringaceae)	Seeds	Ethanolic	[18]
34.	Seeds of *Psidium guajava* (Myrtaceae)	Stems	Ethyl acetate	[19]
35.	Leaves of *Newbouldia laevis* (Bignoniaceae)	Leaves	Ethyl acetate	[19]
36.	Fruits of *Lagenaria siceraria* (Cucurbitaceae)	Fruits	Aqueous	[20]
37.	Leaves of *Momordica Charantia* (Cucurbitaceae)	Leaves	Diethyl ether and methanol extracts	[21]
38.	Leaves of *Santalum album* (Santalaceae)	Leaves	Water and ethyl acetate	[22]
39.	Leaves of *Emblica officinalis* (Phyllanthaceae)	Leaves	Water and ethyl acetate	[22]
40.	Leaves of *Butea frondosa* (Fabaceae)	Leaves	Water and ethyl acetate	[23]
41.	Aerial parts of *Achillea talagonica* (Asteraceae)	Aerial parts	Aqueous and methanolic	[24]
42.	Bark of *Madhuca longifolia* (Sapotaceae)	Bark	Methanolic	[25]
43.	Roots of *Boerhaavia diffusa* Nyctaginaceae	Roots	Aqueous/ ethanolic	[26]
44.	Whole plant of *Leucas aspera* Lamiaceae	Whole plant	Ethanolic/ aqueous	[27]
45.	Fruits of *Ogbignya phalerata* Palmae	Fruits	Methanolic	[28]
46.	Roots of *Tripterygium wilfordii* Celastraceae	Roots	Ethanolic	[29]
47.	Bark of *Uncaria tamentosa* Rubiaceae	Bark	Aqueous	[30]
IMMUNOADJUVANTS				
48.	Roots of *Aparagus racemosus* (Asparagaceae)	Root	Aqueous	[31]
49.	Roots of *Glycyrrhiza uralensis* (Fabaceae)	Root	Aqueous	[32]
50.	Leaves of *Azadirachta indica* (Meliaceae)	Leaves	Aqueous	[33]
51.	Leaves of *Butea frondosa* (Fabaceae)	Leaves	Aqueous	[33]
52.	Leaves of *Ficus religiosa* (Moraceae)	Leaves	Aqueous	[33]
53.	Leaves of *Calamus rotang* (Arecaceae)	Leaves	Aqueous	[34]
54.	Bulb of *Allium sativum* (Amaryllidaceae)	Bulb	Aqueous	[35]

CHALLENGES IN THE DELIVERY OF NATURAL IMMUNOMODULATORS

Natural immunomodulators have been considered a part of important therapeutic regimens since ancient times in many countries like India, China and Egypt. These natural products have been shown to benefit patients by providing relief from ailments. Naturally occurring immunomodulators are indigenous, easily available, economical, and associated with cultural beliefs.

Natural immunomodulators exhibit potential activity only when delivered at the target site in optimum concentration. Thus, it becomes extremely important to formulate the drug and administer it in a suitable dosage form so that its pharmacological activity gets enhanced manifold. In order to devise an appropriate drug delivery system, a study of the inherent physicochemical and biological properties of natural immunomodulators is essential. Natural products and phytochemicals isolated from them have large complex molecular structures and intrinsic instability, creating more challenges than success. These drawbacks have prompted researchers to design and develop new formulations that can deliver natural immunomodulators efficiently [36]. Following are the various challenges that limit the clinical utility of natural immunomodulators:

Standardization Challenges

Natural immunomodulators have been extensively used since ancient times for the prophylaxis and treatment of various ailments. Despite widespread use, these compounds are not the primary treatment choice. One of the reasons is the lack of an efficient, well-developed standardization protocol for testing natural immunomodulators [37]. Standardization provides assurance of batch-to-batch uniformity, confirmation dose uniformity unit and standard for comparison to understand any possible degradation during manufacturing. The official monographs, chemical markers and chromatographic specifications of natural immunomodulators are not well documented. Natural products are composed of many constituents and are, therefore, capable of biodiversity. The analytical limits for the active constituents present in natural product formulation cannot be so precise as synthetic chemicals. This is due to the variability of the plant material owing to different conditions of growth, harvesting, drying, and storage. For example, a study on the cultivation of St. John's wort showed that there was significant variation in the content of actives in the plant throughout the growing season, between the same plant species at different locations and also among plants at different sites within the same location. Such variations present a considerable challenge, especially for developing a uniform protocol for standardization. The extraction method, polarity of solvents and stability of phytoconstituents directly influence the composition and quality of extracts.

Standardization of natural immunomodulators requires the selection of appropriate marker compounds. Marker compounds are one or more constituents that occur naturally in the botanical material but may not necessarily be the active constituent. Selection of marker compound depends on factors like stability of the constituents, ease of analysis, amount of time and cost of analysis, potential relevance to therapeutic effects, stability and previous use by other manufacturers or researchers. However, there exists a lot of ambiguity in the selection of markers. For example, some of the *E. purpurea* products are standardized to specific citric acid content, while others are standardized to "total phenolic" content. Discrepancies in choice and evaluation of marker content exist since some natural immunomodulators like P. ginseng products are claimed to have been standardized to contain anywhere from 7 to 70 percent ginsenosides. Lack of sophisticated testing facility, lack of marker compounds, non-uniformity in the formulation of natural immunomodulators, presence of known and unknown adulterants, presence of microbes and aflatoxins and questionable safety-efficacy data of natural immunomodulators all contribute to challenges in the development of a proper standardization protocol [38, 39].

Formulation Challenges

Many natural immunomodulators, despite their extraordinary potential *in-vitro* findings, often demonstrate poor results in preclinical experimentation due to their low lipid solubility and permeability, resulting in poor bioavailability. A major challenge in developing the formulation of natural immunomodulators is the low yield of active components *versus* the substantial amount needed for research and development and for ultimate clinical use. Therefore, there is a constant need to improve pre-existing techniques or develop new methods for extraction, isolation, and high throughput screening. For example, it took around 30 years from the first discovery of the activity of *Taxus brevifolia* extracts till the development of paclitaxel formulations to clinical trials [40]. Even after extraction, the purification process of the active may require variable time depending on the presence of related and other unrelated compounds that may interfere with the separation and identification processes [37, 41, 42].

The preparation of extracts from plants is often non-reproducible. This creates a need for robust quality assurance methods when preparing crude extracts from plants. Most often, many plant extracts used traditionally by people have been prepared using either water or dilute aqueous ethanol. For example, Artemisia annua aqueous extracts are used as anti-malarial locally in Malawi. The main active compound artemisinin in pure form is insoluble in water. When researchers examined the aqueous extract of the plant, they found that a therapeutically relevant quantity of artemisinin was present in the extract. Later they attributed this to the presence of surfactant-type components in the plant that may have acted as natural solubilizers.

Cultivation of natural immunomodulatory plants is also another challenge in itself. The cultivation of such plants can be difficult since collection time, location, season, climate, weather, method of cultivation and environment can have an impact on the quantity of active compounds. Thus, cultivation of these plants requires careful handling, good manufacturing practice, and expertise in procedure, especially when some plants have slow growth and low concentration of actives. Also, isolation, identification, and testing of each compound need to be studied to understand the immunomodulatory mechanism of action and proper use; product quality and efficacy need to be guaranteed [43].

Administration Challenges

The route of administration of a therapeutic moiety is a significant factor affecting drug efficacy, biodistribution and pharmacokinetic profile. Most of the active phytoconstituents extracted from natural article-titles have high molecular weight and are susceptible to enzyme degradation. Thus, parenteral administration becomes the primary and undoubtedly most suitable delivery route for such drug molecules. However, parenteral administration has its own drawbacks, such as the requirement of medical intervention, invasive nature of the delivery mode, frequent dosing in case of drugs with short plasma half-life, long-term therapy and the possibility of fluctuating drug concentration in blood. These aspects are critical in case of management of autoimmune diseases and chronic diseases like cancers. In order to improve the convenience of patients and their compliance with the treatment regime, various formulation approaches have been explored to deliver natural immunomodulators *via* noninvasive modes like oral, transdermal, pulmonary, and nasal routes of administration.

Successful noninvasive delivery of natural immunomodulators still remains a challenge since each route presents its own distinct problems. Oral administration is most of the preferred mode of drug delivery because of its convenience and acceptability to patients. However, factors like large molecular size, hydrophilicity, inherent instability, limited intestinal permeability, low bioavailability, and susceptibility to degradation in the gastric and proteolytic enzymatic gastrointestinal environment limit the clinical use of natural products. These aspects eventually pose a major obstacle to successful oral delivery [44].

Skin delivery of drugs is also a convenient and noninvasive route of administration that addresses the major drawbacks of oral and parenteral delivery.

However, the stratum corneum, the outermost layer of skin, acts as an impermeable barrier, allowing this route to permeate only a few molecules. The required set of physicochemical characteristics for an active moiety to undergo diffusion through the skin include low molecular weight (<500 Dalton), a balance of lipophilicity (log P = 1–3) and water solubility (>1 mg/mL), a modest melting point (<200°C) and a low dose of less than 1000mg. Since most natural immunomodulators are large molecular weight compounds with some compounds being hydrophilic in nature and have high melting points, transdermal delivery of such immunomodulators may also seem a farfetched and difficult approach.

Regulatory Concerns

Although herbal remedies are safer to use since they are obtained from natural article-titles, toxicity can emerge from some inherent properties of herbal constituents, which can induce major adverse responses, or from interactions with conventional drugs. Toxicity may also be caused by misuse, abuse, and overuse of products like Cannabis sativa and by adulteration of products or misidentification of plants [45]. Often, the safety profile and article-title of toxicity of natural products may be unknown [46]. Thus, there is increasing worldwide concern about the safety of herbal products, with the accent lying on appropriate quality control and proper labeling of ingredients [47].

NOVEL APPROACHES FOR DELIVERY OF NATURAL IMMUNOMODULATORS

Since ancient times, herbal drugs and natural products have been used to relieve ailments and diseases. The effectiveness of natural products depends on the supply of active compounds Table **1**. These pharmacologically active compounds of extracts such as flavonoids, terpenoids, tannins, *etc.*, have excessively large molecular size, low absorption, cannot cross plasma membranes and hence show low bioavailability and efficacy. One of the possible ways postulated to potentiate the activity of natural immunomodulators is to deliver them to the site of action by conjugating them to nanocarrier-based delivery systems [48]. Delivery of natural immunomodulators by using nanosized drug delivery systems can have the following advantages:

1. Nanocarriers are nanosized drug delivery systems that work on the principle of Enhanced Permeability and Retention (EPR effect). By virtue of their size (10-1000nm); they can easily permeate into vasculatures and target tissue
2. They have high drug loading capacity and can deliver a high concentration of natural immunomodulators to their site of absorption
3. Since they deliver natural products at the site of action, any unwanted systemic

absorption of drugs is avoided, thus reducing side effects
4. Lesser amount of dose is required as compared to conventional delivery
5. Nanocarriers can be modulated for both active targeting and passive targeting of immunomodulators
6. Due to their small size, these delivery systems persist for longer times at the absorption site before getting cleared off.

Many nanocarriers like liposomes, nanoparticles, micelles, nanoemulsions *etc.*, have been reported to deliver natural immunomodulators [46, 51 - 56]. The advantages and limitations of each nanocarrier will be discussed in the upcoming section:

Nanoparticles

Nanoparticles are particles in the nanosize range (1-1000nm) with unique magnetic, optical, electrical and thermal properties. These particles can be synthesized from various materials such as polymers, lipids and metals like platinum, gold, silver and silica [55]. The drugs can be either loaded on the surface of nanoparticles or inside the core of particles. These nanoparticles can also be conjugated with a ligand such as hyaluronic acid, polysaccharides, glutathione, peptides and antibodies for better targetability [56]. The advantages of using nanoparticles as a drug delivery system are:

- Controlled and sustained release for natural immunomodulators
- Increase in therapeutic activity
- Decreased toxicity
- Site-specific targeting
- Use of polymers to achieve biocompatibility
- Can be used for various routes of administration, including oral, topical, ophthalmic, nasal, vaginal, parenteral *etc* [57].

Polymeric Nanoparticless

Polymeric nanoparticles are colloidal particles that are synthesized using biocompatible and biodegradable polymers. Owing to their size and long circulation time, they have been investigated for their use as carriers for immunomodulators or adjuncts in vaccines. Polymers used for these nanoparticles should be water soluble, biodegradable, non-immunogenic, inexpensive, non-toxic and easy to synthesize. Natural hydrophilic polymers and synthetic polymers can be used to prepare polymeric nanoparticles. Natural polymers used are gelatin, albumin, legumin, alginate, dextran, lecithin, chitosan, pullulan and agarose. One disadvantage that limits the clinical utility of natural polymers is difficult batch-to-batch reproducibility; thus, introducing the need for synthetic polymers like polylactic acid and polyalkylacrylates are introduced polycaprolactone, poly lactide-co-glycolides *etc.* Ionic gelation, nanoprecipitation, salting out, spray drying and emulsion cross-linking are some methods commonly used to synthesize polymeric nanoparticles. Polymeric nanoparticles consist of nanospheres (drug in the polymeric matrix) and nanocapsules (drug in cavity lined with polymeric membrane). The main routes of administration of polymeric nanoparticles can be intravenous, subcutaneous, intramuscular, ophthalmic, peroral or topical [57 - 60].

Polymeric nanoparticles have been reported to deliver many immunomodulatory agents like Coumarin-6, Curcumin, Paclitaxel, geraniol, ginsenosides, propolis extract and essential oils like Palmarosa oil, thyme oil, lavender oil, bergamot oil, orange oil and rosemary oil. Curcumin, a polyphenolic compound is a potent immunomodulator. However, clinical use of Curcumin is limited because of its rapid metabolism, insolubility, instability, poor tissue distribution and thus low bioavailability. Many studies have shown that polymeric nanoparticles can be used to overcome these limitations of Curcumin. Khan *et al.* formulated Curcumin entrapped poly lactic-co-glycolic acid (PLGA) nanoparticles. It was observed that entrapping curcumin not only increased the solubility of curcumin tenfold but also increased the distribution potential to a target site in comparison to free curcumin [61]. Shaikh *et al.* attempted to formulate curcumin nanoparticles with a view to improving their aqueous-phase solubility [62]. Curcumin nanoparticles were found to be freely dispersible in water in the absence of any surfactants and much more effective than curcumin against *Staphylococcus aureus, Bacillus subtilis, Escherichia coli, Pseudomonas aeruginosa, Penicillium notatum,* and *Aspergillus niger.* PLGA nanoparticles of curcumin enhanced the relative oral bioavailability of curcumin by 563% compared to the unformulated curcumin. The increased bioavailability was due to the inhibition of the P-gp-mediated efflux mechanism, allowing for an increase in permeability and absorption of curcumin in the blood [63].

Gingkolides and bilobalides are active constituents of Gingko biloba. These constituents show excellent cardioprotective, anticancer, neuroprotective and anti-inflammatory activity. The half-life of these constituents, when administered parenterally, is very less. Thus, poly lactide-co-glycolide and monomethoxy polyethylene glycol nanoparticles were synthesized and loaded with ginkgolides and bilobalide. Encapsulation efficiency was 79% and mean particle size was 123nm. The half-life time of the ginkgo compounds was moreover considerably increased by loading into the polymeric nanoparticles [64]. Wang T formulated Ginkgo biloba-loaded starch nanosphere to improve solubility, bioavailability, biocompatibility, and biodistribution *In vitro* to enhance the therapeutic efficacy of actives [65].

After systemic administration, polymeric nanoparticles have also been evaluated for their capability to cross the blood-brain barrier (BBB). Nerodilol-loaded nanospheres showed enhanced permeation in BBB and accumulation in brain tissue. Nerolidol was used to eliminate Trypanosoma evansi from the central nervous system in mice model after oral gavage [66]. Salvianolic acid B, an active constituent of *Salvia miltiorrhiza L.,* is neuroprotective in nature and can prevent nervous degeneration in various animal models. However, its poor chemical stability and low bioavailability severely limit its use. Poly ethylcyanoacrylate nanoparticles loaded with Salvianolic acid showed a modified release of Salvianolic acid B, distribution of nanoparticles within the injected hemisphere and their interaction with microglial cells. The encapsulation efficacy of Salvianolic acid B was about 99%, and the size was less than 200nm for easy penetrability. In another recent study, albumin nanoparticles loaded with andrographolide were evaluated for anti-Alzheimer activity in a mice model. The size of the nanoparticles was about 160 nm. When tagged with the probe, the nanoparticles were traced in the brain parenchyma, evidencing their ability to cross the BBB and could penetrate both undamaged and damaged brain tissues [67].

The above studies are some examples of research involving the use of polymeric nanoparticles as a promising strategy for the delivery of immunomodulators.

Mesoporous Silica Nanoparticles

Mesoporous silica nanoparticles are one of the well-studied inorganic nanocarriers for the delivery of drugs. These nanoparticles possess some unique characteristics, such as:

- Large surface area,
- selective surface functionality,
- high pore volume and porosity,
- adjustable size and surface potential,
- high loading capacity,
- tunable pore size and
- good biocompatibility

The synthesis of MSNs is simple, low-cost, and scalable. MSNs are synthesized using sodium silicate or tetraethyl orthosilicate as precursors under basic conditions in an alcoholic solution using a surfactant. Since MSNs have high drug loading capacity and effective cellular targeting, the drugs have minimal systemic toxicity and enhanced bioavailability [68 - 71]. Many natural immunomodulators have been entrapped on MSNs to achieve desired pharmacokinetic outcomes. Curcumin was loaded on folic acid–conjugated MSN for treatment of cervical carcinoma [72]. These nanoparticles displayed higher cellular uptake and sustained intracellular release. In order to prevent destruction by the Reticuloendothelial system (RES) Curcumin and Paclitaxel-loaded lipid bilayer-coated MSNs were formulated by coating with PEG. These particles showed a high degree of dispersity that could enable the intravenous administration of a hydrophobic drug, improve stability and dissolution ability and provide sustained release *in vitro* [73].

Ursolic acid, a natural triterpenoid found in many vegetables and fruits, is known for its anti-oxidant, anti-inflammatory and anti-carcinogenic activity. Ursolic acid-loaded MSN displayed high loading capacity, high cellular uptake and sustained release with improved bioavailability. The particles showed improved *In vitro* cytotoxicity and apoptotic activity in carcinoma cells [74]. Silybin, another immunomodulatory flavolignans isolated from milk thistle (Silybum marianum), is known for its hepatoprotective activity [75].

Lipid Nanoparticles

Lipid-based nanocarriers have gained considerable interest in a couple of decades. Lipid nanoparticles are sometimes preferred over polymeric nanoparticles due to the use of biocompatible and biodegradable lipids. Polymeric nanoparticles are often associated with toxicity and large-scale production difficulty. Lipid nanoparticles are easier to synthesize on a large scale, and biocompatible lipids make them preferable over polymer-based systems. Solid lipid nanoparticles (SLN) and Nanostructured Lipid Carriers (NLC) are two types of lipid nanocarriers. Such particles are known to improve solubility, absorption, penetrability, and residence time and help molecule cross biological membranes. Solid lipid nanoparticles (SLNs) are synthesized by enclosing drugs in a solid lipid core. These particles are in the size range of 10-100nm, and particles with a size less than 200 nm can even bypass liver and spleen filtration. Since drug molecules are entrapped in low mobility solid lipid matrix, these particles help achieve sustained release over other formulations.

Solid lipids such as monoacid triglycerides (tristearin, tripalmitin), steroids (cholesterol), fatty acids (stearic acids), waxes and fats are commonly used. Surfactants or surface-active agents like polysorbates, poloxamers, lecithin, phospholipids and phosphatidylcholines are used to stabilize these particles. SLNs may or may not contain other additives like cryoprotectants, preservatives and charge modifiers. Nanostructured lipid carriers (NLCs) are second-generation

SLNs. In NLCs, the liquid lipid is used along with solid lipid to create a less ordered matrix which can increase drug loading efficiency and prevent drug leaching or oxidation, a common drawback of SLN. High-energy methods like high-pressure homogenization, ultrasonication, and supercritical fluid technique and low-energy methods like double emulsion, phase inversion and microemulsion-based techniques are some commonly used methods for the preparation of lipid nanoparticles. Organic solvent-based methods like solvent injection, evaporation and diffusion are also used but not preferred owing to the possibility of residual organic solvents and interaction of organic solvents with drug molecules [76 - 82].

Some advantages of using SLNs and NLCs as drug delivery vehicles for immunomodulators are:

- SLNs and NLCs can be used for lipophilic and hydrophilic drugs
- Production yield is high, thus making industrial scale-up feasible
- SLNs and NLCs can control the release profile of entrapped molecules
- Since natural immunomodulators are entrapped in the solid matrix or solid-liquid lipid matrix, the molecules have improved stability
- Lipids used are similar in nature to biological lipids, hence more biocompatible in nature
- Particle size and surface charge can be easily modulated.
- Ligands can be anchored on the surface of lipid nanoparticles for easy targeting [76, 82].

SLNs and NLCs are considered vehicles of choice for the delivery of phytoconstituents, natural products and natural immunomodulators to help overcome absorption problems, low bioavailability and stability issues. Tryptanthrin, curcumin, citral, and thymoquinone are some natural immunomodulators that were envisaged for nanocarrier-mediated delivery [83].

One of the most widely used examples is Puerarin-loaded SLNs. Puerarin is an isoflavone immunomodulator found in various plants and herbs. It has a wide spectrum of pharmacological activities, including cardioprotection, antioxidant, anti-inflammation, vasodilation, pain attenuation and bone formation. With an attempt to accumulate Puerarin in higher concentrations in some tissues, the drug was formulated as SLN. Puerarin-loaded SLN showed rapid absorption, improved bioavailability and increased tissue concentrations in the heart and brain. SLNs formulated with stearic acid, lecithin and Myrj 52 and loaded with curcumin were investigated for efficacy in a rat model by intraperitoneal injection. SLNs had a mean average diameter of 190 nm, with 75% drug entrapment efficiency. Enhanced plasmatic and tissue curcumin concentrations, especially in the lung and liver, were obtained with the solid lipid nanoparticles when compared with free curcumin [84].

Triptolide, a natural product from the Chinese herb Tripterygium wilfordii, is known to cause irritation to the gastrointestinal (GI) tract. Thus triptolide-loaded SLN was formulated to improve solubility, and reduce toxicity, hyperemia, and irritation to the gastrointestinal tract by minimizing direct contact with the mucosal surface, gradual drug-releasing, and avoiding high local drug concentration [85].

Another example is andrographolide, formulated in nanoparticles based on compritol 888 ATO, glyceryl monostearate ATO lecithin and Tween-80, with entrapment efficiency of about 91% and drug loading of about 3.5%. Its bioavailability and antihyperlipidemic activity were improved in comparison to the free andrographolide, by increasing its solubility and stability in the intestine. Andrographolide was also formulated for brain-targeted parenteral delivery using Brij and compritol. SLNs were detected in brain parenchyma outside the vascular bed, confirming their ability *in vivo* to cross the blood-brain barrier [86].

Cantharidin, Noscapine and Terandrine are herbal immunomodulators isolated from Cantharis vesicatoria, Papaver somniferum, and Stephania terandra. Cantharidin-loaded SLNs showed a sustained release profile (half-life in circulation) without a burst effect and higher bioavailability after oral administration in rats induced with gastric mucus membrane irritation [87]. Noscapine SLNs could easily cross the blood-brain barrier and penetrate brain tissues for the treatment of glioblastoma with improved half-life and longer circulation [88].

Immunomodulators like Silymarin, tripterine, triptolide, curcumin *etc.*, are loaded on NLCs to overcome limitations like low solubility, permeability, and bioavailability. There are many examples to demonstrate how NLCs, by their size, lipid components and surfactant contents, have enhanced the absorption of these natural products [83]. One important example is the loading of Cardamom essential oil on NLCs. Cocoa butter was used as solid lipid, and Olive oil was a liquid lipid. Cardamom oil could not be used in the flavoring of aqueous foods, but with increased solubility ensured by NLC, using cardamom oil, NLC could be used as a food flavoring with good physical and chemical stability [89]. Thymoquinone, a monoterpene molecule found abundantly in seeds of *Nigella sativa*, is an immunomodulatory and cancer inhibitory agent. Thymoquinone-loaded NLCs showed improved oral bioavailability and enhanced anti-oxidant power in paracetamol-induced liver injury [90]. Similarly, Zerumbone (Zingiber zerumbet) and Citral (Cymbogon citratus) loaded NLCs showed enhanced water solubility, bioavailability, sustained release and low systemic toxicity [91 - 93].

Silymarin, from seeds of Silybum marianum, was proposed for protective activity in type 2 diabetes. In order to increase water solubility and bioavailability, Piazzini *et al.* loaded Silymarin onto NLCs synthesized using Stearic acid, capryol 90 and Brij S20. *In vivo* studies showed that silymarin-loaded NLCs increased the bioavailability of silymarin 2 folds as compared to silymarin suspension [94].

Metal Nanoparticles

Over the years, metal nanoparticles have been increasingly used to develop not only drug delivery systems but also for bioimaging, detection, photoablation and photothermal-based therapy. Many metals like gold, silver, platinum, iron, zinc oxide, selenium *etc.*, are used to synthesize metallic nanoparticles. Metal nanoparticles can be modulated into different sizes, shapes and morphology. The optical and magnetic properties of these particles can be put to use while delivering drug moiety for localized treatment. By virtue of their size and other properties, metallic nanoparticles can easily be functionalized with various ligands, antibodies, peptides and nucleic acids for drug delivery. Lack of reproducibility, low yield and toxicity are some factors that limit the use of metal nanoparticles. These nanoparticles gain their noncovalent interaction or covalent conjugation drug-loading capacity due to their surface plasmon resonance (SPR) ability, structural diversity, poor toxicity, and high biocompatibility. Thus, they can be utilized for achieving intracellular drug delivery and controlled release [95, 96].

Licocalcone A was loaded on hollow gold (HAuNPs) nanoparticles. The HAuNPs showed improved stability, solubility, biocompatibility, biodegradability and release of the compound and potential to be used as anticancer drug delivery carriers. This is because surface plasmon resonance is a unique property of gold nanoparticles which helps these nanoparticles to target specific tissue with the help of photothermal energy [97].

When a transitioning metal oxide like iron oxide is used to synthesize nanoparticles, the developed particle is magnetic in nature. Such magnetic nanoparticles can be used for various biomedical applications, such as magnetic resonance imaging, hyperthermia, drug delivery, tissue repair, cell and tissue targeting and transfection. One important advantage of the magnetic nanoparticle is its ability to reduce the concentration of drugs in healthy organs and diminish drug-related side effects. With the help of an external magnetic field, the release and uptake of these particles can be controlled. Gambogic acid from Garcinia hanburyi, a brownish orange resin, was loaded on iron oxide magnetic nanoparticles. These particles improved the water solubility of gambogic acid and halted the proliferation-migration of pancreatic cancer cells [98]. Another example of a magnetic nanoparticle would be the loading of gallic acid on iron oxide nanoparticles. Gallic acid is prone to thermal degradation, but gallic acid nanoparticles showed enhanced thermal stability and improved release of drugs from nanocarriers [99].

Some more examples of metal nanoparticles used for the delivery of immunomodulators are mentioned in Table **3**.

Table 3. Reported metal nanoparticles used for delivery of immunomodulators.

Immunomodulators	Metal Nanocarrier	References
Pod extract of *Amaranthus caudata*	Silver	[100]
Extract of *Camellia sinensis*	Palladium	[101]
Curcumin	Iron oxide	[102]
Brown seaweed *Sargassum muticum*	Zinc oxide	[103]
Argemone Mexicana leaf extract	Iron oxide	[104]
Ocimum basilicum mucilage	Iron oxide	[105]
Panax Ginseng	Silver, gold	[106, 107]

Liposomes and Niosomes

Liposomes and Niosomes are vesicular drug delivery systems that have been used to improve the therapeutic index of drugs by modifying their absorption, prolonging biological half-life and reducing metabolism and toxicity. Liposomes are made of amphiphilic molecules that, when placed in water, form a bilayered vesicle with hydrophobic segments away from the water. Liposomes can be used to entrap both hydrophobic and hydrophilic drug molecules. Phospholipids and sphingolipids are primary lipids used in the synthesis of liposomes. These vesicles can be easily coupled with site-specific ligands for active targeting. The size of vesicles varies from 25 nanometers to 2.5 micrometers. Based on the number of bilayers, liposomes can be classified as small unilamellar and large multilamellar systems. Niosomes are similar to liposomes but made up of lipids and non-ionic surfactants like spans and tweens. Niosomes are also made of lipids like phosphatidylcholine or cholesterol, which form a bilayer in an aqueous environment. Non-ionic surfactants provide stability to vesicles which makes Niosomes and hence makes them less prone to oxidation as compared to liposomes. Both Niosomes and Liposomes are flexible, biodegradable, non-toxic, biocompatible and non-immunogenic in nature. Since the structure of liposomal and niosomal bilayer is similar to biological membranes, liposomes can easily penetrate through the plasma membrane and into the cells. Thus, these systems are increasingly used to deliver large molecules and natural immunomodulators across cell membranes into tissues [108 - 110].

Naringenin is a flavonoid obtained from citrus fruits like orange and grapefruit. It has diverse pharmacological activities like anti-obesity, anti-diabetic, antifibrotic, anti-dyslipidemic and anticancer. However, on oral administration, it gets degraded into an active aglycone by the action of certain intestinal bacterial enzymes. Thus, with a view to stabilize the immunomodulator, Naringenin was formulated as liposomes. The size of liposomes was less than 70nm. Enhanced bioavailability (about 14-fold) of naringenin after oral administration was also observed by *in vivo* studies [111]. Berberine is anti-neoplastic in nature. Nanoliposomes of berberine and tariquidar (efflux pump inhibitor) displayed enhanced berberine chloride intracellular concentration in doxorubicin-resistant human erythroleukemia cells (K562/ DOXO) [112]. Some studies have also shown that essential oils can be loaded inside liposomes. The essential oil isolated from *Artemisia annua* L. was loaded in conventional liposomes and its anti-fungal activity was evaluated against 10 different drug-resistant Candida strains. The minimum fungicidal concentration of Artemisia annua essential oil loaded in liposomes, ranging 5 to 10 mg/mL, was much inferior than that of free essential oil [113 - 115].

Surface functionalization of liposomes helps to improve their pharmacokinetic profile and effectiveness. Artemisinin, a sesquiterpene lactone from the Artemisia annua L, was loaded on pegylated long-circulating liposomes. Conventional and long-circulating liposomes, with sizes of 130–140 nm and encapsulation efficacy higher than 70%, were injected in healthy mice. Free artemisinin was quickly cleared from plasma, and it was almost no more detectable 1 hour after the injection. By contrast, artemisinin was still detectable after 3 and 24 hours when formulated in conventional or pegylated liposomes, respectively. A metabolite of artemisinin, dihydroartemisinin, was also loaded on conventional and pegylated liposomes and studied for cell uptake, it was observed that Higher internalization occurred for conventional liposomes rather than for stealth liposomes, probably due to the hydrophilic steric barrier of polyethylene glycol molecules [116].

Niosomal formulations tend to show prolonged circulation, skin retention and sustained release when administered topically. Resveratrol-loaded niosomes were formulated for skin cancers using Gelot 64 (G64) as surfactant, and two skin-compatible unsaturated fatty acids (oleic and linoleic acids) as penetration enhancers. Ethanol injection modified method was used to synthesize niosomes (size about 400 nm). Resveratrol penetration was enhanced in the epidermis and dermis (EDD), with values up to 21% for both penetration enhancers [117]. More examples of natural immunomodulator-loaded liposomes and niosomes are mentioned in Table **4**.

Table 4. Reported liposomes and niosomes for delivery of natural immunomodulator.

Immunomodulator	Summary	References
	LIPOSOMES	
Verbacoside	Particle size was 120 nm, and 83% encapsulation efficiency. Prolonged anti-inflammatory and wound healing activity achieved	[118]
Curcumin	Curcumin-loaded pluronic liposomes showed slower *in vitro* release of curcumin as compared to free drug.	[119]
Serenoa repens L.	Enhanced anti-inflammatory activity anti-androgen and anti-proliferative response	[120]
Salvia triloba L. and *Rosmarinus officinalis* L	Stability, antibacterial activity and anti-inflammatory activity of liposomal essential oils improved	[121]
Salvianolic acid B w	The antihyperalgesic activity prolonged for 30 min after administration, and lasted for 45 min	[122]
Paclitaxel from *Taxia Brevifolia*	Enhanced solubility, biodistribution, cellular uptake and stability	[123]
Polydatin from *Polgonum cuspidum*	Improved solubility, sustained release and prolonged circulation time	[124]
Baicalein from *Scrutelleria baicalensis*	Improved solubility, sustained-release behavior, and better drug permeability	[125]
	NIOSOMES	
Rosemarinic acid from *Rosamarinus officnalis*	Sustained delivery and enhanced antimicrobial and anti-inflammatory activity	[126]
Embelin from *Embelia ribes*	Improved drug stability, sustained release of drug, bioavailability	[127]
Nerium oleander	Improved cell penetration, tolerability and *in vitro* cytotoxicity	[128]
Lawsone from *Lawsonia intermis*	Improved stability, sustained release, bioavailability, and permeability *In vitro*.	[129]
Spermacoce hispida	Improved stability, sustained release, bioavailability, and permeability *In vitro*	[130]

Polymeric Micelles

Micelles are polymeric core-shell structures in a nano-size range that are formed by the self-association of amphiphilic block copolymers in an aqueous environment. Several advantages like low toxicity, core-shell arrangement, biocompatibility, size, morphology, control-release property, high stability, tissue-penetration capability, high and versatile loading capacity, conjugation ability with ligands for targeting and high concentration at target site render polymeric micelles beneficial for drug delivery. Generally, three types of polymers are used in the synthesis of micelles. First, di-block copolymers, like polystyrene and poly (ethylene glycol) (PEG); second, triblock copolymers, like poly (ethylene oxide); and lastly, graft copolymers, like stearic acid and G-chitosan. The hydrophilic exterior of micelles helps to protect the entrapped drug from nonspecific uptake by the reticuloendothelial system. Thus, polymeric micelles exhibit several unique features that favor the delivery of natural immunomodulators [131 - 134].

Gou *et al.* conducted a study wherein curcumin was loaded on a polymeric micelle synthesized using monomethoxy poly (ethylene glycol)-poly(--caprolactone) (MPEG-PCL) micelles. Curcumin being a lipophilic molecule, conventionally cannot cross physiological barriers and penetrate colon cancer cells. However, curcumin micelles selectively accumulated in the colon tissue and exhibited cytotoxicity against colon cancer cells without affecting regular cells [135]. In another study by Abdelmoneem and team, berberine from Berberis plants and diosmin from citrus plants have exhibited good anticancer activity against Hep G2 liver cancer cells. However, they are not efficiently taken up by the cells. Berberine and diosmin-loaded casein micelles not only have improved solubility and targeted delivery but also higher cellular uptake against cancer cells [136].

Many other immunomodulators like camptothecin (*Camptothecin acuminata*), Shikonin (*Lithospermum erythrorhizon*) and *Sesbania Grandiflora* have been incorporated in polymeric micelles to improve solubility, biodegradability, cellular internalization, stability and sustained release [137 - 139].

Dendrimer

During the last few decades, it has been observed that dendrimers have been used to deliver a variety of anti-inflammatory, anticancer and antimicrobial drugs *via* various routes of administration. Dendrimers are the emerging polymeric hyper-branched architectures (size 1-100nm) that are known for their defined structures, versatility in drug delivery and high functionality whose properties resemble biomolecules. Their defined structure consists of core, branches and terminal groups attached to branches. The arrangement is such that there are many internal cavities for the encapsulation of drug molecules. Dendrimers have shown the potential to entrap or conjugate high molecular weight hydrophilic/hydrophobic moieties by various interactions and covalent bonding, respectively. The high ratio of surface groups to molecular volume has made them a promising synthetic vector for the delivery of both hydrophilic-hydrophobic natural products. PAMAM or polyamidoamine is a dendrimer class that is made up of repetitively branched amide and amine subunits. PAMAMs have a sphere-like shape overall, and are typified by an internal molecular architecture consisting of tree-like branching, with each outward 'layer', or generation, containing exponentially more branching points [140]. Recently, spherical-shaped dendrimers (150 nm) in diameter were prepared using polyamidoamine (PAMAM) and loaded with curcumin in order to increase its solubility and bioavailability. Curcumin solubility was enormously increased, and it was 415 times more soluble than free curcumin [141]. PAMAM dendrimers had shown positive potential for solubility enhancement and dual release profile when quercetin was loaded on PAMAM dendrimers to confirm their activity against inflammation [142]. PAMAM-loaded natural immunomodulators, which have been reported till now, are mentioned in Table **5**.

Table 5. Reported studies of dendrimers loaded with natural immunomodulators.

Immunomodulators	Article-title	Effect of loading on PAMAM dendrimers	References
Puerarin	*Pueraria lobata*	Improved oral bioavailability	[143, 144]
Silybin	*Milk thistle*	Solubility, sustained release and improved bioavailability	[145]
Anthocyanin	*Dacus Carota*	Improved stability, solubility, sustained release, and cytotoxicity	[146]
Liquiritin	*Glycyrrhiza glabra*	Improved biocompatibility, solubility, permeability, and stability.	[147]

Nanoemulsion And Microemulsions

Nanoemulsions and microemulsions are thermodynamically unstable, kinetically metastable dispersion of two immiscible liquids. These emulsions are of two types: oil in water (o/w) or water in oil (w/o). Multiple emulsion systems can also be developed, such as the water-in-oil-in-water (w/o/w) and oil-in-water-in-oil (o/w/o) emulsions. In contrast to conventional emulsions, nanoemulsions and microemulsions use surfactants to ensure the emulsification of one liquid into another. Surfactants/ emulsifiers stabilize the emulsion systems by reducing the interfacial tension resulting in the formation of small and stable emulsions. The size of nanoemulsions is usually less than 200 nm, and that of microemulsions is more than 200 nm to several microns. Both hydrophilic and hydrophobic drugs can be entrapped inside the droplets of emulsion.

Microemulsions and nanoemulsions have been proposed as drug delivery systems to enhance the absorption of natural immunomodulators across biological membranes. Some of the advantages include increased solubility and stability of drugs, ease and economical scale-up. Like every other delivery system, emulsions have some limitations:

1. Premature leakage/release of incorporated drug
2. Phase inversion problem
3. Many of the effective surfactants and/or cosurfactants do not have a pharmaceutically acceptable toxicity profile
4. Microemulsion and nanoemulsions systems often require the development of complex systems that may be time-consuming [148 - 150]

Recently Gupta and their team formulated a microemulsion loaded with green tea catechins and caffeine using Labrasol (oil phase), Cremophor EL (surfactant), glycerol (co-surfactant) and water. The studies extensively proved that microemulsions could well-preserve the antioxidant properties of the loaded constituents, and the formulation was also safe for mammalian cells [151]. In order to improve the oral absorption of extracts of *Vitex agnus-castus* L. and *Silybum marianum* L., Piazzini *et al.* formulated oil in water nanoemulsion (10-20nm) using Labrasol, Cremophor EL, Labrafil and water. The study proved that nanoemulsions improved the permeation of the characteristic constituents of the extracts, when compared with the unformulated extracts [152]. Self-micro emulsifying drug delivery systems (SMEDDS) are closely related to microemulsions. These systems typically consist of a mixture of surfactant, oil, and drug, that emulsify on being introduced into the body, in the form of droplets with approximately the same size range as observed in microemulsion systems [153, 154]. A self-microemulsifying drug delivery system, formulated with castor oil, Cremophor EL and 1,2-propanediol, was loaded in sustained-release pellets, for the oral administration of puerarin. The pharmacokinetic profiles and the bioavailability of loaded drugs were assessed in beagle dogs. The absolute bioavailability of puerarin loaded in the innovative formulation increased 2.6-fold, when compared with that obtained using a conventional formulation, while the relative bioavailability was found to be 259.7% [155]. Some of the studies formulated with natural products are summarized in Table **6**.

Table 6. Microemulsions, nanoemulsions and self-microemulsifying drug delivery systems for delivery of natural immunomodulators.

Natural Immunomodulator	System	Immuno-Modulatory Activity	Inference	Ref
Salicis cortex L. extract (40 mg/mL)	Microemulsion Triacetin, Tween 20, Labrasol and water	Anti-inflammatory, anti-angiogenesis, anti-apoptosis	Enhanced permeation observed in Caco-2 cells.	[156]

(Table 6) cont.....

Natural Immunomodulator	System	Immuno-Modulatory Activity	Inference	Ref
Serenoa repens CO_2 extract	Microemulsion	Anti-oxidant and anti-inflammatory	Enhanced oral absorption and improved stability in the simulated stomach and intestinal conditions	[157]
Serenoa repens CO_2 extract	SMEDDS	Anti-oxidant and anti-inflammatory	Enhanced oral absorption and improved stability of these nanocarriers in the simulated stomach and intestinal conditions	[157]
Tuscan unripe olives (*Olea europaea* L.), characterized by oleuropein (ca. 31%), ligstroside (ca. 3%) and verbascoside (ca. 2.5%)	Microemulsion Capryol 90, Cremophor EL, Transcutol and water	Anti-neoplastic, anti-inflammatory	Permeability was twice in comparison to unformulated olive extract. Better permeation in Caco-2 cells	[158]
Hydroxy-safflor yellow A (from *Carthamus tinctorius*)	Nanoemulsion	Immunomodulator	Improved bioavailability, stability and enhanced systemic absorption	[159]
Quercetin	Nanoemulsion	Immunostimulant, Anti-neoplastic Neuroprotective Anti-inflammatory	Increase in cutaneous permeability with lower skin retention	[160]
Basil oil	Nanoemulsion	Antibacterial	Enhanced antibacterial activity against pure *E. coli* culture	[161]
Curcumin	SMEDDS	Anti-neoplastic, anti-inflammatory	Improved solubility, stability, bioavailability, drug release and absorption *In vitro* Caco-2 cells	[162]

(Table 6) cont.....

Natural Immunomodulator	System	Immuno-Modulatory Activity	Inference	Ref
Camptothecin	SMEDDS	Anti-cancer	Improved solubility and stability. Lower toxicity in HeLa cells, MCF-7 and HL-60 cells.	[163]
Lutein	SMEDDS	Anti-inflammatory	Improved absorption and distribution	[164]
Curcumin	Nanoemulsion Medium-chain-triglycerides and natural soy phospholipid and poloxamer 188	Antiangiogenesis and antitumor activity	Curcumin nanoemulsion improved drug concentration at the target site and protection against degradation	[165]
Camptothecin	Nanoemulsion	Anti-cancer	The camptothecin-loaded nanoemulsions showed cytotoxicity of 60% against cervical cancer cells with encapsulation of > 90% camptothecin	[166]

Transferosome

Transferosomes are newer vesicular drug carrier systems composed of phospholipids and edge activator (EA), which is a membrane-softening agent (such as Tween 80, Span 80 and sodium cholate) that facilitates the ultra-deformable property of the transferosomes. Transferosomes consist of an aqueous core surrounded by a lipid bilayer. The bilayer makes transferosomes so flexible and elastic that they can easily squeeze in through the membranes and vessels. Compared to conventional liposomes, transferosomes are more deformable, smaller in size and with more permeation efficiency [167 - 169]. Natural immunomodulators can be easily loaded on the transferosomes irrespective of their size, structure, molecular weight or polarity. Over the years, transferosomes have been extensively used for the delivery of natural immunomodulators like curcumin, capsaicin, resveratrol, Epigallocatechin-3-gallate (EGCG) and colchicine. Natural immunomodulator, method of preparation, formulation and details of reported studies are discussed in Table **7**.

Table 7. Reported studies on delivery of natural immunomodulators using transferosomes.

Drug	Method of Preparation	Formulation	Inference	Ref
Resveratrol	High-pressure homogenization	Phosphatidylcholine, Tween 20, Plantacare® 1200 UP, Tween 80	Enhanced bioavailability, solubility, absorption and stability	[170]
Curcumin	Modified handshaking method	Ethanol:chloroform (1:1), lecithin, Tween 80 and Span 80, lecithin:surfactant ratio, solvents (ethanol, isopropyl alcohol), PBS (pH 7.4)	Potent anti-inflammatory properties and better permeation and bioavailability	[171]
Capsaicin	Thin film hydration method	Phospholipon 90G, tween 80, hydrated with distilled water, sonicated by bath sonicator	Reduction in arthritis and better tolerability	[172]
Epigallocatechin-3-gallate (EGCG)	Modified thin film hydration method+ high-pressure homogenization	chloroform:methanol (4:1 v/v), Soya phosphatidylcholine and sodium cholate	High skin permeation and deposition of EGCG	[173]
Colchicine	Rotary evaporation sonication method	Chloroform:methanol (2:1), Soy phosphatidylcholine, Cholesterol, Span 80, Span 60	Showed a 6-fold increase in transdermal flux and better and sustained antigout activity in rats.	[174]

Ethosomes

Ethosomes are lipid nanovesicular formulated using high concentrations of phospholipids and ethanol (50%) and water. Soya phosphatidylcholine, egg phosphatidylcholine, dipalmitoyl phosphatidyl choline (DPPC), and distearyl phosphatidyl choline (DSPC) are commonly used to form ethosomal vesicles. Ethosomes are capable of entrapping the molecules of a drug with different physicochemical characteristics like lipophilic, hydrophilic and amphiphilic nature. Ethosomes are vesicular systems preferred for topical and transdermal drug delivery because of their high permeability potential as compared to conventional liposomes. The presence of high ethanol concentration in ethosomes helps to penetrate into intercellular lipids by decreasing the density of lipid multilayer of the cell membrane and increasing the fluidity of cell membrane lipids. Ethosomes also have better compatibility with barriers as compared to ultra-flexible liposomes [175 - 177]. Many natural immunomodulators like colchicine, apigenin, ginsenoside, tanshinone C, and Berberi's extract were loaded into ethosomes for improved stability, bioavailability, and enhanced permeation and, in some cases, better transdermal diffusion [83]. Some of these studies are discussed in the following sections.

Tetrandrine is an alkaloid extracted from the roots of Stephania tetrandra S. (Menispermaceae family). Tetrandrine exhibits varied pharmacological activities such as anti-inflammatory, antioxidation, antisilicosis, antitumor, antiallergic reaction, and antiplatelet aggregation. The phytoconstituent has also been clinically used for the treatment of edema, rheumatic disorders, and inflammatory diseases. Commercially available conventional dosage forms of Tetradine, like conventional tablets and injections, are associated with drawbacks like low bioavailability, low patient compliance, hepatic and renal toxicity and intestinal damage. With a view to developing a novel delivery system for topical delivery of tetrandrine through the skin, Fan C *et al.* developed ethosomes of tetrandrine using phosphatidylcholine, cholesterol and ethanol. The mean diameter of tetrandrine-loaded ethosomes was 78.03 ± 0.24 nm with 52.87% entrapment efficiency. Unlike conventional liposomes, ethosomes were shown to permeate through the stratum corneum barrier and possessed significantly higher transdermal flux in comparison with tetrandrine liposomes [178].

Colchicine (from dried corn and seeds of plants of the genus Colchicum) was formulated as transethosomal gel with the purpose to improve stability, solubility, and bioavailability and enhancing skin diffusion and permeation of colchicine [179].

Many other novel drug delivery systems like phytosomes, cubosomes, nanocrystals, nanofibers, nanotubes, polymersomes and hybrid nanoparticles have also been investigated for delivery of natural immunomodulators. A summary of these nanocarriers, along with reported studies, is briefly discussed in Table **8**.

Table 8. Summary of studies on delivery of natural immunomodulators using nanocarriers

Natural Immunomodulator	Activity	Study	References
PHYTOSOMES Phytosomes or phyto-phospholipid complexes are lipid vesicular systems used for the encapsulation of drugs and plant-derived nutraceuticals such as polyphenolic compounds [180 - 183].			

(Table 8) cont.....

Natural Immunomodulator	Activity	Study	References
Epigallocatechin gallate	Anti-inflammatory	Nanophytosomal formulation of EGCG and egg phospholipid complex had lower particle size (100-250nm) and high drug loading capacity (90%). Phytosomal EGCG showed significantly better anti-inflammatory activity against acute paw edema as compared to free drugs.	[184]
Rutin	Anti-oxidant, anti-inflammatory, anti-thrombotic	Phytosomes of rutin were prepared to increase the oral bioavailability and transdermal permeation of rutin. The particle size of rubin Phytosomes was 266.4nm with an encapsulation efficiency of 95.61%.	[185]
Gingerol	Anti-viral	Phytosomes were prepared by blending gingerol with soya lecithin in organic solvent and then loading the solution in chitosan. Encapsulation efficiency was around 85%, and gingerol Phytosomes showed potent *In vitro* antioxidant activity.	[186]
CUBOSOMES Cubosomes are self-assembled liquid crystalline nanoparticles formed from the lipid cubic phase and outer corona stabilized by a polymer [187, 188].			
Curcumin	Anti-microbial	Curcumin-loaded cubosomes had a particle size of the formulation of about 75.2 nm and zeta potential -24 mv. The developed curcumin-loaded cubosomal hydrogel enhanced curcumin anti-bacterial activity in topical drug delivery.	[189]
Piperine	Anti-vitiligo therapy	Piperine cubosomes prepared using poloxamer and glyceryl monooleate were able to target up to 88.03% in the deep epidermis and could achieve better tissue drug bioavailability at the target site	[190]
Hinokitiol	Anti-microbial, anti-neoplastic	Permeation studies showed that the flux of HKL loaded in cubosome was much higher than in the case of HKL dissolved in water.	[191]
POLYMERSOME Polymersomes are bilayered vesicular structures formed by the self-assembly of amphiphilic block copolymers in solution. They have a hydrophilic inner core and lipophilic bilayer. This makes them a suitable candidate for loading both hydrophilic and lipophilic drugs [192 - 195].			

(Table 8) cont.....

Natural Immunomodulator	Activity	Study	References
Oxymatrine	Anti-hepatic fibrotic effect	Oxymatrine polymersome could overcome short elimination half-life and poor distribution of the drug.	[196]
Paclitaxel	Anti-cancer	Paclitaxel polymersomes were found to be more stable, more toxic than free drugs and accumulated in malignant lesions as compared to the conventional formulation	[197]
Bacosides	Epigenetic modulator	Polymersomes could cross BBB *via* receptor-mediated endocytosis and reverse the epigenetic changes of scopolamine-induced amnesic mouse brain	[198]
NANOCRYSTAL Nanocrystals are pure crystals of drugs within the nano size range. They have a high drug-loading capacity and excellent stability that render them to be widely used to deliver poorly soluble and hydrophilic materials in the form of a colloidal dispersion [83, 199].			
Curcumin	Anti-bacterial	Curcumin nanocrystals were prepared using high-pressure homogenization, to improve their solubility in acidic or neutral conditions and improve stability in alkaline pH.	[200]
Apigenin	Anti-oxidant, anti-inflammatory	Apigenin nanocrystals resulted in more rapid dissolution of apigenin from nanocrystals than from coarse powder with better plasma concentration	[201]
Quercetin	Neuroprotective	The dissolution profile of the quercetin nanocrystals was much higher than that of the pure drug at pH 6.8 and 1.2. The antioxidant activity and reducing the power of the quercetin nanocrystals were more effective than the drug itself.	[202]
NANOFIBERS Nanofibres are spun using the electrospinning method to give solid polymer fibers with diameters of 10–1000 nm that have a large surface area with a small pore size [203, 204]			
Lycium barbarum polysaccharide (LBP)	Neuroprotective	LBP nanofibers enhanced both proliferation and neuronal differentiation of PC12 cells induced by NGF, thus proving to be promising in nerve recovery	[205]

(Table 8) cont.....

Natural Immunomodulator	Activity	Study	References
Curcumin	Wound healing	Curcumin-loaded electrospun zein–silk fibroin–chitosan (ZSFC) nanofibers enhanced cell proliferation and adhesion, and they do not have any cytotoxic effect on HGF-1 cells.	[206]
Aloe vera	Anti-inflammatory	Aloe vera and PCL nanofibers were fabricated to enhance the regeneration of periodontium tissues.	[207]
Sophora flavescens	Anti-microbial	The nanofiber-loaded filters possessed 99.99% filtration efficiency and 99.98% antimicrobial activity against Staphylococcus epidermidis.	[208]
NANOTUBES Nanotubes are hollow tubes constructed from 2 different dimensional structures (tetrahedral and octahedral). Nanotubes have a high surface area, biocompatibility and loading capacity [83, 209, 210]			
Silibinin	Anti-cancer	Silibinin was loaded on carboxylated multi-walled carbon nanotubes and investigated for its cytotoxicity, which showed enhanced cytotoxicity to human cancer cell lines in comparison with free drugs. The release was pH dependent, and the maximum percentage release of SB from the nanocarrier reached approximately 96.6% within 1000 minutes when exposed to pH 7.4	[211]
Thyme oil	Anti-microbial	Thyme oil encapsulated in a capsule developed using halloysite nanotubes was effective in inhibiting E. coli, mesophilic aerobic bacteria, and molds and yeasts on fresh produce	[212]
Curcumin	Anti-cancer	Curcumin single-walled carbon nanotubes had a size of 170.4nm and a zeta potential of -12.5mV. In PC-3 cells, improved inhibition efficacy was achieved by curcumin nanotubes compared with free curcumin.	[213]
HYBRID NANOCARRIER (HN) Hybrid nanocarriers are composed either of the combinations of 2 different organic materials or a combination of an organic with an inorganic material to ensure enhanced drug delivery performance [83, 214].			

(Table 8) cont.....

Natural Immunomodulator	Activity	Study	References
Panax notoginsenoside-loaded core-shell HN (PNS-HLV)	Stop or slow down bleeding	Novel Panax notoginsenoside-loaded core-shell hybrid liposomal vesicles (PNS-HLV) were developed to resolve the restricted bioavailability of PNS and to enhance its protective effects *in vivo* on oral administration. PNS-HLV was stable for 12 months and was able to significantly inhibit the edema of the brain and reduce the infarct volume.	[215]

CONCLUSION

Since ancient times, traditional natural immunomodulators have always shown exceptional therapeutic potential to be used clinically. In fact, many actives isolated from botanical herbs have been used in various pharmaceutical preparations. One of the major shortcomings of the therapeutic use of natural immunomodulators is poor aqueous solubility and limited bioavailability. Also, their large molecular weight, degradation in the gastrointestinal environment, the requirement of high doses to elicit therapeutic effect, and inability to cross physiological membrane challenge their use in modern medicine. Thus, several novel drug delivery systems and nanotechnology are being used to alter the physicochemical properties of natural products in order to improve the targetability, control their release and alter their pharmacokinetic profile to suit the therapeutic requirement. Many nanocarriers encapsulated plant extracts are being explored and envisaged in pre-clinical or clinical phases setup to ensure safe and effective disease management. Thus, by virtue of their unique characteristics, Nanocarriers can help circumvent traditional limitations of natural products and be used as economic, patient compliant and therapeutically relevant drug carrier systems.

CONSENT FOR PUBLICATION

Not applicable.

CONFLICT OF INTEREST

The authors declare no conflict of interest, financial or otherwise.

ACKNOWLEDGEMENTS

The authors of this chapter would like to acknowledge SVKM'S Dr. Bhanuben Nanavati College of Pharmacy, Mithibai Campus, Vile Parle (W), Mumbai-400056, India

REFERENCES

[1] Nagoba B, Davane M. Natural Immunomodulators 2018.http://www.imedpub.com/

[2] Sharma P, Kumar P, Sharma R, Gupta G, Chaudhary A. Immunomodulators: Role of medicinal plants in immune system. Natl J Physiol Pharm Pharmacol 2017; 7(6): 552-556 [http://dx.doi.org/10.5455/njppp.2017.7.0203808032017]

[3] Kumar D, Arya V, Kaur R, Bhat ZA, Gupta VK, Kumar V. A review of immunomodulators in the Indian traditional health care system. J Microbiol Immunol Infect 2012; 45(3): 165-84. [http://dx.doi.org/10.1016/j.jmii.2011.09.030] [PMID: 22154993]

[4] https://www.ncbi.nlm.nih.gov/books/NBK27123/

[5] Baxter D. Active and passive immunity, vaccine types, excipients and licensing. Occup Med (Lond) 2007; 57(8): 552-6. [http://dx.doi.org/10.1093/occmed/kqm110] [PMID: 18045976]

[6] Singh N, Tailang M, Mehta SC. A review on herbal plants as immunomodulators. Int J Pharm Sci Res 2016; 7(9): 3602. [http://dx.doi.org/10.13040/IJPSR.0975-8232.7 (9).3602-10]

[7] Chaplin DD. Overview of the immune response. J Allergy Clin Immunol 2010; 125(2) (Suppl. 2): S3-S23. [http://dx.doi.org/10.1016/j.jaci.2009.12.980] [PMID: 20176265]

[8] Coffman RL, Sher A, Seder RA. Vaccine adjuvants: putting innate immunity to work. Immunity 2010; 33(4): 492-503. [http://dx.doi.org/10.1016/j.immuni.2010.10.002] [PMID: 21029960]

[9] Shukla S, Bajpai VK, Kim M. Plants as potential sources of natural immunomodulators. Rev Environ Sci Biotechnol 2014; 13(1): 17-33. [http://dx.doi.org/10.1007/s11157-012-9303-x]

[10] Ortuño-Sahagún D, Rawat AKS, Zänker K. Natural Immunomodulators 2018. J Immunol Res 2019; 2019: 1-3. [http://dx.doi.org/10.1155/2019/4341698] [PMID: 31781677]

[11] Mohan Sahoo B. Medicinal Plants: Source for Immunosuppressive Agents 2018.

[12] Mohamed S I A, Jantan I, Haque M A. Naturally occurring immunomodulators with antitumor activity: An insight on their mechanisms of action Int Immunopharma 2017; 50. [http://dx.doi.org/10.1016/j.intimp.2017.07.010]

[13] Amirghofran Z. Herbal Medicines for Immunosuppression 2012.http://journals.tums.ac.ir/

[14] Jantan I, Ahmad W, Bukhari S N A. Plant-derived immunomodulators: An insight on their preclinical evaluation and clinical trials front Plant Sci. front Plant Sci. 2015;6. [http://dx.doi.org/10.3389/fpls.2015.00655]

[15] Nfambi J, Bbosa GS, Sembajwe LF, Gakunga J, Kasolo JN. Immunomodulatory activity of methanolic leaf extract of Moringa oleifera in Wistar albino rats. J Basic Clin Physiol Pharmacol 2015; 26(6): 603-11. [http://dx.doi.org/10.1515/jbcpp-2014-0104] [PMID: 26103628]

[16] Rungkat FZ, Nurahman N, Prangdimurt EP, Tejasari T. Antioxidant and Immunoenhancement Activities of Ginger (Zingiber officinale Roscoe) Extracts and Compounds in *In vitro* and *In Vivo* Mouse and Human System. Prev Nutr Food Sci 2003; 8(1): 96-104. [http://dx.doi.org/10.3746/jfn.2003.8.1.096]

[17] Zimmermann-Klemd AM, Reinhardt JK, Morath A, *et al.* Immunosuppressive Activity of *Artemisia argyi* Extract and Isolated Compounds. Front Pharmacol 2020; 11: 402. [http://dx.doi.org/10.3389/fphar.2020.00402] [PMID: 32322200]

[18] Mahajan SG, Mehta AA. Immunosuppressive activity of ethanolic extract of seeds of Moringa oleifera Lam. in experimental immune inflammation. J Ethnopharmacol 2010; 130(1): 183-6. [http://dx.doi.org/10.1016/j.jep.2010.04.024] [PMID: 20435128]

[19] Ujam NT, Ajaghaku DL, Okoye FBC, Esimone CO. Antioxidant and immunosuppressive activities of extracts of endophytic fungi isolated from Psidium guajava and Newbouldia laevis. Phytomedicine Plus 2021; 1(2): 100028. [http://dx.doi.org/10.1016/j.phyplu.2021.100028]

[20] https://www.researchgate.net/publication/284816453_Immunosuppressive_activity_of_aqueous_extract_of_Lagenaria_siceraria_standley_in_mice

[21] Mahamat O, Flora H, Tume C, Kamanyi A. Immunomodulatory Activity of *Momordica charantia* L. (Cucurbitaceae) Leaf Diethyl Ether and Methanol Extracts on *Salmonella typhi* -Infected Mice and LPS-Induced Phagocytic Activities of Macrophages and Neutrophils. Evid Based Complement Alternat Med 2020; 2020: 1-11. [http://dx.doi.org/10.1155/2020/5248346] [PMID: 32256648]

[22] Anti-inflammatory and immunosuppressive activities of flavonoids from medicinal plants. https://www.researchgate.net/publication/322366107_Anti-inflammatory_and_immunosuppressive_activities_of_flavonoids_from_medicinal_plants (accessed Nov. 01, 2021).

[23] Gupta A, Chaphalkar SR. Anti-inflammatory and immunosuppressive activities of flavonoids from medicinal plants. J Herbmed Pharmacol. 2016; 5: 120-124. http://herbmedpharmacol.com/Article/JHP_1011_20160323162817

[24] Immunosuppressive principles from Achillea talagonica, An endemic species of Iran. https://www.researchgate.net/publication/235418450_Immunosuppressive_principles_from_Achillea_talagonica_An_endemic_species_of_Iran (accessed Nov. 01, 2021).

[25] V C, Ganesh D, Shrinivas S. Study of the immunosuppressive activity of methanolic extract of Madhuca longifolia (Koenig). Orient Pharm Exp Med 2010; 10(3): 150-4. [http://dx.doi.org/10.3742/OPEM.2010.10.3.150]

[26] Mehrotra S, Mishra KP, Maurya R, Srimal RC, Singh VK. Immunomodulation by ethanolic extract of Boerhaavia diffusa roots. Int Immunopharmacol 2002; 2(7): 987-96. [http://dx.doi.org/10.1016/S1567-5769(02)00031-0] [PMID: 12188040]

[27] Evaluation of Leucas aspera extracts for immunomodulatory activity | Request PDF. https://www.researchgate.net/publication/301514072_Evaluation_of_Leucas_aspera_extracts_for_immunomodulatory_activity (accessed Nov. 01, 2021).

[28] Pereira da Silva B, Paz Parente J. An anti-inflammatory and immunomodulatory polysaccharide from Orbignya phalerata. Fitoterapia 2001; 72(8): 887-93. [http://dx.doi.org/10.1016/S0367-326X(01)00338-0] [PMID: 11731113]

[29] Shao D, Dunlop W D, Lui E M K, Bernards M A. Immunostimulatory and Anti-inflammatory Polysaccharides from Tripterygium wilfordii.: Comparison with Organic Extracts 2008. Pharma Bio 2008;46(1-2). [http://dx.doi.org/10.1080/13880200701729588]

[30] Domingues A, Sartori A, Valente LMM, Golim MA, Siani AC, Viero RM. Uncaria tomentosa

aqueous-ethanol extract triggers an immunomodulation toward a Th2 cytokine profile. Phytother Res 2011; 25(8): 1229-35.
[http://dx.doi.org/10.1002/ptr.3549] [PMID: 21656603]

[31] Gautam M, Diwanay S, Gairola S, Shinde Y, Patki P, Patwardhan B. Immunoadjuvant potential of Asparagus racemosus aqueous extract in experimental system. J Ethnopharmacol 2004; 91(2-3): 251-5.
[http://dx.doi.org/10.1016/j.jep.2003.12.023] [PMID: 15120447]

[32] Xie YC, Dong XW, Wu XM, Yan XF, Xie QM. Inhibitory effects of flavonoids extracted from licorice on lipopolysaccharide-induced acute pulmonary inflammation in mice. Int Immunopharmacol 2009; 9(2): 194-200.
[http://dx.doi.org/10.1016/j.intimp.2008.11.004] [PMID: 19071231]

[33] Immunoadjuvant potential of Azadirachta indica, Butea frondosa and Ficus religiosa against Swine flu vaccine antigen. https://www.researchgate.netpublication322366425_Immunoadjuvant_potential_of_Azadirachta_indica_Butea_frondosa_and_Ficus_religiosa_against_Swine_flu_vaccine_antigen

[34] Gupta A, Shaikh AC, Chaphalkar SR. Aqueous extract of Calamus rotang as a novel immunoadjuvant enhances both humoral and cell mediated immune response. J Herbmed Pharmacol. 2017;6: 43-48. http://herbmedpharmacol.com/Article/JHP_1011_20160716111049

[35] Chandrashekar PM, Venkatesh YP. Fructans from aged garlic extract produce a delayed immunoadjuvant response to ovalbumin antigen in BALB/c mice. Immunopharmacol Immunotoxicol 2012; 34(1): 174-80.
[http://dx.doi.org/10.3109/08923973.2011.584066] [PMID: 21631395]

[36] Spreafico F. Problems and Challenges in the Use of Immunomodulating Agents A General Introduction 1985.

[37] Siri Sindhura D K, Jain V. Challenges in formulating herbal cosmetics. Int J Appl Pharm 2018; 10(6): pp. 47–53, 2018.
[http://dx.doi.org/10.22159/ijap.2018v10i6.27377]

[38] Kumar Malik M, Malik B R, Singh Thind B, Prakash D. Challenges in standardization in Traditional Medicine / Herbal Drugs. 2009.

[39] Silpavathi L, Das M K, Das A D. Challenges and prospective solutions in non-classical herbal formulations: A review. Indian J Pharm Sci 2019; 81 (6): 981-987.
[http://dx.doi.org/10.36468/pharmaceutical-sciences.595]

[40] Jachak S.M, Saklani A. Challenges and opportunities in drug discovery from plants. Curr Sci 2007; 92(9): pp. 1251-1257. https://www.jstor.org/stable/24097892

[41] Silpavathi L, Das M K, Das A D. Challenges and prospective solutions in non-classical herbal formulations: A review . Indian J Pharm Sci 2019; 81 (6): 981-987.
[http://dx.doi.org/10.36468/pharmaceutical-sciences.595]

[42] Vanan T. Challenges, Constraints and Opportunities in Herbal Medicines-A Review A review about herbs in siddha medicine which having inhibitory effect on RNA types of virus View project Challenges, Constraints and Opportunities in Herbal Medicines-A Review. Int J Herb Med 2014; 2 (1): 21-24. https://www.researchgate.net/publication/269106753

[43] Woods N, *et al.* Natural Vaccine Adjuvants and Immunopotentiators Derived From Plants, Fungi, Marine Organisms, and Insects. in Immunopotentiators in Modern Vaccines: Second Edition, Elsevier Inc., 2017, pp. 211–229.
[http://dx.doi.org/10.1016/B978-0-12-804019-5.00011-6]

[44] Homayun B, Lin X, Choi HJ. Challenges and Recent Progress in Oral Drug Delivery Systems for Biopharmaceuticals. Pharmaceutics 2019; 11(3): 129.
[http://dx.doi.org/10.3390/pharmaceutics11030129] [PMID: 30893852]

[45] Sahoo N, Manchikanti P. Herbal drug regulation and commercialization: an Indian industry

perspective. J Altern Complement Med 2013; 19(12): 957-63. [http://dx.doi.org/10.1089/acm.2012.0275] [PMID: 23829812]

[46] WHO guidelines on safety monitoring of herbal medicines in pharmacovigilance systems. 2013.

[47] Ann Liebert M, Stephen Forte J, Raman A. Regulatory Issues Relating to Herbal Products-Part 2: Safety and Toxicity 2000.

[48] Bonifácio BV, Silva PB, Ramos MA, Negri KM, Bauab TM, Chorilli M. Nanotechnology-based drug delivery systems and herbal medicines: a review. Int J Nanomedicine 2014; 9: 1-15. [PMID: 24363556]

[49] Silva P, Bonifácio B, Ramos M, Negri K, Maria Bauab T, Chorilli M. Nanotechnology-based drug delivery systems and herbal medicines: a review. Int J Nanomedicine 2013; 9(1): 1-15. [http://dx.doi.org/10.2147/IJN.S52634] [PMID: 24363556]

[50] Ansari SH, Sameem M, Islam F. Influence of nanotechnology on herbal drugs: A Review. J Adv Pharm Technol Res 2012; 3(3): 142-6. [http://dx.doi.org/10.4103/2231-4040.101006] [PMID: 23057000]

[51] Patra J K, *et al.* Nano based drug delivery systems: Recent developments and future prospects 10 Technology 1007 Nanotechnology 03 Chemical Sciences 0306 Physical Chemistry (incl. Structural) 03 Chemical Sciences 0303 Macromolecular and Materials Chemistry 11 Medical and Health Sciences 1115 Pharmacology and Pharmaceutical Sciences 09 Engineering 0903 Biomedical Engineering Prof Ueli Aebi, Prof Peter Gehr. J Nanobiotech 2018; 16 (1). [http://dx.doi.org/10.1186/s12951-018-0392-8]

[52] Sandhiya V, Ubaidulla U. A review on herbal drug loaded into pharmaceutical carrier techniques and its evaluation process. Fut J Pharmaceut Sci 2020; 6(1): 51. [http://dx.doi.org/10.1186/s43094-020-00050-0]

[53] Wani K, Tarawadi K, Kaul-Ghanekar R. Nanocarriers for delivery of herbal based drugs in breast cancer-an overview. J Nano Res 2015; 34: 29-40. [http://dx.doi.org/10.4028/www.scientific.net/JNanoR.34.29]

[54] Gupta S, Gupta MK. Possible role of nanocarriers in drug delivery against cervical cancer. Nano Rev Exp 2017; 8(1): 1335567. [http://dx.doi.org/10.1080/20022727.2017.1335567] [PMID: 30410707]

[55] Khan I, Saeed K, Khan I. Nanoparticles: Properties, applications and toxicities. Arab J Chem 2019; 12(7): 908-31. [http://dx.doi.org/10.1016/j.arabjc.2017.05.011]

[56] Serrano-Sevilla I, Artiga Á, Mitchell SG, de Matteis L, de la Fuente JM. Natural polysaccharides for siRNA delivery: Nanocarriers based on chitosan, hyaluronic acid, and their derivatives Mol 2019; 24(14). [http://dx.doi.org/10.3390/molecules24142570]

[57] Jawahar N, Meyyanathan SN. Polymeric nanoparticles for drug delivery and targeting: A comprehensive review. Int J Health Allied Sci 2012; 1(4): 217. [http://dx.doi.org/10.4103/2278-344X.107832]

[58] Zielinska A, *et al.* Polymeric Nanoparticles: Production, Characterization, Toxicology and Ecotoxicology. Mol 2020; 25(16). [http://dx.doi.org/10.3390/molecules25163731]

[59] Owens D III, Peppas N. Opsonization, biodistribution, and pharmacokinetics of polymeric nanoparticles. Int J Pharm 2006; 307(1): 93-102. [http://dx.doi.org/10.1016/j.ijpharm.2005.10.010] [PMID: 16303268]

[60] Nabila M, Jahan N, Penheiro DE. Polymeric nanoparticles for targeted delivery in cancer treatment: An overview Int. J Pharm Sci Rev Res 2018; 52 (1). http://globalresearchonline.net/journalcontents/v52-1/19.pdf%0Ahttp://ovidsp.ovid.com/ovidweb.cgi?T=JS&PAGE=reference&D=emexa&NEWS=

N&AN=624202638

[61] Khan MN, Haggag YA, Lane ME, McCarron PA, Tambuwala MM. Polymeric Nano-Encapsulation of Curcumin Enhances its Anti-Cancer Activity in Breast (MDA-MB231) and Lung (A549) Cancer Cells Through Reduction in Expression of HIF-1α and Nuclear p65 (Rel A). Curr Drug Deliv 2018; 15(2): 286-95.
[http://dx.doi.org/10.2174/1567201814666171019104002] [PMID: 29065834]

[62] Shaikh J, Ankola DD, Beniwal V, Singh D, Kumar MNVR. Nanoparticle encapsulation improves oral bioavailability of curcumin by at least 9-fold when compared to curcumin administered with piperine as absorption enhancer. Eur J Pharm Sci 2009; 37(3-4): 223-30.
[http://dx.doi.org/10.1016/j.ejps.2009.02.019] [PMID: 19491009]

[63] Xie X, Tao Q, Zou Y, *et al.* PLGA nanoparticles improve the oral bioavailability of curcumin in rats: characterizations and mechanisms. J Agric Food Chem 2011; 59(17): 9280-9.
[http://dx.doi.org/10.1021/jf202135j] [PMID: 21797282]

[64] Han L, Fu Y, Cole AJ, Liu J, Wang J. Co-encapsulation and sustained-release of four components in ginkgo terpenes from injectable PELGE nanoparticles. Fitoterapia 2012; 83(4): 721-31.
[http://dx.doi.org/10.1016/j.fitote.2012.02.014] [PMID: 22414318]

[65] Wang T, Wu C, Fan G, Li T, Gong H, Cao F. Ginkgo biloba extracts-loaded starch nano-spheres: Preparation, characterization, and *In vitro* release kinetics. Int J Biol Macromol 2018; 106: 148-57.
[http://dx.doi.org/10.1016/j.ijbiomac.2017.08.012] [PMID: 28780415]

[66] Baldissera MD, Souza CF, Grando TH, *et al.* Nerolidol-loaded nanospheres prevent hepatic oxidative stress of mice infected by *Trypanosoma evansi*. Parasitology 2017; 144(2): 148-57.
[http://dx.doi.org/10.1017/S0031182016001803] [PMID: 27748203]

[67] Grossi C, Guccione C, Isacchi B, *et al.* Development of Blood-Brain Barrier Permeable Nanoparticles as Potential Carriers for Salvianolic Acid B to CNS. Planta Med 2016; 83(5): 382-91.
[http://dx.doi.org/10.1055/s-0042-101945] [PMID: 27002395]

[68] Pednekar PP, Godiyal SC, Jadhav KR, Kadam VJ. Mesoporous silica nanoparticles: a promising multifunctional drug delivery system. Nanostructures for Cancer Therapy 2017; (Jan): 593-621.
[http://dx.doi.org/10.1016/B978-0-323-46144-3.00023-4]

[69] Bharti C, Gulati N, Nagaich U, Pal AK. Mesoporous silica nanoparticles in target drug delivery system: A review. Int J Pharm Investig 2015; 5(3): 124-33.
[http://dx.doi.org/10.4103/2230-973X.160844] [PMID: 26258053]

[70] Vallet-Regí M. Mesoporous Silica Nanoparticles: Their Projection in Nanomedicine. ISRN Materials Science 2012; 2012: 1-20.
[http://dx.doi.org/10.5402/2012/608548]

[71] Tang F, Li L, Chen D. Mesoporous silica nanoparticles: synthesis, biocompatibility and drug delivery. Adv Mater 2012; 24(12): 1504-34.
[http://dx.doi.org/10.1002/adma.201104763] [PMID: 22378538]

[72] Thulasidasan AKT, Retnakumari AP, Shankar M, *et al.* Folic acid conjugation improves the bioavailability and chemosensitizing efficacy of curcumin-encapsulated PLGA-PEG nanoparticles towards paclitaxel chemotherapy. Oncotarget 2017; 8(64): 107374-89.
[http://dx.doi.org/10.18632/oncotarget.22376] [PMID: 29296172]

[73] Gao J, Fan K, Jin Y, *et al.* PEGylated lipid bilayer coated mesoporous silica nanoparticles co-delivery of paclitaxel and curcumin leads to increased tumor site drug accumulation and reduced tumor burden. Eur J Pharm Sci 2019; 140: 105070.
[http://dx.doi.org/10.1016/j.ejps.2019.105070] [PMID: 31518679]

[74] Li T, Chen X, liu Y et al., pH-Sensitive mesoporous silica nanoparticles anticancer prodrugs for sustained release of ursolic acid and the enhanced anti-cancer efficacy for hepatocellular carcinoma cancer. Eur J Pharmaceut Sci 2017; 96: 456-63.

[http://dx.doi.org/10.1016/j.ejps.2016.10.019]

[75] Nasr S S, Nasra M M A, Hazzah H A, Abdallah O Y. Mesoporous silica nanoparticles, a safe option for silymarin delivery: preparation, characterization, and *in vivo* evaluation. 2019; 9(5): 968-79. [http://dx.doi.org/10.1007/s13346-019-00640-3]

[76] Dhiman N, Awasthi R, Sharma B, Kharkwal H, Kulkarni G T. Lipid Nanoparticles as Carriers for Bioactive Delivery. Front Chem. 2021; 9: 23. [http://dx.doi.org/10.3389/fchem.2021.580118]

[77] Sandhiya V, Ubaidulla U. A review on herbal drug loaded into pharmaceutical carrier techniques and its evaluation process. Fut J Pharmaceut Sci 2020; 6(1): 1-16. [http://dx.doi.org/10.1186/s43094-020-00050-0]

[78] Ansari SH, Sameem M, Islam F. Influence of nanotechnology on herbal drugs: A Review. J Adv Pharm Technol Res 2012; 3(3): 142-6. [http://dx.doi.org/10.4103/2231-4040.101006] [PMID: 23057000]

[79] Vijayanand P, Jyothi V, Aditya N, Mounika A. Development and Characterization of Solid Lipid Nanoparticles Containing Herbal Extract: *In Vivo* Antidepressant Activity. J Drug Deliv 2018; 2018: 1-7. [http://dx.doi.org/10.1155/2018/2908626] [PMID: 29973993]

[80] Mukherjee S, Ray S, Thakur RS. Solid lipid nanoparticles: A modern formulation approach in drug delivery system. Indian J Pharm Sci 2009; 71(4): 349-58. [http://dx.doi.org/10.4103/0250-474X.57282] [PMID: 20502539]

[81] Scioli Montoto S, Muraca G, Ruiz ME. Solid Lipid Nanoparticles for Drug Delivery: Pharmacological and Biopharmaceutical Aspects. Front Mol Biosci 2020; 7: 587997. [http://dx.doi.org/10.3389/fmolb.2020.587997] [PMID: 33195435]

[82] Chuang S Y, Lin C H, Huang T H, Fang J Y. Lipid-Based nanoparticles as a potential delivery approach in the treatment of rheumatoid arthritis. Nanomater 2018; 8(1). [http://dx.doi.org/10.3390/nano8010042]

[83] Rahman HS, Othman HH, Hammadi NI, *et al.* Novel drug delivery systems for loading of natural plant extracts and their biomedical applications. Int J Nanomedicine. 2020; 15: 2439-2483. [http://dx.doi.org/10.2147/IJN.S227805]

[84] Luo CF, Chen M-S, Professor Yuan , *et al.* Metabolic profile of puerarin in rats after intragastric administration of puerarin solid lipid nanoparticles. Int J Nanomedicine 2013; 8: 933-40. [http://dx.doi.org/10.2147/IJN.S39349] [PMID: 23486407]

[85] Zhang C, Gu C, Peng F, *et al.* Preparation and Optimization of Triptolide-Loaded Solid Lipid Nanoparticles for Oral Delivery with Reduced Gastric Irritation. Molecules. 2013; 18 (11): 13340–13356. [http://dx.doi.org/10.3390/molecules181113340]

[86] Graverini G, Piazzini V, Landucci E, *et al.* Solid lipid nanoparticles for delivery of andrographolide across the blood-brain barrier: *In vitro* and *in vivo* evaluation. Colloids Surf B Biointerfaces 2018; 161: 302-13. [http://dx.doi.org/10.1016/j.colsurfb.2017.10.062] [PMID: 29096375]

[87] Dang Y-J, Zhu C-Y. Oral bioavailability of cantharidin-loaded solid lipid nanoparticles Chinese Med 2013; 8(1). [http://dx.doi.org/10.1186/1749-8546-8-1]

[88] Madan J, Pandey RS, Jain V, Katare OP, Chandra R, Katyal A. Poly (ethylene)-glycol conjugated solid lipid nanoparticles of noscapine improve biological half-life, brain delivery and efficacy in glioblastoma cells. Nanomedicine 2013; 9(4): 492-503. [http://dx.doi.org/10.1016/j.nano.2012.10.003] [PMID: 23117045]

[89] Keivani Nahr F, Ghanbarzadeh B, Hamishehkar H, Samadi Kafil H. Food grade nanostructured lipid

carrier for cardamom essential oil: Preparation, characterization and antimicrobial activity. J Funct Foods 2018; 40: 1-8.
[http://dx.doi.org/10.1016/j.jff.2017.09.028]

[90] Ong YS, Saiful Yazan L, Ng WK, *et al.* Thymoquinone loaded in nanostructured lipid carrier showed enhanced anticancer activity in 4T1 tumor-bearing mice. Nanomedicine (Lond) 2018; 13(13): 1567-82.
[http://dx.doi.org/10.2217/nnm-2017-0322] [PMID: 30028248]

[91] Nordin N, Yeap SK, Zamberi NR, *et al.* Characterization and toxicity of citral incorporated with nanostructured lipid carrier. PeerJ 2018; 6(1): e3916.
[http://dx.doi.org/10.7717/peerj.3916] [PMID: 29312812]

[92] Mohamad NE, Abu N, Rahman HS, *et al.* Nanostructured lipid carrier improved *in vivo* anti-tumor and immunomodulatory effect of Zerumbone in 4T1 challenged mice. RSC Advances 2015; 5(28): 22066-74.
[http://dx.doi.org/10.1039/C5RA00144G]

[93] Rasedee A, Abdul AB, Zeenathul NA, *et al.* Zerumbone-loaded nanostructured lipid carrier induces G2/M cell cycle arrest and apoptosis *via* mitochondrial pathway in a human lymphoblastic leukemia cell line. Int J Nanomedicine 2014; 9(1): 527-38.
[http://dx.doi.org/10.2147/IJN.S54346] [PMID: 24549090]

[94] Piazzini V, Micheli L, Luceri C, *et al.* Nanostructured lipid carriers for oral delivery of silymarin: Improving its absorption and *in vivo* efficacy in type 2 diabetes and metabolic syndrome model. Int J Pharm 2019; 572: 118838.
[http://dx.doi.org/10.1016/j.ijpharm.2019.118838] [PMID: 31715362]

[95] Luo YH, Chang LW, Lin P. Metal-Based Nanoparticles and the Immune System: Activation, Inflammation, and Potential Applications. BioMed Res Int 2015; 2015: 1-12.
[http://dx.doi.org/10.1155/2015/143720] [PMID: 26125021]

[96] Patra J K, *et al.* Nano based drug delivery systems: Recent developments and future prospects 10 technology 1007 nanotechnology 03 chemical sciences 0306 physical chemistry (incl. structural) 03 chemical sciences 0303 macromolecular and materials chemistry 11 medical and health sciences 1115 pharmacology and pharmaceutical sciences 09 engineering 0903 biomedical engineering prof ueli aebi, prof peter gehr. J Nanobiotech 2018; 16 (1).
[http://dx.doi.org/10.1186/s12951-018-0392-8]

[97] Sun YW, Wang LH, Meng DL, Che X. A green and facile preparation approach, licochalcone A capped on hollow gold nanoparticles, for improving the solubility and dissolution of anticancer natural product. Oncotarget 2017; 8(62): 105673-81.
[http://dx.doi.org/10.18632/oncotarget.22387] [PMID: 29285282]

[98] Chen B, Cailian W, Zhang H, Shi F, Chen B. Gambogic acid-loaded magnetic Fe_3O_4 nanoparticles inhibit Panc-1 pancreatic cancer cell proliferation and migration by inactivating transcription factor ETS1. Int J Nanomedicine 2012; 7: 781-7.
[http://dx.doi.org/10.2147/IJN.S28509] [PMID: 22393285]

[99] Dorniani D, Kura AU, Ahmad Z, Halim Shaari A, Hussein MZ, Fakurazi S. Preparation of Fe3O4 magnetic nanoparticles coated with gallic acid for drug delivery. Int J Nanomedicine 2012; 7: 5745-56.
[http://dx.doi.org/10.2147/IJN.S35746] [PMID: 23166439]

[100] Azeez L, Lateef A, Adebisi S A. Silver nanoparticles (AgNPs) biosynthesized using pod extract of Cola nitida enhances antioxidant activity and phytochemical composition of Amaranthus caudatus Linn. Appl Nanosci 2017; 7(1).
[http://dx.doi.org/10.1007/s13204-017-0546-2]

[101] Azizi S, Mahdavi Shahri M, Rahman H, Abdul Rahim R, Rasedee A, Mohamad R. Green synthesis palladium nanoparticles mediated by white tea (*Camellia sinensis*) extract with antioxidant, antibacterial, and antiproliferative activities toward the human leukemia (MOLT-4) cell line. Int J

Nanomedicine 2017; 12: 8841-53.
[http://dx.doi.org/10.2147/IJN.S149371] [PMID: 29276385]

[102] Danafar H, Sharafi A, Askarlou S, Manjili H. Preparation and Characterization of PEGylated Iron Oxide-Gold Nanoparticles for Delivery of Sulforaphane and Curcumin. Drug Res (Stuttg) 2017; 67(12): 698-704.
[http://dx.doi.org/10.1055/s-0043-115905] [PMID: 28738425]

[103] Namvar F, Rahman HS, Mohamad R, *et al.* Cytotoxic effects of biosynthesized zinc oxide nanoparticles on murine cell lines. Evid Based Complement Alternat Med 2015; 2015: 1-11.
[http://dx.doi.org/10.1155/2015/593014] [PMID: 25784947]

[104] Arokiyaraj S, Saravanan M, Udaya Prakash NK, Valan Arasu M, Vijayakumar B, Vincent S. Enhanced antibacterial activity of iron oxide magnetic nanoparticles treated with Argemone mexicana L. leaf extract: An *In vitro* study. Mater Res Bull 2013; 48(9): 3323-7.
[http://dx.doi.org/10.1016/j.materresbull.2013.05.059]

[105] Allafchian A, Jalali SAH, Hosseini F, Massoud M. Ocimum basilicum mucilage as a new green polymer support for silver in magnetic nanocomposites: Production and characterization. J Environ Chem Eng 2017; 5(6): 5912-20.
[http://dx.doi.org/10.1016/j.jece.2017.11.023]

[106] Singh P, Kim YJ, Wang C, Mathiyalagan R, Yang DC. The development of a green approach for the biosynthesis of silver and gold nanoparticles by using *Panax ginseng* root extract, and their biological applications. Artif Cells Nanomed Biotechnol 2015; 44(4): 1-8.
[http://dx.doi.org/10.3109/21691401.2015.1011809] [PMID: 25771716]

[107] Castro-Aceituno V, Ahn S, Simu S Y, *et al.*, Anticancer activity of silver nanoparticles from Panax ginseng fresh leaves in human cancer cells, Biomed & Pharmacotherapy 2016; 84.
[http://dx.doi.org/10.1016/j.biopha.2016.09.016]

[108] Gharbavi M, Amani J, Kheiri-Manjili H, Danafar H, Sharafi A. Niosome: A Promising Nanocarrier for Natural Drug Delivery through Blood-Brain Barrier, Adv Pharmacolog Sci 2018; 2018.
[http://dx.doi.org/10.1155/2018/6847971]

[109] Çağdaş M, Sezer AD, Bucak S. liposomes as potential drug carrier systems for drug delivery. in application of nanotechnology in drug delivery, intech, 2014.
[http://dx.doi.org/10.5772/58459]

[110] Akbarzadeh A, *et al.* Liposome: classification, preparation, and applications 2013. http://www.nanoscalereslett.com/content/8/1/10210.1186/1556-276X-8-102

[111] Wang Y, Wang S, Firempong CK, *et al.* Enhanced Solubility and Bioavailability of Naringenin *via* Liposomal Nanoformulation: Preparation and *In vitro* and *In Vivo* Evaluations. AAPS PharmSciTech 2017; 18(3): 586-94.
[http://dx.doi.org/10.1208/s12249-016-0537-8] [PMID: 27151135]

[112] Vanti G, Coronnello M, Bani D, Mannini A, Bergonzi MC, Bilia AR. Co-delivery of berberine chloride and tariquidar in nanoliposomes enhanced intracellular berberine chloride in a doxorubicin-resistant K562 cell line due to P-gp overexpression. Pharmaceutics 2021; 13(3): 306.
[http://dx.doi.org/10.3390/pharmaceutics13030306] [PMID: 33652886]

[113] Risaliti L, *et al.* Development of Artemisia annua essential oil liposomes with antifungal activity against Candida species. 67th International Congress and Annual Meeting of the Society for Medicinal Plant and Natural Product Research (GA) in cooperation with the French Society of Pharmacognosy AFERP vol. 85. 2019.
[http://dx.doi.org/10.1055/s-0039-3399727]

[114] Risaliti L, Pini G, Ascrizzi R, *et al.* Artemisia annua essential oil extraction, characterization, and incorporation in nanoliposomes, smart drug delivery systems against Candida species. J Drug Deliv Sci Technol 2020; 59: 101849.
[http://dx.doi.org/10.1016/j.jddst.2020.101849]

[115] Das S, Vörös-Horváth B, Bencsik T, *et al.* Antimicrobial Activity of Different *Artemisia* Essential Oil Formulations. Molecules 2020; 25(10): 2390.
[http://dx.doi.org/10.3390/molecules25102390] [PMID: 32455592]

[116] Isacchi B, Arrigucci S, Marca G, *et al.* Conventional and long-circulating liposomes of artemisinin: preparation, characterization, and pharmacokinetic profile in mice. J Liposome Res 2011; 21(3): 237-44.
[http://dx.doi.org/10.3109/08982104.2010.539185] [PMID: 21158702]

[117] Pando D, Matos M, Gutiérrez G, Pazos C. Formulation of resveratrol entrapped niosomes for topical use. Colloids Surf B Biointerfaces 2015; 128: 398-404.
[http://dx.doi.org/10.1016/j.colsurfb.2015.02.037] [PMID: 25766923]

[118] Sinico C, Caddeo C, Valenti D, Fadda A M, Bilia A R, Vincieri F F. Liposomes as Carriers for Verbascoside: Stability and Skin Permeation Studies J Liposome Res 2008; 18 (1): 83-90.
[http://dx.doi.org/10.1080/08982100801894067]

[119] Z. ling Li *et al.*, Pluronics modified liposomes for curcumin encapsulation: Sustained release, stability and bioaccessibility. Food Res Int 2018;108:246-253.
[http://dx.doi.org/10.1016/j.foodres.2018.03.048]

[120] Vanti G, Camilla Bergonzi M, Rita Bilia A. Development of Nanoliposomes Loaded with Carbon Dioxide *Serenoa repens* (Saw Palmetto) Extract. J Nanosci Nanotechnol 2021; 21(5): 2943-5.
[http://dx.doi.org/10.1166/jnn.2021.19045] [PMID: 33653463]

[121] Risaliti L, Kehagia A, Daoultzi E, *et al.* Liposomes loaded with *Salvia* triloba and Rosmarinus officinalis essential oils: *In vitro* assessment of antioxidant, antiinflammatory and antibacterial activities. J Drug Deliv Sci Technol 2019; 51: 493-8.
[http://dx.doi.org/10.1016/j.jddst.2019.03.034]

[122] I. B *et al.*, Salvianolic acid B and its liposomal formulations: anti-hyperalgesic activity in the treatment of neuropathic pain. Eur J Pharm Sci 2011;44 (4):552-8.
[http://dx.doi.org/10.1016/j.ejps.2011.09.019]

[123] Crosasso P, Ceruti M, Brusa P, Arpicco S, Dosio F, Cattel L. Preparation, characterization and properties of sterically stabilized paclitaxel-containing liposomes. J Control Release 2000;63 (1-2):1--30.
[http://dx.doi.org/10.1016/S0168-3659 (99)00166-2]

[124] Guan Q, chen , hu , Wang X, Li L. Novel nanoliposomal delivery system for polydatin: preparation, characterization, and *in vivo* evaluation. Drug Des Devel Ther 2015; 9: 1805-13.
[http://dx.doi.org/10.2147/DDDT.S77615] [PMID: 25848217]

[125] Fang CL, Wang Y, Tsai KHY, Chang HI. Liposome-Encapsulated Baicalein Suppressed Lipogenesis and Extracellular Matrix Formation in Hs68 Human Dermal Fibroblasts. Front Pharmacol 2018; 9(MAR): 155.
[http://dx.doi.org/10.3389/fphar.2018.00155] [PMID: 29559910]

[126] Budhiraja A, Dhingra G. Development and characterization of a novel antiacne niosomal gel of rosmarinic acid. Drug Deliv 2015; 22(6): 723-30.
[http://dx.doi.org/10.3109/10717544.2014.903010] [PMID: 24786487]

[127] Shamsir A MD, Ahad A, Abidin L, Aqil M, Rasool S M, Mujeeb M. Embelin-loaded oral niosomes ameliorate streptozotocin-induced diabetes in Wistar rats. Biomed Pharmacother 2018; 97:1514-1520.
[http://dx.doi.org/10.1016/j.biopha.2017.11.073]

[128] Gunes A, Guler E, Un RN, *et al.* Niosomes of Nerium oleander extracts: *In vitro* assessment of bioactive nanovesicular structures. J Drug Deliv Sci Technol 2017; 37(37): 158-65.
[http://dx.doi.org/10.1016/j.jddst.2016.12.013]

[129] Barani M, Mirzaei M, Torkzadeh-Mahani M, Nematollahi MH. Lawsone-loaded Niosome and its antitumor activity in MCF-7 breast Cancer cell line: a Nano-herbal treatment for Cancer. Daru 2018;

26(1): 11-7.
[http://dx.doi.org/10.1007/s40199-018-0207-3] [PMID: 30159762]

[130] Anghore D, Kulkarni GT. Development of Novel Nano Niosomes As Drug Delivery System of *Spermacoce hispida* Extract and *In vitro* Antituberculosis Activity. Curr Nanomater 2017; 2(1).
[http://dx.doi.org/10.2174/2405461502666170314151949]

[131] Yadav HKS, Almokdad AA. S. I. M. shaluf, and M. S. Debe, "Polymer-Based Nanomaterials for Drug-Delivery Carriers. 2019; 531-56.
[http://dx.doi.org/10.1016/B978-0-12-814033-8.00017-5]

[132] Galetti M, Rossi S, Caffarra C, Gerboles A G, Miragoli M. Chapter 9 - Innovation in nanomedicine and engineered nanomaterials for therapeutic purposes. Exposure to Engineered Nanomaterials in the Environment, pp. 235–262, May 2019.
[http://dx.doi.org/10.1016/B978-0-12-814835-8.00009-1]

[133] Rana V, Sharma R. Recent advances in development of nano drug delivery. Appl Target Nano Drugs and Deliver Syst 2019;93-131.
[http://dx.doi.org/10.1016/B978-0-12-814029-1.00005-3]

[134] Sarisozen C, Joshi U, Mendes LP, Torchilin VP. Stimuli-responsive polymeric micelles for extracellular and intracellular drug delivery. Advanced Nanocarriers for Therapeutics 2019; (Jan): 269-304.
[http://dx.doi.org/10.1016/B978-0-08-101995-5.00012-X]

[135] Gou M, Men K, Shi H, *et al.* Curcumin-loaded biodegradable polymeric micelles for colon cancer therapy *In vitro* and *in vivo.* Nanoscale 2011; 3(4): 1558-67.
[http://dx.doi.org/10.1039/c0nr00758g] [PMID: 21283869]

[136] Abdelmoneem MA, Mahmoud M, Zaky A, *et al.*, Dual-targeted casein micelles as green nanomedicine for synergistic phytotherapy of hepatocellular carcinoma. J Control Release 2018; 287: 78-93.
[http://dx.doi.org/10.1016/j.jconrel.2018.08.026]

[137] Anantaworasakul P, Okonogi S. Encapsulation of Sesbania grandiflora extract in polymeric micelles to enhance its solubility, stability, and antibacterial activity. J Microencapsul 2017; 34 (1): 73-81.
[http://dx.doi.org/10.1080/02652048.2017.1284277]

[138] Su Y, Huang N, Chen D, *et al.* Successful *in vivo* hyperthermal therapy toward breast cancer by Chinese medicine shikonin-loaded thermosensitive micelle. Int J Nanomedicine 2017; 12: 4019-35.
[http://dx.doi.org/10.2147/IJN.S132639] [PMID: 28603416]

[139] Wu H, Yu T, Tian Y, Wang Y, Zhao R, Mao S. Enhanced liver-targeting *via* coadministration of 10-Hydroxycamptothecin polymeric micelles with vinegar baked Radix Bupleuri. Phytomedicine 2018; 44: 1-8.
[http://dx.doi.org/10.1016/j.phymed.2018.04.022] [PMID: 29895488]

[140] Mignani S, Rodrigues J, Tomas H, *et al.* Dendrimers in combination with natural products and analogues as anti-cancer agents. Chem Soc Rev 2018; 47(2): 514-32.
[http://dx.doi.org/10.1039/C7CS00550D] [PMID: 29154385]

[141] Falconieri M, Adamo M, Monasterolo C, Bergonzi M, Coronnello M, Bilia A. New Dendrimer-Based Nanoparticles Enhance Curcumin Solubility. Planta Med 2016; 83(5): 420-5.
[http://dx.doi.org/10.1055/s-0042-103161] [PMID: 27002394]

[142] Madaan K, Lather V, Pandita D. Evaluation of polyamidoamine dendrimers as potential carriers for quercetin, a versatile flavonoid. Drug Deliv 2016; 23(1): 254-62.
[http://dx.doi.org/10.3109/10717544.2014.910564] [PMID: 24845475]

[143] Gu L, Wu Z H, Qi X, *et al.* Polyamidomine dendrimers: an excellent drug carrier for improving the solubility and bioavailability of puerarin. Pharmaceut Develop Technol 2013; 18(5).
[http://dx.doi.org/10.3109/10837450.2011.653822]

[144] Kambhampati SP, Kannan RM. Dendrimer nanoparticles for ocular drug delivery. J Ocul Pharmacol

Ther 2013; 29(2): 151-65.
[http://dx.doi.org/10.1089/jop.2012.0232] [PMID: 23410062]

[145] Diaz C, Guzmán J, Jiménez VA, Alderete JB. Partially PEGylated PAMAM dendrimers as solubility enhancers of Silybin. Pharm Dev Technol 2018; 23(7): 689-96.
[http://dx.doi.org/10.1080/10837450.2017.1315134] [PMID: 28368674]

[146] Yesil-Celiktas O, Pala C, Cetin-Uyanikgil EO, Sevimli-Gur C. Synthesis of silica-PAMAM dendrimer nanoparticles as promising carriers in Neuro blastoma cells. Anal Biochem 2017; 519: 1-7.
[http://dx.doi.org/10.1016/j.ab.2016.12.004] [PMID: 27939389]

[147] Qu WJ, Li HF, Su YY, Dong ZQ, Ge YR. Absorption enhancing effects and safety of PAMAM dendrimers on liquiritin. Zhongguo Zhongyao Zazhi 2017; 42(9): 1766-71.
[http://dx.doi.org/10.19540/J.CNKI.CJCMM.2017.0070] [PMID: 29082704]

[148] Simonazzi A, Cid AG, Villegas M, Romero AI, Palma SD, Bermúdez JM. Nanotechnology applications in drug controlled release. Drug Targeting and Stimuli Sensitive Drug Delivery Systems.2018; 81-116.
[http://dx.doi.org/10.1016/B978-0-12-813689-8.00003-3]

[149] Singh Y, *et al.* Meher J G, Raval K, *et al.* Nanoemulsion: Concepts, development and applications in drug delivery. J Control Release 2017; 252.
[http://dx.doi.org/10.1016/j.jconrel.2017.03.008]

[150] Jaiswal M, Dudhe R, Sharma P K. Nanoemulsion: an advanced mode of drug delivery system. 3 Biotech. 2015; 5(2): 123–127.
[http://dx.doi.org/10.1007/s13205-014-0214-0]

[151] Gupta S, Bansal R, Ali J, Gabrani R, Dang S. Development and characterization of polyphenon 60 and caffeine microemulsion for enhanced antibacterial activity. BioMed Res Int 2014; 2014: 1-7.
[http://dx.doi.org/10.1155/2014/932017] [PMID: 25050379]

[152] Piazzini V, Monteforte E, Luceri C, Bigagli E, Bilia AR, Bergonzi MC. Nanoemulsion for improving solubility and permeability of *Vitex agnus-castus* extract: formulation and *In vitro* evaluation using PAMPA and Caco-2 approaches. Drug Deliv 2017; 24(1): 380-90.
[http://dx.doi.org/10.1080/10717544.2016.1256002] [PMID: 28165811]

[153] Rani ER, Radha GV. Insights into novel excipients of self-emulsifying drug delivery systems and their significance: an updated review. Crit Rev Ther Drug Carrier Syst 2021; 38(2): 27-74.
[http://dx.doi.org/10.1615/CritRevTherDrugCarrierSyst.2020034975] [PMID: 33639067]

[154] Čerpnjak K, Zvonar A, Gašperlin M, Vrečer F. Lipid-based systems as a promising approach for enhancing the bioavailability of poorly water-soluble drugs. Acta Pharm 2013; 63(4): 427-45.
[http://dx.doi.org/10.2478/acph-2013-0040] [PMID: 24451070]

[155] Zhang Y, Wang R, Wu J, Shen Q. Characterization and evaluation of self-microemulsifying sustained-release pellet formulation of puerarin for oral delivery. Int J Pharm 2012; 427(2): 337-44.
[http://dx.doi.org/10.1016/j.ijpharm.2012.02.013] [PMID: 22366381]

[156] Piazzini V, Bigagli E, Luceri C, Bilia AR, Bergonzi MC. Enhanced Solubility and Permeability of Salicis cortex Extract by Formulating as a Microemulsion. Planta Med 2018; 84(12/13): 976-84.
[http://dx.doi.org/10.1055/a-0611-6203] [PMID: 29689586]

[157] Guccione C, Bergonzi M, Awada K, Piazzini V, Bilia A. Lipid Nanocarriers for Oral Delivery of Serenoa repens CO2 Extract: A Study of Microemulsion and Self-Microemulsifying Drug Delivery Systems. Planta Med 2018; 84(09/10): 736-42.
[http://dx.doi.org/10.1055/a-0589-0474] [PMID: 29544228]

[158] Cecchi L, Piazzini V, D'Ambrosio M, *et al.* Formulation of a Phenol-Rich Extract from Unripe Olives (*Olea europaea* L.) in Microemulsion to Improve Its Solubility and Intestinal Permeability. Molecules 2020; 25(14): 3198.
[http://dx.doi.org/10.3390/molecules25143198] [PMID: 32668791]

[159] Zhao F, Wang P, Jiao Y, Zhang X, Chen D, Xu H. Hydroxysafflor Yellow A: A Systematical Review on Botanical Rearticle-titles, Physicochemical Properties, Drug Delivery System, Pharmacokinetics, and Pharmacological Effects. Front Pharmacol 2020; 11: 579332.
[http://dx.doi.org/10.3389/fphar.2020.579332] [PMID: 33536906]

[160] Gokhale JP, Mahajan HS, Surana SJ. Quercetin loaded nanoemulsion-based gel for rheumatoid arthritis: *In vivo* and *In vitro* studies. Biomed Pharmacother 2019; 112: 108622.
[http://dx.doi.org/10.1016/j.biopha.2019.108622] [PMID: 30797146]

[161] da Silva Gündel S, Velho MC, Diefenthaler MK, *et al.* Basil oil-nanoemulsions: Development, cytotoxicity and evaluation of antioxidant and antimicrobial potential. J Drug Delivery Science and Technology 2018; 46: 378-83.
[http://dx.doi.org/10.1016/j.jddst.2018.05.038]

[162] Cui J, Yu B, Zhao Y, *et al.* Enhancement of oral absorption of curcumin by self-microemulsifying drug delivery systems. Int J Pharm 2009; 371(1-2): 148-55.
[http://dx.doi.org/10.1016/j.ijpharm.2008.12.009] [PMID: 19124065]

[163] Dhumal DM, Akamanchi KG. Self-microemulsifying drug delivery system for camptothecin using new bicephalous heterolipid with tertiary-amine as branching element. Int J Pharm 2018; 541(1-2): 48-55.
[http://dx.doi.org/10.1016/j.ijpharm.2018.02.030] [PMID: 29462684]

[164] Yoo J, Baskaran R, Yoo BK. Self-nanoemulsifying drug delivery system of lutein: physicochemical properties and effect on bioavailability of warfarin. Biomol Ther (Seoul) 2013; 21(2): 173-9.
[http://dx.doi.org/10.4062/biomolther.2013.011] [PMID: 24009877]

[165] Jiang T, Liao W, Charcosset C. Recent advances in encapsulation of curcumin in nanoemulsions: A review of encapsulation technologies, bioaccessibility and applications. Food Res Int 2020; 132: 109035.
[http://dx.doi.org/10.1016/j.foodres.2020.109035]

[166] Fang JY, Hung CF, Hua SC, Hwang TL. Acoustically active perfluorocarbon nanoemulsions as drug delivery carriers for camptothecin: Drug release and cytotoxicity against cancer cells. Ultrasonics 2009; 49(1): 39-46.
[http://dx.doi.org/10.1016/j.ultras.2008.04.009] [PMID: 18554679]

[167] Cheng YC, Li TS, Su HL, Lee PC, Wang HMD. Transdermal Delivery Systems of Natural Products Applied to Skin Therapy and Care. Molecules 2020; 25(21): 5051.
[http://dx.doi.org/10.3390/molecules25215051] [PMID: 33143260]

[168] Obeid M A, al Qaraghuli M M, Alsaadi M, Alzahrani A R, Niwasabutra K, Ferro V A. Delivering natural products and biotherapeutics to improve drug efficacy.Ther Deliv 2017; 8 (11): 947-956
[http://dx.doi.org/10.4155/tde-2017-0060]

[169] Opatha S A T, Titapiwatanakun V, Chutoprapat R. Transfersomes: A promising nanoencapsulation technique for transdermal drug delivery. Pharmaceutics. 2020; 12(9): 855.
[http://dx.doi.org/10.3390/pharmaceutics12090855]

[170] Wu PS, Li YS, Kuo YC, Tsai SJ, Lin CC. Preparation and Evaluation of Novel Transfersomes Combined with the Natural Antioxidant Resveratrol. Molecules 2019; 24(3): 600.
[http://dx.doi.org/10.3390/molecules24030600] [PMID: 30743989]

[171] https://www.researchgate.net/publication/41394963_Development_and_Characterization_of_Curcumin_Loaded_Transfersome_for_Transdermal_Delivery

[172] Sarwa K K, Mazumder B, Rudrapal M, Verma V K. Potential of capsaicin-loaded transfersomes in arthritic rats. Drug Deliv 2015; 22(5): 638-46.
[http://dx.doi.org/10.3109/10717544.2013.871601]

[173] Avadhani KS, Manikkath J, Tiwari M, *et al.* Skin delivery of epigallocatechin-3-gallate (EGCG) and hyaluronic acid loaded nano-transfersomes for antioxidant and anti-aging effects in UV radiation

induced skin damage. Drug Deliv 2017; 24(1): 61-74.
[http://dx.doi.org/10.1080/10717544.2016.1228718] [PMID: 28155509]

[174] Rai S, Pandey V, Rai G. Transfersomes as versatile and flexible nano-vesicular carriers in skin cancer therapy: the state of the art. Nano Rev Exp 2017; 8(1): 1325708.
[http://dx.doi.org/10.1080/20022727.2017.1325708]

[175] Development and characterization of curcumin loaded transfersome for transdermal delivery. https://www.ijddr.in/drug-developmentethosomes-a-potential-carries-for-trans-ermal-drugdelivery.php?aid=5392

[176] Godin B, Touitou E. Ethosomes: new prospects in transdermal delivery. Crit Rev Ther Drug Carrier Syst 2003; 20(1): 63-102.
[http://dx.doi.org/10.1615/CritRevTherDrugCarrierSyst.v20.i1.20] [PMID: 12911264]

[177] Abdulbaqi IM, Darwis Y, Khan NAK, Assi RA, Khan AA. Ethosomal nanocarriers: the impact of constituents and formulation techniques on ethosomal properties, *in vivo* studies, and clinical trials. Int J Nanomedicine 2016; 11: 2279-304.
[http://dx.doi.org/10.2147/IJN.S105016] [PMID: 27307730]

[178] Fan C, Li X, Zhou Y, *et al.* Enhanced topical delivery of tetrandrine by ethosomes for treatment of arthritis. BioMed Res Int 2013; 2013: 1-13.
[http://dx.doi.org/10.1155/2013/161943] [PMID: 24062995]

[179] Abdulbaqi IM, Darwis Y, Abou Assi R, Abdul Karim Khan N. Transethosomal gels as carriers for the transdermal delivery of colchicine: statistical optimization, characterization, and *ex vivo* evaluation. Drug Des Devel Ther 2018; 12: 795-813.
[http://dx.doi.org/10.2147/DDDT.S158018] [PMID: 29670336]

[180] Kumar S, Baldi A, Sharma DK. Phytosomes: A Modernistic Approach for Novel Herbal Drug Delivery - Enhancing Bioavailability and Revealing Endless Frontier of Phytopharmaceuticals. J Dev Drugs 2020; 9(2): 1-8.
[http://dx.doi.org/10.35248/2329-6631.20.9.195]

[181] Anjana R, Sunil K, Hitender S, K KR. Phytosome drug delivery of natural products: A promising technique for enhancing bioavailability. Int J of Drug Delivery Technology 2017; 7(3): 157-65.
[http://dx.doi.org/10.25258/ijddt.v7i03.9559]

[182] Alharbi W S, *et al.* Phytosomes as an emerging nanotechnology platform for the topical delivery of bioactive phytochemicals. Pharmaceutics 2021; 13(9): 1475.
[http://dx.doi.org/10.3390/pharmaceutics13091475]

[183] Matias D, Rijo P, Pinto Reis C. Phytosomes as Biocompatible Carriers of Natural Drugs. Curr Med Chem 2017; 24(6): 568-89.
[http://dx.doi.org/10.2174/0929867323666161028160855] [PMID: 27804877]

[184] H Shariare M, Afnan K, Iqbal F, *et al.* Development and Optimization of Epigallocatechin-3-Gallate (EGCG) Nano Phytosome Using Design of Experiment (DoE) and Their *In Vivo* Anti-Inflammatory Studies. Molecules 2020; 25(22): E5453.
[http://dx.doi.org/10.3390/molecules25225453] [PMID: 33233756]

[185] Nguyễn K. Preparation of Rutin Phytosome Complex. VNU J Sci Med Pharmaceut Sci 2018; 34(2).
[http://dx.doi.org/10.25073/2588-1132/vnumps.4123]

[186] Singh RP, Gangadharappa HV, Mruthunjaya K. Phytosome complexed with chitosan for gingerol delivery in the treatment of respiratory infection: *In vitro* and *in vivo* evaluation. Eur J Pharm Sci 2018; 122: 214-29.
[http://dx.doi.org/10.1016/j.ejps.2018.06.028] [PMID: 29966737]

[187] Garg G, Saraf S, Saraf S. Cubosomes: An Overview. Biol Pharm Bull 2007; 30(2): 350-3.
[http://dx.doi.org/10.1248/bpb.30.350] [PMID: 17268078]

[188] Gaballa S, el Garhy O, Abdelkader H. Cubosomes: composition, preparation, and drug delivery

applications. J Adv Biomed Pharmaceu Sci 2020; 3(1): 1-9.
[http://dx.doi.org/10.21608/jabps.2019.16887.1057]

[189] Archana A, Sri KV, Madhuri M, Kumar CA. Curcumin loaded nano cubosomal hydrogel: preparation, *in vitro* characterization and antibacterial activity. Chem Sci Trans. 2015; 4(1): 75-80. 2015.
[http://dx.doi.org/10.7598/cst2015.913]

[190] Tiwari A, Mahadik KR, Gabhe SY. Piperine: A comprehensive review of methods of isolation, purification, and biological properties. Medicine in Drug Discovery 2020; 7: 100027.
[http://dx.doi.org/10.1016/j.medidd.2020.100027]

[191] Kwon T K, Kim J-C. Preparation and *in vitro* skin permeation of cubosomes containing hinokitiol. J Dispersion Sci Tech 2010; 31(7): 1004-1009.
[http://dx.doi.org/10.1080/01932690903224862]

[192] Aguilar ZP. Targeted drug delivery. Semin Oncol 2013; 20(1): 181-234.
[http://dx.doi.org/10.1016/B978-0-12-385089-8.00005-4] [PMID: 8475405]

[193] Alibolandi M, Shahriari M, Ramezani M. Smart polymersomes as intelligent nanomedicines in cancer treatment. In: Polymeric nanoparticles as a promising tool for anti-cancer therapeutics 2019.
[http://dx.doi.org/10.1016/B978-0-12-816963-6.00016-9]

[194] Madkour LH. Advanced drug delivery systems: New nanomedication technologies. 2019; 1-29.
[http://dx.doi.org/10.1016/B978-0-12-819777-6.00001-9]

[195] Zhang X, Zhang P. Polymersomes in Nanomedicine - A Review. Curr Nanosci 2017; 13(2): 124-9.
[http://dx.doi.org/10.2174/1573413712666161018144519]

[196] Yang J, Dai G, Hou Y, *et al.* Quantification of oxymatrine in rat plasma by UPLCMS/MS to support the pharmacokinetic analyses of oxymatrineloaded polymersomes. Anal Methods 2014; 6(6): 1811-7.
[http://dx.doi.org/10.1039/C3AY42294A]

[197] Simón-Gracia L, Hunt H, Scodeller PD, *et al.* Paclitaxel-Loaded Polymersomes for Enhanced Intraperitoneal Chemotherapy. Mol Cancer Ther 2016; 15(4): 670-9.
[http://dx.doi.org/10.1158/1535-7163.MCT-15-0713-T] [PMID: 26880267]

[198] Goyal K, Konar A, Kumar BSH, Koul V. Lactoferrin-conjugated pH and redox-sensitive polymersomes based on PEG-S-S-PLA-PCL-OH boost delivery of bacosides to the brain. Nanoscale 2018; 10(37): 17781-98.
[http://dx.doi.org/10.1039/C8NR03828G] [PMID: 30215650]

[199] Müller R, Junghanns . Nanocrystal technology, drug delivery and clinical applications. Int J Nanomedicine 2008; 3(3): 295-309.
[http://dx.doi.org/10.2147/IJN.S595] [PMID: 18990939]

[200] Rachmawati H, Shaal LA, Müller RH, Keck CM. Development of curcumin nanocrystal: physical aspects. J Pharm Sci 2013; 102(1): 204-14.
[http://dx.doi.org/10.1002/jps.23335] [PMID: 23047816]

[201] Zhang J, Huang Y, Liu D, Gao Y, Qian S. Preparation of apigenin nanocrystals using supercritical antisolvent process for dissolution and bioavailability enhancement. Eur J Pharm Sci 2013;48 (4-5):740-7
[http://dx.doi.org/10.1016/j.ejps.2012.12.026]

[202] NG Sahoo. Preparation and characterization of quercetin nanocrystals. J Pharm Sci 2011;100(6):2379-90.
[http://dx.doi.org/10.1002/jps.22446]

[203] Vasita R, Katti DS. Nanofibers and their applications in tissue engineering. Int J Nanomedicine 2006; 1(1): 15-30.
[http://dx.doi.org/10.2147/nano.2006.1.1.15] [PMID: 17722259]

[204] Nemati S, Kim S, Shin Y M, Shin H. Current progress in application of polymeric nanofibers to tissue

engineering. Nano Converg 2019; 6: 36.
[http://dx.doi.org/10.1186/s40580-019-0209-y]

[205] Wang, J., Tian, L., He, L. *et al.* Lycium barbarum polysaccharide encapsulated Poly lactic-co-glycolic acid Nanofibers: cost effective herbal medicine for potential application in peripheral nerve tissue engineering. Sci Rep 2018; 8.
[http://dx.doi.org/10.1038/s41598-018-26837-z]

[206] Akrami-Hasan-Kohal M, Tayebi L, Ghorbani M. Curcumin-loaded naturally-based nanofibers as active wound dressing mats: morphology, drug release, cell proliferation, and cell adhesion studies. New J Chem 2020; 44(25): 10343-51.
[http://dx.doi.org/10.1039/D0NJ01594F]

[207] Carter P, Rahman SM, Bhattarai N. Facile fabrication of aloe vera containing PCL nanofibers for barrier membrane application. J Biomater Sci Polym Ed 2016; 27(7): 692-708.
[http://dx.doi.org/10.1080/09205063.2016.1152857] [PMID: 26878323]

[208] Choi J, Yang BJ, Bae GN, Jung JH. Herbal Extract Incorporated Nanofiber Fabricated by an Electrospinning Technique and its Application to Antimicrobial Air Filtration. ACS Appl Mater Interfaces 2015; 7(45): 25313-20.
[http://dx.doi.org/10.1021/acsami.5b07441] [PMID: 26505783]

[209] Liu M, Cao X, Liu H, Yang X, Zhou C. Halloysite-based polymer nanocomposites. Nanomaterials from Clay Minerals: A New Approach to Green Functional Materials, pp. 589–626, Jan. 2019.
[http://dx.doi.org/10.1016/B978-0-12-814533-3.00012-0]

[210] Marti ME, Sharma AD, Sakaguchi DS, Mallapragada SK. Nanomaterials for neural tissue engineering. Nanomaterials in Tissue Engineering: Fabrication and Applications, pp. 275–301, 2013.
[http://dx.doi.org/10.1533/9780857097231.2.275]

[211] Tan JM, Karthivashan G, Arulselvan P, Fakurazi S, Hussein MZ. Characterization and *In vitro* sustained release of silibinin from ph responsive carbon nanotube-based drug delivery system. J Nanomater 2014; 2014: 1-10.
[http://dx.doi.org/10.1155/2014/439873]

[212] Lee MH, Seo HS, Park HJ. Thyme Oil Encapsulated in Halloysite Nanotubes for Antimicrobial Packaging System. J Food Sci 2017; 82(4): 922-32.
[http://dx.doi.org/10.1111/1750-3841.13675] [PMID: 28272803]

[213] Li H, Zhang N, Hao Y, *et al.* Formulation of curcumin delivery with functionalized single-walled carbon nanotubes: characteristics and anticancer effects *In vitro*, Drug delivery 2014; 21(5): 379-87.
[http://dx.doi.org/10.3109/10717544.2013.848246]

[214] Madni A, Tahir N, Rehman M, *et al.* Hybrid Nano-carriers for Potential Drug Delivery. Advanced Technology for Delivering Therapeutics 2017.
[http://dx.doi.org/10.5772/66466]

[215] Zhang J, Han Z, Li X, *et al.*, Coreshell hybrid liposomal vesicles loaded with panax notoginsenoside: preparation, characterization and protective effects on global cerebral ischemia/reperfusion injury and acute myocardial ischemia in rats. Int J Nanomedicine 2012; 7: 4299-310.
[http://dx.doi.org/10.2147/IJN.S32385]

CHAPTER 10

Marketing Strategy & Regulatory Perspective for Natural Immunomodulators

Alveera Ansari[1], **Namrata Nailwal**[1], **Sujata Sawarkar**[2] and **Gaurav Doshi**[1,*]

[1] *Department of Pharmacology, SVKM'S Dr.Bhanuben Nanavati College of Pharmacy, Mithibai Campus, Vile Parle (W), Mumbai-400056, India*

[2] *Department of Pharmaceutics, SVKM's Dr. Bhanuben Nanavati College of Pharmacy, V. M. Road, Vile Parle (W), Mumbai-400056, Maharashtra, India*

Abstract: Many natural products, such as *Azardicaindica*, *Curcuma longa*, and *Ocimumsanctum*, are often used as immunomodulators. The increased prevalence of chronic diseases, along with the negative effects of synthetic immunomodulators, has resulted in the establishment of a global natural immunomodulator market. For researchers, complementary and alternative medicine provides a new target for drug discovery approaches and medication development. Ayurveda, Homeopathy, Naturopathy, and the Chinese medicine system are examples of complementary and alternative medicine approaches. Phytoconstituents with therapeutic action are included in the Complementary and Alternative Medicine (CAM) categories of natural goods. In Europe, natural immunomodulators are considered food supplements, while in the United States, they are utilized as dietary supplements. In India, it is controlled by the Ministry of AYUSH (Ayurveda, Yoga & Naturopathy, Unani, Siddha and Homeopathy). With the help of the literature findings, we understand that even natural phytoconstituents also require and must undergo well-defined regulatory approval processes to launch in the market. But the regulation slightly differs as per the country and region. With the help of all the findings, one can conclude that the regulation of natural immunomodulators is equally important to set its marketing strategies as well as for its post-marketing surveillance as compared to the synthetic molecules. With this objective, the primary goal of this chapter is to draw more attention to the regulatory aspects of natural immunomodulators by comprehending the information on natural immunomodulator marketing strategy as well as the legislation that governs it.

Keywords: Guidelines, Legislation, Marketing Strategies, Natural Immunomodulators, Regulatory Agencies.

[*] **Corresponding author Gaurav Doshi:** Department of Pharmacology, SVKM'S Dr. Bhanuben Nanavati College of Pharmacy, Mithibai Campus, Vile Parle (W), Mumbai-400056, India; E-mail: gaurav.pharmacology@gmail.com

Vandana S. Nikam, Sujata P. Sawarkar, Girish B. Mahajan and Supriya G. Jagtap (Eds.)

INTRODUCTION

Immunomodulators can help combat and mitigate diseases and illnesses caused by immunodeficiencies [1 - 6]. Several metabolites that decrease immune responses may be effective in the treatment of autoimmune illnesses [7, 8]. Reactivation of latent Tuberculosis (TB) is another documented unfavorable effect, particularly in association with new-generation immunomodulatory medicines [9, 10].

Pharmaceutical drug laws, commonly called pharmaceuticals regulatory guidelines, are a collection of authorized, procedural, and technical requirements used by government agencies to guarantee patient safety, drug efficacy, and purity, as well as the reliability of the product. The word "regulation" encompasses comprehensive elements (for example, rules, recommendations, processes and policies) with varied legal bases and jurisdictions [3, 4]. This is achieved by a variety of regulatory processes performed throughout the life cycle of drug discovery and development, which includes premarket screening and analysis of new medicines, an inspection of manufacturing facilities, legislation, marketing, and post-market surveillance. Each country has unique rules that govern invention, production, screening, advertising, and post-marketing research. The goal is to keep drug standards high at all times to meet the needs of health maintenance of each country [5].

In India, the regulatory bodies are the Central Drug Standard Control Organization (CDSCO), the Indian Council of Medical Research (ICMR), and the Ministry of Health and Family Welfare (MoHFW). The CDSCO is responsible for carrying out the tasks delegated by the Central Government under the jurisdiction of the Drugs and Cosmetics Act. It is responsible for guaranteeing the quality, usefulness, and purity of medications distributed to the public at both the federal and state levels. CDSCO is in charge of drug importation, new drug authorization, clinical trials, and meetings of the Drugs Technical Advisory Board (DTAB) and Drugs Consultative Committee (DCC). The CDSCO plays a key role in approving specific licenses through the Central Licensing Approval Committee. ICMR is considered one of the oldest clinical study organizations in the world and the best framework in India to design, coordinate, and promote biomedical studies. The organization is supported by the Government of India through the Department of Health and Family Welfare [6, 7]. The Union Health Minister is in charge of the governing body. The Scientific Advisory Board comprising notable professionals in the field of life sciences and biomedical areas, advises the CDSCO on technical and scientific concerns [8, 9].

The US Department of Health and Human Services (HHS) is the primary organization in charge of preserving the health of all Americans and providing basic humanitarian assistance. HHS has 11 operational departments, including eight US public health services agencies and three human services agencies. These departments offer a wide range of health and human services, as well as life-saving scientific studies. The Food and Drug Administration (FDA) is among 11 agencies within the Department of Health and Human Services responsible for ensuring that the product is healthy and genuine. FDA authenticates the quality and confirms that animal and human medicament, biopharmaceuticals, and surgical instruments are medically beneficial, and computerized devices emitting radiation are harmless. The FDA is divided into five offices that handle various functions: Medical Products and Tobacco, Foods and Veterinary Medicine, Global Regulatory Operations and Policy, Operations and Policy, and Planning, Legislation, and Analysis.

The Centre for Drug Evaluation and Research (CDER) is a department of the Division of Medical Products that regulates biological therapeutics and generic pharmaceuticals. The CDER plays an important role in public health by ensuring that safe and effective medications available to help people in the United States live healthier lives. CDER regulates over-the-counter and prescription pharmaceuticals, including biological therapies and generic drugs, as part of the US Food and Drug Administration (FDA). CDER The Center for Drug Evaluation and Research has twelve separate offices. There are several types of the department, each of which has its subsection. To sell medicinal products or drugs in the United States, pharmaceutical companies must first obtain the product cleared by the US FDA. Each product must go through a rigorous certification process established by the Centre for Drug Evaluation and Research to receive approval [10, 11].

Apart from India and America, “The Pharmaceutical and Food Safety Bureau” (PFSB) of the Ministry of Health, Labour, and Welfare (MHLW) is the pharmaceutical regulating authority of Japan. The Pharmaceuticals and Medical Devices Evaluation Center (PMDEC) is the decision body concerned with new drug approvals [12, 20]. The Organization for Pharmaceutical Safety and Research (OPSR), often known as “KIKO or “the DO” (Drug Organization), is an independent entity affiliated with MHLW, responsible for negotiating drug development projects with companies. The GCP (Good Clinical Practice) guideline will improve the ethical and scientific quality of studies conducted in Japan. It may also improve relationships between medical professionals and patients if the requirement for explicit informed consent in clinical trials leads to the provision of a comparable level of patient information in routine care and changes physicians' traditional paternalistic attitude toward patients. The GCP guideline was implemented in Japan in 1997. International Council for Harmonization-Efficacy guidelines (ICH-E6), sometimes known as “the new

GCP" in Japan, had and has a significant and almost revolutionary impact on the Japanese legislative framework. Unlike other ICH principles that are simply translated into Japanese, the ICH-E6 was published in three separate documents; the most important of which is Ministry Order # 28. The English version of the Japanese GCP is available [11, 13, 14]. The agreement to compile all Quality, Safety, and Efficacy information in a standard format (known as the CTD - Common Technical Document) has revolutionised regulatory review processes, resulting in harmonised electronic submissions and the implementation of excellent review methods. It has eliminated the requirement for industries to reformat material for submission to various ICH regulatory bodies. The Common Technical Document specifies the procedures for submitting applications for the approval of pharmaceuticals intended for use in Japan, Europe, and the United States. Now it is a uniform framework for preparing new drug proposals for submission to global regulatory agencies. Numerous regulatory bodies throughout the world are establishing and drafting policies and laws to ensure the proper functioning of drug commercialization approval.

This chapter provides insights into the regulations and marketing strategies related to pharmaceuticals and natural products. The chapter opens with an overview of the scope, purpose, and goals of natural product global market access rules. The significant cost trade-offs connected with these goals are identified and mentioned in the chapter.

The pharmaceutical regulatory framework encompasses several interconnected actions intended to promote and safeguard community health. The extent and execution vary from place to place, however in general, the objectives are Licensing the production, import, export, distribution, promotion, and marketing of medicines; Evaluating the safety, efficacy, and purity of medicines; and providing regulatory approval for specific products; Inspection and monitoring of pharmaceutical makers, importers, dealers, and dispensers; Overseeing medicine quality available in the market; Regulating the advertising and marketing of pharmaceuticals responsible for monitoring the safety of marketed drugs, including the collection and analysis of side - effect reports; Providing unbiased information on medications to experts and the general population [15 - 17].

Connections with numerous stakeholders (*e.g.*, manufacturers, dealers, customers, medical practitioners, academicians, and government bodies) whose financial, ethical, and political agendas are affected by legal and regulatory framework intentions may varied, making regulatory execution both politically and technically difficult. The administrative aspect of medicine regulation is crucial, but the scientific base is significantly more important. All drugs must meet three criteria: they must be of high quality, effective, and useful. Decisions about the purity, quality, and effectiveness of medicines should be based on strong evidence. Several general and specific variables contribute to (national regulatory authority) NRAs' effective regulation [18 - 20]. The details of the countries with regulatory agencies as been depicted in Table **1**.

Table 1. List of regulatory agencies of various countries.

S. No.	Country	Regulatory Abbreviations	Regulatory Authority	References
1.	United States of America (USA)	USFDA	The Food and Drug Administration	[21]
2.	India	CDSCO	Central Drugs Standard Control Organisation	[22]
3.	Australia	TGA	Therapeutic Goods Administration	[23]
4.	United Kingdom (UK)	MHRA	Medicines and Healthcare products Regulatory Agency	[24]
5.	Canada	HC	Health Canada	[25]
6.	Europe	EMA	European Medicines Agency	[26]
7.	Denmark	DKMA	Danish Medicines Agency	[27]
8.	New Zealand	Medsafe	New Zealand Medicines and Medical Devices Safety Authority	[28]
9.	Ireland	IMB	Irish Medicines Board	[29]
10.	Brazil	ANVISA	Agencia Nacional de Vigilancia Sanitaria	[30]
11.	Thailand	Thai FDA	Thai Food and Drug Administration	[31]
12.	Sweden	MPA	Medical Products Agency	[32]
13.	Italy	AIFA	Italian Medicines Agency	[33]
14.	Germany	BfArM	Federal Institute for Drugs and Medical Devices (BundesinstitutfürArzneimittel und Medizinprodukte)	[34]
15.	China	SFDA	State Food and Drug Administration	[35]
16.	Korea	KFDA	Korean Food and Drug Administration	[36]
17.	Switzerland	Swissmedic	Swiss Agency for Therapeutic Products	[37]
18.	Hongkong	DH	Department of Health	[38]
19.	France	ASNM	National Agency for the Safety of Medicines and Health Products	[39]
20.	Nigeria	NAFDAC	National Agency for Food and Drug Administration and Control	[40]
21.	Uganda	UNCST	Uganda National Council for Science and Technology	[41]
22.	Malaysia	NPRA	The National Pharmaceutical Regulatory Agency	[42]

(Table 1) cont.....

S. No.	Country	Regulatory Abbreviations	Regulatory Authority	References
23.	Netherlands	MEB	Medicines Evaluation Board	[43]
24.	Singapore	HSA	Health Science Authority	[44]
25.	Japan	MHLW	Ministry of Health, Labour and Welfare of Japan	[45]
26.	Saudi Arabia, Kuwait, the United Arab Emirates, Qatar, Bahrain, Oman	GCC	Gulf Cooperation Council	[46]
27.	South Africa	SAHPRA	South African Health Products Regulatory Authority	[47]
28.	Armenia, Azerbaijan, Belarus, Georgia, Kazakhstan, Kyrgyzstan, Turkmenistan Moldova, Russia, Tajikistan, Ukraine, Uzbekistan	CIS	The Common wealth of Independent States	[48]
29.	Vietnam, Thailand, Singapore, Philippines, Brunei, Cambodia, Indonesia, Laos, Malaysia, Myanmar	ASEAN	Association of South Asian Nations	[49]

UNITED STATES OF AMERICA (USA)

The FDA is mandated by law to publish its rules in the Federal Register, the federal government's primary publication for informing the public about a variety of agency activities. Federal rules are either required or authorised by statute. Some, like the FDA's egg safety laws, are centralised or procedural in character, while others, like citizen petition regulations, address a specific issue or acknowledged health hazard. The policymaking practices are based on US law, Presidential Executive Orders (EOs) and memos, and FDA regulations. A pharmaceutical commercial enterprise seeking FDA clearance to commercialize a brand new prescription drug needs to undergo a five-step procedure, which incorporates discovery/concept, preclinical research, scientific research, FDA review, and FDA post-marketplace protection monitoring. After evaluating the medicine, the manufacturer submits a new drug application (NDA) to the FDA, which must include the following information: The results of the drug's tests, Manufacturing data to demonstrate the company's ability to manufacture the medicine correctly, Data obtained during animal investigations and clinical trials in humans, the drug's proposed label, which lists the uses for which it has been demonstrated to be beneficial, potential hazards, and how to use it, according to the manufacturer. The drug study and labelling instructions on how to use the drug are next reviewed by FDA physicians and scientists. The drug is approved and can be marketed in the United States if the findings show that the treatment's benefits outweigh its known risks — and that the drug can be manufactured in a way that ensures a quality product. Following approval, the FDA will continue to monitor the medicine. Before making a decision, the FDA does not actually test the medicine. However, as part of the approval process, the FDA inspects the facility where the medicine is being manufactured [50]. The FDA's regulatory jurisdiction is extraordinarily extensive. The FDA's responsibilities are linked with the responsibilities of a number of different federal agencies. Customers are frequently irritated and dubious when it comes to locating the right regulatory employer to contact. The following is a compilation of some of the generally recognized marketplace sectors that come below the legislative control of the FDA; although the list is not exhaustive. In general, the FDA controls marketing approval of the following:

- Nutritional Supplements
- Packaged Water
- Food Additives
- Infant Foods
- Other food items (although the U.S. Department of Agriculture plays a lead role in regulating aspects of some meat, poultry, and egg products).

Drugs & Biological Products

- Prescription medications (both brand-name and generic) and non-prescription (over-the-counter) drugs.
- Human vaccinations, as well as blood and blood products, are examples of biologics. Pharmaceutical items for cellular and gene therapy
- Tissue and tissue-related goods.

Medical Devices, including:

- Simple goods such as tongue depressors and bedpans, advanced technologies such as heart pacemakers, dental instruments, prosthetic limbs, and surgical implants.

Electronic products that emit radiation, such as:

- Microwave ovens, x-ray machines, laser products, ultrasonic therapy equipment, mercury vapor lamp, sunlamps

Cosmetics include:

- Colour pigments included in makeup and other hygiene products, skin creams and washes, nail polish, and cologne

Veterinary Products, such as:

- Animal feeds, pet foods, and veterinary medicines and devices

Tobacco products, such as:

- Cigarettes, cigarette tobacco, wrap tobacco, and smokeless tobacco.

Advertising:

The Federal Trade Commission is a federal organization in charge of regulating all sorts of advertising. The FTC protects consumers by prohibiting unfair, misleading, or misleading business activities in the marketplace [51].

INDIA

The national regulatory authority (NRA) of India is the Central Drugs Standard Control Organisation (CDSCO) which comes under the purview of the Directorate General of Health Services, Ministry of Health & Family Welfare, Government of India. CDSCO headquarters are located at FDA Bhawan, New Delhi, and it has 6 zonal offices, four sub zonal offices, thirteen port offices, and seven laboratories dispersed across the country. The Drugs and Cosmetics Act of 1940 and the Rules of 1945 delegated many drug and cosmetics-related tasks to critical and national authorities. The law aims to protect patients' safety, rights, and health by regulating prescription medications and cosmetics in accordance with the requirements of the Act and the Rules issued thereunder. CDSCO is usually striving to enhance openness, accountability, and consistency in its offerings to make certain the safety, efficacy, and high-satisfactory of scientific merchandise made, imported, and dispensed withinside the country. Furthermore, CDSCO, in collaboration with nation regulators, is liable for granting licenses for a few unique classes of critical capsules, which include blood and blood merchandise, intravenous fluids, vaccines, and sera [52]. All medicines intended for internal or external use for or in the diagnosis, treatment, mitigation, or prevention of disease or disorder in humans or animals, and prepared only in accordance with the formulae, are considered Ayurvedic, Siddha, and Unani drugs. The principal class of Ayurveda, Siddha, or Unani (ASU) drugs covered in Indian regulations are: Classical ASU drugs as described in authoritative books of ASU system drugs, which are created and called according to the formulations stated in authoritative sources. Unless the drug is intended for a new indication, in which case proof of effectiveness is necessary, a licence to manufacture is issued based on citation in reputable books and published literature. Patent or proprietary medicine uses substances included in authoritative books' formulae, but with intellectual intervention, innovation, or invention to create medicines that are distinct from classical medicine. In India, ASU medications are regulated by the Department of AYUSH. The gazette notification establishes regulatory provisions for phytopharmaceuticals, as well as regulatory submission requirements for scientific data on quality, safety, and efficacy, in order to evaluate and allow the marketing of herbal drugs in the same way that synthetic, chemical moieties are marketed [53].

AUSTRALIA

The Therapeutic Goods Administration (TGA) is regulating agency of Australia for healthcare products such as medications, blood products, and tissues, and medical equipment. It also assures public access to novel therapeutic goods and safeguards public health through the Therapeutic Goods Act of 1989. (The Act). The TGA is a branch of the Australian Department of Health and Ageing. The Advisory Committee on Medical Devices (ACMD), earlier referred to as the Medical Device Evaluation Committee, advises the TGA on medical device safety, quality, and performance (MDEC) [54]. The TGA monitors the current benefits and risks of pharmaceuticals when they are approved for use and has the authority to intervene if the benefits are not fulfilled, or additional dangers emerge. Little participation, like labelling changes, to the withdrawal of the pharmaceutical product from the market are among the regulatory steps performed [55].

UNITED KINGDOM

In the United Kingdom, the Medications and Healthcare products Regulatory Agency (MHRA) controls medicines, medical devices, and blood components for transfusion. The MHRA is a government organization that is funded by the Department of Health and Social Care. The agency plays a leadership role in safeguarding and enhancing public health, as well as support for the project through scientific research.

The agency comprises of three centers: Clinical Practice Research Datalink (CPRD), a record studies carrier geared toward enhancing public fitness through using anonymized NHS scientific records. The National Institute for Biological Standards and Control (NIBSC), a worldwide pioneer in organic scientific standardization and control The Medicines and Healthcare Regulatory Agency (MHRA) is vital to guarantee the safety, purity, and efficacy of medicines, scientific devices, and organic fluids for transfusion withinside the United Kingdom [56].

CANADA

Health Canada is the federal agency in charge of regulating, analyzing, and overseeing the safety, efficacy, and quality of pharmaceutical and diagnostic products sold in Canada. These items include drugs, medical equipment, disinfectants, and sanitizers with a disinfectant claim. The agency analyses the information presented in the clinical trial application before the start of a clinical trial in Canada. The findings of preclinical studies, production processes, dosage form, and details on the investigators who will be performing the study are all included in a clinical trial application. When a sponsor intends to commercialize a drug in Canada, the company submits a "New Drug Submission" with the HPFB of Health Canada.This submission document contains information about the safety, efficacy, and quality of the drug. The document includes the results of preclinical and clinical trials, either conducted in Canada or in other regions, as well as information on the drug's manufacturing process, packaging, and labeling criteria, as well as therapeutic claims and side effects. The HPFB performs a thorough review of the information supplied, which may include the involvement of consultants not associated with the agency and advisory bodies.The HPFB assesses the potential advantages of the drug and risks by evaluating its safety, effectiveness, and quality data. The HPFB examines the drug information that the sponsor intends to disclose to physicians and patients (*e.g.*, the label, product brochure), analyzes the risk-to-benefit ratio, and eventually, the drug is given approval by issuing a Notice of Compliance (NOC) and a Drug Identification Number (DIN), allowing the sponsor to market the drug in Canada. Furthermore, before and after a biological product is approved for sale in Canada, Health Canada laboratories may analyze it. The company's Lot Release Process is used to keep track of the products' safety, efficacy, and quality. If there is insufficient data to substantiate the drug's safety, effectiveness, or quality claims, the HPFB will deny marketing permission. All pharmaceuticals granted marketing authorization in Canada are subjected to a review to ensure that they meet the rules of the Food and Drugs Act. If the HPFB declines to grant marketing approval, the sponsor may provide further information, resubmit its application at a later date with supplementary supporting data, or request that the HPFB re-examine its judgment [57].

The Food and Drugs Act (the Act) (official title An Act respecting food, medications, cosmetics, and therapeutic devices) is a Canadian law that governs the production, import, export, cross-provincial transportation, and sale of food, drugs, contraceptive devices, and cosmetics (including personal cleaning products such as soap and toothpaste). The rule and regulations of the act establish the requirements for licensing and manufacturing pharmaceuticals in Canada. The bill authorizes the Minister of Health to cancel or suspend licenses of enterprises that fail to meet the conditions. The producer is required to comply with all the conditions before selling the drug in the market. Health advocates call for post-approval monitoring to look for unanticipated concerns [58].

Following the recent expansion of its duty to cover the regulation of non-prescription and disinfection medications in addition to natural health goods, the Natural Health Products Directorate (NHPD) has changed its name to the Natural and Non-prescription Health Products Directorate (NNHPD). The Natural Health Products Regulations, which went into effect on January 1, 2004, apply to all natural health products (NHPs) sold in Canada. The Regulations make it easier for Canadians to choose safe, effective, and high-quality natural health products. After extensive conversations with Canadian consumers, academics, health care practitioners, and industry stakeholders, the Natural Health Products Regulations were developed. All natural health products must have a product licence to be lawfully sold in Canada, and the Canadian sites that produce, package, label, and import these goods must have site licences. Specific labelling and packaging criteria must be satisfied, good manufacturing procedures must be followed, and adequate safety and efficacy evidence must be produced to get product and site licences. The Natural Health Products Regulations impose licence requirements on anyone who makes, packages, labels, or imports NHPs for commercial sale in Canada. They do not apply to healthcare professionals who compound goods for their patients on an individual basis, nor to NHP retailers. Before natural health products can be sold in Canada, they must first get a product licence. Applicants must provide Health Canada with thorough information about the product, including medicinal ingredients, source, dose, potency, non-medicinal constituents, and suggested usage, in order to obtain a licence.

After Health Canada has evaluated a product and determined that it is safe, effective, and of high quality, it grants a product licence, which includes an eight-digit Natural Product Number (NPN) or Homeopathic Medicine Number (DIN-HM) that must be displayed on the label. This number indicates that Health has reviewed and approved the product [59].

EUROPE

The European Medicines Agency (EMA) is a centralized European Union (EU) agency that is in charge of the scientific review, monitoring, and safety data of medicines in the EU. An autonomous Management Board governs EMA. EMA workers, who are directed by the EMA's Executive Director, were in charge of the organization's day-to-day operations. The European Medicines Agency (EMA) is a collaborative institution that hires various specialists from around Europe in its operations. These professionals perform the tasks of the EMA's scientific committees. In March 2020, the EMA adopted organizational adjustments to ensure that it functions effectively to deliver high-quality results for public and animal health. The primary modifications are as follows: Combining efforts in the field of human therapeutics into a single division, forming four mission-critical task forces to assist the veterinary and human medicine divisions, and bringing professionals together to create restructuring in high-priority areas. The redesign takes into account the fast-changing scenario in the field of pharmaceutical research and development, so that the regulators design policies that are abreast with the developments in science and technology.

The Management Board is made up of 36 individuals who have been assigned to operate in the public interest and are not affiliated with any central regulatory body, organization, or sector. The Board establishes the Agency's economy, approves the annual work program, and is in charge of making sure that the Agency functions correctly and productively with partner organizations throughout the EU and beyond. The Executive Director is the prosecutor of the agency. The person is in charge of all operational risks, staffing issues, and developing the year work schedule. The Agency's personnel assist the Executive Director in carrying out his duties, which include legal and procedural aspects of EU law relating to the assessment and safety monitoring of medicines in the EU. The European Medicines Agency (EMA) includes seven scientific committees that review drugs throughout their lifespan, from early phases of development to marketing approval and safety data after they are available for the public.

Furthermore, the Agency maintains several working parties and allied groups with which the committees can communicate on scientific matters about their specific field of specialization. These bodies are made up of European experts who are provided by the national competent authorities of the EU Member States, who collaborate closely with the EMA in the European pharmaceuticals regulation network [60].

Traditional herbal medicine companies seeking market access in European Union (EU) the Member States must follow national processes. Applicants may, however, seek scientific support and guidance from the European Medicines Agency's (EMA) Committee on Herbal Medicinal Products (HMPC). On scientific and regulatory elements of applications, national competent authorities of Member States can contact the HMPC. Applicants should review the questions and answers section before submitting a request to determine whether their question has previously been answered [61].

DENMARK

The Danish Medicines Act governs the authorization and control of pharmaceutical items, as well as the companies that manufacture, store, or otherwise handle pharmaceutical products. It also establishes guidelines for reporting adverse reactions to pharmaceutical items and advertising pharmaceutical products. The Act also governs the authorization of human clinical research. In a multitude of places, the Danish Medicines Agency can seek advice from various committees and councils comprised of either experts in the relevant field or representatives from interested parties. The panels and forums are self-governing bodies, and their role is to provide advice to the Danish Medicines Agency.The Danish Medicines Agency can reach people with committees and councils [62]. To offer pharmaceuticals, company authorization is required. Company authorizations are granted by the Danish Medicines Agency.

Retail distribution of natural medical items and traditional medicines is subject to additional regulations. A product is evaluated to confirm if it is a medicinal product. Two factors are used to determine whether a product is a medical product: Product presentation – Is the remedy marketed as a suitable medicinal product for the treatment or prevention of diseases in humans or animals. Product function – can the product be used to restore, rectify, or modify physiological functioning in humans or animals. In general, a product is deemed as a medicinal product if it fits in one of the criteria listed above. Under the Medicines Act, the Ministry of Health issued Executive Order No. 790 on herbal medicines on September 21, 1992. The Executive Order specifies the conditions that must be completed for the covered preparations to be granted marketing permission.

Herbal medications that aren't covered by the executive order must be applied under the Medicines Act's general provisions, which often need bibliographic documentation. Herbal medications may only be sold in Denmark if the Danish Medicines Agency has previously granted a marketing license. An application case processing period is limited to a total of 180 days. The applicant receives initial remarks on the application from the Danish Medicines Agency within 120 days. Following then, the applicant may submit supplementary material in support of the initial application for a maximum of 6 months. If the case processing is repeated (for a maximum of 60 days), more material can be submitted upon request, and the case processing can be restarted in a maximum of 6 months. In exceptional circumstances, the deadline can be extended by up to 6 months. Following that, the case can only be reopened with a fresh application and payment of a new fee [63].

NEW ZEALAND

The New Zealand Medicines and Medical Devices Safety Authority is known as Medsafe. The agency is under the purview of the Ministry of Health and is in charge of medicinal product regulation in New Zealand. The headquarter of Medsafe is located in Wellington. The administrative managing duties of Medsafe include product approval and setting standards for the approval of drugs. It is also answerable to pharma companies for projects sponsored by industry funds. Medsafe is incharge of enforcing the Medicines Act 1981 and Regulations 1984. Medsafe is responsible for implementing a framework of controls aimed to guarantee that therapeutic goods accessible in New Zealand have more benefits than risks when used responsibly. This is accomplished by pre-marketing product approval and post-marketing surveillance. Pre-marketing authorization is required for new and modified medications. New drugs cannot be commercialized in New Zealand without the Minister of Health's approval. Medicines that have undergone alterations cannot be marketed without the decision of the Director-General of Health. Before consent may be granted, data that establishes the product's quality, safety, and efficacy for the purposes for which it is to be used must be provided for examination. Medsafe does not fund drugs; this is the responsibility of PHARMAC. Both Medsafe and PHARMAC, on the other hand, are dedicated to ensuring that New Zealanders have access to safe and effective drugs. Post-marketing monitoring keeps track of the safety of medications and medical devices in use. Products that are shown to be hazardous are banned from usage, and practitioners are informed about new product safety information. Post-marketing monitoring is accomplished by initiatives such as:tracking adverse drug reactions in New Zealand, as well as monitoring international literature and other information sources;comparing the quality of marketed medicines to product specifications;taking care of grievances and investigations, and inspecting and licensing pharmaceutical manufacturers [64].

IRELAND

The Irish Medicines Board (IMB) is a regulatory body in Ireland. The IMB is committed to the implementation and ongoing improvement of a defined quality management system. The system is based on legislative, regulatory, and ISO 9000:2000 criteria; it also incorporates guidelines, standards, and best practices from Irish and international agencies.Through the regulation of medications, medical devices, and healthcare items, organizations can protect and improve public and animal health.The IMB's goal is to ensure, to the greatest extent feasible, the purity, safety, and efficacy of medicines available in Ireland, under current medical and scientific knowledge, and to involve in the systems meant to do so throughout the European Union. Before a medicine can be used, an application must be submitted to the IMB, which must include all of the relevant facts confirming its quality, safety, and efficacy [65]. The Irish Medicines Board (IMB) was rechristened as Health Products Regulatory Authority on July 1, 2014. (HPRA). The IMB name has served well since its establishment in 1996. Moreover, in the last 18 years, the government mandate has grown to include other health products as well as a variety of health-related substances. Medical equipment, regulated pharmaceuticals, clinical trials, blood products and components, tissues and cells, cosmetic items, the protection of animals used in experimental investigations, and organs intended for transplant surgery are among the sectors it now regulates. The Traditional Herbal Medicinal Products Directive (2004/24/EC) was implemented in Ireland on July 23, 2007. (S.I. No. 540 of 2007). The Directive established a regulatory clearance process for herbal medicines in the EU. Traditional herbal remedies that can be used without medical supervision must be registered in each EU Member State. This is a streamlined registration method for herbal medicines with a long history of use and approved safety and quality. TR numbers are assigned to products that have been approved for traditional-use registration.Even if a herbal medical product does not meet the criteria for registration as a traditional herbal medicinal product (THMP), it can nevertheless be awarded a marketing authorization in the same way that non-herbal medicines are.Products that make therapeutic claims or include ingredients that are likely to affect the body are considered medications and will require marketing authorization from the HPRA. The marketing authorization is accompanied by a Product Authorisation (PA) number, which appears on the medicine box/container. Individuals or businesses interested in learning more about the procedures for licensing human medicines in Ireland should read the essential materials, including guides and forms, as well as the explanatory information given [66].

BRAZIL

Brazil, South America's largest country, has grown to become the world's second-largest pharmaceutical market in the emerging world The Brazilian Health Surveillance Agency, abbreviated from the Portuguese "Agencia Nacional de Vigilancia Sanitaria," (ANVISA) is the country's food and drug regulatory agency. ANVISA was established in 1999 and is affiliated with the Ministry of Health, with the fundamental purpose of protecting and promoting public health surveillance over Brazilian products and services. ANVISA is in charge of drug registration and licensing of pharmaceutical laboratories and other companies involved in the pharmaceutical manufacturing process. The agency is also in charge of developing clinical trial regulations (in terms of drug Chemistry, Manufacturing, and Control (CMC) and subject safety). ANVISA collaborates with the Chamber of Drug Market Regulation (CMED) to govern drug pricing in collaboration with the Health Ministry and other ministry members. Ethical human clinical trials are governed by an Ethics Committee (EC) affiliated with the Ministry of Health. The agency is also in charge of health control at ports, airports, and borders, as well as developing relationships with the Ministry of Foreign Affairs and foreign entities and institutions to handle international health monitoring issues. ANVISA has been approved as a new regulatory member of the International Council on Harmonization of Technical Requirements for Pharmaceuticals for Human Use (ICH). As part of its goal to broaden its worldwide reach, ICH invited ANVISA from Brazil and the Ministry of Food and Drug Safety (MFDS) from South Korea as the very first new regulatory Members in November 2016, together with the Biotechnology Innovation Organization (BIO) as a new member of an industry association There are now 13 members and 22 observers on the board [67].

The Brazilian Health Regulatory Agency (Anvisa) is an autarchy related to the Ministry of Health that serves as the coordinator of the Brazilian Health Regulatory System (SNVS), which is present throughout the national territory.

Anvisa's role is to enhance population health protection by carrying out sanitary control of the manufacture, marketing, and use of health-regulated products and services, including relevant settings, processes, substances, and technology, as well as control at ports, airports, and borders. The Medicine Market Regulation Chamber (CMED) is the inter-ministerial organization in charge of economic regulation of the Brazilian pharmaceutical market, and Anvisa serves as the Chamber's Executive Secretariat.

CMED sets medicine price restrictions, creates rules to promote competition in the sector, monitors sales, and imposes fines when its rules are not followed. It is also in charge of establishing and maintaining the mandatory minimum discount for public purchases.

Anvisa classifies drugs as follows: new synthetic drugs, generic drugs, similar drugs (a generic drug marketed under a brand name), potentized medicines (homeopathic, anthroposophic, and antigenotoxic), specific medicines, notified medicines (low risk), OTC (over-the-counter) drugs, herbal medicines, medicinal gases, biological products, and radiopharmaceuticals. The maximum timelines for

Anvisa to make a final judgment on pre-market approvals for medications are specified by Law 13,411/2016: 120 days from the submission date of the prioritizing request for drugs in the prioritized category and 365 days for drugs in the ordinary category. The above-mentioned periods may be extended by no more than one-third.

Pre-market approvals are valid for five years from the date they are published in the Brazilian Official Gazette, and they can be renewed for equal and subsequent periods. Foreign corporations cannot make administrative arrangements with Anvisa to issue market authorizations directly. Foreign enterprises must have a legal partner in Brazil who is legally accountable for the products brought into and distributed on Brazilian territory.

According to Resolution RDC 57/2009, APIs generated in Brazil or imported from other countries cannot be industrialized, exposed to sale, or promoted in Brazil without necessary pre-market authorization by Anvisa. The active pharmaceutical ingredient, on the other hand, will be employed for scientific or technological research, as well as formulation research and development. The APIs present in the imported drug composition, whether a semi-elaborated or final product, are thus subject to Anvisa's pre-market approval. Anvisa does not currently require pre-market approval for APIs of vegetable origin, but their manufacturer must adhere to the current GMP. To gain pre-market approval for a final drug product, Anvisa must also provide pre-market approval to the API. Nonetheless, there are two distinct permission processes: each request must be submitted independently, following the submission guidelines, and each will have its authorization number. The API submission may be made before the request for market approval for the finished medicinal product.

Resolution RDC 09/2015 and Resolution RDC 205/2017 are the regulations that standardize the filing of clinical studies using pharmaceuticals and biological products to Anvisa for approval (special procedure for rare diseases) [68].

THAILAND

The Thailand Food and Drug Administration (Thai FDA) is the regulatory authority in charge of regulating the import of medications for research purposes, as well as indirectly regulating drug clinical studies in people. The Thai FDA is a regulatory agency within the Ministry of Public Health (MOPHCluster)'s of Public Health Service Support, as stated in the DrugAct, THA-33, and THA-49, and is given control by the MOPH to protect consumer health. The agency is also in charge of ensuring the quality, safety, and efficacy of health items in Thailand, such as meals, pharmaceuticals, cosmetics, and medical devices. Furthermore, under the 2019 revisions to the DrugAct and THA-6, the MOPH has the jurisdiction to establish and/or amend drug research-related processes, regulations, and conditions through Government Gazette announcements. The Secretary-General of the Thai FDA is also authorized to control drug research study activities by issuing temporary suspensions, requests for specific modifications, or ending a study that fails to conform with the Minister's published criteria.The Thai FDA's Medicines Regulation Division is a member of the Drug Board, as stated in the DrugAct and THA-32 (also referred to as the Drug Committee in the English translation of the drug). The Medicines Regulation Division was once called the Bureau of Drug Control, according to an in-country subject matter expert. The board shall include five to nine drug experts, as well as MOPH departmental directors-general and members from relevant organizations. The Minister of Public Health appoints the Committee, which is headed by the MOPH's Permanent Secretary, every two years. The board's 14 members have formed 20 subcommittees to help the board in its role of advising the Minister on regulatory matters and guaranteeing drug control. The subcommittee on permission to produce or import pharmaceuticals for clinical research is the most directly involved with clinical trial and drug import registration.

The drug also directs the board to form a subcommittee to investigate the drug review and approval process. The following people should be on the subcommittee: an official representative and Office of Consumer Protection Board representatives, including representatives from associations, foundations, and the pharmaceutical sector, whose aim is to manufacture, sell, import, or order medications for use in Thailand THA-32 has the most recent list of subcommittees, which includes the subcommittee on review and approval for the registration of modern pharmaceuticals for human use and the subcommittee on approval of producing or importing medications for clinical research. THA-49 goes on to say that the Medicines Regulation Division is in charge of reviewing licenses to import or order drugs into the country that are not subject to drug formulation registration, issuing licenses to produce a sample drug for registration, and issuing a permit to import or prescribe drug samples into the country. The International Affairs and Investigational New Drug Section of the Thai FDA's Medicines Regulation Division is in charge of application examination and approval recommendations. According to the ClinDrugReqsDetails and the Thai FDA's organizational structure indicated in THA-33, the final decision to approve the application is made by the Secretary-General of the Thai FDA [69].

SWEDEN

The Medical Products Agency is in charge of regulating and monitoring the creation, manufacture, and distribution of pharmaceuticals and other medicinal products. The Agency's mission is to ensure that both individual patients and healthcare practitioners have access to safe and effective pharmaceutical goods that are used rationally and cost-effectively. The acquisition of a license to sell pharmaceutical products in Sweden and the EU is governed by uniform EU rules. Approved items have a five-year marketing authorization that must be renewed at least once. All approved pharmaceutical goods in Sweden, as well as ones that have been withdrawn, can be found in the database Läkemedelsfakta. Only pharmaceutical items intended for marketing in Sweden can be authorized through the national procedure. A nationwide application for marketing authorization can be filed to the Swedish Medical Products Agency without requesting a time slot in advance. After the application is filed, a 14-day validation process begins. The application is checked in, and the Swedish Medical Products Agency (Swedish MPA) checks that it is complete before proceeding with the procedure. The operation is broken down into three stages, with a total processing time of 210 calendar days.

- Round one:

Once the application is approved, the procedure begins on day 0.

The primary assessment is completed on day 110, and the Swedish MPA sends the applicant a request for additional information. The deadline for responses is 90 days. If no response is received within the specified term, the Swedish MPA may decide on the application.An extended response deadline can only be granted in extreme circumstances, and only if the request is received enough in advance of the scheduled response date.

- Round two:

When a complete response is submitted, the operation is reopened. This is the 111th day of the year. Responses to the Swedish MPA must be complete; partial responses sent at different periods will not be accepted. When the responses are received, a new round is started because they are presumed to be complete. Day 165 marks the end of the secondary assessment. If the application is not approved, the Swedish MPA will send the applicant a request for additional information. The deadline for responses is in 40 days. The applicant's second response should only include answers to inquiries and clarifications; new extensive data is not acceptable at this stage. The premise is the same as in decentralized and centralized procedures.

- Round three:

When a complete response is submitted, the operation is reopened. This is the 166th day of the year. If the application is still not approved on day 190 following the third evaluation, the Swedish MPA sends a notice of likely rejection, giving the company the option to withdraw the application or communicate the relevant difficulties to the applicant. The applicant is expected to respond to any unresolved issues that may arise during the third round as soon as possible. All unresolved concerns must be handled by day 195 for approval to be granted by day 210. There will be no more rounds with extended response deadlines. The Swedish MPA draughts the decision after day 195, which is sent by day 210. If final labeling has not been agreed upon by day 195, the approval may be issued without final labeling. In that instance, the permission is conditional, thus, marketing can begin only after the labeling is approved.

An application for marketing authorization may be denied if, for example, negative risk-benefit balance, GxP documentation is lacking, inadequate impurity level qualification, inadequate methods of analysis, and gaps in process validation. During the evaluation, the applicant may provide additional information in response to unresolved questions in the assessment report. The application may be rejected if the supplemental information is deemed insufficient or is not supplied on time. In the event of a refusal, a Public Assessment Report (PAR) is issued, which briefly describes the grounds for the refusal.

Herbal medical medicines for human use can be approved for marketing in one of three ways:

Marketing authorization by the documents in Chapter 3 of the MPA's provisions (LVFS 2006:11) on marketing authorization for medicinal products, (Article 8 of Directive 2001/83/EC), a so-called “Full application” in which efficacy and safety are demonstrated by data from product-specific clinical and preclinical trials in the same way that conventional drugs are.

Marketing authorization under the documents in Chapter 5, Section 6 and 7 of the Swedish MPA's provisions LVFS 2006:11 (Article 10a of Directive 2001/83/EC), where data from clinical and preclinical trials can be replaced by information on “well-established medicinal use” in the EEA for at least ten years, supported by scientific literature.

Registering as a traditional herbal medicinal product by the documents in the MPA's provisions (LVFS 2006:3) on traditional herbal medicinal products for human use (Article 16c of Directive 2001/83/EC), where the efficacy and safety are based on evidence that the product has been in "traditional use" for at least 30 years, of which at least 15 years in the EE. Published scientific literature or product-specific data can be used to demonstrate safety. Traditional herbal medical items are only for human use and are constrained to self-medication, which does not require a practitioner's diagnosis, prescription, or treatment supervision. However, for some symptoms, it may be necessary to rule out other serious underlying illnesses. Only oral administration, external application, and/or inhalation may be permitted for the items.

Authorized herbal medicinal items may be sold as either prescription-only or over-the-counter medications (OTC). OTC herbal medicinal items that are authorized can be sold in locations other than pharmacies if they are on the list of OTC products that can be sold in places other than pharmacies [70].

ITALY

The Italian Medicines Agency - AIFA - is a public entity that operates under the principles of autonomy, openness, and efficiency, reporting to the Ministry of Health and being overseen by the Ministry of Health and the Ministry of Economy. AIFA collaborates with the States, the Italian National Institute of Health (ISS), Scientific Institutes for Research, Hospitalisation, and Health Care, patient associations, healthcare professionals and educational organizations, the manufacturing and distribution industries, and the world of research and development. Asa health-protection tool, AIFA ensures access to medicines as well as their safe and appropriate usage. Following the Regions ensures national unity of the pharmaceutical system, allows for the management of pharmaceutical expenditure in the framework of economic and financial compatibility, as well as the pharmaceutical industry's competitiveness, assures innovation, efficiency, and simplicity of registration procedures, particularly to enable faster access to novel medications and medicines for rare disorders, develops relationships with foreign agencies, the European Medicines Agency (EMA), and other international organizations. Encourages and motivates R&D investments in Italy by publicizing lucrative innovation discussions and communicating with the community of patient organizations, the medical and scientific world, and production and distribution companies to enhance knowledge and awareness of medicines, as well as the collection and evaluation of international best practices.

AIFA is organized into six management departments (five scientific-technical departments, namely the Pre-Authorisation Department, the Medicinal Products

Authorisation Department, the Post-Marketing Surveillance Department, the Economic Strategy of Pharmaceutical Products Department, the Inspection and Certification Department, and the Administration Department) and cross-functional supporting structures [71].

GERMANY

The German medical device regulating authority is the Federal Institute for Drugs and Medical Devices (BundesinstitutfürArzneimittel und Medizinprodukte, or BfArM). The BfArM is an independent authority under the Federal Ministry of Health that deals with the authorization of medications and medical devices under the German Medicines Act (Arzneimittelgesetz, AMG), oversees legal narcotics trade, and assesses possible risk. The BfArM is divided into nine divisions, with the ninth department solely dedicated to medical device management.

One of the BfArM's primary responsibilities is the authorization of completed medicinal products under the Medicinal Products Act (Arzneimittelgesetz, AMG). During these licensing procedures, the health benefit, *i.e.*, efficacy, safety, and pharmaceutical quality of the medical items, is evaluated. Furthermore, the BfArM performs critical responsibilities related to drug licensing on a European level. The BfArM either registers homeopathic medications without a statement of indications or licenses them with indications. A marketing authorization or registration is required before a pharmaceutical product can be placed on the market. Pharmaceutical entrepreneurs must submit the necessary applications to the BfArM for these to be granted. Various sorts of marketing authorization applications are accessible, depending on the nature of the project. The pages that follow provide information about the relevant requirements. Section 22(3)(1) of the German Medicines Act (AMG) and Article 10a of Directive 2001/83/EC both specify a particular type of marketing authorization application. Data for Modules 1–3 must therefore be submitted, but it is possible to replace pre-clinical and clinical trial results with comprehensive references to published scientific literature if it can be demonstrated that the active ingredients of a medicinal product in the stated therapeutic indication have been in well-established medicinal use within the Union for at least ten years, with identified efficacy. This data must be supported by a comprehensive scientific bibliography that covers all relevant preclinical and clinical features of the pharmaceutical product. As a result, this type of application is often known as a "bibliographical application." This data must be supported by a comprehensive scientific bibliography that covers all relevant preclinical and clinical features of the pharmaceutical product. As a result, this type of application is often known as a "bibliographical application."

Aside from the content, the nature of the literary sources is also important, as the submitted literature must be freely available in the public domain and published by a credible source. As a result, data from personal preclinical and clinical experiments may be excluded from the discussion of a bibliographic application. It should be noted that assessment reports such as the EPAR for EU marketing authorizations or comparable summary reports from competent authorities inside and outside the EU that are made publicly available for transparency reasons by competent authorities cannot be considered.

The German Medicines Act clearly states that the features of "specific treatment systems" must be respected, based on the concept of pluralism in pharmacotherapy. As a result, the legislator has created specific commissions (Commission C for anthroposophic medicinal products, Commission D for homeopathic medicinal products, and Commission E for herbal medicinal products) to assist the BfArM's work by providing medical expertise in the respective therapeutic fields. Division 5 of the BfArM is responsible for the management and scientific assistance of the aforementioned commissions and the Commission under 109a (3) AMG for traditional medicinal items.

Division 4 is in charge of conducting scientific evaluations of the efficacy, safety, and pharmaceutical quality of medical goods related to "specific treatment systems" as well as traditional medicinal remedies. Responsibilities include preparing medical and pharmaceutical assessments, as well as managing the full administrative project, including the issuance of marketing authorization based on successful licensing, simplified registration, or review procedures. Assessments are frequently prepared at the request of other divisions in procedural variations or renewals, European licensing procedures for herbal medicinal products, legal proceedings, and pharmacovigilance issues. Core data are developed to reflect the current state of the art in pharmacotherapy, and to standardize patient information pamphlets and information aimed at health professionals. Furthermore, at the request of pharmaceutical corporations, scientific assistance is offered before the start of licensing procedures [72, 73].

CHINA

The State Food and Drug Administration (SFDA) is based on the State Drug Administration. SFDA reports directly to the People's Republic of China's State Council and is in charge of comprehensive oversight on the safety management of food, health food, and cosmetics, as well as being the competent body for drug control in mainland China.

- Primary responsibilities:

Coordinate the relevant authorities to create laws and regulations for the management of food safety, healthy foods, and cosmetics; Organize the competent authorities to formulate a comprehensive supervision strategy and work plan and monitor its implementation.

Carry out comprehensive monitoring of the safety management of food, health food, and cosmetics under applicable laws; Planning and coordination of the supervisory work of the authorities responsible for food safety, food, and cosmetics.

To organize and carry out investigations and punish serious accidents in the field of food safety, food, and cosmetics; as delegated by the State Council to organize, coordinate, and conduct specific law enforcement campaigns across the country for food safety, healthy food, and cosmetics; and the organization, coordination, and cooperation with the competent authorities in the implementation of emergency rescue tasks in the event of serious accidents related to food, healthy food, and cosmetics.

Design and supervise the implementation of laws and regulations for the administration of medical devices; be responsible for the registration and regulation of medical devices; Elaboration of relevant national standards, development and revision of technical standards for medical devices and manufacturing processes; and monitor its implementation.

Responsible for the registration of drugs, development, modification, and dissemination of national pharmaceutical standards; Developing criteria for the approval of natural food products; and reviewing and approving healthy foods. Create a classification system for prescription and over-the-counter drugs; Creation and improvement of an ADR monitoring system; be responsible for drug re-evaluation, review of drugs to be discontinued, and develop a national essential drug list. To develop and revise best practices for medication research, production, distribution, and use, as well as to monitor their implementation. Controlling the quality of drugs and medical devices in manufacturers, distributors, and medical institutions; publishing a national quality bulletin on drugs and medical devices regularly; investigating and punishing illegal activities such as producing and selling counterfeit and inferior drugs and medical devices by the law.

Radioactive medicines, narcotics, toxins, psychotropics, and other prohibited substances and equipment must be regulated in line with the legislation.

Creating and improving a qualifying system for licensed pharmacists, as well as supervising and directing the registration of qualified pharmacists. To direct national drug regulation and thorough oversight of food, health food, and cosmetics safety management.

Exchanging information and cooperating with foreign governments and international organizations on drug control, and pertinent safety management of food, health food, and cosmetics.

To carry out various tasks delegated by the State Council. Pharmaceutical substances made and exported by chemical businesses are not regulated by the State Food and Drug Administration. This regulatory gap, which has resulted in significant negative international news coverage of China, has been recognized for a decade, but the reluctance of Chinese regulatory authorities to collaborate has precluded effective regulation [74].

SOUTH KOREA

The South Korean government body in charge of overseeing food, medicines, medical devices, and cosmetics is the Food and Drug Administration (KFDA). It was founded in 1996 and reformed in 2005 with the addition of the Medical Devices Management Division and the Bioproduct Technical Support Division, only to be renamed and elevated to a ministry in 2013. Medical device approval, GMP standards, and pre- and post-market monitoring of the medical device category process are all handled by the MFDS. The Medical Device Safety Bureau is the MFDS division in charge of medical devices, and it is divided into the following divisions: Division of Medical Device Policy, Division of Medical Device Management, Division of Medical Device Quality.

A new medication is a pharmaceutical with a completely different chemical structure or original composition than a previously approved pharmaceutical in Korea, or multiple preparations, including a novel material as an active drug substance, as designated by the Minister of Food and Drug Safety. (Article 2 Subparagraph 8 of the Pharmaceutical Affairs Act) The term "pharmaceutical necessary for data submission" refers to a pharmaceutical that is required for safety and efficacy testing rather than a novel medicine. (Article 2 Subparagraph 8 of the Regulation on Pharmaceutical Approval, Notification, and Review (MFDS Notification)) Pharmaceuticals with improved efficacy, novel composition, increased/decreased active drug substance strength, and pharmaceuticals with a different route of administration are only a few examples.

A generic medicine is a pharmaceutical that is equivalent to a new drug in terms of the active component, dose form, and potency (reference drug). (Regulation on

Pharmaceutical Safety (Ordinance of the Prime Ministerial) Article 9) Data Requirements for New Drug Approval.

(Drug Evaluation Department review) Data on safety and efficacy, specifications and test techniques, Drug Master Files (DMF), manufacture and marketing certificates (Imported Pharmaceutical) Data such as the name and address of active pharmaceutical ingredient manufacturers (Review by Other Departments) Data from the evaluation of Good Manufacturing Practices (GMP).

Data on Substances

Structure identification data

Physical and chemical property data

Data about manufacturing processes

Details about specifications and testing techniques are provided.

Specifications and test procedures are supported by data.

Information on test results

Reference standards, reagents, and test solutions data

Container and packaging material information

Pharmaceutical data submission is required: Selectively submit data for safety and effectiveness evaluations when submitting data for new medicines.

Throughout the drug review and approval process, including submission, pre-review, supplementation, approval, and amendment for each product, consult with the Central Pharmaceutical Affairs Advisory Committee (CPAC).

Pre-review system: PM assesses the accuracy of submission data as well as the data requirements' sufficiency.

Product Briefing, (Priority) new pharmaceutical, IMD, and when requested by a civil petitioner, Review Division, Pharmaceutical Policy Division, (Participants) civil petitioner, Improve the speed and predictability of the review and approval process by increasing mutual understanding between the reviewer and the petitioner of a product subject to approval. Update on Drug Approval

Weekly exclusions, monthly clearances, approval reports (NDA),. safety and efficacy evaluation findings (pharmaceuticals required for data submission) [75].

SWITZERLAND

Swissmedic, or the Swiss Agency for Therapeutic Products, is a Swiss government-run public agency. It's part of the Federal Department of Home Affairs. Swissmedic is governed by the Federal Act on Medicinal Products and Medical Devices (Therapeutic Products Act - TPA).Swissmedic began operations on January 1, 2002, when the TPA went into effect. The International Office for the Control of Medicines and the Therapeutic Products Section of the Swiss Federal Office of Public Health merged to become the Agency. The new area of responsibility takes into account the expanding international demand for health protection and quality requirements. Swissmedic is funded through fees, contributions from the Federal Government in exchange for public-interest services, and services supplied to third parties. The public services are outlined in a Federal Council service mandate and an annual service agreement with the Federal Department of Home Affairs. The Agency is managed by acceptable business practices to ensure the efficiency of its control operation.

The Agency publishes a Swiss Public Assessment Report (SwissPAR) summary evaluation report for all human pharmaceutical products containing a new active component, as well as transplant products, based on Art. 67 para. 1 TPA and the implementing provisions of Art. 68 para. 1 let. e TPO. It also publishes a supplementary report for accepted or refused applications relating to additional indications for human medical products for which a SwissPAR has been published as a result of the new authorization. The SwissPAR contains the review results of a human medical product's application for new authorization or additional indication, but not the applicant's commercial or manufacturing secrets or personal data. TheSwissPAR is primarily intended for use by healthcare professionals, industry representatives, and other national and international authorities. Swissmedic publishes the SwissPAR in English, employing specific technical terms.

At a Round Table on Regulatory Affairs (referred to below as the "Round Table"), Swissmedic and the pharmaceutical sector meet regularly to discuss topics connected to the regulation of medical products. The Round Table allows the parties to express their concerns to respond to regulatory and technological signals in a timely and suitable manner if needed. In some situations, Swissmedic must consult with representatives of the pharmaceutical sector before making a change in the regulation of medical products, so that practical aspects of operational execution can be properly taken into account and communicated effectively to the target audience. The Round Table is made up of representatives from the pharmaceutical sector and its associations, as well as top representatives from Swissmedic's Authorisation section. Over the years, direct communication between Swissmedic and the pharmaceutical sector has shown to be a fruitful approach to developing a mutual understanding of the parties' issues, as well as efficient planning and implementing regulatory, process-related, and technical changes. Separate Round Tables have been formed to address concerns about veterinary pharmaceutical goods, as well as complementary and herbal medicines. The Round Table will include a maximum of 12 pharmaceutical industry representatives who are familiar with operational challenges in the pharmaceutical business due to their day-to-day work or many years of expertise. They will also need to be well-versed in legislation, the political environment, and Swissmedic's working practices.

The Swiss federal parliament approved the new Article 9b as part of the amendment of the Therapeutic Products Act (TPA-2) on March 18, 2016. Art. 9b (new) Temporary authorization for use and restricted placing on the market. According to Article 9, paragraph 2 letter d, the Agency may, for a short time, allow specific individuals or groups of individuals to utilize medical products outside the scope of clinical studies. To give a temporary authorization to use medical products on January 1, 2019, by Article 9b paragraph 1 TPA.This means that patients may be treated with an unapproved product outside of the scope of a clinical trial. This authorization, which is granted by Swissmedic, is subject to several conditions outlined in Section 5 of the updated MPLO (Medicinal Products Licensing Ordinance). Complementary and herbal therapies are commonly utilized in Switzerland and are well-accepted by the general public. Swissmedic verifies that the primary approval conditions are met for these product types. According to the general rules of the ordinance on the simplified authorization of supplementary and herbal medicinal products, a simplified authorization procedure is available for all categories of these medicinal products. In each scenario, quality, safety, and efficacy must be guaranteed [76].

HONGKONG

The Boards and Councils Office (B&C Office) provides secretariat support to 15 healthcare-related statutory Boards and Councils, including the Medical Council of Hong Kong, Dental Council of Hong Kong, Nursing Council of Hong Kong, Midwives Council of Hong Kong, Supplementary Medical Professional Council, and five Boards established under the Council (*i.e.*, Medical Laboratory Technologists Board, Occupational Telecommunications Board, Occupational Telecommunications Board, and Occupational Telecommunications Board). The Central Registration Office under the B&C Office provides support to respective Boards and Councils on the registration of healthcare professionals and related issues.The Department of Health was reorganized on October 1, 2019, to better handle society's public health challenges.

The Regulatory Affairs function, led by the Controller, Regulatory Affairs, has been redefined as a result of the reorganization. The Controller, Regulatory Affairs is in charge of overseeing the operation of seven services, as well as directing the enforcement of public health legislation and the development of regulatory strategies capable of responding to new challenges posed by the evolving landscape of medical and health services.The Department of Health's Chinese Medicine Regulatory Office is responsible for executing the Chinese Medicine Ordinance, which was passed by the Legislative Council on July 14, 1999. The Ordinance regulates the use, manufacture, and sale of Chinese medicines, as well as the, practice of Chinese medicine practitioners. The Chinese Medicine Council of Hong Kong, which was established in September 1999 under the Chinese Medicine Ordinance, is responsible for implementing Chinese medicine rules, establishing the Government Chinese Medicines Testing Institute (GCMTI) to specialize in testing and scientific research on Chinese medicines, providing professional input for the investigation and management of adverse events related to the use of Chinese medicines, communicating and collaborating with stakeholders in the Chinese medicine field for disease prevention and control, and providing public education on Chinese medicine [77].

FRANCE

The National Agency for the Safety of Medicines and Health Products is the public actor that allows access to health products in France on behalf of the state and ensures their safety throughout their life cycle. They are at the heart of the health system, serving patients and ensuring their safety with health professionals and in consultation with their respective representatives.

They facilitate access to innovative products through authorization procedures tailored to each stage of the drug's life before and after it hits the market. They ensure that the health goods provided in France are safe, effective, accessible, and well-used through assessments, expertise, and policy monitoring. There are 900 workers split over three locations: Saint-Denis, Lyon, and Montpellier-Vendargues. They rely on a network of national, European, and worldwide knowledge and monitoring under ethical and transparent values [78].

NIGERIA

The National Agency for Food and Drug Administration and Control (NAFDAC) was established by Decree No. 15 of 1993, as revised by Decree No. 19 of 1999, and is now recognized as the National Agency for Food and Drug Administration and Control Act Cap N1 Laws of the Federation of Nigeria (LFN) 2004. Its mission is to regulate and control the production, importation, exportation, distribution, advertisement, sale, and use of food, drugs, and cosmetics (collectively known as regulated products). The Agency was initially founded in October 1992. The Director General's Office and eighteen Directorates that carry out the Agency's tasks make up the NAFDAC organization: The Agency also has six Zonal Offices, as well as the FCT and Lagos State Offices, all of which are led by Directors.

The Governing Council of the National Agency for Food and Drug Administration and Control (NAFDAC) in the exercise of the powers conferred on it by Sections 5 and 30 of the NAFDAC Act Cap N1 LFN 2004 and Section 12 of the Food, Drugs, and Related Products (Registration, *etc*.,) Act Cap F33 LFN 2004, and all other specialized on it in that regard, THE GOVERNING COUNCIL OF THE NATIONAL AGENCY FOR FOOD AND DRUG ADMINISTRATION AND CONTROL -These Regulations control the registration of pharmaceuticals and associated commodities manufactured, imported, exported, advertised, sold, distributed, or utilized in Nigeria(1) No drug product may be made, imported, exported, advertised, sold, distributed, or used in Nigeria unless it has been registered according to these Regulations. (2) Irrespective of provisions of Regulation 2(1) of this Regulation, the National Agency for Food and Drug Administration and Control (NAFDAC) may issue a permit for the import of goods or manufacture of a sample of a drug product for the following purposes: (a) registration (b) clinical trial (c) service drug scheme (d) use in an emergency due to disease outbreaks. (e) All humanitarian aid donations, as well as importation and production, must be made as per the permit's restrictions. (3) No person who has been issued a certificate of registration under these Regulations may lend, hire, sell, transfer, or otherwise dispose of the certificate of registration without the Agency's consent.

1) An application for registration of a drug product is made by filing a final registration form, which must be accompanied by the required paperwork as recommended by the Agency from time to time, and must: (a) contain the standards and characterization of the drug product for which the application is made; and (b) be accompanied by such fee as the Agency may prescribe from time to time.

2) The drug product particulars and description must be precise enough to include all administrative and technical information necessary for the Agency to make an educated decision regarding the product. (3) When evaluating an application, the Agency may: (a) request more information from the applicant to decide on the application; and (b) satisfy itself that the drug product needs to be registered in Nigeria. (c) The drug product may be registered under the provisions of the Food, Drug, and Related Products (Registration, *etc*.) Act section F33 LFN 2004. (4) A drug product's registration under these Regulations is valid for five years unless

terminated earlier and may be renewed. (5) The Agency shall, periodically, publish on the Agency's official website a list of registered drugs or drug products, informing the registration of a drug product. (6) The Agency may deny or disapprove any application form if: (a) the procedure, amenities, or limits used in the manufacturing process, processing, and packaging of the drug product are insufficient to regularly ensure and preserve its identity, strength, quality, and purity; or (b) the method, facilities, or controls used in the manufacture, processing, and labeling of the drug product are inadequate to guarantee and preserve its identity, strength, quality, and purity; or (c) the method, facilities, or controls used in the product manufacturing, (a) The laboratory report for the product is insufficient. (a) The good manufacturing practice inspection report is inadequate. (d) product labelling violates the 2019 Drug and Related Products Act.

TECHNICAL INFORMATION SUBMISSION TEMPLATE (TIST) NATIONAL AGENCY FOR FOOD AND DRUG ADMINISTRATION AND CONTROL HERBAL MEDICINES 1. GENERAL DESCRIPTION OF EACH PLANT COMPONENT CONTAINED IN THE PRODUCT a. Scientific Name with Authority and Photograph b. Synonyms c. Family d. Vernacular Names (Hausa, Igbo, Yoruba) e. Common names g. Herbal medicinal raw material harvesting and management h. Botanical description i. Plant parts used j. Official Plant Substitute (if any)

2. CHEMICAL CONSTITUENTS AND RECORD OF USE OF THE PLANT OR POLYHERBAL (IF MORE THAN ONE PLANT) a. Chemical Constituents (Literature) b. Herbarium Specimen c. *Major Uses d. *Other Uses e. *Claims Verification (Testimonials, Anecdotal) 3. IDENTIFICATION (PHYTO-CHEMISTRY) AND STANDARDIZATION OF HERBAL MEDICINAL PRODUCT a. Organoleptic Properties b. Fourier Transform Infra-red Identification of plant (powder or liquid) c. Macroscopic Description d. Microscopic Description e. Moisture Content f. Extraction Method g. Thin Layer Chromatography (Literature or Lab Acquired) 4. PHARMACOLOGICAL PROPERTIES a. *In Vitro* Experiments (Literature or Experimental Record) b. *In Vivo* Animal Experiments (Literature or Experimental Record) 5. SAFETY DATA OF EACH PLANT COMPONENT IN THE PRODUCT a. Traditional Use Safety Records 3 b. Acute Toxicity Literature (or Pass Down History) c. Sub-chronic and Chronic Toxicity (Literature or Otherwise) d. Reproductive Toxicity (Literature if any) e. Mutagenic Potentials (literature if any) f. Carcinogenic Potentials (literature if any) * 6. FORMULATION g. Formula and Ingredients (Plant and Excipients/Non-active Ingredients and Properties Organoleptic Properties Fourier Transform Infra-red Identification of the plant (powder or liquid) Macroscopic and Microscopic Description Moisture Content h. Method of

Preparation/ Manufacturing Process *7. LABELLING INFORMATION (PACKAGE INSERT/ LEAFLET) i. Dosage and Frequency of Administration j. Route of Administration k. Contraindications l. Side Effects and Adverse Effects m. Pregnancy and Lactation (Statement of exclusion) n. Overdose and Antidote (if any) o. Drug-Herb Interaction (Record if any) p. Children below 12 years (Statement of exclusion)- Except formulation meant for children q. Storage condition 4 8. HERBAL MEDICINE VIGILANCE (SAFETY MONITORING – LITERATURE IF ANY) 9. CLINICAL SAFETY DATA (QUOTED LITERATURE) [79].

UGANDA

UgandaNational Council for Science and Technology (UNCST) since 1995, UNCST has been a member. The Uganda National Council for Science and Technology was founded in 1990 to advise on and coordinate the creation of national policy in all disciplines of science and technology, as well as to aid in the promotion and development of indigenous science and technology. It builds and operates institutions for scientific and technological research and development, as well as disseminates R&D findings. The Council works closely with various organizations engaged in scientific and technological endeavors. The Council's operations are organized around three major areas of work. Knowledge-for-policy is a program that encourages and supports international scientific research and study, as well as communicates science that is relevant to international policy challenges. Policy-for-science aspires to promote innovations that will enable science to contribute more effectively to critical public-policy issues around the world. Scientific autonomy and the obligation to preserve ethical and responsible scientific practice Through a variety of co-sponsored international research programs, networks, and committees, the Council's activities cover a wide range of issues, including global sustainability, poverty, urban health and wellbeing, and disaster risk reduction, as well as data, observing systems, and science advice to governments [80].

MALAYSIA

The National Pharmaceutical Regulatory Agency (NPRA), originally known as the National Pharmaceutical Control Bureau (NPCB), was established in October 1978 as part of the Pharmacy and Supply Programme's quality control operation. This organization was created to ensure the quality of pharmaceutical products. The infrastructure and facilities were developed to accommodate testing and quality control activities. Beginning in 1985, the National Pharmaceutical Registration and Licensing Agency (NPRA) was tasked with guaranteeing the quality, efficacy, and safety of medications through registration and licensing structure. This is accomplished by evaluating scientific data and conducting laboratory tests on all items before they are sold. The NPRA also organizes courses and training for drug regulatory employees from other nations, such as Sri Lanka, Bangladesh, Myanmar, Mongolia, and Vietnam. The World Health Organization (WHO) designated NPRA as a "WHO Collaborating Centre for Regulatory Control of Pharmaceuticals" in 1996. This accolade is from WHO in acknowledgment of NPRA's contribution to the field of regulatory affairs.

- **Roles & Functions**

To put the drug registration / cosmetic notification process into action by evaluating technical data, laboratory analysis, research, and information from foreign authorities. Conducting analytical, pharmaceutical, microbiological, and pharmacological tests on medications and cosmetics to determine their quality, efficacy, and safety. Implementing a regulatory regime for the quality of pharmaceutical items on the market by random sampling and analytical testing. To put in place a licensing structure for pharmaceutical makers, importers, and distributors, as well as a clinical trial licensing scheme. To encourage and support local pharmaceutical firms in raising their production standards to levels similar to the World Health Organization's Good Manufacturing Practice guidelines (WHO). Manage the Adverse Drug Reaction Monitoring Program and take part in the WHO International Adverse Drug Reaction Monitoring Program. To oversee the product recall plan for pharmaceutical products that are deemed to be inferior or hazardous to customers. To disseminate information on Drug Control Authority (DCA) policies/news through the newsletter "BeritaUbat-ubatan," as well as to give service in the form of explaining to the public the process of online registration, information on registered items, and other NPRA-related queries. Conduct methodology and basic research to evaluate the quality, efficacy, and safety of drugs/cosmetics. To provide training for pharmaceutical regulatory officers, as well as other professional and semi-professional officials, through a local training program or an international cooperation program [81].

NETHERLANDS

Anyone who utilizes medications should be able to put their trust in them. That is what the Medicines Evaluation Board (MEB) works on every day in the Netherlands and throughout Europe. They evaluate medicines to decide whether they can be placed on the market, monitor adverse reactions and hazards, and promote proper medication use: this is the heart of their work. The (statutory) duties of the Medicines Evaluation Board (MEB) are broadly classified into three categories: reviewing medicines, monitoring adverse reactions and dangers, and promoting proper medication usage. Another significant statutory responsibility is to provide scientific advice to pharmaceutical corporations. People who take medicines in the Netherlands have access to around 20,000 licensed items. All of these medications must meet stringent criteria. For example, the effect of a medicine must be balanced against the hazards, the quality must be acceptable, and the patient information leaflet must be comprehensive. As the Netherlands' medicines authority, the MEB evaluates each medicine that enters the market to ensure that it meets all legal requirements. They continue to monitor a medicine once it is on the market. They monitor the safety of the medicine and take action if there is any danger, for example, based on reported adverse reactions and other information.

The MEB's administrative regulations refer to the Advisory Board. The Advisory Board's position, tasks, and working procedures are established in the "MEB Advisory Board administrative regulations 2013". The Advisory Board must include at least five members. The MEB appoints the members after the Chairperson of the Board and the Director of the Secretariat nominate them. Members come from a variety of social backgrounds. They have specific knowledge of the MEB's areas of specialization. At least twice a year, the Advisory Board meets. Following the national procedure, applicants will be issued a marketing authorization that is only valid in the Netherlands. Furthermore, the national procedure is not available for medicinal product dossiers where the same applicant has already obtained marketing authorization in one of the other EU/EEA Member States or has already submitted an application for marketing authorization in one of the other EU/EEA Member States and the application is being considered. Applicants that intend to proceed through a national procedure must submit a marketing authorization dossier to the MEB. When the marketing authorization is obtained, the Summary of Product Characteristics, packaging leaflet, and label text (including layout) will be decided if the decision is favorable. Decisions to award national marketing authorizations are kept in a medicinal product register. Applicants who plan to use a national procedure must submit a marketing permission dossier to the MEB. If the marketing authorization is granted, the Summary of Product Characteristics, package leaflet, and label text (including layout) will be determined. A medicinal product register keeps track of decisions to grant national marketing authorizations [82].

SINGAPORE

The Singapore Food Agency is responsible for food and food supplements (SFA).Pharmaceutical Administration Center. The Health Products Act (HPA) and its rules, particularly the Health Products (Therapeutic Products) Regulations 2016, govern therapeutic products in Singapore. Before manufacturing, importing or supplying medicinal items, enterprises must get a dealer's license. All therapeutic goods will need to be registered before they can be sold in Singapore.

Before conducting clinical trials of therapeutic items in Singapore, it is mandatory to apply for a Clinical Trial Authorisation or submit a Clinical Trial Notification. Registration of therapeutic products. Before selling medicinal products in Singapore, candidates must first register them. Registration requirements will vary based on whether the candidate submitted a new drug application or a generic medication application and the registration evaluation path. Traditional medicines (TM) in the local context relate to Malay and Indian traditional medicinal products. They are finished goods comprising materials whose applications are documented in relevant TM references.

HSA does not require permissions or licensing for the importing, manufacturing, or sale of TM. The inclusion of pharmaceutical compounds, such as steroids, in TM is prohibited by the HSA. The HSA also places rigorous limitations on the amount of harmful heavy metals in these items. Before supplying TM to Singapore, dealers (importers, producers, wholesale dealers, and retailers) must guarantee that their products are neither dangerous nor unsafe and that they fulfill the guidelines [83].

JAPAN

The Pharmaceutical Affairs Law (PAL) and associated ordinances govern clinical trials and the approval of new drugs in Japan. The Ministry of Health, Labour and Welfare (MHLW) is the government agency in charge of enacting pharmaceutical laws. The MHLW takes the ultimate decision on whether to discontinue studies for which investigational new drug notifications (INDs) have been made, as well as whether to approve medications for which New Drug Applications (NDAs) have been submitted. The Pharmaceuticals and Medical Devices Entity (PMDA) is a law-enforced semi-government agency that performs scientific reviews of INDs and NDAs through internal review teams. With recent advancements in worldwide regulatory harmonisation and the need for cooperation between the regulator and the sector, the PMDA's position as a review agency has become crucial in pharmaceutical research and development efforts. The PMDA also offers clinical development consultancy services comparable to those offered by the US Food and Drug Administration. Japanese rules have developed over time by progressively incorporating Western regulatory elements into pre-existing ones. Despite the fact that most fundamental regulatory systems are comparable to those in Western nations, there are some major variations, such as the application of INDs. Encountered with a recent drop in the number of domestic trials, the MHLW has taken several steps to encourage them, including grants to train hospital staff. However, the decline is unusual to be reversed quickly because it is linked to a decline in demand for Japanese trials as a result of globalisation of pharmaceutical research and development [45].

GULF COUNTRIES (SAUDI ARABIA, KUWAIT, THE UNITED ARAB EMIRATES, QATAR, BAHRAIN, OMAN)

Regulatory Agencies of the Gulf Cooperation Council

The Gulf Central Committee for Drug Registrations (GCC-DR) is a body that oversees the registration of drugs; it was approved in May 1999. Located in Riyadh, Saudi Arabia, the Executive Office for Health Ministers. Drug registration is divided into two stages:

Procedure for Centralised Registration

After confirming that all registration criteria have been met and the following documents have been fully filled out, the executive office of GCC-DR accepts receipt of registration files: The registration form of a pharmaceutical company. A registration form for a pharmaceutical chemical substance or preparation. Each chemical entity must submit eight full files and 17 samples to the executive office, with two samples sent to each nation along with the registration file. Every nation must examine the registration files sent to it and then submit them to the committee with its recommendations. The corporation must also provide a laboratory for the investigation of standard materials, procedures, and other items. The executive office sends chemical entity samples to a reference-accredited laboratory for examination. Following central approval of a company's or chemical entity's registration, the remaining authentication and paperwork, as well as costs, are concluded on a country-by-country basis, in accordance with their prescribed and established regulations. The registration certificate is issued by the executive office.

Companies have two months from the date of GCC-DR notification of their registration to file a dispute with the executive office. Centralising medication registration is not required in the GCC. However, registration through the centralised method is required for some groups of medications. The following are some of them: Inhalable medications and several nasal inhalers are examples of generic pharmaceuticals for which bioequivalence tests are not possible. Drugs that are supported by biotechnology but require clinical or pharmacodynamic investigations since bioequivalence studies are not possible. Orally given drugs with a restricted therapeutic range.

Procedure for Registration that is not Centralised

Regulations on registration in the GCC's main nations. Although medication registration in GCC nations is centralised and rather uniform, the regulatory procedures of a few large countries, such as Saudi Arabia and the United Arab Emirates, are distinct. These countries have a well-developed regulatory structure that is enforced [84].

SOUTH AFRICA

SAHPRA is a division of the National Department of Health that was established by the South African government to guarantee that human and animal health is prioritised. The Medicines Control Council (MCC) and the Directorate of Radiation Control (DRC), both of which were situated under the National Department of Health (NDoH), were taken over by SAHPRA. SAHPRA was established as an autonomous body that reports to the National Minister of Health through its Board of Directors.

To be assessed by SAHPRA, all new medication applications must meet rigorous standards. New registration applications must follow current rules and be submitted in either the eCTD or eSubmission formats. Applicants are obliged to provide all needed papers in the appropriate areas. Appendix A offers a list of all applicable guidelines that should be followed when putting together a new medication registration application. The rest of this section goes through how to create fresh registration applications in more detail.

Application Number

Before submitting an application to SAHPRA, one needs to request an application number. If the application contains several strengths, they should be compiled into a single dossier.

Electronic Entries

SAHPRA requires that all applications for medication registration be filed electronically (eCTD or eSubmission). The CTD standards, the ICH granularity document, and the ICH file naming conventions should all be followed for both types of submissions.

The sequence 0000 should always be used in new drug registration applications submitted to SAHPRA.

Models of Reliance

For eligible applicants, SAHPRA will deploy dependence models. The General Information Guideline offers the most up-to-date information on SAHPRA's evaluation paths, Recognised Regulatory Authorities (RRAs), and collaborative/work-sharing methods. The General Information Guideline is the major source of information on dependence, with the Clinical Guidelines and the Quality and Bioequivalence Guideline providing further details.

GMP

Prior to the filing of the relevant application, all manufacturing and quality control facilities influencing the application must be GMP compliant. As proof of GMP compliance, a GMP certificate or comparable manufacturing license is necessary.

Document SCoRE

The Summary of Critical Regulatory Elements (SCoRE) document is intended to provide a top-down summary-driven approach to reviews, shortening overall application processing time [47].

ARMENIA, AZERBAIJAN, BELARUS, GEORGIA, KAZAKHSTAN, KYRGYZSTAN, TURKMENISTAN, MOLDOVA, RUSSIA, TAJIKISTAN, UKRAINE, UZBEKISTAN (THE COMMONWEALTH OF INDEPENDENT STATES)

The Commonwealth of Independent States (CIS), sometimes known as the Russian Commonwealth or the old CIS region, is a confederation comprising nine member countries and two associate members. The Commonwealth of Independent States (CIS) was established in 1991 as a regional organisation whose member nations are former Soviet republics following the disintegration of the Union of Soviet Socialist Republics (USSR). The Commonwealth of Independent States (CIS) was founded following the disintegration of the Soviet Union and included the majority of former Soviet republics. Armenia, Azerbaijan, Belarus, Kazakhstan, Kyrgyzstan, Moldova, Russia, Tajikistan, and Uzbekistan are CIS members, as is Georgia, who withdrew from the organisation in 2008. Turkmenistan and Ukraine are two associate member nations that have not approved the CIS membership. Mongolia is occasionally assigned to the area, despite having no direct relationship with the CIS.

In CIS nations, regulatory processes are directed and controlled by Regulatory Agencies that work closely with or within the individual Ministries of Health. Individual registration rules have been created in each of the CIS nations. In

RUSSIA, registration is a nationwide practice. The operation is expected to take up to 24 months. Documentation is completed in Russian and in a manner that complies with Russian regulations. The recommended submission of a bioequivalence study is carried out at authorized research organisations on the territory of the Russian Federation. Both original and generic products go through the same registration process. Both original and generic products undergo the same registration process. Original goods must go through all registration processes, whereas generic drugs are free from certain of them. In Russia, for example, the original product must go through clinical studies. Bio-equivalence tests for generic products can be undertaken in any country, not just in Russia [48].

VIETNAM, THAILAND, SINGAPORE, PHILIPPINES, BRUNEI, CAMBODIA, INDONESIA, LAOS, MALAYSIA, MYANMAR (ASSOCIATION OF SOUTH ASIAN NATIONS)

For licensing drugs, the Association of Southeast Asian Nations (ASEAN) has a variety of regulatory procedures. Despite regional harmonisation attempts, the regulatory procedure for acquiring Marketing Authorizations (MAs) for medications in the ASEAN area remains mainly country-specific. While most ASEAN nations adopt the International Council for Harmonization (ICH) and European Medicines Agency (EMA) guidelines, country-specific restrictions must be met for effective MA approval by health authorities (HA). The Common Technical Document (CTD) is a useful resource for most local MA applications, although it is not necessary for its entirety.

The ASEAN region is made up of ten countries: Malaysia, Indonesia, Thailand, the Philippines., Singapore, Brunei, Vietnam, Laos, Cambodia, and Myanmar. The ASEAN organisation was founded on August 8, 1967, in Bangkok, Thailand. Malaysia, Indonesia, Thailand, the Philippines, and Singapore were the first five nations to join. Brunei, Cambodia, Laos, Myanmar, and Vietnam were later admitted to ASEAN. ASEAN's first trade endeavour was the formation of the ASEAN Free Trade Area (AFTA) in 1992, to promote economic development and improve competitiveness *via* the removal of trade obstacles.

The ASEAN area has established the ASEAN Common Technical Requirements (ACTRs), which are similar to Notice to Applicants (NtAs) and give standards for the development of drug dossiers.

ASEAN Common Technical Document (ACTD) and ASEAN Common Technical Requirements are led by the following countries:

Indonesia - High Quality (Q)

Thailand – Effectiveness (E)

Philippines - Security (S)

Malaysia - Administrative information, product details, and a glossary. After the patent for an innovator medication/original drug expires, generic pharmaceuticals may be marketed in ASEAN nations. A patent is only valid for 20 years and cannot be extended. In Malaysia, there is a data exclusivity clause that states that the period of data exclusivity shall not exceed: five years for a new drug product containing a new chemical entity; three years for a second indication of a registered drug product; the period of data exclusivity is only for the data concerning the second indication. For paediatric medicine, no extra data exclusivity is supplied [49].

CONCLUSION

Immunomodulators are natural or manufactured substances that can inhibit, activate, or modify the immune system, including both adaptive and innate immunity. The rising frequency of chronic diseases, along with the undesirable effects of synthetic immunomodulators, has resulted in the formation of an international market for natural immunomodulators. Herbal medicine presents a fresh target for drug discovery methodologies and medication development for researchers. The word "regulation" refers to a wide range of items with varying legal bases and authority (for example, rules, recommendations, processes, policies, and so on). Pharmaceutical regulation aims to ensure the safety, usefulness, and quality of medications made available to the general population. Several regulatory activities accomplish this throughout a drug's life cycle, including premarket screening and analysis of novel medications, an inspection of manufacturing facilities, legislation, marketing, and post-market surveillance. Every country has different rules governing invention, production, inspection, advertising, and post-marketing surveillance. The aim is to maintain drug standards high for the better health of the country's patients. In this chapter, we have discussed the importance of natural immunomodulators, regulatory bodies of different countries, and the process of market approval for drugs.

CONSENT FOR PUBLICATION

Not applicable

CONFLICT OF INTEREST

The authors declare no conflict of interest, financial or otherwise.

ACKNOWLEDGEMENTS

The authors of this chapter would like to acknowledge SVKM's Dr.BhanubenNanavati College of Pharmacy, V.M. Road, Vile Parle (W), Mumbai-400056, India.

REFERENCES

[1] Billiau A, Matthys P. Modes of action of Freund's adjuvants in experimental models of autoimmune diseases. J Leukoc Biol 2001; 70(6): 849-60. [http://dx.doi.org/10.1189/JLB.70.6.849] [PMID: 11739546]

[2] Juyal P. Parasitology LS-ID of V, 2001 undefined. Herbal immunomodulatory and therapeutic approaches to control parasitic infection in livestock. HillagricAcIn n.d.

[3] Introduction LP-L. Int Coop Converg Harmon Pharm Regul 2014; 1–5 [http://dx.doi.org/10.1016/B978-0-12-800053-3.00001-X]

[4] Olson MK. Regulation of Safety, Efficacy, and Quality. Encycl Heal Econ 2014; pp. 240-8. [http://dx.doi.org/10.1016/B978-0-12-375678-7.01202-5]

[5] Olson MK. Regulation of Safety, Efficacy, and Quality. Encycl Heal Econ 2014; pp. 240-8. [http://dx.doi.org/10.1016/B978-0-12-375678-7.01202-5]

[6] Kirtikumar N. and DM-J of pharmaceutical science, 2014 undefined. Documentation requirements for generic drug application to be marketed in india-a review. JpsbrCom 2014; 4: 237-42.

[7] Agarwal NB, Karwa M. Pharmaceutical Regulations in India. Pharm Med Transl Clin Res 2017: 215–31. [http://dx.doi.org/10.1016/B978-0-12-802103-3.00013-4]

[8] Andrade C, Shah N. The new patent regime: Implications for patients in India. Indian J Psychiatry 2007; 49(1): 56–59. [http://dx.doi.org/10.4103/0019-5545.31520]

[9] Imran M, Najmi A, Rashid M, Tabrez S, Shah M. Clinical research regulation in India-history, development, initiatives, challenges and controversies: Still long way to go. J Pharm Bioallied Sci 2013; 5(1): 2-9. [http://dx.doi.org/10.4103/0975-7406.106553] [PMID: 23559817]

[10] Narang S. Pharmaceutical Regulations in the United States: An Overview. Pharm Med Transl Clin Res 2018; 157-74. [http://dx.doi.org/10.1016/B978-0-12-802103-3.00011-0]

[11] Naito C. Necessity and requirements of bridging studies and their present status in Japan. Int J Clin Pharmacol Ther 2000; 38(2): 80-6. [http://dx.doi.org/10.5414/CPP38080] [PMID: 10706195]

[12] Nagata R, Fukase H, Rafizadeh-Kabe JD. East-West development: understanding the usability and acceptance of foreign data in Japan. Int J Clin Pharmacol Ther 2000; 38(2): 87-92. [http://dx.doi.org/10.5414/CPP38087] [PMID: 10706196]

[13] Nagata R, Raflzadeh-Kabe J-D. Japanese pharmaceutical and regulatory environment. Dialogues Clin Neurosci 2002; 4(4): 470-4. [http://dx.doi.org/10.31887/DCNS.2002.4.4/rnagata] [PMID: 22034129]

[14] Picano E. Risk of cancer from diagnostic X-rays. Lancet 2004; 363(9424): 1909-10. [http://dx.doi.org/10.1016/S0140-6736(04)16373-3]

[15] 991 International guidelines for ethical review of epidemiological studies n.d. 2002.

[16] Handbook for good clinical research practice (gcp) guidance for implementation 2002.

[17] Handbook for good clinical research practice (gcp) guidance for implementation 2003.

[18] Rägo L, Santoso B. Rägo L, Santoso B. Drug Regulation: History, Present and Future 1 2008.

[19] Guidelines for the Regulatory Assessment of Medicinal Products for use in Self-Medication n.d 2002.

[20] Permanand G, Mossialos E, McKee M. Regulating medicines in Europe: the European Medicines Agency, marketing authorisation, transparency and pharmacovigilance. Clin Med (Lond) 2006; 6(1): 87-90.
[http://dx.doi.org/10.7861/clinmedicine.6-1-87] [PMID: 16521363]

[21] U.S. Food and Drug Administration n.d. https://www.fda.gov/

[22] Medicines and Healthcare products Regulatory Agency - GOV.UK n.d. https://www.gov.uk/government/organisations/medicines-and-healthcare-products-regulatory-agency (accessed September 30, 2021).

[23] Therapeutic Goods Administration (TGA) | Australian Government Department of Health n.d. https://www.tga.gov.au/ (accessed September 30, 2021).

[24] H n.d. home n.d. https://cdsco.gov.in/opencms/opencms/en/Home/ (accessed October 4, 2021).

[25] Health Products and Food Branch - Canada.ca n.d. https://www.canada.ca/en/health-canada/corporate/about-health-canada/branches-agencies/health-products-food-branch.html (accessed October 1, 2021).

[26] European Medicines Agency | n.d. https://www.ema.europa.eu/en (accessed October 1, 2021).

[27] Frontpage - Danish Medicines Agency n.d. https://laegemiddelstyrelsen.dk/en/ (accessed October 1, 2021).

[28] Current Regulatory Guidelines n.d. ovt.nz/regulatory/current-guidelines.asp (accessed October 1, 2021).

[29] Medicines Authorisation n.d. http://www.hpra.ie/homepage/medicines/regulatory-information/medicines-authorisation (accessed October 1, 2021).

[30] Página inicial — Português (Brasil) n.d. https://www.gov.br/anvisa/pt-br (accessed October 1, 2021).

[31] Pages - Main n.d. https://www.fda.moph.go.th/sites/fda_en/Pages/Main.aspx (accessed October 1, 2021).

[32] Marketing authorisation | Swedish Medical Products Agency n.d. https://www.lakemedelsverket.se/en/permission-approval-and-control/marketing-authorisation (accessed October 1, 2021).

[33] Italian Medicines Agency n.d. https://www.aifa.gov.it/en/web/guest/home (accessed October 1, 2021).

[34] BfArM - Homepage n.d. https://www.bfarm.de/EN/Home/_node.html (accessed October 1, 2021).

[35] China SFDA Approval and Registration for Medical Devices, SFDA Registration Agent service n.d. http://www.sfda.com/ (accessed October 1, 2021).

[36] Welcome to the Ministry of Food and Drug Safety | Minisry of Food and Drug Safety n.d. https://www.mfds.go.kr/eng/index.do (accessed October 1, 2021).

[37] Homepage n.d. https://www.swissmedic.ch/swissmedic/en/home.html (accessed October 4, 2021).

[38] Pharmaceutical services n.d. https://www.health.nsw.gov.au/pharmaceutical/Pages/default.aspx (accessed October 1, 2021).

[39] The French Agency for the Safety of Health Products n.d. https://www.emergobyul.com/resources/europe/french-agency-safety-health-products (accessed October 1, 2021).

[40] Product Registration & Regulation – NAFDAC n.d. https://www.nafdac.gov.ng/our-services/ product-

registrationevaluation/ (accessed October 1, 2021).

[41] Uganda National Council for Science and Technology – UNCST – Science,Technology and Innovation n.d. https://uncst.go.ug/ (accessed October 1, 2021).

[42] National Pharmaceutical Regulatory Agency (NPRA) - Home n.d. https://www.npra.gov.my/index.php/en/ (accessed October 1, 2021).

[43] Home | Medicines Evaluation Board n.d. https://english.cbg-meb.nl/ (accessed October 1, 2021).

[44] Health Sciences Authority (HSA) n.d. https://www.hsa.gov.sg/ (accessed October 1, 2021).

[45] Ono S. Ministry of Health, Labour and Welfare (MHLW, Japan). Wiley Encycl Clin Trials 2007. [http://dx.doi.org/10.1002/9780471462422.eoct344]

[46] Pateriya S, Janodia MD, Deshpande PB, *et al.* Regulatory aspects of pharmaceuticals' exports in gulf cooperation council countries. J Young Pharm 2011; 3(2): 155-62. [http://dx.doi.org/10.4103/0975-1483.80305] [PMID: 21731362]

[47] Product registration process - sahpra n.d.https://www.sahpra.org.za/product-registration-process/# (accessed November 20, 2021).

[48] Handoo S, Khera D, Nandi PK, Sahu SK, Arora V. A comprehensive study on regulatory requirements for development and filing of generic drugs globally. Int J Pharm Investig 2012; 2(3): 99-105. [http://dx.doi.org/10.4103/2230-973X.104392] [PMID: 23373001]

[49] The Drug Regulatory Landscape in the ASEAN Region | RAPS n.d. https://www.raps.org/news-an--articles/news-articles/2018/1/the-drug-regulatory-landscape-in-the-asean-region (accessed November 20, 2021).

[50] FDA Approval - Process of Approving Drugs & Medical Devices n.d. https://www.drugwatch.com/fda/ approval-process/ (accessed September 3, 2021).

[51] FDA Rules and Regulations | FDA n.d. https://www.fda.gov/regulatory-information/fda-rules--nd-regulations (accessed September 3, 2021).

[52] CDSCO n.d. ov.in/CDSCO/homepage (accessed September 4, 2021).

[53] Bhatt A. Phytopharmaceuticals: A new drug class regulated in India. Perspect Clin Res 2016; 7(2): 59-61. [http://dx.doi.org/10.4103/2229-3485.179435] [PMID: 27141470]

[54] Australia's Therapeutic Goods Administration n.d. https://www.emergobyul.com/resources/australia/therapeutic-goods-administration (accessed September 4, 2021).

[55] Australia H. Therapeutic Goods Administration (TGA) 2019.

[56] What is the Medicines and Healthcare products Regulatory Agency? - Medicines and Healthcare products Regulatory Agency (MHRA) - Patient Safety Learning - the hub n.d. https://www.pslhub.org/learn/organisations-linked-to-patient-safety--k-and-beyond/regulators-and-their-regulations/system-and--roduct-regulators/mhra/what-is-the-medicines-and-healthcare-products-regulatory-agency-r527/ (accessed September 4, 2021).

[57] How Drugs are Reviewed in Canada - Canada.ca n.d. https://www.canada.ca/en/health-canada/services/drugs-health-products/drug-products/fact-sheets/drugs-reviewed-canada.html (accessed September 8, 2021).

[58] Branch LS. Consolidated federal laws of canada, Food and Drugs Act. Laws-LoisJusticeGcCa n.d.

[59] About Natural Health Product Regulation in Canada - Canada.ca n.d. https://www.canada.ca/en/health-canada/services/ drugs-health-products/natural--on-prescription/regulation.html#a1 (accessed November 20, 2021).

[60] What we do | European Medicines Agency n.d. https://www.ema.europa.eu/en/about-us/what-we-do

(accessed September 8, 2021).

[61] Herbal medicines: regulatory and scientific support | European Medicines Agency n.d. https://www.ema.europa.eu/en/human-regulatory/herbal-products/herbal-medici-es-regulatory-scientific-support (accessed November 20, 2021).

[62] The Danish Medicines Act n.d. https://laegemiddelstyrelsen.dk/en/about/targets-an--tasks/legislation/the-danish-medicines-act/ (accessed September 12, 2021).

[63] Guidance on marketing authorization for herbal medicines n.d. https://laegemiddelstyrelsen.dk/da/godkendelse/godkendelse-af-medicin/markedsfoeringstilladelse/ansoegning--m-markedsfoeringstilladelse/markedsfoeringstilladelse-til-naturlaegemidler/ (accessed September 24, 2021).

[64] About Medsafe n.d. ovt.nz/other/about.asp (accessed September 13, 2021).

[65] PharmaBoardroom | Irish Medicines Board (IMB) n.d. https://pharmaboardroom.com/directory/irish-medicines-board-imb/ (accessed September 13, 2021).

[66] Medicines Information n.d. http://www.hpra.ie/homepage/medicines/medicines-information (accessed September 13, 2021).

[67] Huynh-Ba K, Beumer Sassi A. ANVISA: an introduction to a new regulatory agency with many challenges. AAPS Open 2018 41 2018;4:1–6. [http://dx.doi.org/10.1186/s41120-018-0029-x]

[68] Brazilian Health Regulatory Agency (Anvisa) — Português (Brasil) n.d. https://www.gov.br/anvisa/pt-br/english

[69] Clinical Research Regulation For Thailand | ClinRegs n.d. https://clinregs.niaid.nih.gov/country/thailand#_top (accessed September 14, 2021).

[70] Swedish Medical Products Agency | Start n.d. https://www.lakemedelsverket.se/en (accessed September 19, 2021).

[71] Legislation - Italian Medicines Agency | Italian Medicines Agency n.d. https://www.aifa.gov.it/en/web/guest/normativa-di-riferimento-agenzia-italiana-del-farmaco (accessed September 21, 2021).

[72] Germany's Federal Institute for Drugs and Medical Devices n.d. https://www.emergobyul.com/resources/europe/germany-federal-institute-drugs-medical-devices (accessed September 21, 2021).

[73] BfArM - Homepage n.d. https://www.bfarm.de/EN/Home/_node.html (accessed September 21, 2021).

[74] sFDA CHINA « New Drug Approvals n.d. https://newdrugapprovals.org/sfda-china/ (accessed September 21, 2021).

[75] Approval Process|Drugs|Our Works|Minisry of Food and Drug Safety n.d. https://www.mfds.go.kr/eng/wpge/m_17/denofile.do (accessed September 22, 2021).

[76] Agency Council n.d. https://www.swissmedic.ch/swissmedic/en/home/about-us/organisation/agenc--council.html (accessed September 24, 2021).

[77] Department of Health - Legislative Council Business n.d. https://www.dh.gov.hk/english/legislative/legislative.html (accessed September 24, 2021).

[78] In brief - ANSM n.d. https://ansm.sante.fr/qui-sommes-nous/ (accessed September 24, 2021).

[79] NAFDAC – National Agency for Food & Drug Administration & Control n.d. https://www.nafdac.gov.ng/ (accessed September 24, 2021).

[80] Uganda National Council for Science and Technology – UNCST – Science,Technology and Innovation n.d. https://www.uncst.go.ug/ (accessed September 25, 2021).

[81] National Pharmaceutical Regulatory Agency (NPRA) - Home n.d. https://www.npra.gov.my/index.php/en/ (accessed September 25, 2021).

[82] Home | Medicines Evaluation Board n.d. https://english.cbg-meb.nl/ (accessed September 26, 2021).

[83] HSA | Regulatory overview of traditional medicines n.d. https://www.hsa.gov.sg/traditional-medicines/regulatory-overview-of-traditional-medicines (accessed September 30, 2021).

[84] Regulatory Aspects of Pharmaceuticals' Exports in Gulf Cooperation Council Countries n.d. https://www.ncbi.nlm.nih.gov/pmc/articles/PMC3122046/ (accessed November 20, 2021).

CHAPTER 11

Natural *vs.* Synthetic Immunomodulators

Girish B Mahajan[1,*] and **Lakshmi Balachandran**[2]

[1] *HiMedia Laboratories Pvt Ltd, Maharashtra, India*

[2] *Freelance Medical Writer, Maharatshtra, India*

Abstract: Immunomodulators are key components in deciding immunity status and development in an individual. The topic has been under more emphasis, especially during and after the COVID-19 pandemic phase. Several plants with medicinal potentials are appreciated in traditional medicines for their healing perspective and have been technically examined for their immunomodulation potential. A number of plant-based bioactive compounds have been extracted and purified with such bioactivities that can rationalise their usage in conventional medication in the past and can stimulate further research in the future as well. Synthetic immunomodulators are significant for generating remedial or prophylactic formulations with defined chemical ingredients from regulatory perspectives. The review highlights the key immunomodulators, both synthetic and natural, until 2020. It also emphasises on market potential and commercial aspects of these. We have explained and listed several plants and their active scaffolds having immunomodulation activities along with synthetic compounds with similar bioactivity. We envisage the review to be an organised compilation and comparison of natural and synthetic immunomodulators and also focus on new chemical immunomodulator scaffolds.

Keywords: Adjuvant, Antibody-Mediated Immunity, Cell-Mediated Immunity, COVID-19, Humoral, Immunity, Immunology, Immunomodulators, Innate Immunity, Immuno-Stimulants, Plant Extracts, Synthetic Immunomodulator, Synthetic Immunomodulator, Traditional Medicine.

INTRODUCTION

The Nature of the Immune Response

In a world where we are faced with an environment that is host to innumerable microbes and toxic molecules, a functional immune system is paramount to homeostasis and good health. The environment is inhabited by commensals, parasites, toxins and various pathogens, and the pathogens continuously evolve

* **Corresponding author Girish B Mahajan:** HiMedia Laboratories Pvt Ltd., Maharashtra, India; E-mail: girishbm2000@gmail.com

Vandana S. Nikam, Sujata P. Sawarkar, Girish B. Mahajan and Supriya G. Jagtap (Eds.)

with their myriad mechanisms to invade, replicate, spread, and affect the normal host functions. Phagocytic cells, like macrophages & neutrophils, cytokines, interferons, natural killer cells, and complements comprise the primary wall of our defence. These are non-specific or generalised defence mechanisms, aimed at localizing the foreign elements and eliminating them. The second wall of defence assumes some specificity. Lymphocytes and other substances such as cytokines and antibodies, and the macrophages present the antigens to two distinct types of cells: Thymus derived cells (T-cells) and Bursa derived cells (B-cells). Each lymphocyte recognizes an Immunogen. The combination of cell and antibodies-mediated immunity together accounts for combating the majority of microbes, such as fungi (both spores & mycelia), bacteria, viral particles, many parasites, cancer-induced cells, *etc.* The tertiary wall of immunity is the concerted action of innate immune responses and the products of particular acquired immunity activities.

Widely touted as the "Drugs of the 90s" immunomodulators are biological response modulators [1]. Optimum health depends on the ability of the defence mechanism to discriminate between "self (own)" and "non-self (foreign)" molecules, cells as well as tissues. The human immune response is a systematic, organized, three-layered defence mechanism comprising of both cellular and humoral immune responses.

An immunomodulator can be any substance of natural or man-made origin that can kindle, subdue, or modify the immune reaction. This includes the innate response and the adaptive reactions, too [2]. Immunosuppressants are antagonists of the immune system [3], and help prevent the rejection of implanted organs and tissues, and in controlling autoimmune disorders [4]. Many implant centers use multiple drugs, each targeted at a specific location in the T-cell activation cascade. They can generally be classified as transcription inhibitors, nucleotide synthesis inhibitors, growth factor signal inhibitors, and differentiation inhibitors. Polyclonal anti-lymphocyte antibodies, monoclonal antibodies targeted to the T-cell antigen receptor complex (OKT3, TIOB9), and monoclonal antibodies targeted to more cellular antigens, including interleukin-2 receptor alpha, which pay special attention to immune cell responses and are used as ingestion therapy and/or antidepressants, in clinical practice [5]. Immunoadjuvants are specific immune stimulants that improve immunity, especially for vaccine's efficacy [3]. They promise to be a true module for the immune response. Immunostimulants activate both innate, innate arms and flexible responses. They play a dual role depending on a person's immune system. In healthy people, they act as immunopotentiators, and in those with weak immune responses, they act as immunotherapeutic agents. Immunostimulators, in particular, are responsible for the antigen-dependent stimulation of granulocyte and macrophages, and have a positive effect on their function [6 - 8].

NATURAL IMMUNOMODULATORS (NI)

The immune response can be altered by the host's natural resources or by external products from various sources.

Natural immunomodulators of exogenous types have been used to modulate immune response since antiquity. Traditionally, ancient Indian medicine uses plant products to modulate the immune response, as immunostimulants as well as immunosuppressors. For the past few decades, new healthcare challenges have emerged in the form of multidrug resistance of pathogens, against empirically used antibiotics. This "dark age" of antibiotics has propelled new research on immunomodulatory agents from plant, fungal, and microbial origin.This has negated the beneficial effects of the "golden era of antibiotics". It is believed that there were ample forebodings of this situation, even before the discovery of the "Selman Waksman" antibiotics. It is disappointing to note that modern techniques in drug modelling and design have not impacted the pipeline in a massive way, as compared to the number of anti-microbial agents discovered around half a century ago. The future of combination therapy was evident much before [9].

Natural immunomodulators possess a low level of clarity in their action as compared to antibiotics. However, the current worldview is in favor of combination therapy that targets two or more specific sites in the immune system. Around 75% of the global population depends on traditional healthcare remedies. Traditional medicine relies mainly on natural sources as therapeutic and healing agents. Currently, many phytochemicals with therapeutic potential have been identified and used as immunomodulators [10].

Rasayana [10]

The word Rasayana, a combination of two words (*rasa* and *ayana*), refers to nutrition and its transportation throughout the body. Rasayana therapy enhances the qualities of rasa, enriching it with nutrients so one can attain longevity, improved memory and intelligence, freedom from disorder, youthfulness, excellence of hair, complexion and voice, optimum development of the physique and sense organs, mastery over phonetics and brilliance. As a dedicated stream of medication for immune promotion, antidegenerative and rejuvenating health care, the Rasayana therapy of Ayurveda is known to prevent the effects of ageing and improve the quality of life for healthy as well as diseased individuals. Rasayana is helpful to improve immunity and is normally advised during the degenerative phase of life, which starts from around 45 years in both males and females [10].

This rasayan laid the foundation of the isolation or synthesis of chemical modulators.

CHEMICAL NATURE OF NATURAL IMMUNOMODULATORS

Many other types of natural compounds found in the foods and additives we use to have at least some scientific evidence that they have an immunomodulation function. Many of these ingredients are found in plants and can be easily eaten in food and nutritional supplements. Examples include omega-3 and omega-6 polyunsaturated fatty acids (PUFA), such as linoleic acid and oleic acid, which are proposed to have anti-inflammatory effects in humans. The most common fatty acids, docosahexaenoic acid (DHA) and eicosapentaenoic acid (EPA), have been studied for many biological effects, including immunomodulation and are found mainly in marine animals. Plant-extracted polyphenols such as curcumin and quercetin have been tested in human studies for immunomodulatory (usually anti-inflammatory) and other biological effects. Natural immunomodulators have a very wide range of chemical nature &properties. The vast variety can be summarized based on the molecular weight difference Table **1** and Fig. **1**.

Table 1. Key representatives of Natural products classes with immunomodulatory potential based on molecular masses.

Chemical Class	Examples
Immunomodulators with a Low Molecular Mass	
Terpenoids	Sesquiterpene lactones, diterpenes, triterpenes
Phenolics	Flavonoids, coumarins, quinones, tannins, caffeic, ferulic, and p-coumaric acids
Alkaloids	Cocaine, Berberine, Vincristine, Chelerythrine
Immunomodulators with a High Molecular Mass	
Lectins	Concanavalin A, ArtinM, Banlec
Nucleotides	Poly I:C
Polysaccharides	Glucans, fructans, xlyans, pectinsgalactans, mannans and fucoidans

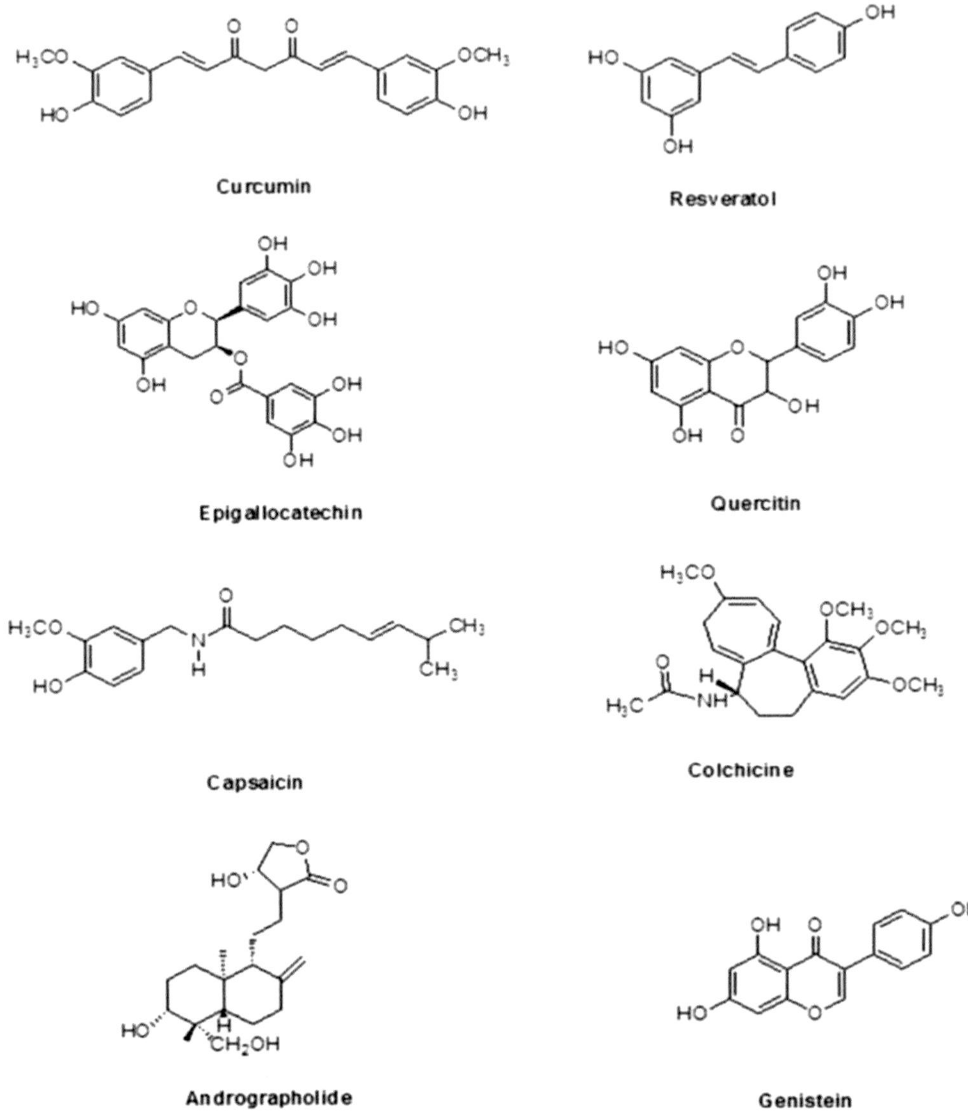

Fig (1). Chemical structures of key immunomodulators derived from plants which are in clinical trials [10].

Propionibacterium Species as an Immunomodulator

Conventional *Propionibacteria* is found in raw milk. It was reported from the studies that a dose of 1.0–1.3 × 10^4 cfu ml^{-1} in French raw milk, and average contamination of 7 × 10^2 cfu ml^{-1} & 2.5 × 10^2 cfu ml^{-1} in raw milk used for Italian Grana cheese & in Swiss raw milk, respectively. The presence of propionibacteria in raw milk leads to their development in certain types of cheeses, where they can reach levels of 10^9 cfu g^{-1} of cheese. They are predominantly found in Swiss-type cheese because the temperature of the long ripening (several weeks at about 24°C), the low salt concentration and the relatively high pH (5.2) favor their growth. *Propionibacterium* species are reported to activate the macrophages, phagocytic action, and activation of T-cells and B-lymphocytes [11].

Glucan

Beta-glucan occurs naturally in the majority of different types of fungi, including yeasts and mushrooms. Moreover, they are also reported in some bacteria, algae and plants (cereal grains). The ß-glucans produced by these diverse organisms vary in molecular structure depending on which organism/microorganism has synthesized it. It has been vividly established that the bioactivity of a ß-glucan observed in the human body is linked to its specific chemical structure [12]. In the milieu of this structure-activity relationship (SAR) inherent in ß-glucan biology, it is essential to recognize the exact source and apt chemical structure of a ß-glucan when investigating an immunomodulator food ingredient since not all ß-glucans have similar immunomodulatory properties.

There are a number of scientific studies reported in literature that explains the effects of yeast's ß-glucan on the immune system. Some representative and important ones are mentioned herewith:

- an increase in the production of the innate immune system's chemical units, such as reactive oxygen species [13]
- an enhancement in the production capacity of cytokines which are important in response to active immunity [14]
- an augmented speed and directionality of innate immunity cells migrating towards a disease-causing germ's challenge [15]
- boosted ability of phagocytosis of extraneous (non-self) challenges [16]
- reversal of technically-induced immune suppression [17]
- improves the body's ability to produce innate body cells [18]

Curcumin [19]

Curcumin is a natural diarylheptanoid compound found in the rhizome of Curcuma longa and related species. The therapeutic benefits of curcumin have been known for centuries. A variety of biological and pharmacological properties of curcumin have been reported, including anti-cancer, anti-oxidant, pro-apoptotic, anti-proliferative, anti-angiogenic, *etc.* Curcumin is one of the most widely studied ingredients among the many immunomodulatory studies. Curcumin reduces the inflammatory response by inhibiting the production of NO, cyclooxygenase-2 (COX-2), nuclear factor-kappa B (NK-kB), and inducible nitric oxide synthase (NOS), and lipoxygenase in NK and IFN-γ cells, or TNF-α activated macrophages.

Jurenka (2009) reviewed pre-clinical trials and curcumin treatments performed at various locations [20]. Among these, majorities of the studies were based on the anti-inflammatory properties of curcumin. As such curcumin has low bioavailability; nevertheless significant developments have been made to solve this problem through chemical and technical ways [21]. Though some fine and coherent studies are required for Curcumin, one good outcome until now demonstrates that Curcumin has a good and non-toxic safety profile. Moreover, it is well tolerated in the human system [21].

Esculetin (6, 7-dihydroxycoumarin) is a coumarin derivative that is reported to be isolated from many plants such as *Artemisia capillaries, Citrus limonia* and *euphorbia lathyris*. The compound showed pleiotropic biological activities, including lipoxygenase-curbing activity, free radical scavenger activity, inhibitory activity on oxidative damage to DNA, tyrosinase-inhibition, as well as being cancer chemopreventive and antitumor activities. Cytotoxic coumarins were reported to be obtained from the root of *Angelica dahurica*.

Resveratrol

Resveratrol, which is chemically known as (5-[(E)-2-(4-hydroxyphenyl) ethenyl] benzene-1,3-diol), is a derived of stilbene and phytoalexin. It occurs in various dietary products and plants, including grapevines, red wine and peanuts. Resveratrol was found to employ a range of pharmacological activities such as anti-microbial, chemopreventive, anticancer/proapoptotic, anti-inflammatory, and anti-oxidant traits. The inflammatory molecules generated in the body are sturdily repressed by resveratrol. The immunomodulatory & pharmacological activities mentioned above are assigned to their range of mechanisms of the inhibition of NF-κB in PMA, LPS or TNF-α-mediated macrophages, epithelial (HeLa), Jurkat, myeloid (U-937) and dendritic cells. NF-κB activation was inhibited by resveratrol *via* inhibition of IκB kinase [22]. Thus, Resveratrol is a powerful natural immunomodulator.

Moreover, Resveratrol was also found to curtail the production of inflammatory cytokines and C5a-stimulated neutrophil recruitment and/ or migration in C5a-stimulated acute peritonitis mouse model [23]. The cell adhesion molecule's expression was also reported to be curbed by this compound. The IL-6-stimulated ICAM-1 expression in endothelial cells was also decreased by it [24]. The compound also inhibits *Porphyromonas gingivalis* LPS-induced endothelial dysfunction in human microvascular endothelial cells. It was reported to block the expression of ICAM-1 and VCAM-1 on human microvascular endothelial cells by inhibition of NF-κB activation [25].

Considering the multifaceted activities of Resveratrol, the scientific community has put in a lot of effort into revealing the exact mechanism of action of each activity. Inspite of the excellent immunomodulation properties revealed for this compound, there are no substantial efforts in translating this knowledge into an approved clinical remedial formulation. More than 40 clinical trials on resveratrol are mentioned in PubMed for a range of disorders and diseases such as coronary artery disease (CAD), obesity, diabetes, and more. The majority of these reports were to either investigate & infer inflammation-based parameters in blood cells and in plasma/serum or to echo functional parameters like the standing of the endothelium [26]. Several trials persuasively showed that these parameters are usefully influenced by resveratrol. Though, if this amended inflammatory status of the patients indeed leads to a clinically relevant improvement of the severity of the diseases or, most significantly, in a decreased incidence of disease-specific life-threatening events has not been studied yet. At present, 99 such studies are reported or ongoing. Forty-nine studies have been completed, while 28 clinical trials on Resveratrol are currently recruiting or planned. Among these, 27 studies are concerned with the anti-inflammatory actions of resveratrol. The promising field of interest is its activity against metabolic syndrome/type 2 diabetes, followed by mild cognitive impairment, non-alcoholic fatty liver disease, and polycystic ovary syndrome (POS). The molecule has a future, and more rigorous studies on its immunomodulation properties are also required.

Glycosides [27]

These are the polysaccharide materials of plants, animal, and microbial origin, which yield the same or different types of sugar on enzyme or acid hydrolysis. To be more precise chemically, they are the acetals or ethers moieties of sugar, produced by the interaction of the hydroxyl functional groups of the sugar and non-sugar moieties, with the release of a water (H_2O) molecule (dehydration). Dendroside A and dendronobilosides B were found to excite the proliferation of murine T and B lymphocytes *in vitro*, while dendronobiloside B showed inhibitory activity in this similar assay.

Flavonoids [28]

Flavonoids, a group of natural chemicals with diverse phenolic chemical structures, are found in fruits, vegetables, grains, barks, roots, stems, and flowers, as well as common beverages like tea and wine. These natural chemicals are well known for their beneficial effects on health, and efforts are being made to isolate the ingredients, so-called flavonoids. Flavonoids are considered as an indispensable component in a variety of nutraceutical, pharmaceutical, medicinal and cosmetic uses. Flavonoids are part of the polyphenol class of phytonutrients. Chemically, flavonoids have a fifteen-carbon skeleton (C6- C3-C6) which consists of two phenyl rings connected by a three-carbon bridge. Flavonoids consist of flavones, anthocyanidins, flavonones, isoflavones, flavonols, and flavonols. Several types of flavonoids employ immunomodulatory actions, including apigenin, oligomeric proanthocyanidins, isoflavonoids, flavones, and anthocyanidins. Such immunomodulatory flavonoids are found in *Terminalia arjuna*.

Sapogenins

Sapogenins are the aglycones, or non-saccharide, portions of the family of natural products known as saponins.

Sapogenins [29], such as triterpenoid saponins and diterpenes, express a variety of immunomodulatory activities. Classic examples of such sapogenins synthesizers are *Gymnema sylvestre*, *Chlorophytum borivilianum*, *Boswellia* spp. and *Randia dumetorum.* They contain steroid or other triterpene frameworks as their key organic feature. For example, steroidal sapogenins such as tiggenin, neogitogenin, and tokorogenin were isolated from the tubers of *Chlorophytum arundinaceum.*

Alkaloids

Alkaloids are a class of basic, naturally occurring organic compounds that contain at least one nitrogen atom. These organic compounds are normally heterocyclic, of limited distribution and have specific physiological actions on the human or animal body. *Achillea millefolium*, *Murraya koenigii*, *Cissam pelospareira* and *Actinidia macrosperma*are the examples of alkaloids [30]. This group also encompasses some closely related compounds with neutral and even weakly acidic properties. Some synthetic compounds of similar structures can also be termed alkaloids. They have varying immunomodulatory activities.

Thiosulfinates

Thiosulfinate esters are formed in the condensation reaction of two sulfenic acids or *via* oxidation of disulfides. They are also an intermediate in the reduction of sulfinic acids *via* ATP-dependent sulfiredoxin (Srx)-catalyzed pathways. Thiosulfinate esters are biologically reactive species. These compounds demonstrate potent immunomodulatory and adaptogenic [31] properties, *e.g.*, from *Allium hirtifolium.*

Volatile Oils and Terpenoids [32]

The term terpene denotes the unsaturated hydrocarbons (C5H8), while terpenoids include the hydrocarbon as well as their oxygenated derivatives. Terpenes and terpenoids are all low boiling point oils of plant or animal origin. Many plant constituents with terpene moiety exhibit immunomodulatory activity, *e.g.*, eugenol from *Ocimum sanctum*, diterpene from *Achillea millefolium, Androgra phispaniculata, Alternan theratenella,* triterpenes from *Ganoderma lucidum*, lupeol and amyrine in *Bauhinia variegate* (Table **2**). Several plant-origin immunomodulators have been described in Table **3**.

Table 2. Natural Immunomodulators classes based on their chemical nature.

Compound	Species
Aliphatic	
Organosulfer compounds	*Allium spp.* Alliaceae
Phenolics	
Coumarins	-
7-hydroxycoumarins	-
Scopoletin (coumarin compound)	*Artemisia feddei*
Oxypeucedanin	*Citrus hystric*
Oleuropein	*Oliea europaea*
Saponins	
Virgaurea saponins	*Solidago virgaurea*
Ginseng saponins	*Panax ginseng*
Saikosapponins	*Bupleurum chinense*
Esculentoside	*Phytolacca Americana*
Bryostatins	*Bugula neritina*
Glycoproteins	
Viscotoxins	*Viscum album*
Ginsans	*Panax ginseng*

Table 3. Plant-derived immunomodulators.

Botanical Name	Function	Constituents	References
Abutilon Indicum	Diuretic, antibacterial	Flavonoids, triterpenoids	[65]

(Table 3) cont.....

Botanical Name	Function	Constituents	References
Acacia catechu	Treatment of asthma, cough, bronchitis, colic, diarrhea, dysentery, boils, skin afflictions, sores and for stomatitis, hypoglycemic, astringent	Flavonoids, quercetin; Effect on DTH reactions & peritoneal macrophages	[66-69]
Acantho panax sessliflorus	Lympho-proliferative activity	Biopolymers	[70]
Achillea millefolium	Anti-inflammatory, antispasmodic, antipyretic, diuretic.	Flavonoids, alkaloids, polyacetylenes, coumarins, triterpenes	[71]
Achille awilhelmsii	Irritable Bowel Syndrome	Flavonoids, terpenoids, saponins, and some alkaloids	[72, 73]
Actinidi amicrosperma	Antileprotic	Alkaloids, saponins	[74]
Agelas mauritianus	Phagocytic activity	Glycolipid(α-galactosylceramide)	[75]
Allium hirtifolium	Antirheumatic, anti-inflammatory	Thiosulfinates, flavonoids	[76]
Allium sativum	Immunomodulatory	Sulfur-containing compounds, polynoids, flavonoids	[77]
Aloe vera Tourn, ex Linn	Purgative, emmenagogue, emollient, anti-inflammatory	Anthraquinone glycosides	[78-80]
Alternanthera tenella	Antitumor, anti-inflammatory.	Flavonoids, triterpenes	[81]
Andrographis paniculata Nees	Hepatoprotective, antispasmodic, blood purifier, febrifuge	Diterpenes	[82]
Aphanothece halophytica	Inhibits influenza virus	Exopolysaccharide	[83]
Bidens Pilosa	Anti-inflammatory	Flavonoids, coumarins	[84]
Artemisia annua	Immunosuppressive	Artemisinin	[85]
Asparagus recemosus	Ulcer healing agent, nervine tonic, anti-gout	Saponins, sitosterols	[68, 86]
Azadiratcha indica	Immunomodulatory, anti-inflammatory, anto-carcinogenic, anti-viral, antihyperglyceamic	Nimbin, Nimbinene, 6-deacetylnimbeine, Nimbandiol, Nimbolide, Quercetin	[87]
Bauhinia variegate	Antifungal, astringent	Flavonoids, beta-sitosterol, lupeol	[88]
Bidens Pilosa	Anti-inflammatory, immunosuppressive, antibacterial and antimalarial	Polyacetylenes	[89]

(Table 3) cont.....

Botanical Name	Function	Constituents	References
Boerhaavia diffusa	Immunostimulatory	Alkaloid	[90]
Boswellia sp.	Hypoglycaemic	Triterpenes, ursanes	[91]
Botryllus schlosseri	Antioxidant, antiviral, antimicrobial and antitumoral	Cytokines	[92]
Bugula neritina	Immunomodulator	Macrocyclic lactones	[93]
Byrsonima crassa	Anti-microbial. Anti-oxidant	Flavonoids, tannins, terpenes	[94]
Calendula officinalis	Antitumor antiviral activity, anti-HIV properties	Polysaccharides, proteins, fatty acids, carotenoids, flavonoids, triterpenoids	[95]
Camellia sinensis	Anticancer activity, lipid-lowering activity, anticataract activity, hepatoprotective and anti-oxidant	(−)Epigallocatechingallate, quercetin, gallicacid	[96]
Chlorophytum borivilianum	Antifungal	Sapogenins	[97]
Cissampelos pareira	Antipyretic, analgesic, antilithic	Hayatine alkaloids	[98]
Citrus natusdaidai	Anti-oxidant	Auraptene, flavonoids	[99]
Cleome gynandra	Anti-inflammatory	Hexacosanol, kaempferol	[100]
Cordiasuperba`	Anti-inflammatory, anti-microbial	Alpha-amyrin	[101]
Couroupita guianensis	Antifungal	Steroids, flavonoids, phenolics	[102]
Curcuma longa	Used in the treatment of various chronic diseases (Diabetes mellitus)	TNF- blocker	[103]
Cynodon dactylon	Used in a wide variety of conditions	Cynodin, beta-carotene, hydrocyanic acid, and Triticin are powerful anti-oxidants	[104, 115]
Dioscorea japonica	Immunomodulatory	Saponin steroid	[105]
Gelsemium elegans	Immunomodulatory	Alkaloids	[106]
Ganoderma lucidum	Anti-oxidant	Flavonoids, triterpenes	[107]
Genus Ardisia	Antimetastatic drug, anti-HIV property	Peptides, saponins, Isocoumarins, quinones and alkyl phenols	[108]
Genus Aristolochia	Antiangiogenic, employed in prostate cancer	Aristolochic acid	[109]
Genus Aspergillus	Antifungals	Polyene, triazoles	[110]

(Table 3) cont.....

Botanical Name	Function	Constituents	References
Gymnema sylvestre	Antidiabetic, diuretic, antibilious	Sapogenins	[111]
Heraclium persicum	Anti-microbial	Flavonoids, furanocoumarins	[112]
Hibiscus rosasinensis	Antidiarrheal, anti-inflammatory	Cyclopropanoids	[100]
Hyptis suaveolens	Carminative, antispasmodic	Lupeol, beta-sitosterol	[113]
Jatropha curcas	Immunomodulatory	Glycosides	[114]
Lagenaria siceraria	Purgative, emetic	Cucurbitacin, beta-glycosidase	[115]
Leonarus japonicas	Immunomodulatory	Terpenoids, alkaloids, flavonoids,glycosides, peptides	[116]
Morus alba	Expectorant, hypocholesterolaemic, diuretic	Flavonoids, anthocyanins	[117]
Murraya koenigii	Antifungal, insecticidal, insecticidal.	Coumarin, carbazole alkaloids, glucoside	[118]
Nycanthesarbor-tristis	Anti-inflammatory, antispasmodic	Iridoid glucosides	[119]
Ocimum sanctum	Carminative, hepatoprotective, antispasmodic, anti-histaminic	Essential oils such as eugenol, cavacrol, derivatives of ursolic acid, apigenin	[68, 120-122]
Panex ginseng	Adaptogenic properties, antiarrhythmic.	Saponins such as ginsenosides, panaxdiol, panaxtriole and oleanolic acid	[123]
Picrorhiza scrophulariiflora	Antioxidant	Iridoid glycosides, amphicoside	[124]
Piper longum	Anti-inflammatory, anti-microbial, anti-obesity, antifungal, anti-pyretic	Alkaloids, flavonoids, steroids, essential oils	[125]
Pteridium aquilinum	Imunomodulatory	Polysaccharide	[126]
Randia duometorum	Chlorosis, antiarthritic	Saponins, triterpenes	[127]
Tinospora cordifolia	Hypoglycaemic agent, antipyretic	Alkaloidal constituents such as berberine, tinosporic acid	[39, 68]
Terminalia arjuna	Cardiotonic, diuretic, prescribed for hypertension	Flavonoids, oligomeric proanthocyanidins, tannins	[128]
Urenalobata	Diuretic, emollient, antispasmodic	Flavonoids	[129]

MECHANISM OF NATURAL IMMUNOMODULATORS

Natural immunomodulators have a wide variation in their mechanism of action, similar to their chemical nature.

As mentioned earlier, "Rasayana" are stimulants, and nutritional supplements and have powerful anti-oxidant activities. They also act as antagonists on oxidative stressors, leading to the formation of different free radicals [33]. They are mainly used to combat the effects of aging, atherosclerosis, cancer, diabetes, rheumatoid arthritis, autoimmune disease and Parkinson's disease. Rasayana herbs appear to be effective in immunostimulant, immunoadjuvant, and immunosuppressant activities or by affecting the active arm of the immune system. Immunomodulation mechanisms occur mainly by reactivating phagocytosis, activation of macrophages, the effect of the immune system on peritoneal macrophages, stimulation of lymphoid cells, improvement of immune function and indirect effect of the cellular immune system, cell proliferation specific immunoglobulin and increase the production of non-spec immunoglobulin, reduce chemical leukopenia, and increase the number of circulating white cells and interleukin-2 levels [33].

Modification of immune responses through stimulating or stressful phyto-extract activity has been found to maintain a healthy state in normal or unhealthy people [34]. Agents that activate immune systems where there is a defective immune response may provide supportive treatment to conventional chemotherapy. High levels of cell proliferation make bone marrow a critical issue, especially in various cytotoxic drugs [35]. In fact, the bone marrow is the most affected organ in the course of any immunosuppression treatment with this class of drugs [35]. Loss of stem cells and the ability of bone marrow to regenerate new blood cells causes thrombocytopenia and leucopenia [35]. Phytoconstituents such as triterpenoid saponins or steroidal glycosides have been proven to be important phytoconstituents that have various pharmacological functions, such as antiallergic, antiphlogistic, cytotoxic antitumour, antiviral, anti-inflammatory, immunomodulating, molluscicidal, and antifungal activity [37]. Recently, three diosgenylsaponins isolated from *Paris polyphylla* have been reported to have immunostimulant properties in relation to phagocytosis, respiratory failure, and nitric oxide production in RAW 264.7 cells [36].

Macrophages play an important role in regulating immunological reactions through a variety of functions, including the phagocytic elimination of foreign or denatured substances and the release of cytokines and reactive oxygen species (ROS). Stimulation of macrophages leads to phagocytosis, respiratory failure, and nitric oxide (NO) production. Macrophage phagocytosis is an important means of protecting cells from foreign matter, which are not isolated and used as an important indirect immunity parameter to test immune function. It is acknowledged that phagocytes are capable of producing superoxide anion and its active discovery during a period of intense oxygen consumption consumption is called as respiratory explosion. Respiratory explosions that play an important role in microbicidal activity can be considered an effective test of immune system tests at the cellular and physiological levels. In macrophages, NO is synthesized from L-arginine in the presence of nitric oxide synthase (NOS), which is involved in a variety of biological processes, including inflammation and immunity. In addition, lymphocyte regenerative tests were performed on eight cycloartane saponins isolated from the *Astragalus melanophrurius* plant, indicating their potential role, in acting as active immunomodulating saponins [37].

It was reported that *Panax ginseng* showed continuous improvement in immune function at week four and a statistically significant difference at week eight, evidenced by the development of PMN cell chemotaxis, phagocytosis, and the total number of T-helper and T-suppressor cells [38].

Excerpt from *Tinospora cordifolia* Miers. in the Menispermiaceae family, suggests that it improves phagocyte function without affecting the joint and humoral immune system and results in inhibition of the C3 convertase classical complement pathway, which is why it acts as an immunomodulator [39].

Further details are summarized in Tables **3** and **4**.

Table 4. Plant-derived (natural) immunomodulators.

Immunomodulator	MOA	Reference
Astralagus	Stimulates IL-2, IL-4, & IFN-γ production & cytotoxic lymphocytes	[130]
Reservatrol	Stimulates lymphocytes &NK cells, and stimulates cytokine production	[131]
Curcumin	Has strong anti-oxidant qualities & cancer growth	[132, 133]
Pterostilbene	Stimulates macrophages and keratinocytes	[134]
Ellagic Acid	Stimulates apoptysis& inhibits melanoma cell growth	[135]
Vitamin C	Modulates macrophages & immune parameters	[136, 137]
Chlorella	Enhances NK cells & cytokine production	[138]
Cat's Claw	Increases antibody formation	[139]
Glucan #300	Stimulates macrophages, cytokines, NK cell activity, antibody response, reduces stress, & cholesterol levels	[140]
Echinacea	Activates the phagocyte system	[141]

SYNTHETIC IMMUNOMODULATORS (SI)

Immunomodulators, some of which are well-defined in chemistry and some are complex systems, exhibit a wide variety of chemical properties that are briefly reviewed.

Bacillus Calmette-Guerin (BCG)

Much evidence available so far suggests the need for advanced mycobacterial vaccines given early in life, through alternative therapies, especially mucosal vaccines. Since T-helper type 2 immune response by inserting T-type 1 helper cannot explain the basic mechanisms for making mycobacterial antigens, it may be useful to investigate whether T-regulatory cells are formed in response to different mycobacterial adjuvants. BCG is a synthetic immunostimulator obtained from bacterial species after stepwise purification. The BCG vaccine is made from an attenuated strain of *Mycobacterium bovis* [40], a bacterium closely related to *M. tuberculosis*, which is the actual causative agent of the disease. It activates the macrophages (APC), natural killer (NK) cells and B lymphocytes.

Muramyl Dipeptide (MDP)

Muramyl dipeptide (MDP) is a synthetic immunoreactive peptide that binds N-acetyl muramic acid linked to a short series of amino acids L-Ala-D-isoGln [41]. It was first identified in the bacterial cell wall peptidoglycan as an active component in Freund's complete adjuvant. In the cell, MDP is secreted by NOD2, a cytoplasmic receptor located in the human reproductive system. NOD2 mutations are often seen in patients with Crohn's disease, an autoimmune disorder, which raises the importance of the MDP-NOD2 approach to immune function. For this reason, modifications to the structure of MDP and its derivatives have been studied extensively in an effort to increase adjuvant activity and improve the immune response effectively for clinical use in the treatment of cancer and other diseases.

Lipopolysaccharide (LPS) [42]

Lipopolysaccharide is an important component of the outer layer of all gram-negative bacteria that can also function as a virulence factor. LPS has a unique chemical structure depending on the biological environment, with a variety of biological and energy functions. The three major domains of LPS are lipid A or endotoxin backbone, a key phosphorylated oligosaccharide, and repetitive oligosaccharide chain chains. LPS can be prepared with TCA, phenol, or phenol-chloroform, petroleum ether (heavy type) background. The TCA released by lipopolysaccharides is similar in structure to phenol extract. Their electrophoretic pattern and endotoxicity are similar.

Levamisole

Levamisole is a heterocyclic compound that is an effective antihelminthic agent and also immunoregulatory [43]. Levamisole is an antihelminthic drug that was commonly used to treat infections caused by viruses, bacteria and viruses. Produced by Janssen and first used in 1969 as a deworming agent. Levamisole was approved by the FDA in 1990 as an adjuvant treatment for colon cancer. Prior to this, levamisole was used as an antirheumatic treatment in the 1970's and 1980's in patients with rheumatoid arthritis.

Because of its immunomodulatory effects, the drug has been studied in the treatment of various autoimmune diseases, with some studies showing positive results. This drug has also been used in combination with other drugs to treat various cancers.

Levamisole was withdrawn from the American market in 2000 because of its ability to cause serious side effects, including agranulocytosis. Interestingly, levamisole has been found to be a cocaine addict and can lead to a variety of side effects in people who use the drug [44].

Isoprenosine

Inosine pranobex is a synthetic product, also known as isoprinosine or inosine acedobene dimepranol [45], with anti-viral properties that are thought to be related to its effect on T-cell-mediated immune system rather than directing antiviral activity. Experiments have been performed on many bacterial infections as well as rheumatoid arthritis, multiple sclerosis, and alopecia. However, clinical trials have generally shown modest or no therapeutic benefits, and there are no adverse effects or reactions, other than an increase in uric acid concentration in serum, indicating metabolic mechanisms of purines.

Pyrimidine Derivatives [46]

Other antiproliferative drugs show immunodepressive potential, acting on a level of different subpopulations of non-immunocompetent cells, *i.e.* antimetabolite compounds compounds such as methotrexate, folic acid analog.

Purine Derivatives [47]

Thioguanine, mercaptopurine and azathioprine are the main representatives of this class of compounds.

Nitrogen Mustard Alkylating Agents [48]

Chlorambucil, cyclophosphamide, uramucil and melphalan show significant bioactivity for immunomodulation.

Synthetic Corticosteroids [49]

Predsolone and its derivatives, dexamethasone and triamcinolone, are also immunodepressors, while lynestrol exhibits immunosuppressive properties.

Heterocyclic Structures

Heterocyclic compounds with two interlocking rings are represented in several promising products. Brenidin, a microbial immunosuppressive agent [50] (4-carbomoyl-1-/~-D-ribofuranosyl-imidazolium-5-olate) and cimetidine, an antagonist of histamine H2, directly inhibits the activity of T-lymphocyte suppressor and 5-mercaptopyridoxine, which are protective substances. Thiabendazole is a compound of benzimidazole, which works on the development and differentiation of lymphoid and hemopoietic cells.

Aromatic Compounds

Lobenzarit [51] has been reported to suppress adjuvant arthritis and prevent the development of autoimmune kidney disease, possibly by activating suppressed T-cells, while Tilorone is an effective interferon inducer.

Simple Non-cyclic Chemicals

Mercapto-2-ethanol, Mercaptopropionylglycine, 2-mercapto-2-methylpropan-yl-L-cysteine (SA 96), D-penicillamine, avridine (CP 20961), diethyldithio-carbamate(DTC), synthetic fatty acylated D-glucosamine or D- glucose derivatives, [52].

Azathioprine, chlorambucil, cyclophosphamide and corticoids are currently used inclinical immunodepression.

MECHANISM OF SYNTHETIC IMMUNOMODULATORS

Immunomodulation activity is primarily mediated through the activation of phagocytes, macrophages, and lymphoid cells, which results in an increase in circulating complete white cell counts (WBCs) and interleukin-2 quantums. Nonspecific and specific immune responses, cell-mediated and antibody-mediated immune responses, activation and repression of immunocompetent cells, and the impact of endocrine and additional systems all play a role in immunological defence. The immunostimulant's primary targets are thymus-derived (T) or bursa-derived (B) cells, and it plays a critical role in immunostimulation. [53] The activation of lymphocytes &macrophages, which could be done directly or indirectly *via* macrophages, is the second most critical role in T lymphocyte stimulation.

MARKET ANALYSIS [54-56]

In the middle of the COVID-19 crisis, the world market for Immunomodulators was around at US$167.9 Million in the year 2020. It is envisaged to be US$244.6 Million by 2027, increasing at a CAGR of 5.5% over 7 years. Immunosuppressant, a key sector among the immunomodulators is projected to record 5.3% CAGR and reaches US$133.4 Million by the end of the 2027. After an early analysis of the business implications of the pandemic and its induced economic crisis, growth in the Immunostimulants segment is readjusted to a revised 5.7% CAGR for the next 7-year period.

The Immunomodulators market in the U.S. was at US$45.2 Million in 2020. China, the world`s second-largest economy, is forecast to reach an expected market size of US$53 Million by the year 2027 at a CAGR of 8.9% over the period 2020 to 2027. Among other notable local markets are Japan and Canada, each forecast will grow by 3% and 4.4%, respectively, over the period 2020-2027. In Europe, Germany is expected to grow at about 3.9% CAGR.

The global impact of COVID-19 has been unprecedented and shocking, with Immunomodulators proving to shocking demand in all regions during the epidemic.

SIGNIFICANCE OF NATURAL IMMUNOMODULATORS AND SYNTHETIC IMMUNOMODULATORS

Role of Immunomodulators in Human Health and Animal Health

The immune system is a highly flexible immune system that has developed to protect animals from pathogenic microorganisms and cancer-related diseases. In addition, the immune system is able to detect the subtle chemical differences that distinguish one virus from another. In addition, the system is able to distinguish between foreign molecules as well as body cells and proteins. The efficiency and effectiveness of the immune system may be influenced by a variety of external factors that contribute to the suppression of the immune system or to the strengthening of the immune system. Several agents tasked with adapting or correcting pathophysiological processes are called immunomodulatory agents.

Depression often causes an overdose of glucocorticoids [57]. Increased glucocorticoid levels lead to suppression of immune function in humans and animals [57]. Natural stress plays an important role in lowering the level of glucocorticoid in the blood, which suppresses both natural and acquired immune function and makes it easier to treat diseases [57]. These days, there is overwhelming evidence that stress responses can cause immune and immune disorders [58]. The term immunity implies resistance to injury, particularly by poisons, foreign proteins and invading pathogens.

In addition, both immunostimulation and immunosuppression need to be addressed in order to regulate normal immunological functioning. Therefore, both immunostimulation and immunosuppressing agents have their own ranks and are looking for better agents, making these functions a field of great interest worldwide [59]. Natural adjuvants, synthetic agents and antibody reagents are used as immunosuppressive and immunostimulative agents. However, there are major limitations in the normal use of these agents, such as the increased risk of infection and general effect on all immune systems.

In recent years, there has been an increase in the clinical use of traditional drugs due to relief from harmful toxic effects and better performance. In addition, the proliferation of antibiotics and the side effects of synthetic drugs have prompted scientists to seek out herbal immunomodulators to treat various ailments. Herbal medicines are believed to enhance the body's natural resistance to infection, and their immune functions have been reported in many plants [59].

Indian medicinal plants and various 'Rasayanas' are said to have an immune function [60]. The medicines of the Rasayana group are believed to promote health, immunity and longevity [60]. According to Ayurveda, they strengthen all body tissues, prevent aging, promote intelligence and prevent disease. Historically, herbs have been the mainstay of drug treatment and are currently receiving attention as sources of synergistic combination.

COMPARATIVE SIDE EFFECTS OF IMMUNOMODULATORS CONSIDERING THEIR NATURAL & SYNTHETIC ORIGIN [61]

There are several side effects of chemical and/or synthetic drugs such as immunotherapy. A major side effect of these chemical or synthetic drugs, such as cyclosporine, is kidney failure/toxicity. Nephrotoxicity can occur in about 75% of patients. Other toxins include high blood pressure, hepatotoxicity, hirsutism, gingival hyperplasia, stomach poisoning (nausea, vomiting, diarrhea, anorexia and abdominal pain), neurotoxicity such as headaches, insomnia, and pain, heart poisoning, poisoning be-metabolic (hyperkalemia, hyper kalemia, hypo magnesaemia *etc.*). Contra-indication of chemical compounds, including azathioprine, also affects rapidly growing cells, including bone marrow and intestinal cells leading to leucopoenia, thrombocytopenia and gastrointestinal toxicity.

Some chemical or synthetic drugs cause bleeding cystitis and severe pancytopenia. High levels of toxins are caused by anti-thymocyte globulin, which is considered a protein, leading to serum sickness and nephritis. Other toxic symptoms of chemical agents include fever, leukopoenia, thrombocytopenia and skin rashes. In some cases, chemical agents lead to infertility due to the destruction of testicular and ovarian cells.

INDUSTRIAL MANUFACTURERS [62, 63]

Roche, Amgen Inc., Abbott, Johnson and Johnson, Novartis AG, Eli Lilly and Company, Bristol-Myers Squibb Company, Merck and Co. Inc., Biogen, Pfizer Inc., are key leaders in R&D and the production of immunomodulators worldwide.

By 2020, the COVID-19 epidemic has had a profound impact on the development of biotechnology in the world, and in Russia, in particular. The need for effective vaccines and effective drugs has led to a high level of cooperation, that is, strategic agreements in the development and production of biotechnology, which has led to the growth of their shares in world trade. At the same time, the feature of 2020 is that the transaction that took several years took place in a few months.

For example, Vir Biotechnology, which has acquired two antibodies from the COVID-19 virus spike protein, has entered into agreements with other companies Wuxi, Alnylam, Xencor, NIH and Biogen for immune development, methods of RNA therapies and vaccines, as well as recent agreement with Glaxosmithkline affect two leading MAb against spike protein VIR7831 and VIR-7832. Recent developments in the field of COVID-19 have made Vir Biotechnology a leading player in the biotechnology market, which also led to a 3-fold increase in corporate shares by the end of 2020, with market capitalization reaching $ 3.5 billion (Mega Trends). In 2020, a strategic alliance was established between X biotech and the Bio bridge, as well as Amgen and Adaptive, to search for inactive antibodies in COVID-19 patients in order to obtain anti-retroviral drugs. The strategic alliance between Ethris & Neurimmune seeks to obtain the information needed to develop mRNA therapies [64].

CONCLUSION

The idea of immunomodulation was first developed by Edward Jenner in 1796 with reference to the first vaccination program. The success there prompted massive work in discovering and developing large scaffolds having immunomodulation capacity. The quest for an ideal immunomodulator is on. In addition to efficacy data, the real challenge, especially for synthetic immunomodulators, lies in getting safe (non-toxic, non-pyrogenic, non-carcinogenic, non-teratogenic *etc.*) immunomodulators. It is also well reported that there exists a close interaction between the immune and nervous systems. Communication between the neuroendocrine and immune systems is indispensable to maintain the fine balance in the body. Any variation in these interactive relations can lead to boosted susceptibility of the body to various infectious, inflammatory, or autoimmune diseases. From the several hundreds of immunomodulatory compounds broth, both natural & synthetic origin, plant extracts, and herbal products, it is good to notice that natural immunomodulators seem to have good activity and better safety data as compared with the majority of synthetic immunomodulators. Many herbal medicines are reported to enhance the body's natural resistance to microbial infection. Among the three key kinds of immunomodulators, such as immunosuppressants, immunoadjuvants, and immunostimulators, the market for immunoadjuvants is several times higher over the other two types. The global impact of COVID-19 has been exceptional and shocking, with an alarmingly huge demand for Immunomodulators across all regions.

CONSENT FOR PUBLICATION

Not applicable.

CONFLICT OF INTEREST

The authors declare no conflict of interest, financial or otherwise.

ACKNOWLEDGEMENTS

Special thanks to Mr. Manoj Dev, ICT, Mumbai for his help.

REFERENCES

[1] Takx-Köhlen BC. Immunomodulators. Future prospects. Pharm Weekbl Sci 1992; 14(4A): 245-52. [PMID: 1437506]

[2] Hesham El Enshasy. Immunomodulators. Industrial Application [2nd Edition] Springer-Verlag Berlin Heidelberg; 2010. [cited 2021 Jul 31]. 165p.

[3] Nagoba B, Davane M. Nagoba, B.; Davane, M. Natural Immunomodulators. J Immunol Microbiol 2018; (2): 1-2.

[4] Fireman M, DiMartini AF, Armstrong SC, Cozza KL. Immunosuppressants. Psychosomatics 2004; 45(4): 354-60. [http://dx.doi.org/10.1176/appi.psy.45.4.354] [PMID: 15232051]

[5] Suthanthiran M, Morris RE, Strom TB. Immunosuppressants: Cellular and molecular mechanisms of action. Am J Kidney Dis 1996; 28(2): 159-72.

[http://dx.doi.org/10.1016/S0272-6386(96)90297-8] [PMID: 8768909]

[6] Kumar D, Arya V, Kaur R, Bhat ZA, Gupta VK, Kumar V. A review of immunomodulators in the Indian traditional health care system. J Microbiol Immunol Infect 2012; 45(3): 165-84. [http://dx.doi.org/10.1016/j.jmii.2011.09.030] [PMID: 22154993]

[7] Singh N, Tailang M, Mehta SC. A review on herbal plants as immunomodulators. Int J Pharm Sci Res 2016; 7: 3602-10.

[8] Billiau A, Matthys P. Modes of action of Freund's adjuvants in experimental models of autoimmune diseases. J Leukoc Biol 2001; 70(6): 849-60. [PMID: 11739546]

[9] Sadgrove N J, Jones G L. From Petri Dish to Patient: Bioavailability Estimation and Mechanism of Action for Antimicrobial and Immunomodulatory Natural Products. Front Microbiol. 2019; 10: 2470. [http://dx.doi.org/10.3389/fmicb.209.02470]

[10] Kumar D, Arya V, Kaur R, Bhat ZA, Gupta VK, Kumar V. A review of immunomodulators in the Indian traditional health care system. J Microbiol Immunol Infect 2012; 45(3): 165-84. [http://dx.doi.org/10.1016/j.jmii.2011.09.030] [PMID: 22154993]

[11] Bascones-Martinez A, Mattila R, Gomez-Font R, Meurman J H. Immunomodulatory drugs: oral and systemic adverse effects. Med Oral Patol Oral Cir Bucal 2014, 19(1), e24-e31. [http://dx.doi.org/10.4317/medoral.19087]

[12] https://khni.kerry.com/news/what-are-immunomodulators-how-do-they-work/

[13] Paiva CN, Bozza MT. Are reactive oxygen species always detrimental to pathogens? Antioxid Redox Signal 2014; 20(6): 1000-37. [http://dx.doi.org/10.1089/ars.2013.5447] [PMID: 23992156]

[14] Arango Duque G, Descoteaux A. Macrophage cytokines: involvement in immunity and infectious diseases. Front Immunol 2014; 5: 491. [http://dx.doi.org/10.3389/fimmu.2014.00491] [PMID: 25339958]

[15] Sato T, Iwabuchi K, Nagaoka I, *et al.* Induction of human neutrophil chemotaxis by Candida albicans-derived -1,6-long glycoside side-chain-branched -glucan. J Leukoc Biol 2006; 80(1): 204-11. [http://dx.doi.org/10.1189/jlb.0106069] [PMID: 16670126]

[16] Rubin-Bejerano I, Abeijon C, Magnelli P, Grisafi P, Fink GR. Phagocytosis by human neutrophils is stimulated by a unique fungal cell wall component. Cell Host Microbe 2007; 2(1): 55-67. [http://dx.doi.org/10.1016/j.chom.2007.06.002] [PMID: 18005717]

[17] Novakovic B, Habibi E, Wang SY, *et al.* β-Glucan Reverses the Epigenetic State of LPS-Induced Immunological Tolerance. Cell 2016; 167(5): 1354-1368.e14. [http://dx.doi.org/10.1016/j.cell.2016.09.034] [PMID: 27863248]

[18] Patchen ML, Liang J, Vaudrain T, *et al.* Mobilization of peripheral blood progenitor cells by Betafectin PGG-Glucan alone and in combination with granulocyte colony-stimulating factor. Stem Cells 1998; 16(3): 208-17. [http://dx.doi.org/10.1002/stem.160208] [PMID: 9617896]

[19] Jantan I, Ahmad W, Bukhari SNA. Plant-derived immunomodulators: an insight on their preclinical evaluation and clinical trials. Front Plant Sci 2015; 6: 655. [http://dx.doi.org/10.3389/fpls.2015.00655] [PMID: 26379683]

[20] Jurenka JS. Anti-inflammatory properties of curcumin, a major constituent of Curcuma longa: a review of preclinical and clinical research. Altern Med Rev 2009; 14(2): 141-53. [PMID: 19594223]

[21] Anand P, Kunnumakkara AB, Newman RA, Aggarwal BB. Bioavailability of curcumin: problems and promises. Mol Pharm 2007; 4(6): 807-18. [http://dx.doi.org/10.1021/mp700113r] [PMID: 17999464]

[22] Holmes-McNary M, Baldwin AS Jr. Chemopreventive properties of trans-resveratrol are associated with inhibition of activation of the IkappaB kinase. Cancer Res 2000; 60(13): 3477-83. [PMID: 10910059]

[23] Issuree PDA, Pushparaj PN, Pervaiz S, Melendez AJ. Resveratrol attenuates C5a-induced inflammatory responses *in vitro* and *in vivo* by inhibiting phospholipase D and sphingosine kinase activities. FASEB J 2009; 23(8): 2412-24. [http://dx.doi.org/10.1096/fj.09-130542] [PMID: 19346296]

[24] Wung BS, Hsu MC, Wu CC, Hsieh CW. Resveratrol suppresses IL-6-induced ICAM-1 gene expression in endothelial cells: Effects on the inhibition of STAT3 phosphorylation. Life Sci 2005; 78(4): 389-97. [http://dx.doi.org/10.1016/j.lfs.2005.04.052] [PMID: 16150460]

[25] Park HJ, Jeong SK, Kim SR, *et al.* Resveratrol inhibits Porphyromonas gingivalis lipopolysaccharide-induced endothelial adhesion molecule expression by suppressing NF-κB activation. Arch Pharm Res 2009; 32(4): 583-91. [http://dx.doi.org/10.1007/s12272-009-1415-7] [PMID: 19407977]

[26] Bakker GCM, van Erk MJ, Pellis L, *et al.* An antiinflammatory dietary mix modulates inflammation and oxidative and metabolic stress in overweight men: a nutrigenomics approach. Am J Clin Nutr 2010; 91(4): 1044-59. [http://dx.doi.org/10.3945/ajcn.2009.28822] [PMID: 20181810]

[27] Zhao W, Ye Q, Tan X, *et al.* Three new sesquiterpene glycosides from Dendrobium nobile with immunomodulatory activity. J Nat Prod 2001; 64(9): 1196-200. [http://dx.doi.org/10.1021/np0102612] [PMID: 11575955]

[28] González-Gallego J, García-Mediavilla MV, Sánchez-Campos S, Tuñón MJ. Anti-inflammatory and immunomodulatory properties of dietary flavonoids. Polyphenols in human health and disease. 2014; 435-52.

[29] Khajuria A, Gupta A, Garai S, Wakhloo BP. Immunomodulatory effects of two sapogenins 1 and 2 isolated from Luffa cylindrica in Balb/C mice. Bioorg Med Chem Lett 2007; 17(6): 1608-12. [http://dx.doi.org/10.1016/j.bmcl.2006.12.091] [PMID: 17270438]

[30] Gharibi S, Rahimmalek M, Mirlohi A, Majidi MM, *et al.* Assessment of genetic diversity in Achillea millefolium subsp. millefolium and Achillea millefolium subsp. elbursensis using morphological and ISSR markers. J Med Plants Res 2011; 5(11): 2413-23.

[31] Mikaili P, Maadirad S, Moloudizargari M, Aghajanshakeri S, Sarahroodi S. Therapeutic uses and pharmacological properties of garlic, shallot, and their biologically active compounds. Iran J Basic Med Sci 2013; 16(10): 1031-48. [PMID: 24379960]

[32] Da Silva SL, Figueiredo PMS, Tomomasa Y. Chemotherapeutic potential of the volatile oils from Zanthoxylumrhoifolium Lam leaves. Eur J Pharmacol. 20017; 576(1-3): 180-8.

[33] Chulet R, Pradhan P. A Review on Rasayana. Phcog Rev 2009; 3(6): 229-34.

[34] Hase K, Basnet P, Kadota S, Namba T. Immunostimulating activity of Celosian, an antihepatotoxic polysaccharide isolated from Celosia argentea. Planta Med 1997; 63(3): 216-9. [http://dx.doi.org/10.1055/s-2006-957656] [PMID: 9225602]

[35] Bafna AR, Mishra SH. Immunostimulatory effect of methanol extract of Curculigo orchioides on immunosuppressed mice. J Ethnopharmacol 2006; 104(1-2): 1-4. [http://dx.doi.org/10.1016/j.jep.2005.06.048] [PMID: 16207521]

[36] Zhang X, Cui Y, Huang J, *et al.* Immuno-stimulating properties of diosgenyl saponins isolated from Paris polyphylla. Bioorg Med Chem Lett 2007; 17(9): 2408-13. [http://dx.doi.org/10.1016/j.bmcl.2007.02.039] [PMID: 17350838]

[37] Shukla S, Bajpai VK, Kim M. Plants as potential sources of natural immunomodulators. Rev Environ Sci Biotechnol 2014; 13(1): 17-33.
[http://dx.doi.org/10.1007/s11157-012-9303-x]

[38] Panax ginseng. Monograph. Altern Med Rev 2009; 14(2): 172-6.
[PMID: 19594226]

[39] Sinha K, Mishra N P, Singh J, Kanjua S P S. Tinosporacordifolia, a reservoir plant for therapeutic applications: A review. 2004.

[40] Andersen CAS, Rosenkrands I, Olsen AW, *et al.* Novel generation mycobacterial adjuvant based on liposome-encapsulated monomycoloyl glycerol from Mycobacterium bovis bacillus Calmette-Guérin. J Immunol 2009; 183(4): 2294-302.
[http://dx.doi.org/10.4049/jimmunol.0804091] [PMID: 19620310]

[41] Souvannavong V, Brown S, Adam A. The synthetic immunomodulator muramyl dipeptide (MDP) can stimulate activated B cells. Mol Immunol 1988; 25(4): 385-91.
[http://dx.doi.org/10.1016/0161-5890(88)90033-8] [PMID: 3260989]

[42] https://www.wakopyrostar.com/blog/post/immunomodulation-by bacterial lipopolysaccharides /#

[43] Symoens J, Rosenthal M, De Brabander M, Goldstein G. Immunoregulation with levamisole. 1980; 195-214.

[44] https://go.drugbank.com/drugs/DB00848

[45] Lasek W, Janyst M, Wolny R, Zapała Ł, Bocian K, Drela N. Immunomodulatory effects of inosine pranobex on cytokine production by human lymphocytes. Acta Pharm 2015; 65(2): 171-80.
[http://dx.doi.org/10.1515/acph-2015-0015] [PMID: 26011933]

[46] Vadlamani S, Poosarla BKA, Bapatla VK. Immunomodulatory Activity of Ethanolic Leaf Extract of Terminaliachebula. Int Lett Nat Sci 2015; 47: 82-8.

[47] Conta AC, Stelzner DJ. Immunomodulatory effect of the purine nucleoside inosine following spinal cord contusion injury in rat. Spinal Cord 2008; 46(1): 39-44.
[http://dx.doi.org/10.1038/sj.sc.3102057] [PMID: 17406376]

[48] Jawed SI, Myskowski PL, Horwitz S, Moskowitz A, Querfeld C. Primary cutaneous T-cell lymphoma (mycosis fungoides and Sézary syndrome). J Am Acad Dermatol 2014; 70(2): 223.e1-223.e17.
[http://dx.doi.org/10.1016/j.jaad.2013.08.033] [PMID: 24438970]

[49] Cain DW, Cidlowski JA. Immune regulation by glucocorticoids. Nat Rev Immunol 2017; 17(4): 233-47.
[http://dx.doi.org/10.1038/nri.2017.1] [PMID: 28192415]

[50] El-Helw EAE, Morsy ARI, Hashem AI. Evaluation of some new heterocycles bearing 2-oxoquinolylmoiety as immunomodulator against highly pathogenic avian influenza virus (H5N8). J Heterocycl Chem 2021; 58(4): 1003-14.
[http://dx.doi.org/10.1002/jhet.4233]

[51] González R, Remírez D. Current views on the pharmacological properties of the immunomodulator, lobenzarit disodium. J Investig Allergol Clin Immunol 1997; 7(2): 77-82.
[PMID: 9161931]

[52] Horwitz LD. Bucillamine: a potent thiol donor with multiple clinical applications. Cardiovasc Drug Rev 2003; 21(2): 77-90.
[http://dx.doi.org/10.1111/j.1527-3466.2003.tb00107.x] [PMID: 12847560]

[53] Kayser O, Masihi KN, Kiderlen AF. Natural products and synthetic compounds as immunomodulators. Expert Rev Anti Infect Ther 2003; 1(2): 319-35.
[http://dx.doi.org/10.1586/14787210.1.2.319] [PMID: 15482127]

[54] https://www.fortunebusinessinsights.com/immunomodulators-market-104692

[55] https://www.verifiedmarketresearch.com/product/immunomodulators-market/

[56] https://www.globenewswire.com/news release/2021/01/25/2163337/0/en/Immunomodulators-Marke--worth-USD-285-01-Billion-at-6-3-CAGR-Enhancement-of-Supply-Chain-to--oost-Growth-amid-COVID-19-reports-Fortune-Business-Insights.html

[57] Srikumar R, Jeya Parthasarathy N, Sheela Devi R. Immunomodulatory activity of triphala on neutrophil functions. Biol Pharm Bull 2005; 28(8): 1398-403. [http://dx.doi.org/10.1248/bpb.28.1398] [PMID: 16079482]

[58] Jacobs R, Pawlak CR, Mikeska E, *et al.* Systemic lupus erythematosus and rheumatoid arthritis patients differ from healthy controls in their cytokine pattern after stress exposure. Rheumatology (Oxford) 2001; 40(8): 868-75. [http://dx.doi.org/10.1093/rheumatology/40.8.868] [PMID: 11511755]

[59] Patwardhan B, Kalbag D, Patki PS, Nagsampagi BA. Search of immunomodulatory agents. Rev Ind Drug 1990; 28: 348-58.

[60] Atal CK, Sharma ML, Kaul A, Khajuria A. Immunomodulating agents of plant origin. I: Preliminary screening. J Ethnopharmacol 1986; 18(2): 133-41. [http://dx.doi.org/10.1016/0378-8741(86)90025-5] [PMID: 3560991]

[61] https://www.cancer.org/treatment/treatments-and-side-effects/treatm-nt-types/immunotherapy/immunomodulators.html

[62] https://www.biospace.com/article/immunomodulators-market-latest-technological-advances--tudy-analysis/

[63] https://www.researchandmarkets.com/ reports/ 5417332/

[64] Reichert JM. Antibodies to watch in 2015. MAbs 2015; 7(1): 1-8. [http://dx.doi.org/10.4161/19420862.2015.988944] [PMID: 25484055]

[65] Dashputre NL, Naikwade NS. Immunomodulatory activity of Abutilon indicum Linn. on albino mice. IJPSR 2010; 1(3): 178-84.

[66] Sunil MA, Sunitha VS, Radhakrishnan EK, Jyothis M. Immunomodulatory activities of Acacia catechu, a traditional thirst quencher of South India. J Ayurveda Integr Med 2019; 10(3): 185-91. [http://dx.doi.org/10.1016/j.jaim.2017.10.010] [PMID: 29502869]

[67] Khare CP. Indian Medicinal Plants.An illustrated dictionary. 2007. [http://dx.doi.org/10.1007/978-0-387-70638-2]

[68] K.M. Nadkarni, A.K. Nadkarni. Indian Materia medica. (3rd ed.), Popular Prakashan, Mumbai (2005).

[69] Ismail S, Asad M. Immunomodulatory activity of Acacia catechu. Indian J Physiol Pharmacol 2009; 53(1): 25-33. [PMID: 19810573]

[70] Jeong SC, Jeong YT, Yang BK, Song CH. Chemical characteristics and immuno-stimulating properties of biopolymers extracted from Acanthopanax sessiliflorus. J Biochem Mol Biol 2006; 39(1): 84-90. [PMID: 16466642]

[71] Sharififar F, Pournourmohammadi S, Arabnejad M. Immunomodulatory activity of aqueous extract of Achillea wilhelmsii C. Koch in mice. Indian J Exp Biol 2009; 47(8): 668-71. [PMID: 19775073]

[72] Derakhshande P, Navabi SJ, Shokoohinia Y, *et al.* Efficacy and safety of Achillea wilhelmsii C. Koch capsules on symptom severity and quality of life in patients with irritable bowel syndrome: a randomized, placebo-controlled clinical trial. J Complement Integr Med 2019; 16(4). [http://dx.doi.org/10.1515/jcim-2018-0123]

[73] Sharififar F, Pournourmohammadi S, Arabnejad M, Rastegarinzadeh R, *et al.* Immunomodulatory

activity of aqueous extract of Achilleawilhelmsii, C. Koch in mice. Iran J Pharm Res 2009; 8(4): 287-92.

[74] Lu Y, Fan J, Zhao Y, *et al.* Immunomodulatory activity of aqueous extract of Actinidia macrosperma. Asia Pac J Clin Nutr 2007; 16(1) (Suppl. 1): 261-5.
[PMID: 17392116]

[75] Hung LC, Lin CC, Hung SK, *et al.* A synthetic analog of α-galactosylceramide induces macrophage activation *via* the TLR4-signaling pathways. Biochem Pharmacol 2007; 73(12): 1957-70.
[http://dx.doi.org/10.1016/j.bcp.2007.03.006] [PMID: 17445776]

[76] Jafarian A, Ghannadi A, Elyasi A. The effects of Allium hirtifolium Boiss.on cell-mediated immune response in mice. IJPR 2003; 2: 51-5.

[77] Moutia M, Habti N, Badou A. *In vitro* and *In vivo* Immunomodulator activities of *Allium sativum* L. Evid. Based. Complementary. Altern. Med Evid Based Complement Alternat Med 2018; 2018: 4984659.
[http://dx.doi.org/10.1155/2018/4984659]

[78] Sikarwar SM, Patil MB, Sharma S, Bhat V. Aloe vera: plant of immortality. IJPSR 2010; 1: 7-10.

[79] Hamman J. Composition and applications of Aloe vera leaf gel. Molecules 2008; 13(8): 1599-616.
[http://dx.doi.org/10.3390/molecules13081599] [PMID: 18794775]

[80] Cooper JC, Turcasso N. Immunostimulatory effects of β-1,3 glucan and acemannan. JANA 1999; 2: 5-11.

[81] Guerra RNM, Pereira HAW, Silveria LMS, Olea RSG. Evaluation of immunomodulatory and anti-inflammatory effects and phytochemical screening of Alternantheratenella Colla (Amaranthaceae) aqueous extract. Braz J Med Biol Res 2003; 36: 1215-9.
[http://dx.doi.org/10.1590/S0100-879X2003000900011] [PMID: 12937788]

[82] Varma A, Padh H, Shrivastava N. Andrographolide: a new plant-derived antineoplastic entity on horizon. Evid Based Complement Alternat Med 2011; 2011: 1-9.
[http://dx.doi.org/10.1093/ecam/nep135] [PMID: 19752167]

[83] Zheng W, Chen C, Cheng Q, Wang Y, Chu C. Oral administration of exopolysaccharide from Aphanothece halophytica (Chroococcales) significantly inhibits influenza virus (H1N1)-induced pneumonia in mice. Int Immunopharmacol 2006; 6(7): 1093-9.
[http://dx.doi.org/10.1016/j.intimp.2006.01.020] [PMID: 16714212]

[84] Cherng JM, Chiang W, Chiang LC. Immunomodulatory activities of common vegetables and spices of Umbelliferae and its related coumarins and flavonoids. Food Chem 2008; 106(3): 944-50.
[http://dx.doi.org/10.1016/j.foodchem.2007.07.005]

[85] Noori S, Naderi GA, Hassan ZM, Habibi Z, Bathaie SZ, Hashemi SMM. Immunosuppressive activity of a molecule isolated from Artemisia annua on DTH responses compared with cyclosporin A. Int Immunopharmacol 2004; 4(10-11): 1301-6.
[http://dx.doi.org/10.1016/j.intimp.2004.05.003] [PMID: 15313428]

[86] Bopana N, Saxena S. Asparagus racemosus—Ethnopharmacological evaluation and conservation needs. J Ethnopharmacol 2007; 110(1): 1-15.
[http://dx.doi.org/10.1016/j.jep.2007.01.001] [PMID: 17240097]

[87] Durrani FR, Chand N, Jan M, Sultan A, Durrani Z, Akhtar S. Immunomodulatory and growth promoting effects of neem leaf infusion in broiler chicks. Sarhad J Agric 2008; 24(4): 655-60.

[88] Ghaisas MM, Shaikh SA, Deshpande AD. Evaluation of the immunomodulatory activity of ethanolic extract of the stem bark of *Bauhinia variegata* Linn. Int J Green Pharm 2009; 3(1): 70-4.
[http://dx.doi.org/10.4103/0973-8258.49379]

[89] Chang SL, Chiang YM, Chang CLT, *et al.* Flavonoids, centaurein and centaureidin, from Bidens pilosa, stimulate IFN-γ expression. J Ethnopharmacol 2007; 112(2): 232-6.

[http://dx.doi.org/10.1016/j.jep.2007.03.001] [PMID: 17408892]

[90] Mungantiwar AA, Nair AM, Shinde UA, *et al.* Studies on the immunomodulatory effects of Boerhaavia diffusa alkaloidal fraction. J Ethnopharmacol 1999; 65(2): 125-31. [http://dx.doi.org/10.1016/S0378-8741(98)00153-6] [PMID: 10465652]

[91] Mikhaeil BR, Maatooq GT, Badria FA, Amer MMA. Chemistry and immunomodulatory activity of frankincense oil. Z Naturforsch C J Biosci 2003; 58(3-4): 230-8. [http://dx.doi.org/10.1515/znc-2003-3-416] [PMID: 12710734]

[92] Ballarin L. Immunobiology of compound ascidians, with particular reference to Botryllusschlosseri: state of art. ISJ 2008; 5: 54-74.

[93] Sredni B, Kalechman Y, Albeck M, *et al.* Cytokine secretion effected by synergism of the immunomodulator AS101 and the protein kinase C inducer bryostatin. Immunology 1990; 70(4): 473-7.
[PMID: 2118479]

[94] Bonacorsi C, Raddi MSG, Carlos IZ, Sannomiya M, Vilegas W. Anti-Helicobacter pylori activity and immunostimulatory effect of extracts from Byrsonima crassa Nied. (Malpighiaceae). BMC Complement Altern Med 2009; 9(1): 2.
[http://dx.doi.org/10.1186/1472-6882-9-2] [PMID: 19149866]

[95] Medina EJ, Lora AG, Paco L, Algarra I, *et al.* A new extract of the plant Calendula officinalis produces a dual *in vitro* effect: cytotoxic anti-tumor activity and lymphocyte activation. BMC Complement Altern Med 2006; 6(119): 1-14.

[96] Bhatt RP, Pandya BK, Sheth RN. Camellia sinensis L: the medicinal beverage: a review. IJPSRR 2010; 3(2): 6-9.

[97] Thakur M, Bhargava S, Dixit VK. Immunomodulatory Activity of *Chlorophytum borivilianum* Sant. F. Evid Based Complement Alternat Med 2007; 4(4): 419-23.
[http://dx.doi.org/10.1093/ecam/nel094] [PMID: 18227908]

[98] Bafna A, Mishra S. Bafna, A.; S. Mishra. Anti-oxidant and immunomodulatory activity of the alkaloidal fraction of Cissampelospareira Linn.ÖPhG., 78 2009; 21-31.

[99] Tanaka T, Sugiura H, Inaba R, *et al.* Immunomodulatory action of citrus auraptene on macrophage functions and cytokine production of lymphocytes in female BALB/c mice. Carcinogenesis 1999; 20(8): 1471-6.
[http://dx.doi.org/10.1093/carcin/20.8.1471] [PMID: 10426794]

[100] Gaur K, Kori ML, Nema RK. Comparative screening of immunomodulatory activity of hydro-alcoholic extract of Hibiscus rosa sinensis Linn. and ethanolic extract of Cleome gynandra Linn. GJP 2009; 3(2): 85-9.

[101] Costa JFO, David JPL, David JM, *et al.* Immunomodulatory activity of extracts from Cordia superba Cham. and Cordia rufescens A. DC. (Boraginaceae), plant species native from Brazilian Semi-arid. Rev Bras Farmacogn 2008; 18(1): 11-5.
[http://dx.doi.org/10.1590/S0102-695X2008000100004]

[102] Pradhan D, Panda PK, Tripathy G. Evaluation of immunomodulatory activity of methanolic extract of Couroupitaguianensis Aubl flowers in rat. NPR 2009; 8(1): 37-42.

[103] Karlowicz-Bodalska K, Han S, Freier J, Smolenski M, Bodalska A. Curcuma longa as medicinal herb in the treatment of diabet-ic complications. Acta Pol Pharm 2017; 74(2): 605-10.
[PMID: 29624265]

[104] Nair A, Chattopadhyay D, Saha B. Plant derived Immunomodulators. 2019; 435-99.

[105] Makiya NN, Djati MS. Potency of purple yam (Dioscoreaalata L) as an immunomodulatory agent. BerkalaKedokteran 2018; 14(1): 89-98.

[106] Lin H, Qiu H, Cheng Y, *et al.* *Gelsemium elegans* Benth: Chemical Components, Pharmacological

Effects, and Toxicity Mechanisms. Molecules 2021; 26(23): 7145.
[http://dx.doi.org/10.3390/molecules26237145] [PMID: 34885727]

[107] Habijanic J, Berovic M, Wraber B, Hodzar D, *et al.* Immunostimulatory effects of fungal polysaccharides from Ganoderma lucidum submerged biomass cultivation. Food Technol Biotechnol 2001; 39(9): 327-31.

[108] Kobayashi H, de Mejía E. The genus Ardisia: a novel source of health-promoting compounds and phytopharmaceuticals. J Ethnopharmacol 2005; 96(3): 347-54.
[http://dx.doi.org/10.1016/j.jep.2004.09.037] [PMID: 15619551]

[109] Wang C, Tao W, Wang Y, *et al.* Rosuvastatin, identified from a zebrafish chemical genetic screen for antiangiogenic compounds, suppresses the growth of prostate cancer. Eur Urol 2010; 58(3): 418-26.
[http://dx.doi.org/10.1016/j.eururo.2010.05.024] [PMID: 20605315]

[110] Steinbach WJ, Stevens DA. Review of newer antifungal and immunomodulatory strategies for invasive aspergillosis. Clin Infect Dis 2003; 37(s3) (Suppl. 3): S157-87.
[http://dx.doi.org/10.1086/376523] [PMID: 12975751]

[111] Malik JK, Manvi FV, Nanjwade BK, Alagawadi KR, *et al.* Immunomodulatory activity of Gymnemasylvestre R.Br. leaves on *in vitro* human neutrophils. J Pharm Res 2009; 2(8): 1284-6.

[112] Sharififar F, Pournourmohammadi S, Arabnejad M, Rastegarianzadeh R, *et al.* Immunomodulatory activity of aqueous extract of Heracleumpersicum Desf. in mice. IJPR 2009; 8(4): 287-92.

[113] Jain V, Bhagwat D, Jat RC, Bhardwaj S. The immunomodulation potential of Hyptissuaveolens. IJPRD 2005; 1(11): 1-6.

[114] Mukherjee PK, Nema NK, Bhadra S, Mukherjee D, Braga FC, Matsabisa MG. Immunomodulatory leads from medicinal plants. Indian J Tradit. Knowled 2014; 13(2): 235-56.

[115] Deshpande JR, Choudhari AA, Mishra MR, Meghre VS, Wadodkar SG, Dorle AK. Beneficial effects of Lagenaria siceraria (Mol.) Standley fruit epicarp in animal models. Indian J Exp Biol 2008; 46(4): 234-42.
[PMID: 18512332]

[116] Yue GGL, Liang XX, Li XL, *et al.* Immunomodulatory and antitumour bioactive labdane diterpenoids from *Leonurus japonicus*. J Pharm Pharmacol 2020; 72(11): 1657-65.
[http://dx.doi.org/10.1111/jphp.13348] [PMID: 32757490]

[117] Bharani SER, Asad M, Dhamanigi SS, Chandrakala GK. Immunomodulatory activity of methanolic extract of Morus alba Linn. (mulberry) leaves. Pak J Pharm Sci 2010; 23(1): 63-8.
[PMID: 20067869]

[118] Shah AS, Wakade AS, Juvekar AR. Immunomodulatory activity of methanolic extract of Murraya koenigii (L) Spreng. leaves. Indian J Exp Biol 2008; 46(7): 505-9.
[PMID: 18807753]

[119] Kannan M, Ranjit Singh AJA, Ajith Kumar TT, Jegatheswari P, *et al.* Studies on immuno-bioactivities of Nyctanthesarbortristis (Oleaceae). Afr J Microbiol Res 2007; 1(6): 88-91.

[120] Vaghasiya J, Datani M, Nandkumar K, Malaviya S, *et al.* Comparative evaluation of alcoholic and aqueous extracts of Ocimum sanctum for immunomodulatory activity. Int J Pharm Biol Res 2010; 1(1): 25-9.

[121] Singh S, Taneja M, Majumdar DK. Biological activities of Ocimum sanctum L. fixed oil--an overview. Indian J Exp Biol 2007; 45(5): 403-12.
[PMID: 17569280]

[122] Khare CP. Indian Medicinal Plants. An illustrated dictionary. Springer Publications, New York (2007).
[http://dx.doi.org/10.1007/978-0-387-70638-2]

[123] Panax ginseng. Monograph. Altern Med Rev 2009; 14(2): 172-6.
[PMID: 19594226]

[124] Smit HF. Picrorhizascrophularii flora from traditional use to immunomodulatory activity [doctoral thesis]. Utrecht, Netherlands: University of Utrecht; 2000.

[125] Subramaniam K, Subramaniam SK, Bhargav S, Parameshwari R, *et al.* Review on potential antiviral and immunomodulatory properties of Piper longum. IOP Conf. Ser Mater.Sci. Eng. 2021. DOI: 1145 012099

[126] Song G, Wang K, Zhang H, Sun H, Wu B, Ju X. Structural characterization and immunomodulatory activity of a novel polysaccharide from Pteridium aquilinum. Int J Biol Macromol 2017; 102: 599-604. [http://dx.doi.org/10.1016/j.ijbiomac.2017.04.037] [PMID: 28412343]

[127] Satpute KL, Jadhav MM, Karodi RS, Katare YS, *et al.* Immunomodulatory activity of fruits of Randiadumetorum Lamk. JPP 2009; 1(3): 36-40.

[128] Halder S, Bharal N, Mediratta PK, Kaur I, Sharma KK. Anti-inflammatory, immunomodulatory and antinociceptive activity of Terminalia arjuna Roxb bark powder in mice and rats. Indian J Exp Biol 2009; 47(7): 577-83.
[PMID: 19761042]

[129] Rinku M, Prasanth VV, Parthasarathy G. Immunomodulatory activity of the methanolic extract of Urena lobata Linn. Int J Pharmacol 2009; 1:7. http://www.ispub.com/journal/the_internet_journal_of_pharmacology/volume_7_number_1_27/article/immunomodulatory-activity--f-the-methanolic-extract-of-urena-lobata-linn.html

[130] Du X, Zhao B, Li J, *et al.* Astragalus polysaccharides enhance immune responses of HBV DNA vaccination *via* promoting the dendritic cell maturation and suppressing Treg frequency in mice. Int Immunopharmacol 2012; 14(4): 463-70.
[http://dx.doi.org/10.1016/j.intimp.2012.09.006] [PMID: 23006659]

[131] Yuan J, Lu L, Zhang Z, Zhang S. Dietary intake of resveratrol enhances the adaptive immunity of aged rats. Rejuvenation Res 2012; 15(5): 507-15.
[http://dx.doi.org/10.1089/rej.2012.1321] [PMID: 22950432]

[132] Chang YF, Chuang HY, Hsu CH, Liu RS, Gambhir SS, Hwang JJ. Immunomodulation of curcumin on adoptive therapy with T cell functional imaging in mice. Cancer Prev Res (Phila) 2012; 5(3): 444-52. [http://dx.doi.org/10.1158/1940-6207.CAPR-11-0308] [PMID: 22135043]

[133] Su CC, Yang JS, Lu CC, *et al.* Curcumin inhibits human lung large cell carcinoma cancer tumour growth in a murine xenograft model. Phytother Res 2010; 24(2): 189-92.
[http://dx.doi.org/10.1002/ptr.2905] [PMID: 20077433]

[134] Guo C, Sinnott B, Niu B, Lowry MB, *et al.* Synergistic induction of human cathelicidin anti-microbial peptide gene expression by vitamin D and stilbenoids. Mol Nutr Food Res 2014;58(3):528-536. [http://dx.doi.org/10.1002/mnfr.201300266]

[135] Ren Y, Wei M, Still PC, *et al.* Synthesis and antitumor activity of ellagic acid peracetate. ACS Med Chem Lett 2012; 3(8): 631-6.
[http://dx.doi.org/10.1021/ml300065z] [PMID: 23185648]

[136] Victor VV, Guayerbas N, Puerto M, Medina S, De la Fuente M. Ascorbic acid modulates *in vitro* the function of macrophages from mice with endotoxic shock. Immunopharmacology 2000; 46(1): 89-101.
[http://dx.doi.org/10.1016/S0162-3109(99)00162-9] [PMID: 10665783]

[137] Hesta M, Ottermans C, Krammer-Lukas S, *et al.* The effect of vitamin C supplementation in healthy dogs on antioxidative capacity and immune parameters. J Anim Physiol Anim Nutr (Berl) 2009; 93(1): 26-34.
[http://dx.doi.org/10.1111/j.1439-0396.2007.00774.x] [PMID: 19386005]

[138] Kwak JH, Baek SH, Woo Y, *et al.* Beneficial immunostimulatory effect of short-term Chlorella supplementation: enhancement of Natural Killercell activity and early inflammatory response (Randomized, double-blinded, placebo-controlled trial). Nutr J 2012; 11(1): 53.

[http://dx.doi.org/10.1186/1475-2891-11-53] [PMID: 22849818]

[139] Wang J, Yang J, Chan J, Huang J. Experimental studies on immunocompetence of lophanthus roots. Zhong Yao Cai 1997; 20(9): 470-2.
[PMID: 12572428]

[140] Novak M, Vetvicka V. Glucans as biological response modifiers. Endocr Metab Immune Disord Drug Targets 2009; 9(1): 67-75.
[http://dx.doi.org/10.2174/187153009787582423] [PMID: 19275682]

[141] Roesler J, Emmendörffer A, Steinmüller C, Luettig B, Wagner H, Lohmann-Matthes ML. Application of purified polysaccharides from cell cultures of the plant Echinacea purpurea to test subjects mediates activation of the phagocyte system. Int J Immunopharmacol 1991; 13(7): 931-41.
[http://dx.doi.org/10.1016/0192-0561(91)90046-A] [PMID: 1761359]

CHAPTER 12

Future Path and Perspectives of Immunomodulators

Megha Karne[1], **Supriya G. Jagtap**[2], **Sujata Sawarkar**[3] and **Vandana S. Nikam**[1,*]

[1] *Department of Pharmacology, STES's Smt. Kashibai Navale College of Pharmacy, Kondhwa, S. P. Pune University, Pune, Maharashtra, India*

[2] *Department of Pharmacognosyy, STES's Smt. Kashibai Navale College of Pharmacy, Kondhwa, S. P. Pune University, Pune, Maharashtra, India*

[3] *Department of Pharmaceutics, SVKM'S Dr. Bhanuben Nanavati College of Pharmacy, Mithibai Campus, Vile Parle (W), Mumbai-400056, India*

Abstract: Immunity is the inherent ability of the body to fight against various infections, and foreign invaders. When the host body comes in contact with a foreign body, a series of chemical mediators are released, which collectively elicit an immune response. The biomolecules capable of stimulating, suppressing and modulating innate or acquired immunity, biological or synthetic in origin, are termed as immunomodulators or immunoaugmentors. Limited clinical use of synthetic immunomodulators has attracted the attention of researchers toward immunomodulatory characteristics of natural therapeutics. Though natural immunomodulators render their efficacy in several chronic illnesses, there are challenges that need to be addressed and resolved to make them viable alternate therapeutics. This chapter highlights the challenges and future perspectives of natural immunomodulators.

Keywords: Adaptive Immunity, Future Challenges, Innate Immunity, Immunomodulators, Novel Drug Delivery, Perspective of Immunomodulators.

INTRODUCTION

The immune system is one of the most crucial systems in the body for survival, as stated in previous chapters. It acts as a defensive system to protect the body from harmful agents and infections. It executes its service through coordinated efforts of a wide range of immune cells having specific, defined roles. The immune system discriminates between harmful and benign foreign invaders, eliminating

* **Corresponding author Vandana S. Nikam:** Department of Pharmacology, STES's Smt. Kashibai Navale College of Pharmacy, Kondhwa, S. P. Pune University, Pune, Maharashtra, India; E-mail: vandananikam@sinhgad.edu

Vandana S. Nikam, Sujata P. Sawarkar, Girish B. Mahajan and Supriya G. Jagtap (Eds.)

them from the host system. The immune system is a complicated organ system next to the nervous system in biology.

The complexity of the immune system is observed at many levels. First, the cells of adaptive and innate immunity are interdependent and interconnected. The lymphocytes of the immune system present in a range of differentiated cell states, and they offer adaptive immunity with the help of countless cells of innate immunity.

Second, a complex network of intra- and inter-signaling pathways is operative in immune system functioning. Some of the factors that add to the complexity of the immune system are the process of immune cells education through clonal selection, cell receptors diversity, migration of cells, lymph dissemination throughout the host body, attaining immune homeostasis *via* regulating an ever-changing environment are some add to the complexity of the immune system.

Lastly, lymphocyte specificities, several recognition elements of innate immunity, depict the next level of complexity of the immune system. The feedback mechanism and regulation of immunostains is an intricate, subtle, and complex process and contributes significantly to immunity services.

THE COMPLEXITY OF INNATE AND ADAPTIVE IMMUNITY

The main four networks such as transcriptional, translation, spatiotemporal, and functional, control the overall execution of innate immunity in our body. These networks hold diverse information, including DNA sequence, RNAs, translocation information, spatiotemporal information of protein, subcellular structural details, and signaling process. Moreover, the intercellular communication networks include interactions between host and pathogen, soluble mediators like cytokines channelized linkages between a diverse pool of immune cells and other cells of tissues. The function of the immune system is quite dynamic, resulting in the non-linear behavior of several components, their interactions, feedback regulatory mechanisms, and three-dimensional positioning [1 - 4].

The major hurdles in the quantitative measurement of immune system components are complex and overlapping networks. With the advancement in analytical tools, genomics, proteomics, metabolomics, and cutting-edge technology, it would be possible to reach the depth and girth of the immune system and evaluation of natural immunomodulators. The involvement of sophisticated live and static imaging techniques with novel immunological assay warranted unraveling the complexity in the intracellular networks of the immune system.

Approaches and Challenges in Standardization of Natural Immunomodulators

Natural drugs and their phytoconstituents with potential immunomodulation activity are gaining popularity owing to new immune disorders and illnesses. In addition, complexities in the phytoconstituents have always presented challenges for the standardization of these compounds. It becomes necessary to provide sufficient preclinical data before natural medicines are subjected to clinical trials [5]. These strategies could be promising, allowing the development of new promising bioactive molecules. Within this context, an approach has been illustrated below with the studies conducted on many plant-origin drugs.

A major source of concern is the lack of consistency in pharmacological responses induced by plant extracts. This could be explained by the secondary metabolites' classic reliance on changes in the environment, which could also disrupt the repeatability of the end result with the extracts. Furthermore, the steadiness of therapeutic dose is among the main challenges that researchers face, as the amount of bioactive components generated differs due to the geographic area and ecological elements. Such issues can be resolved if the standardization principles of extracts and enriched fractions are systematically urged for all analytical studies.

The experimental investigation information recorded from immunomodulatory studies of *Phyllanthus* evidences an enthusiasm for identifying new chemical constituents from the available natural assets that can probably adapt to the immune responses of the human system. However, the challenges that are associated with the potential application of extracts of varied *Phyllanthus* species and the bioactive compounds as immunomodulators need to be examined.

The bio-active components of *Phyllanthus* species, namely phyllanthin, hypophyllanthin, ellagic acid, gallic acid, corilagin, niranthin, and geraniin, are highly variable in their expressions of quantity achieved at different elevations, which makes it challenging to retain quality in each batch.

The characterization of bioactive components responsible for the immunomodulation activity of plant extracts, as well as qualitative and quantitative evaluations of the chemical biomarkers for standardization and establishing the basic mechanisms of action, should have been the focus for future investigation into *Phyllanthus* species.

Earlier research studies have reported the contradictory effects of *Phyllanthus* extracts on immunomodulating activity. Very few studies have been performed on the signalling and molecular level for *P. amarus,* and a lot of molecular studies are still required to be performed with other species of the genus *Phyllanthus*.

So, there is a massive scope to study vital events of signalling associated with immunity, which comprises ATF2, TLR4, MyD88, proteomic, and genomic level studies on MAPKs and NF-κB pathways, including the activity of a kinase, to confirm genus *Phyllanthus* as an influential immunomodulation drug. Sufficient data from preclinical has to be produced earlier than the plant samples can be exposed to clinical trials. A small number of clinical studies have been reported on *P. niruri,* which are just a preliminary assessment carried out on a small batch. Studies also confirm that adequate preclinical data has not been reported, so further studies on these plants and their bioactive metabolites can be pursued in preclinical testing before being released to clinical trials [6].

The extract of *Phyllanthus amarus*, as an effective immunosuppressive agent, may be advantageous for the treatment of immune-related illnesses and may be a possible immunotherapeutic agent as a replacement for hazardous conventional therapy treatments. To understand the specific mechanisms behind *P. amarus'* immunomodulatory action, more molecular-based research is needed, which can be done in further studies related to this plant [7].

The immunologic method is an effective solid network of cellular components and chemical products intended to protect the organism's integrity against exterior slurs, and its efficient operation and balance are vital to avoid the incidence of a wide range of ailments. Currently, there has been a high rise in immunological disorders, and much awareness has been emphasized on the development of molecules that can regulate immunity.

Natural plants and their bioactive components have become an imperative resource for clinical therapeutics, and the study of their molecular pharmacology is a huge challenge because it gives a better chemical diversity with numerous pharmacological activities. Natural products, such as curcumin and *Echinacea*, have significant bioactivity that can be used in the design and development of pharmaceutical drugs.

Based on the preparation and research design, there has been scientific proof of both the therapeutic inefficacy and efficacy of *Echinacea* on the immunity system.

Curcumin also has restrictions contributing to its reduced pharmacokinetic and pharmacodynamic properties, being chemically unstable and poor quality.

To resolve these crucial pharmaceutical problems, different methods such as new formulations, modifications in the way of administering, and alternative nanotechnology-based delivery systems like nanoparticles, hydrogels, and liposomes have been implemented.

These methodologies may be challenging to develop a novel chemical entity that should be approved through preclinical studies before being endorsed for clinical trials [8].

As of 2020, the world has now been faced with a serious worldwide pandemic of COVID-19 infection; there have been millions of infections and thousands of deaths worldwide. Because of the virus's sequence alignment from generation to generation, approximately 60% of people are anticipated to become infected for the duration of the pandemic.COVID-19 has been a substantial infection that can lead to pneumonia as well as other problems such as septic shock and multi-organ failure. According to the latest theory, the SARS-COV-2 risk of death is induced by a cytokine storm syndrome in patient populations undergoing hyperinflammatory situations, which results in acute respiratory distress and, eventually, fatality.

Naturally occurring products have long been known for their medicinal value in the treatment of a variety of ailments. Because of the appearance of COVID-19 and being short of targeted therapy, they have started to be widely researched for their immunomodulatory and anti-viral activities. Numerous naturally occurring products were discovered to have immunomodulatory activity, anti-oxidant activity, and anti-viral activity by interfering with various stages of the SARS-CO-2 life cycle.

For example, natural products comprising polyphenols, like chamomile, which consists of quercetin, have anti-inflammatory, anti-oxidant, and anti-viral properties. This polyphenol-rich diet may aid in the reduction of inflammation in COVID-19 patients. Many essential oil-based natural products have been known to have anti-inflammation, immune-modulating, and anti-viral properties. Eucalyptus oil has also been reported as a valuable essential oil because of its promising applications for COVID-19 prevention and treatment [9].

Zinc and lactoferrin have immune-modulatory and anti-viral properties, making them especially promising for the prevention and treatment of COVID-19. Natural drugs are a valuable resource of biodiversity for the implementation of novel anti-viral agents. Even though many research studies on the potent anti-viral activity of natural products are still in the preliminary stages, future prospects on natural immunomodulators include assessing their efficacy and considering their potential use in the treatment of cytokine storm in Covid-19 [9].

Ethanolic extract of *Tinospora crispa* (TC) might increase immunological function; it could be a promising immune-therapeutic drug that can help patients with immune-compromised disorders. The pharmacologically active components in TC, as well as the signalling mechanisms involved in immunostimulation, are still unknown and can be investigated in the future [10].

The immunostimulant activity of the extracts of *Mangifera indica* leaves and *Curcuma domestica* rhizomes would be further explored by identifying, isolating, standardizing and checking the pharmacological activity of the phytoconstituents responsible for the immunostimulant activity. Furthermore, the exact mechanism underlying the activity can also be explored [11].

Further findings can be conducted to discover the dose ceiling limit of *S. suaveolens* root extract (SSRE) for its immunostimulatory activities in order to further confirm this characteristic. To assure a correlation between the immunostimulation activity of SSRE and that of lapachol and dehydro---lapachone, such a study should include isolated and pure compounds of lapachol and dehydro-α-lapachone in its control groups [12].

The immunostimulant activity of *Barleria prionitis* Linn. (BP) must be linked to the immune system's interaction with iridoid fraction (IFBp) (mostly shanzhiside methyl ester and barlerin iridoids), which needs to be further explored for the confirmation of the active constituents involved in the activity. As a result, even in healthy people, using IFBp as an immunomodulator to generate and improve protective immune responses may even be possible [13].

Zingiber zerumbet extract has the potential to operate as an immunomodulator, which could help with the treatment of immune-related disorders. To elucidate the precise mechanisms involved in immunomodulatory effects, comprehensive molecular research is required. Furthermore, more research into the identified bioactive chemical markers in the plant extract is needed to determine if the immunosuppressive effects of this extract were caused by a specific chemical marker or by the synergistic effects of numerous bioactive chemicals [14].

Cytotoxicity and immunomodulating effects on monocytes or macrophages may be a key mechanism and contributing component in the immunosuppression of α-MMC. α-MMC is likely to block the secretion of cytokines from polarised M2 macrophages in the cancer microenvironment, and it is extremely likely to destroy M2 macrophages to restrict tumor growth and metastasis, due to the high prevalence of the LRP1 receptor in monocytes or macrophages. In the future, this is going to be a very promising research direction [14].

The anti-arthritic and immunomodulatory activities of the NDI10218-standardized extract of *Terminalia chebula* fruits were observed, and the immunosuppressive effect of the extract was confirmed. This leads to a confirmed basis for the usefulness of the extract in the treatment of rheumatoid arthritis (RA) in the future as an alternative to the conventional immunosuppressive agents used in the treatment of RA, which has certain toxic effects. *T. chebula's* complex involvement in ulcers, infection, and cancer may provide a useful therapeutic possibility for RA as an alternative or supplemental therapy to currently available RA treatments. Thus, extensive research should be carried out to bring this drug into the market as a new therapy for RA [15].

Using various advanced technologies like cell cultures, tissue cultures, and other biotechnological methods, a quality product can be developed due to the excellent standardization that can be performed on the extracts obtained from the cultured plants due to the development of the plant in a controlled environment as compared to conventionally cultivated plants, which vary according to their growing conditions in all aspects. Also, the phytochemical content is higher in the cultured plants than in the equivalent conventionally cultivated plants. Thus, the drawbacks related to the standardization of conventional plants are overcome in these plants cultivated using advanced technologies. Further research and implementation of these techniques should be done in the future to obtain a high-yield and quality product that is safe and efficacious [16, 17].

In-vitro, *In-vivo* Preclinical Models Development and Translating for Clinical Application

Preclinical models have commonly employed tools for identifying targets, the underlying mechanism of actions, delivery modalities, dose regime and frequency, safety, and toxicological profiling. The transgenic animal models with human HLA types are frequently used in the assessment of biological immunomodulators. However, at a time, the immune phenotype of a single person is grafted and can not have a scale for high throughput screening [18 - 20].

Immunotherapy has emerged as one of the new therapeutic approaches in oncology. Another issue faced with preclinical models used in cancer immunotherapy is the use of cancer cell line implantation, and they do not represent human immune cells and cancer cell interactions [21, 22]. The complexity of immune system interactions involving various steps of priming, activation, and regulation are crucial and hard to translate into clinical settings [22].

Immunomodulatory biologicals render their therapeutic efficacy by harnessing the power of the immune system. However, the adverse reactions associated with them pose a new challenge. It becomes crucial or challenging to keep vigilance on immune-relevant adverse events to deliver safe and efficacious immunomodulatory agents. The preclinical models could be explored to decipher the underlying mechanism of the adverse event observed [23].

Humanised mice presenting the complexity of the immune system are likely to widen the scope of preclinical models in natural immunomodulatory evaluation. Otherwise, a series of preclinical models representing each immune system component needs to be developed, which would be translated into a clinical setting [21]. Another alternative is to turn the clinical experience into a testable hypothesis and test it in a preclinical model to understand the incident of immune-related adverse events [23].

Additionally, developing and implementing standardised biobank concepts concerning immune-related therapeutics and adverse events further widen our scope of clinical understanding [24]. The implementation of cutting-edge methods of data analytics, effective analysis and interpretation will enable us to understand the progression of immune-related diseases and etiology in several chronic illnesses like cancer and autoimmune disorders following immune therapy.

The development of novel assays that mimic the complexity of the immune system and have a capacity for high throughput screening would address the limitations of current preclinical models [25]. New techniques and technologies that more accurately reflect the biology of human cancer immunology are required [26].

Novel Drug Delivery System of Natural Immunomodulators and Challenges, Future Outlook

To date, several scientific reports have suggested that the use of novel drug delivery systems can help overcome pre-existing regulatory, standardization, formulation and administration concerns relating to the delivery of natural immunomodulators.

Nanocarriers like nanoparticles, liposomes, niosomes, micelles, transfersomes, ethosomes *etc.*, have been used to deliver phytoconstituents such as curcumin, resveratrol, puerarin, triptolide *etc.* By virtue of their size, nanocarriers can easily permeate through the cells and be easily retained, thus ensuring better therapeutic efficacy. These unique properties of nanotechnology have led to successful clinical trials of many phytoconstituents. There is an existing gap between the therapeutic potential of natural immunomodulators and their delivery to the target site. Thus, many research initiatives must be undertaken to synthesize more targeted nanotherapeutic delivery systems with high drug payload, better biocompatibility, low toxicity, better cytocompatibility, and high quality for the overall management of various disorders.

The impact of nanotechnology in the delivery of natural immunomodulators is still very limited despite of overwhelming understanding of the future prospect of nanomedicine. Our understanding of the application of nanocarriers will improve with a better understanding of diseases at the molecular level. In this review, we have outlined in brief the known nanomedicines, however, further research would be key for the wider application of nanotechnology for the delivery of natural products. Multidisciplinary research and extensive preclinical studies will help provide valuable data in the potential application of natural immunomodulators. The future involving the use of natural drugs in therapeutics and diagnostics is promising. With gaining popularity, two more areas that would need research inputs are affordability and industrial scale-up of nanotechnology. To be able to deliver natural immunomodulators effectively and safely, well-defined regulations and study protocols to assess the safety and efficacy of nanomedicine should be well established. Due to continuous advances in the field of nanotechnology, the delivery of natural products is not a distant future.

Natural and traditional medicine contribute to a large sector of therapeutic agents. The pharmaceutical industry is developing with improvements in research and development in drug discovery, and the role of natural medicine as an allied and alternative treatment is growing with it. The importance of natural immunomodulators in the regulation of human health has been well-known and documented. The discovery and isolation of more selective natural immunomodulatory have the potential to mitigate synthetic drugs' negative effects and expensive costs [27].

This chapter summarizes the use of bioactive from traditional herbs in the treatment of infections caused by various microorganisms like fungi, bacteria, and viruses in humans and animals. These bioactive include flavonoids, saponins, and alkaloids which exert anti-oxidant, anti-inflammatory, anti-bacterial, anti-viral, and anti-parasitic activity *via* various mechanisms like regulation of cytokines, macrophages, NK cells, and lymphocytes. Certain natural immunomodulators are being studied extensively in clinical trials and may soon be used in traditional treatments effectively.

With the emergence of growing populations being affected by infections, it has become necessary to come up with more safe and cost-effective alternative treatments. In the future, the development of novel drugs will benefit greatly from extensive chemical and pharmacological analyses of traditional formulations and medicinal plants [8].

Currently faced challenges in extraction and production of immunomodulators from natural sources like low bioavailability and standardization have to be overcome. For the effective application of immune-modulating drugs for diverse diseases, these challenges need to be solved by investigating innovative isolation techniques, efficient and targeted drug delivery systems, building standardized quality control measures, and so on. With randomized and controlled clinical studies, further proof regarding the efficacy of herbal treatments is needed. Furthermore, determining the efficacy and safety of traditional treatments may serve as a foundation for their future classification, as well as identifying the potential use of herbal medicines and their processed products in national healthcare systems across the world [8, 28].

Market and Regulatory Perspective of Natural Immunomodulators

Immunomodulators are natural or artificial agents that can activate, inhibit, or modify any function of the immune cells. They are grouped into three types in clinical practice such as immunoadjuvants, immunomodulators, and immunosuppressants. The goal is to keep drug standards high at all times to meet the needs of health maintenance of each country. Pharmaceutical drug laws are a collection of authorized, procedural, and technical requirements used by government agencies to guarantee patient safety, drug efficacy, and purity. Throughout the world, several regulatory authorities are formulating and drafting rules and legislation to ensure the appropriate operation of medication commercialization approval. The scope and execution of pharmaceutical regulation differ from place to location, but the main goals are as follows: Licensing the manufacture, importation, exportation, distribution, promotion, and marketing of pharmaceuticals. Evaluating the safety, effectiveness, and purity of medications, as well as granting regulatory permission for specific goods; Overseeing the quality of accessible medicines on the market; regulating counterfeit pharmaceuticals, and monitoring the safety of marketed products. Strong evidence should be used to make decisions on the purity, quality, and efficacy of medicines [29].

The Central Drug Standard Control Organization (CDSCO), the Indian Council of Medical Research (ICMR), and the Ministry of Health and Family Welfare are the regulatory authorities in India (MoHFW). The CDSCO is in charge of carrying out the responsibilities allocated by the Central Government under the Drugs and Cosmetics Act [30]. ICMR is regarded as one of the world's oldest clinical study organizations, as well as the best framework in India for designing, coordinating, and promoting biological investigations [31]. There are 11 operating departments in the US Department of Health and Human Services. The Food and Drug Administration (FDA) is one of the bodies in charge of guaranteeing the product's safety and authenticity. The FDA verifies the quality of animal and human medications, biopharmaceuticals, and surgical tools [32]. The introduction of the GCP (Good Clinical Practice) guidelines improved the ethical and scientific quality of research undertaken in Japan. It helped in enhancing the interactions between doctors and patients. The commitment to standardize all quality, safety, and efficacy information has transformed regulatory review procedures [33].

Due to the increased prevalence of chronic illnesses, such as multiple sclerosis, allergic disorders, cancer, and asthma, the worldwide market for immunomodulators is predicted to rise exponentially throughout the forecast period. Immunomodulator treatment is a viable option due to its high remission rate and low incidence of organ rejection. The development of sophisticated biological response modulators is accelerating as the global incidence of multiple sclerosis rises [34]. During the projected period of 2022 to 2025, the worldwide immunomodulators market is predicted to grow at a rapid CAGR. Some of the important reasons driving the market include the increasing usage of monoclonal antibodies, the availability of a strong pipeline portfolio, and TNF-alpha inhibitors and B-cell inhibitors. On the other side, obstacles include high patent expiration rates, increased competition from generic and biosimilar pharmaceuticals, adverse drug effects, and the cessation of drugs under development [35].

In 2019, the worldwide immunomodulators market was valued at USD 161.57 billion. COVID-19 has had an unprecedented and devastating worldwide impact, with Immunomodulators seeing a positive demand shock across all areas as a result of the pandemic. The market is expected to increase at a CAGR of 6.3 percent, from USD 186.12 billion in 2020 to USD 285.01 billion in 2027. The abrupt increase in CAGR is due to increased market demand and growth returning to pre-epidemic levels once the pandemic has passed [36].

CONCLUDING REMARKS

The complexity of immune system at many levels makes it challenging to highlight the targets and predict the therapeutic potential with the safety and efficacy of natural immunomodulators.

Although natural immunomodulators have had well-proven traditional uses since ancient times, global acceptance of natural immunomodulators encountered many challenges and needs systematic and scientific evidence.

These are quality and quality control issues, processing and harvesting issues, biodiversity, administrative issues, infrastructure-related issue, pharmacovigilance, conducting globally recognized and harmonized clinical trials, IPR, and biopiracy, irrational use, standardised marker compounds for developing monographs, standard reference compounds, regulatory and market-based analysis, standardization and processing of constituents into modernized dosage forms at large scale.

Resolving all related issues with natural immunomodulators warrant therapeutic efficacy and safety in immune-related diseases and can provide a viable alternative.

CONSENT FOR PUBLICATION

Not applicable.

CONFLICT OF INTEREST

The authors declare no conflict of interest, financial or otherwise.

ACKNOWLEDGEMENTS

The authors of this chapter would like to acknowledge STES's Smt. Kashibai Navale College of Pharmacy, Kondhwa (Bk), Pune411048, Maharashtra, India and SVKM'S Dr. Bhanuben Nanavati College of Pharmacy, Mithibai Campus, Vile Parle (W), Mumbai-400056, India.

REFERENCES

[1] Zak DE, Aderem A. Systems biology of innate immunity. Immunol Rev 2009; 227(1): 264-82. [http://dx.doi.org/10.1111/j.1600-065X.2008.00721.x] [PMID: 19120490]

[2] Gilchrist M, Thorsson V, Li B, *et al.* Systems biology approaches identify ATF3 as a negative regulator of Toll-like receptor 4. Nature 2006; 441(7090): 173-8. [http://dx.doi.org/10.1038/nature04768] [PMID: 16688168]

[3] Elkon R, Linhart C, Halperin Y, Shiloh Y, Shamir R. Functional genomic delineation of TLR-induced transcriptional networks. BMC Genomics 2007; 8(1): 394. [http://dx.doi.org/10.1186/1471-2164-8-394] [PMID: 17967192]

[4] Ramsey SA, Klemm SL, Zak DE, *et al.* Uncovering a macrophage transcriptional program by integrating evidence from motif scanning and expression dynamics. PLOS Comput Biol 2008; 4(3): e1000021. [http://dx.doi.org/10.1371/journal.pcbi.1000021] [PMID: 18369420]

[5] Kunle. Standardization of herbal medicines - A review. Int J Biodivers Conserv 2012; 4(3) [http://dx.doi.org/10.5897/IJBC11.163]

[6] Jantan I, Haque MA, Ilangkovan M, Arshad L. An Insight Into the Modulatory Effects and Mechanisms of Action of *Phyllanthus* Species and Their Bioactive Metabolites on the Immune System. Front Pharmacol 2019; 10: 878. [http://dx.doi.org/10.3389/fphar.2019.00878] [PMID: 31440162]

[7] Ilangkovan M, Jantan I, Mesaik MA, Bukhari SNA. Immunosuppressive effects of the standardized extract of Phyllanthus amarus on cellular immune responses in Wistar-Kyoto rats. Drug Des Devel Ther 2015; 9: 4917-30. [PMID: 26347462]

[8] Catanzaro M, Corsini E, Rosini M, Racchi M, Lanni C. Immunomodulators Inspired by Nature: A Review on Curcumin and Echinacea. Molecules 2018; 23(11): 2778. [http://dx.doi.org/10.3390/molecules23112778] [PMID: 30373170]

[9] Abbas HS, Abd-elhakeem MM, Abd El Galil RM, *et al.* Natural Immunomodulators Treat the Cytokine Storm in SARS-CoV-2. Adv Pharm Bull 2021; 1-16. [http://dx.doi.org/10.34172/apb.2023.006]

[10] Ahmad W, Jantan I, Kumolosasi E, Bukhari SNA. Immunostimulatory effects of the standardized extract of Tinospora crispa on innate immune responses in Wistar Kyoto rats. Drug Des Devel Ther 2015; 9: 2961-73. [PMID: 26089645]

[11] Kumolosasi E, Ibrahim SNA, Ahmad Shukri SM, Ahmad W. Immunostimulant activity of standardised extracts of *Mangifera indica* leaf and *Curcuma domestica* rhizome in mice. Trop J Pharm Res 2018; 17(1): 77-84. [http://dx.doi.org/10.4314/tjpr.v17i1.12]

[12] Maji AK, Samanta SK, Mahapatra S, Banerji P, Banerjee D. *In-vivo* immunomodulatory activity of standardized Stereospermum suaveolens (Roxb.) DC. root extract. Orient Pharm Exp Med 2014; 14(1): 47-54. [http://dx.doi.org/10.1007/s13596-013-0132-4]

[13] Ghule BV, Yeole PG. *In vitro* and *in vivo* immunomodulatory activities of iridoids fraction from Barleria prionitis Linn. J Ethnopharmacol 2012; 141(1): 424-31. [http://dx.doi.org/10.1016/j.jep.2012.03.005] [PMID: 22440262]

[14] Ghazalee NS, Jantan I, Arshad L, Haque MA. Immunosuppressive effects of the standardized extract of *Zingiber zerumbet* on innate immune responses in Wistar rats. Phytother Res 2019; 33(4): 929-38. [http://dx.doi.org/10.1002/ptr.6285] [PMID: 30618097]

[15] Seo JB, Jeong JY, Park JY, *et al.* Anti-Arthritic and Analgesic Effect of NDI10218, a Standardized Extract of Terminalia chebula, on Arthritis and Pain Model. Biomol Ther (Seoul) 2012; 20(1): 104-12. [http://dx.doi.org/10.4062/biomolther.2012.20.1.104] [PMID: 24116282]

[16] Dal Toso R, Melandri F. Echinacea angustifolia cell culture extract. Nutrafoods 2011; 10(1): 19-24. [http://dx.doi.org/10.1007/BF03223351]

[17] Yang X, Lei Z, Yu Y, Xiao L, Cheng D, Zhang Z. Phytochemical characteristics of callus suspension culture of Helicteres angustifolia L. and its *in vitro* antioxidant, antidiabetic and immunomodulatory activities. S Afr J Bot 2019; 121: 178-85. [http://dx.doi.org/10.1016/j.sajb.2018.11.006]

[18] Ishikawa F, Yasukawa M, Lyons B, *et al.* Development of functional human blood and immune systems in NOD/SCID/IL2 receptor γ chainnull mice. Blood 2005; 106(5): 1565-73. [http://dx.doi.org/10.1182/blood-2005-02-0516] [PMID: 15920010]

[19] Pearson T, Greiner DL, Shultz LD. Creation of "humanized" mice to study human immunity. Curr Protoc Immunol. 2008.May;Chapter 15:Unit 15.21:1-21. [http://dx.doi.org/10.1002/0471142735.im1521s81]

[20] King M, Pearson T, Shultz LD, *et al.* A new Hu-PBL model for the study of human islet alloreactivity based on NOD-scid mice bearing a targeted mutation in the IL-2 receptor gamma chain gene. Clin Immunol 2008; 126(3): 303-14. [http://dx.doi.org/10.1016/j.clim.2007.11.001] [PMID: 18096436]

[21] Dranoff G. Experimental mouse tumour models: what can be learnt about human cancer immunology? Nat Rev Immunol 2012; 12(1): 61-6. [http://dx.doi.org/10.1038/nri3129] [PMID: 22134155]

[22] Fridman WH, Pagès F, Sautès-Fridman C, Galon J. The immune contexture in human tumours: impact on clinical outcome. Nat Rev Cancer 2012; 12(4): 298-306.

[http://dx.doi.org/10.1038/nrc3245] [PMID: 22419253]

[23] Chen MS, Lara PN, Dang JHT, Paterniti DA, Kelly K. Twenty Years Post-NIH Revitalization Act: Renewing the Case for Enhancing Minority Participation in Cancer Clinical Trials. Cancer 2014; 120(0 7): 1091-6.

[24] Chapman KL, Andrews L, Bajramovic JJ, *et al.* The design of chronic toxicology studies of monoclonal antibodies: Implications for the reduction in use of non-human primates. Regul Toxicol Pharmacol 2012; 62(2): 347-54. [http://dx.doi.org/10.1016/j.yrtph.2011.10.016] [PMID: 22100994]

[25] Bayless NL, Bluestone JA, Bucktrout S, *et al.* Development of preclinical and clinical models for immune-related adverse events following checkpoint immunotherapy: a perspective from SITC and AACR. J Immunother Cancer 2021; 9(9): e002627. [http://dx.doi.org/10.1136/jitc-2021-002627] [PMID: 34479924]

[26] Hegde PS, Chen DS. Top 10 Challenges in Cancer Immunotherapy. Immunity 2020; 52(1): 17-35. [http://dx.doi.org/10.1016/j.immuni.2019.12.011] [PMID: 31940268]

[27] Mahima null, Rahal A, Deb R, Latheef SK, Abdul Samad H, Tiwari R, et al. Immunomodulatory and therapeutic potentials of herbal, traditional/indigenous and ethnoveterinary medicines. Pak J Biol Sci. 2012; 15(16): 754-4.

[28] Vargason AM, Anselmo AC, Mitragotri S. The evolution of commercial drug delivery technologies. Nat Biomed Eng 2021; 5(9): 951-67. [http://dx.doi.org/10.1038/s41551-021-00698-w] [PMID: 33795852]

[29] Bascones-Martinez A, Mattila R, Gomez-Font R, Meurman JH. Immunomodulatory drugs: Oral and systemic adverse effects. Med Oral Patol Oral Cir Bucal 2014; 19(1): e24-31. [http://dx.doi.org/10.4317/medoral.19087] [PMID: 23986016]

[30] 2022.https://main.mohfw.gov.in/about-us/organisational-set

[31] 2022.https://clinregs.niaid.nih.gov/country/india#_top

[32] Research C for DE and. 2021.https://www.fda.gov/drugs/development-approval-process-drugs

[33] Vijayananthan A, Nawawi O. The importance of Good Clinical Practice guidelines and its role in clinical trials. Biij 2008; 4(1): e5. [http://dx.doi.org/10.2349/biij.4.1.e5] [PMID: 21614316]

[34] Tramacere I, Del Giovane C, Salanti G, D'Amico R, Filippini G. Immunomodulators and immunosuppressants for relapsing-remitting multiple sclerosis: a network meta-analysis. Cochrane Libr 2015; 2015(9): CD011381. [http://dx.doi.org/10.1002/14651858.CD011381.pub2] [PMID: 26384035]

[35] Monaco C, Nanchahal J, Taylor P, Feldmann M. Anti-TNF therapy: past, present and future. Int Immunol 2015; 27(1): 55-62. [http://dx.doi.org/10.1093/intimm/dxu102] [PMID: 25411043]

[36] Immunomodulators Market By Product & Application | Analysis, 2027. 2022 Jan 23. 2022.https://www.fortunebusinessinsights.com/immunomodulators-market-104692

SUBJECT INDEX

A

Acid 94, 96, 141, 142, 144, 151, 152, 220, 230, 260, 383, 402
ascorbic 94, 96
caffeic 155, 157, 158, 249
chebulagic 151, 152, 260
eicosapentaenoic 372
ellagic 141, 142, 144, 220, 230, 260, 383, 402
Glycyrrhetinic 96, 141, 157, 158, 201, 221, 231, 260, 280, 288, 291, 292, 298, 380, 381
hyaluronic 288
hydrocyanic 380
hypochlorous 201
oleanolic 221, 280, 381
orthophosphoric 141
rosmarinic 157, 158
stearic 291, 292, 294, 298
tannic 260
tetrahydrofolic 96
tinosporic 381
ursolic 291, 381
Acquired immuno deficiency syndrome 246
Adaptive immune system 5, 16, 20, 22, 57, 64, 68, 166, 169, 191, 192
Adenosine deaminase 43
Adjuvant therapy 31, 217
Advisory committee on medical devices (ACMD) 332
Agents 67, 77, 99, 165, 166, 167, 169, 172, 200, 203, 244, 245, 370, 382, 387, 388
anti-angiogenic 169
anti-inflammatory 99
chemoprotective 77
chemotherapeutic 67
immunotherapeutic 370
Agranulocytosis 385
Aicardi-Goutieres syndrome 45
Aldrich syndrome 46
Allergic 23, 27, 48, 49, 171, 258
diseases and disorders 48
rhinitis (AR) 23, 27, 48, 49, 171
skin diseases 258
Allergy-related diseases 22
Anaphylaxis reactions 207
Antibacterial 103, 248, 249, 252, 253, 254, 255, 256, 257, 258, 259, 260, 261
activity 248, 249, 252, 253, 254, 255, 256, 257, 258, 259, 260, 261
properties 103, 259
Antibody 128, 199, 369
dependent cellular cytotoxicity 128
forming cells (AFCs) 199
mediated immunity 369
Antifibrinolytic activity 127
Antifilarial activity 128
Antifungal activity 248, 249, 250, 251, 252, 253, 254, 256, 259, 260, 261
Antigen-presenting cells (APCs) 15, 16, 68, 93, 192, 199, 208, 384
Anti-inflammatory 63, 78, 128, 136, 255, 289, 297, 372
activity 78, 128, 289, 297
effects 63, 136, 255, 372
Anti-inflammatory drugs 196, 202
non-steroid 196
Antimicrobial activity 251, 252, 253, 258, 259, 307
Antioxidant proteins 178
Antiparasitic activity 250, 252, 253, 254, 255, 256, 258, 259
Antitumor activities 230, 302, 375
Antiviral efficacy 261
Apoptosis 12, 20, 52, 53, 56, 66, 96, 172, 224, 230, 255
Arthritis 26, 60, 183, 210, 303
chronic 207
collagen-induced 151, 208
mediated autoimmune 207
proteoglycan-induced 210

Asthma 22, 23, 98, 118, 136, 144, 174, 183, 258, 261, 379, 410
bronchial 118
conjunctivitis 22
Atherosclerosis 100, 382
ATM protein 47
Autoimmune 24, 33, 34, 41, 42, 46, 53, 55, 59, 97, 101, 190, 191, 193, 195, 199, 203, 209, 210, 212, 245, 277, 325, 385, 386
diseases (ADs) 41, 42, 53, 55, 190, 191, 193, 209, 210, 212, 245, 277, 385
disorders 33, 34, 53, 55, 59, 97, 101, 190, 195, 199, 203
hemolytic anemia 209
illnesses 210, 325
kidney disease 386
lymphoproliferative syndrome 46
neutropenia 24
thyroiditis 209
Autoimmunity 41, 42, 43, 45, 46, 51, 54, 55, 172
infection-related 55
Auto-inflammatory diseases 33, 43, 60, 61, 62
Autosomal recessive transmission disease 61

B

Bacteria 2, 119, 247, 307
aerobic 307
aerobic spore-forming 119
antibiotic-resistant 247
disease-causing 2
Bechet's disease 64
Betulinic acid 217, 219, 225, 226, 232
Bone marrow-derived macrophages (BMDM) 194
Bradykinesia 58

C

Cancer 31, 33, 34, 41, 65, 66, 67, 68, 83, 84, 171, 176, 199, 217, 218, 222, 224, 225, 231, 245, 380, 385, 406
breast 149, 224
colon 385
hepatic 231
immunotherapy 33, 41, 66, 176, 406
metastatic colorectal 225
prostate 224, 380
Carbonic anhydrase inhibitors 52
Cardiothoracic surgery 47

Cell-mediated 4, 18, 95, 122, 127, 177, 278, 369
immunity (CMI) 4, 18, 95, 122, 127, 177, 278, 369
phagocytosis 127
Chemokines release 27
Chemotaxis 11, 26, 143
Chinese 119, 227, 352
herbal pharmacopoeia 119
medicines 227, 352
Chronic lymphocytic leukaemia 48
Clostridium perfringens 254
Collagen-induced arthritis (CIA) 151, 208
Combination therapy 371
Complementary and alternative medicine (CAM) 249, 324
Coptis chinensis 220, 227
Coronary artery disease (CAD) 376
Coronavirus 176
Corticosteroids, systemic 53
COVID-19 92, 167, 387, 404
crisis 387
infection 404
pandemic 167
vaccines 92
Coxsackie virus 261
Crohn's disease 245, 384
Cytokine(s) 30, 61, 64, 94, 97, 101, 172, 174, 177, 221, 375, 404
anti-inflammatory 30, 64, 97, 172, 174, 221
growth-promoting 167
inflammatory 57, 61, 94, 101, 177, 375
signaling pathways 61
storm syndrome 404
Cytomegalovirus 48, 255

Cytometric bead assay 183
Cytotoxic coumarins 78, 375
Cytotoxicity 25, 193, 194, 195, 200, 217, 218, 219, 221, 298, 299, 307, 405
  and immunomodulating effects on monocytes 405
  antibody-dependent cell-mediated 25
Cytotoxic 14, 383
  lymphocytes 383
  proteins 14

D

Deficiency 43, 122, 246
  immune 122
  immunological 246
  severe combined immune 43
Delayed type hypersensitivity (DTH) 135, 137
Dendritic cells (DCs) 10, 12, 14, 15, 88, 89, 95, 97, 166, 168, 191, 248, 253
Diphtheria disease 32
Disease(s) 77, 209, 218, 387, 407, 411
  cancer-related 387
  cardiovascular 218
  fibrotic 209
  heart 77
  immune-related 407, 411
  lymphoproliferative 209
  modifying anti-rheumatic drug (DMARD) 278
Disorders 30, 33, 42, 43, 44, 45, 46, 47, 56, 68, 138, 261, 304, 405
  congenital 47
  immune-compromised 405
  immune-related 405
  immune system-related 68
  immunodeficiency 42, 43, 44, 45, 46
  metabolic 33
  neurodegenerative 30, 261
  rheumatic 138, 304
  thyroid-affecting 56
Downregulate signaling pathways 170
Droplet counter-current chromatography (DCCC) 180
Drug(s) 47, 48, 64, 96, 110, 111, 118, 190, 224, 28, 244, 245, 262, 278, 288, 289, 290, 291, 295, 299, 303, 306, 330, 332, 333, 334, 339, 341, 347, 359, 385, 405
  allopathic 111
  anti-allergic 190
  anticancer 224, 228
  anti-epileptic 47
  antihelminthic 385
  antiproliferative 385
  chemotherapeutic 48
  chemotherapy 96
  disease-modifying anti-rheumatic 278
  hydrophobic 291, 299
  immune 262
  immune-therapeutic 405
  immunosuppressant 64
  metabolizing enzymes (DMEs) 172
Dysfunction 30, 53, 59, 103, 212, 218
  autonomic 59
  cognitive 212
  sexual 218

E

Ectodermal dystrophy 45
Effects, immune-modulatory 86
EGFR signalling pathways 231
Eholanthrene-induced sarcoma 128
ELISPOT assay 199
Enzymes 66, 77, 97, 100, 122, 173, 255, 376
  drug-metabolizing 172
  hydrolytic 6, 86
  linked immunosorbent assay 151
  lysosomal 10, 23
  mevalonate kinase 61

F

Fever 49, 91
  hay 49
  yellow 91
FHL syndromes 45
Fibrosis, myocardial 210

Folate deficiency 99
FTIR 154, 156
  analysis 154, 156
  spectrometer 154
Functions 61, 76, 96
  immune system's 76
  leukocyte 96
  mitochondrial 61

G

Gas chromatography 115
Gastrointestinal 85, 308
  environment 308
  microflora 85
Genotoxicity 172
Glioblastoma 293
Gut microbiota 85, 99

H

Haemolytic disease 23
Hashimoto's thyroiditis (HT) 56, 208
Heat shock proteins 16, 93, 171
Hepatitis 31, 48, 52, 76, 101, 141, 245, 246, 252, 256
  virus 246
Hepatocellular carcinoma 224
Hepatotoxicity 172, 278, 388
Herbal 336
  medications 336
  Medicinal Products (HMPC) 336, 338, 344, 346, 351
Herpes simplex encephalitis (HSE) 45
High 114, 115, 118, 130, 131, 132, 135, 142, 150, 152, 154, 158, 180, 182
  pressure liquid chromatography (HPLC) 114, 115, 118, 130, 131, 132, 135, 142, 150, 152, 154, 158, 180
  resolution mass spectrometry (HRMS) 182
  speed counter-current chromatography (HSCCC) 180
High-performance 114, 115, 118, 140, 158, 180, 181
  capillary electrophoresis (HPCE) 181
  liquid chromatography 118, 180
  thin layer chromatography (HPTLC) 114, 115, 140, 158, 180
Histiocytosis 48
HPLC technique 145, 147
Human 15, 16, 52, 53, 86
  leukocyte antigen (HLAs) 15, 16, 52, 53
  peripheral blood mononuclear (HPBM) 86
Hydrastis canadensis 227
Hyperglycemia 278

I

Immune 24, 28, 42, 52, 55, 68, 88, 94, 152, 209, 212, 277, 278, 388, 401
  cells migration 152
  checkpoints 68
  diseases 42, 55
  disorders 42, 209, 388
  homeostasis 28, 88, 401
  mediated disease 52, 212
  response, cell-mediated 94, 277, 278
  thrombocytopenia 24
Immune system 41, 58, 247
  acquired 41, 247
  dysregulation 58
Immunity diseases 144
Immuno 68
  checkpoint inhibitors 68
  modulating therapy 68
Immunodeficiency syndromes 42
Immunosuppressive properties 386
Immunotherapy in cancer and autoimmune disorders 34
Inflammation, immune complex-mediated acute 205
Inflammatory 6, 8, 14, 23, 30, 49, 50, 57, 97, 103, 191, 200, 209, 245, 304, 374
  bowel disease (IBD) 30, 97, 245
  diseases 209, 304
  responses 6, 8, 14, 23, 49, 50, 57, 103, 191, 200, 374
Inhibition, tyrosinase 78

Injuries 100, 210, 293
cardiac 210
ischemia-reperfusion 100
paracetamol-induced liver 293
Insomnia 278, 388
Intracellular adhesion molecules (ICAMs) 173
Irritable bowel syndrome 379
Ischemia-reperfusion injury (IRI) 100

J

Japanese encephalitis 256
virus (JEV) 256

K

Kidney transplants 167
Kupffer cells 198

L

Leucopenia 167, 176, 278, 382
Lipopolysaccharide, bacterial 166, 194, 197, 208
Lipoxygenase 248, 375
Liver 124, 175, 183, 251
cirrhosis 175, 183
diseases 124, 251
Lower respiratory tract infection (LRTI) 95, 98, 101
Lycium barbarum polysaccharide (LBP) 306

M

Major histocompatibility complex 15, 52, 53, 192, 208, 211
Methods, spectrophotometry 113
Mitogen-activated protein kinase (MAPK) 219, 231, 256, 403
Mucosal 3, 87, 90
associated lymphoid tissue (MALT) 3
immune system (MIS) 87, 90
Multiple sclerosis (MS) 55, 57, 59, 60, 97, 150, 182, 385, 410
Mycobacterial disease 45

N

Nanoparticles 294, 295
metal 294, 295
metallic 294
Nausea 217, 218, 278, 388
Neurodegenerative diseases 33, 57, 58
Neurological disorders 57
NK cell cytotoxic activity 100
NLRP3 inflammasome 52
Nuclear magnetic resonance (NMR) 182

O

Oil 224, 249, 289, 293, 300, 307
castor 300
lavender 289
olive 224, 293
orange 289
rosemary 289
seed 249
thyme 289, 307
Otosclerosis 209

P

Pain 59, 61, 96, 136, 278, 388
abdominal 61, 278, 388
chest 96
Peptides, antigenic 15, 93
Phagocytic assay 142, 147
Phagocytosis 10, 11, 12, 13, 14, 24, 25, 96, 98, 99, 101, 198, 199, 382, 383
Pharmaceutical affairs 348, 358
act 348
law (PAL) 358
Plant-derived 166, 247, 378
biochemicals 247
immunomodulators 166, 378
Plant materials, medicinal 117

Platelet-activating factor (PAF) 206, 207
Pneumocystis 246
Pneumonia 31, 95, 96, 97, 246, 257, 404
Pneumonitis 218
Polycystic ovary syndrome (POS) 376
Polyendocrinopathy, autoimmune 45
Polygenic autoinflammatory diseases 64
Prostatic acid phosphatase (PAP) 68
Protease inhibitory activity 169
Proteins 221, 224
  metastasis 221
  metastatic 224

R

Reactive oxygen species (ROS) 66, 96, 101, 171, 191, 201, 218, 228, 256, 374, 382
Renal disease 63
Respiratory 31, 98, 99, 138, 253, 257
  syncytial virus (RSV) 31, 98, 138, 253, 257
  tract infections 99
Reversed 135, 142, 144, 205
  passive Arthus reaction 205
  phase HPLC 132, 142, 144
Rhinitis 22, 49
  chronic 49
RhoA-dependent phosphorylation 63
Ribosome-inactivating protein (RIP) 149
RNA 101, 389
  dependent RNA polymerase enzyme 101
  synthesis 101
  therapies 389
Roifman syndrome 44

S

SDS-PAGE gel 150
Secondary 47, 48, 115, 146, 217, 219, 229, 230, 402
  immunodeficiency disorders 47, 48
  metabolites 115, 146, 217, 219, 229, 230, 402
Secretion, inflammatory proteins 12
Severe combined immune deficiency (SCID) 43
Solid lipid nanoparticles (SLNs) 291, 292, 293
Splenectomy 48, 55
Stevens-Johnson syndrome (SJS) 27, 52, 53
Symptoms 78, 212
  hormone-dependent disease 78
  neuropsychiatric 212
Syndrome 44, 45, 46, 47, 48, 61, 62, 127, 376
  nephrotic 47, 48, 127
  polycystic ovary 376
Synovitis, symmetrical 210
Synthetic 41, 48, 60, 167, 176, 203, 209, 211, 245, 258, 384, 386
  corticosteroids 386
  estrogen 176
  immunostimulator 384
  autoinflammatory diseases 60
  auto-inflammatory disorders (SAIDs) 41, 60
  lupus erythematosus (SLE) 48, 167, 203, 209, 211, 245, 258
  sclerosis 209

T

Techniques 179, 201, 209
  colorimetric Griess reaction assay 201
  immunopharmacological 209
  spectroscopic 179
Testing 193, 195
  immunomodulatory activity 193
  of immunological factors 195
Therapies, medicinal plant 110
Thin layer chromatography (TLC) 115, 118, 158, 180, 204, 354
Thrombocytopenia, congenital 44
Thyroidectomy 57
Thyroid gland transplantation 57
Thyroiditis 56
Thyroperoxidase 208
Traditional 77, 109, 111, 165, 171, 181, 218, 258

Chinese medicine (TCM) 77, 109, 111, 165, 171, 218, 258
electrophoresis 181
Indian medicine 178
Traditional herbal 338, 344
medicinal product (THMP) 338, 344
remedies 338
Transcription factors 221
Tumour 14, 24, 51, 53, 59, 65, 95, 100, 200, 202, 218, 229, 232,
destruction 218, 232
heterogeneity 232
microenvironment 229, 232
necrosis factor (TNF) 14, 24, 51, 53, 59, 65, 95, 100, 200, 202
Type IV hypersensitivity reaction 26

U

Ulcers 61, 64, 144, 209
genital 64
oral 61
peptic 144, 209

V

Vascular endothelial growth factor (VEGF) 176, 228, 230
Vomiting 278, 388

W

Wagner's reagent 155
Wiskott-Aldrich syndrome protein (WASP) 63

Z

Zika viruses 257
Zinc deficiency 30